American College of Surgeons
Deutsche Gesellschaft für Chirurgie

Joint Meeting

Munich 1968

Edited by

H. Bürkle de la Camp, F. Linder and M. Trede

Assisted by G. Kolig and K. Junghanns

Section on Gynecology edited by J. Zander

With 313 Figures

Springer-Verlag Berlin Heidelberg GmbH 1969

Proceedings of the Sectional Meeting of the American College of Surgeons in Cooperation with the Deutsche Gesellschaft für Chirurgie June 26—29, 1968, in Munich

ISBN 978-3-642-48259-5 ISBN 978-3-642-48257-1 (eBook)
DOI 10.1007/978-3-642-48257-1

 Library of Congress Catalog Card Number 73-82423. Softcover reprint of the hardcover 1st edition 1969
Title No. 1566

Introduction

This volume contains some hundred papers read before a Sectional Meeting of the American College of Surgeons held in conjunction with the German Surgical Society in Munich from 25th through 29th June 1968. The committee responsible for the scientific program, headed by WILLIAM P. LONGMIRE (Los Angeles) and FRITZ LINDER (Heidelberg) was able to obtain the cooperation of American and European experts in providing a survey of topical problems concerning general and special operative medicine. Thus the subjects range from general surgery with all its specialities, to traumatology and orthopedics, urology as well as gynecology. The response from our colleagues was most gratifying: More than 1200 surgeons from 33 nations, two-thirds of them from the United States and Canada, participated in this international exchange of information, which was supplemented by a series of panel discussions.

We wish to thank Springer-Verlag, Berlin-Heidelberg-New York for publishing these proceedings and thereby contributing to a world wide interest in the improvement of operative therapy. In addition our gratitude has to be expressed to many members of the Surgical Department of Heidelberg University who have given great support and enthusiasm to the preparation of this volume.

The Editors.

Contents

Opening Addresses

Vascular Disease

Cardiac Surgery

Shock and Trauma

Physiology and Surgery of Peptic Ulcer

The Pancreas

Portal Hypertension

Surgery of Infants and Children

Plastic and Reconstructive Surgery

Operative Treatment of Fractures

Urologic Injuries

Renal Stones

Gynecology

List of Participants

Alken, C. E., Profrssor Dr. med., Director of the Urological University Hospital and Medical School of the University at Homburg/Saar

Allgöwer, M., M. D., F. A. C. S., Professor and Chairman of the Department of Surgery, University of Basel, Switzerland

Austen, W. G., M. D., F. A. C. S., Professor of Surgery, Harvard Medical School, Boston

Bailey, R. W., M. D., F. A. C. S., Professor of Surgery, Section of Orthopaedic Surgery, University of Michigan School of Medicine, Ann Arbor

Bauer, K. H., Professor Emeritus of Surgery, Delegate of the Board of Trustees, German Cancer Research Institute, Heidelberg

Beacham, W. D., M. D., F. A. C. S., Professor of Clinical Obstetrics and Gynecology, Tulane University School of Medicine, New Orleans

Bischoff, P., Dr., Professor of Urology and Chief, Department of Urology, St. Elizabeth Hospital and Children's Hospital of Hochallee, Hamburg

Blocker, T. G., Jr., M. D., F. A. C. S., Professor of Surgery and Dean, University of Texas Medical Branch, Galveston

Borst, H.-G., M. D., Professor of Surgery and Director, Surgical University Hospital, Hannover

Boyes, J. H., M. D., F. A. C. S., Clinical Professor of Surgery, University of Southern California School of Medicine, Los Angeles

Bramann, C. von, Dr. med., Specialist in Surgery, Berlin

Brewer, J. I., M. D., F. A. C. S., Professor of Obstetrics and Gynecology, Northwestern University Medical School, Chicago

Bricker, E. M., M. D., F. A. C. S., Professor of Clinical Surgery, Washington University School of Medicine, St. Louis

Brosig, W. J., Dr., Professor of Urology and Director, Urological University Clinic, Free University School of Medicine, Berlin

Buck-Gramcko, D., Dr. med., Chief, Department of Hand Surgery, Traumatology Hospital, Hamburg-Bergedorf

Bürkle de la Camp, H., Dr. med., Professor of Surgery and Secretary of the German Surgical Society, Dottingen

Cave, E. F., M. D., F. A. C. S., Consulting Visiting Orthopaedic Surgeon, Massachusetts General Hospital, Boston

Cockett, A. T. K., M. D., F. A. C. S., Associate Professor of Surgery/Urology, Harbor General Hospital, Torrance, California

Cope, O., M. D., F. A. C. S., Professor of Surgery, Harvard Medical School and Visiting Surgeon, Massachusetts General Hospital, Boston

Culp, D. A., M. D., F. A. C. S., Professor of Urology, State University of Iowa College of Medicine, Iowa City

D'Aubigne, R. Merle, Prof. M. D., F. A. C. S. (Hon.), Professor of Orthopaedic Surgery, University of Paris

Deterling, R. A., Jr., M. D., F. A. C. S., Professor and Chairman, Department of Surgery, Tufts University School of Medicine, Boston

Dingman, R. O., M. D., F. A. C. S., Professor of Surgery and Head, Section of Plastic Surgery, University of Michigan School of Medicine, Ann Arbor

Ekman, C.-A., M. D., Associate Professor, Surgical Department, University of Lund, Sweden

Ericsson, N. O., M. D., Professor of Pediatric Urology, Karolinska Institute, Stockholm

Fikentscher, R., Dr., Professor of Obstetrics and Gynecology and Director of the Hospital for Women No. 2 of the University of Munich

Frey, E. K., Professor Emeritus of Surgery, Munich

Fuchsig, P., Dr., Professor of Surgery and Head of the First Surgical University Hospital, Vienna

Georg, H., Dr., Lecturer in Surgery, University of Heidelberg School of Medicine and Chief, Department of Surgery, Municipal Hospital, Pforzheim

Georgiade, N. G., M. D., F. A. C. S., Professor of Plastic and Maxillofacial Surgery. Department of Surgery, Duke University School of Medicine, Durham

Gerbode, F. L. A., M. D., F. A. C. S., Clinical Professor of Surgery, Stanford University and University of California School of Medicine, San Francisco

Glenn, F., M. D., F. A. C. S., Professor of Surgery, Cornell University Medical College, New York

Gögler, E., Dr. med., Lecturer, Surgical University Hospital, Heidelberg

Goodwin, W. E., M. D., F. A. C. S., Professor of Surgery and Urology, Chief of the Division of Urology, University of California School of Medicine, Los Angeles

Griffith, C. A., M. D., F. A. C. S., Clinical Associate Professor of Surgery, University of Washington School of Medicine, Seattle

Grob, M., Dr., Professor of Pediatric Surgery and Chief, Department of Surgery, Pediatric University Hospital, Zürich

Grözinger, K.-H., Dr., Lecturer, Surgical University Hospital, Heidelberg

Gusberg, S. B., M. D., F. A. C. S., Professor and Chairman of Obstetrics and Gynecology, Mount Sinai School of Medicine, New York

Gütgemann, A., Dr. med., Professor of Surgery and Director, Surgical University Hospital, Bonn-Venusberg

Haller, J. A., Jr., M. D., F. A. C. S., Robert Garrett Professor of Pediatric Surgery, John Hopkins Hospital and University School of Medicine, Baltimore

Hammond, G., M. D., F. A. C. S., Chairman, Orthopaedic Department, Lahey Clinic Foundation, Boston

Hamperl, H., Prof. Dr., Director of the Department of Pathology, University of Bonn

Harrison, E. G., M. D., Consultant in Surgical Pathology and Associate Professor of Pathology, Mayo Clinic and Mayo Graduate School of Medicine, Rochester, Minnesota

Heberer, G., Prof. Dr., Director, Surgical University Hospital, Cologne

Hegemann, G., Dr. med., Professor of Surgery and Director, Surgical University Hospital, Erlangen

Hendren III, W. H., M. D., F. A. C. S., Surgical Chairman, Children's Service of Massachusetts General Hospital, Boston

Huffman, J. W., M. D., F. A. C. S., Professor of Obstetrics and Gynecology, Northwestern University Medical School, Chicago

Johanson, B., Dr., Head of the Plastic Unit, Sahlgrenska Hospital and University, Göteborg

Käser, O., M. D., Professor of Obstetrics and Gynecology, Woman's Hospital of the University of Frankfurt am Main

Kay, A. W., M. D., F. R. C. S., Professor, University Department of Surgery, Western Infirmary, Glasgow

Kern, G., Dr. med., Professor of Obstetrics and Gynecology Women's Hospital of the University of Cologne

Kerr, W. S., Jr., M. D., F. A. C. S., Assistant Clinical Professor of Surgery, Harvard Medical School, Boston

KLOSTERHALFEN, H., Dr. med., Director, Urological University Hospital, Hamburg-Eppendorf

KOLIG, G., Dr. med., Instructor in Surgery, Surgical University Hospital, Heidelberg

LECHNER, F., Dr., Associate Surgeon, Hospital of the Right Bank of the Isar College of Science and Technology, Munich

LEVENTHAL, M. L., M. D., F. A. C. S., Clinical Professor of Obstetrics and Gynecology, Michael Reese Hospital, Chicago

LINDER, F., Dr., M. D., F. R. C. S. (Eng. Hon), F. A. C. S. (Hon.), Professor of Surgery and Chairman, Department of Surgery, University of Heidelberg

LONGMIRE, W. P., JR., M. D., F. A. C. S., Professor and Chairman, Department of Surgery, University of California School of Medicine, Los Angeles

LUTZEYER, W., Dr. med., Professor of Urology, Medical School of Rhein-Westfalen College of Science and Technology, Aachen

LYNCH, J. B., M. D., F. A. C. S., Associate Professor of Plastic and Maxillofacial Surgery, University of Texas Medical Branch, Galveston

MAATZ, R., Prof. Dr. med., Medical Director and Chief of Staff, Auguste-Viktoria City Hospital, Berlin-West

MACKENZIE, W. C., M. D., F. R. C. S. (C), F. A. C. S., Professor of Surgery and Dean of Medicine, University of Alberta Faculty of Medicine, Edmonton

MARBERGER, H., M. D., Head of the Department of Urology, Medical School, University Innsbruck, Austria

MATTHES, T., Prof. Dr. med., Specialist in Thoracic Surgery and Acting Director of the Hospital, German Academy of Science, Berlin, DDR

MAURER, G., Prof. Dr., Director, Surgical University Hospitals, Right Bank of the Isar College of Science and Technology, Munich

MCKEEVER, F. M., M. D., F. A. C. S., Clinical Professor Emeritus of Orthopaedic Surgery, University of Southern California School of Medicine, Los Angeles

MEILING, R. L., M. D., F. A. C. S., Dean of Ohio State University College of Medicine, Columbus

MERCADIER, M., Dr., Professor of Surgery, University of Paris

MOORE, M., JR., M. D., F. A. C. S., Associate Clinical Professor of Orthopaedic Surgery, University of Tennessee College of Medicine and Chief, Orthopaedic Department, Methodist Hospital, Memphis

MORRIS, G. C., JR., M. D., F. A. C. S., Associate Professor of Surgery, Baylor University College of Medicine, Houston

MORRIS, J. M., M. D., F. A. C. S., Professor of Gynecology, Yale University School of Medicine, New Haven, Connecticut

MÜLLER, M. E., Dr., Professor and Chief, Department of Orthopaedic Surgery, University of Bern, Switzerland

MULLER, W. H., JR., M. D., F. A. C. S., Professor and Chairman, Department of Surgery, University of Virginia Medical Center, Charlottesville

MULLIGAN, W. J., M. D., F. A. C. S., Assistant Clinical Professor in Obstetrics and Gynecology, Boston Hospital for Woman, Parkway Division Formerly Free Hospital for Woman, Boston, Brookline

NAHUM, A. M., M. D., F. A. C. S., Assistant Professor of Surgery, University of California School of Medicine, Los Angeles

NARDI, G. L., M. D., F. A. C. S., Associate Clinical Professor of Surgery, Harvard Medical School and Visiting Surgeon, Massachusetts General Hospital, Boston

NAVRATIL, E., M. D., F. A. C. S. (Hon.), Professor of Obstetrics and Gynecology, Hospital of Obstetrics and Gynecology, University of Graz, Austria

Nesbit, R. M., M. D., F. A. C. S., President, American College of Surgeons and Special Assistant to the Dean and Lecturer in Surgery, University of California School of Medicine, Davis, California

Ober, K. G., Dr. med., Professor of Obstetrics and Gynecology, Director, Women's Hospital of the University of Erlangen-Nuremberg

Ochsner, A., M. D., F. R. C. S. (Ire. Hon., Eng. Hon.), F. A. C. S., President, Alton Ochsner Medical Foundation and Professor Emeritus of Surgery, Tulane University School of Medicine, New Orleans

Olsson, O., M. D., Professor of Diagnostic Radiology and Director, Roentgendiagnostic Department, University Hospital, Lund, Sweden

Palmer, R., M. D., Professor at the College of Medicine, Gynecologic Clinic, Broca Hospital, Paris

Park, O. K., M. D., F. A. C. S., Col., U. S. A. F., M. C., Commander, United States Air Force Hospital, Wiesbaden

Parsons, L., M. D., F. A. C. S., Clinical Professor Emeritus of Gynecology, Harvard Medical School, Boston

Patterson, H. A., M. D., F. A. C. S., Chief of Surgery, Roosevelt Hospital, New York

Peacock, E. E., Jr., M. D., F. A. C. S., Professor of Surgery, University of North Carolina School of Medicine Division of Surgical Biology, Chapel Hill

Persky, L., M. D., F. A. C. S., Professor of Urology, Western Reserve University School of Medicine, Cleveland

Peters, P. C., M. D., F. A. C. S., Associate Professor of Surgery, Division of Urology, University of Texas Southwestern Medical School, Dallas

Pickrell, K. L., M. D., F. A. C. S., Chairman and Professor, Division of Plastic and Reconstructive Surgery, Duke University Medical Center, Durham

Pierce, J. M., Jr., M. D., F. A. C. S., Professor and Chairman, Department of Urology, Wayne State University School of Medicine, Detroit

Politano, V. A., M. D., F. A. C. S., Professor of Surgery, Chief, Division of Urology, University of Miami School of Medicine and Jackson Memorial Hospital, Miami

Ponseti, I. V., M. D., F. A. C. S., Professor of Orthopaedic Surgery, State University of Iowa College of Medicine, Iowa City

Pratt, J. H., M. D., F. A. C. S., Professor of Clinical Surgery, Mayo Graduate School of Medicine and Mayo Clinic, Rochester, Minnesota

Priestley, J. T., M. D., F. A. C. S., Head, Section of General Surgery, Mayo Clinic and Professor of Surgery, Mayo Graduate School of Medicine, Rochester, Minnesota

Rehbein, F., Professor Dr., Children's Surgical Hospital, Bremen

Rehn, J., Professor Dr. med., Chief, Surgical Hospital and Policlinic of the Hospitals of the "Bergmannsheil" Employer's Liability Insurance Association, Bochum

Reimers, Th. C., Professor Dr., Chief Surgeon, Municipal Hospital "Ferd.-Sauerbruch," Wuppertal-Elberfeld

Reis, R. A., M. D., F. A. C. S., Professor Emeritus, Gynecology and Obstetrics, Northwestern University Medical School, Chicago

Rhoads, J. E., M. D., F. A. C. S., John Rhea Barton Professor of Surgery and Director of the Harrison Department of Surgical Research, University of Pennsylvania School of Medicine, Philadelphia

Rickham, P. P., M. D., F. R. C. S. (Eng.), Director of Studies in Pediatric Surgery, University of Liverpool and Senior Consultant Pediatric Surgeon, Alder Hey Children's Hospital, Liverpool

Rob, C. G., M. D., F. A. C. S., Professor and Chairman, Department of Surgery, University of Rochester School of Medicine and Denistry, Rochester, New York

Roehl, L., M. D., Professor of Urology, Surgical University Hospital of Heidelberg

Ross, D. N., M. B., Ch. B., F. R. C. S. (Eng.), Consultant Thoracic Surgeon, Guy's Hospital and the National Heart Hospital, London

Roth, R. B., M. D., F. A. C. S., Chief, Department of Urology, St. Vincent Hospital, Erie, Pennsylvania

Scardino, P. L., M. D., F. A. C. S., Chief of Urology, Memorial Hospital of Chatham County, Savannah Urological Clinic, Savannah, Georgia

Schäfer, H., Dr., Associate Surgeon, Surgical Hospital, Right Bank of the Isar College of Science and Technology, Munich

Schettler, G., Dr., Professor of Internal Medicine, Medical Hospital of Heidelberg University

Schink, W., Dr., Professor of Surgery and Director, Second Surgical University Hospital, Cologne

Schlegel, J. U., M. D., F. A. C. S., Professor and Chairman, Section of Urology, Department of Surgery, Tulane University School of Medicine, New Orleans

Schmid, E., M. D., D. D. S., Chief, Department of Facial and Oral Surgery, St. Mary's Hospital, Stuttgart

Schmitz, W., Dr. med., Lecturer, Surgical University Hospital, Heidelberg

Schneider, R., M. D., Chief of Staff, Grosshöchstetten Hospital, Bern, Switzerland

Schuchardt, K., Dr. med. dent., Professor and Director, Northwest German Oral Hospital, State University Hospital Eppendorf, Hamburg

Schwaiger, M., Dr., Professor of Surgery and Director, Surgical University Hospital of the University of Freiburg (Brsg.)

Scott, H. W., Jr., M. D., F. A. C. S., Professor and Chairman, Department of Surgery, Vanderbilt University School of Medicine, Nashville

Scuderi, C. S., M. D., F. A. C. S., Associate Professor of Orthopaedic Surgery, University of Illinois College of Medicine and Chairman of Orthopaedic Surgery, St. Elizabeth and Columbus Hospitals, Chicago

Shires, G. T., M. D., F. A. C. S., Professor and Chairman, Department of Surgery, University of Texas Southwestern Medical School, Dallas

Skoog, T., M. D., F. A. C. S. (Hon.), Professor of Plastic Surgery, University of Uppsala Faculty of Medicine, Sweden

Smith, M. L., M. D., F. A. C. S., Col., U. S. A., M. C., Surgical Consultant, United States Army, Europe and Seventh Army, Heidelberg

Spence, H. M., M. D., F. A. C. S., Clinical Professor of Urology and Chairman, Division of Urology, University of Texas Southwestern Medical School, Dallas

Spencer, F. C., M. D., F. A. C. S., Professor and Chairman, Department of Surgery, New York University Medical Center, New York

Starr, A., M. D., F. A. C. S., Professor of Surgery and Chief of Cardiopulmonary Surgery, University of Oregon Medical School, Portland

Turner-Warwick, R. T., M. D., F. R. C. S. (Eng.), Chief of Urology, Institute of Urology and the Middlesex Hospital, London

Vollmar, J., Dr., Lecturer, Surgical University Hospital, Heidelberg

Voorhees, A. B., Jr., M. D., F. A. C. S., Associate Professor of Clinical Surgery, Columbia University College of Physicians and Surgeons and Columbia-Presbyterian Medical Center, New York

Vossschulte, K., Professor Dr. med., President, German Surgical Society and Professor of Surgery, Surgical University Hospital, Giessen

Wachsmuth, W., Dr. med., Professor of Surgery and Chairman, Department of Surgery, Surgical University Hospital, Würzburg

Warren, W. D., M. D., F. A. C. S., Professor of Surgery and Dean, University of Miami School of Medicine, Miami

Welch, C. E., M. D., F. A. C. S., Clinical Professor of Surgery, Harvard Medical School and Visiting Surgeon, Massachusetts General Hospital, Boston

Wenz, W., Dr., Lecturer, Surgical University Hospital, Heidelberg

Willenegger, H., M. D., Professor of Surgery, University of Basle and Head of the Surgical Hospital of Kanton, Liestal, Switzerland

Wilson, J. C., Jr., M. D., F. A. C. S., Clinical Professor of Orthopaedic Surgery, University of Southern California School of Medicine and Head, Division of Orthopaedic Surgery, Children's Hospital of Los Angeles

Wilson, P. D., Jr., M. D., F. A. C. S., Associate Professor of Orthopaedic Surgery, Cornell University Medical College Hospital for Special Surgery, New York

Witt, A. N., Professor Dr., Director, Orthopaedic Hospital and Policlinic, Free University of Berlin

Wylie, E. J., M. D., F. A. C. S., Professor of Surgery and Chief of Vascular Surgery, University of California School of Medicine, San Francisco

Zander, J., Dr. med., Professor of Obstetrics and Gynecology and Chairman, Department of Obstetrics and Gynecology, University of Heidelberg

Zenker, R., Dr. M. D., F. A. C. S. (Hon.), Professor of Surgery and Director, Surgical University Hospital, Munich

Zollinger, R. M., M. D., F. A. C. S., Professor and Chairman, Department of Surgery, Ohio State University Medical Center, Columbus

Zuidema, G. D., M. D., F. A. C. S., Professor and Director, Department of Surgery, Johns Hopkins University School of Medicine, Baltimore

Zukschwerdt, L., Dr. med., Professor of Surgery and Director, Surgical University Hospital, Hamburg-Eppendorf

Opening Addresses

H. Bürkle de la Camp

May the festive music of *Ludwig van Beethoven* today keep away the restlessnes and rush of our everyday life, may it open the door for a friendly American-German Surgical Meeting and may it ease us into 4 days of scientific exchange in peace and with an open mind, — in a harmonic atmosphere and in a common experience and enjoyment of our stay in this beautiful region of Germany.

I am honoured to welcome all of you on behalf of the Presidential Board and of the members of the German Surgical Society. I perform this responsibility with particular pleasure.

This 4-day meeting of the American College of Surgeons with us here in Munich is intended for the exchange of scientific ideas in various fields of surgery. It includes many topics which also cover the border areas.

Thus it is a cause of particular pleasure to the German surgeons to see so many colleagues from overseas and from Europe with members of their families in our city.

I extend a warm welcome to the surgeons and their families from the United States of America and from Canada who constitute the American College of Surgeons which is highly regarded throughout the world.

I extend the same warm welcome to all congress visitors from many countries of the world: from Africa and Australia, from Austria, Belgium, France, from Great Britain, Greece, Holland, Hungary, Italy, from the Scandinavian Countries, Switzerland and from the Near and Far East.

The multitude of the countries presented here proves that the Sectional Meeting of the American College of Surgeons in cooperation with the German Surgical Society is a pleasant attraction. It is particularly regrettable that the surgeons from the eastern part of our divided country were not able to participate in our congress. We regret that politics do not stop for science.

This is the fourth occasion that the American College of Surgeons holds a Sectional Meeting in a foreign country: 1954 in London, 1958 in Stockholm, 1961 in Mexico City and now here in Munich. The fact that Germany was selected for this meeting and that our German Surgical Society could arrange this congress is a great honour for us.

Does this choice not represent a recognition of German Surgery? I believe I can answer this in the affirmative. And we German surgeons feel that this is the case.

At the end of the last century and until the First World War German surgery was one of the sources from which knowledge and ability spread to the world. — Thanks to our old masters, on whose shoulders we are standing.

And "Thanks to our old Masters" is also the title of our historical booklet which you will receive tomorrow.

The political events since that time changed the conditions to our disadvantage and after World War II we were reduced to acceptors and thankful receivers. — In the first presentations tomorrow we will hear about these changing relationships from a qualified source.

We have attempted to regain lost ground. If we had not achieved this, our American friends would not be here now.

Since the end of World War II we are unfortunately unable to use our own house and our own congress-building in the eastern part of Berlin, the Langenbeck-Virchow-House. We have selected the congresshall of the German Museum in Munich as the location of our annual congresses. Here we found a home and for the last 18 years we have felt at home here in Munich.

May all of you experience this soothing and joyful feeling which we always associate with Munich.

May this meeting fulfil the expectations of all participants.

May you all, Ladies and Gentlemen, during these days learn to love and to hold in high regard Munich, Bavaria and Germany. But our congress may not only serve advanced science. We want to get to know another more closely, we want to learn to think and to live together, we want to approach one another and to completely understand one another.

We want to be friends under the seals of our two societies and to remain friends when, after these short 4 days, we once again depart in all directions.

We German surgeons meet you with an open mind and an open heart.

In this sense I extend to you our greetings: a warm welcome to all of you.

K. Vossschulte

It seems superfluous to stress once again that science does not accept boundaries. We all know that it offers its blessings most abundantly and generously whenever it is based on humanistic ideals. The course of history has demonstrated over again that humanitarian principles have been the prime stimulus for scientific meetings.

The surgeons of my days grew up at a time when the interchange of surgical knowledge depended almost entirely on information gathered from the medical literature. As we all know even these tenuous bonds broke down altogether during a most unfortunate period of our history — a catastrophe that we physicians find difficult to comprehend. It is all the more gratifying that this meeting, serving our common surgical interests, has been convened.

On behalf of the German Surgical Society I am very pleased to welcome most heartily the members of the American College of Surgeons. I wish to thank, our American colleagues first of all for coming to Germany and for their cooperation and interest in our common surgical task. I also wish to thank most cordially all guests who have come from so many countries to support the work of our Congress.

We feel confident that this joint meeting of our two Surgical Colleges will ultimately benefit our patients. We do not speak the same language, but we do feel the same responsibilities. We have to work under widely differing conditions, but we certainly work with the same sense of duty. We may not always have the same success in curing our patients — and we are here to find the reasons for this. We do not always employ the same operative techniques, but by comparing our results it should be possible to find new and optimum methods of therapy.

It seems to me that medicine as a science is increasingly trying to establish the functional and morphological pattern of life by the application of statistics and mathematics. But as we all know this is anything but a simple problem of arithmetics. Valuable as the theoretical results of statistics may be, they require clinical experience to be put into praxis successfully. The blending of these two approaches is one of the prime tasks of our meeting.

Both journalists and physicians cannot ignore the growing public interest in medical progress. Whilst fully realizing the difficulties of scientific and medical reporting we welcome every genuine effort at objective information. Let me stress again that the German Surgical Society is always ready to cooperate in this matter. We consider it part of the surgeons' duty to help and serve.

Recently I came across a paper in the Archives of Surgery by EMERICK SZILAGY. It was entitled "The Physician: savant, saint or servant" — one of those picturesque alliterations which are found so frequently in the English language. Let me remind you of an old illustration depicting a physician as a saint. It is a Byzantine icon in which Hippocrates is pictured wearing a halo — certainly a pardonable glorification by subsequent admirers. It sometimes seems that our own world holds us in similar esteem in relation to our humanitarian tasks. It is our duty to justify this conception by constant improvement of our work through scientific research. Only those living up to these ideals are capable of fulfilling the task so excellently defined by the American College of Surgeons: "For the benefit of humanity by advancing the science of surgery and the ethical and competent practice of its art".

R. M. NESBIT

The German Society of Surgeons has honored the American College of Surgeons in asking us to come to Munich to collaborate in holding this Surgical Congress. We deeply appreciate your invitation and we hope that you will recognize that the large attendance of American and Canadian Fellows at this meeting is an indication to you of their enthusiastic acceptance of your generous offer of hospitality.

The ACS was founded with just one unselfish and humanitarian objective: namely, to bring about better surgical care for human beings. To that end alone, the College has carried out its many activities and programs at home. It has also encouraged the achievement of this objective abroad by granting Fellowship to qualified, ethical surgeons throughout the entire world; and by holding meetings such as this one, periodically, in foreign countries. These meetings provide a forum for the sharing of scientific ideas with our neighbors in foreign countries on their own soil.

You come overseas to visit us from time to time to get acquainted with us and our people: we welcome this occasion for getting better acquainted with you in this beautiful setting. We thank you.

The Influence of German Surgery on American Surgery*

ALTON OCHSNER

I first became aware of the tremendous influence that Germanic surgery exerted on American surgery while in medical school and externing at Augustana Hospital in Chicago under the direction of Dr. A. J. OCHSNER, who was my father's cousin. Because his own son did not study medicine, I became his medical protégé, and I am indebted to him for everything I may have achieved in medicine. Although he was born in Baraboo, Wisconsin, he was early exposed to a distinct Germanic influence because his father had come from Switzerland and only German was spoken in their home. As a matter of fact, Dr. A. J. always spoke with a German accent. In addition, a considerable part of his education was obtained in Germany or was under the direction of Germantrained teachers.

While an undergraduate student at the University of Wisconsin, where he completed a 4 year course in 3 years, graduating first in his class, A. J. OCHSNER came under the influence of Prof. EDWARD A. BIRGE. Prof. BIRGE had recently completed several years of graduate study in histology and embryology at the University of Leipzig. OCHSNER became intensely interested and extremely proficient in microscopy. For his medical education, he chose Rush Medical College because he could give private courses in histology and embryology to special students there. After graduating in 1886, he began interning at Presbyterian Hospital in Chicago.

In the spring of 1887 he took a 9 month leave of absence to study surgery in Vienna under BILLROTH and pathology under KOLASKAO and PALTAUF. Upon returning to Chicago, he taught microscopy at Rush Medical College and completed his internship. In April 1888 he went to Berlin to study pathology under VIRCHOW, bacteriology under KOCH, surgery under von BERGMANN, and gynecology under OHLSHAUSEN and MARTIN. He then returned to Chicago, where he became assistant to CHARLES T. PARKES, Professor of Surgery at Rush. After PARKES' death, he became assistant to NICHOLAS SENN, a fellow Swiss, who succeeded PARKES. OCHSNER's life was strongly influenced by SENN and CHRISTIAN FENGER, a Dane, who had received his training in Europe, studying pathologic anatomy and surgery for a period of time in Vienna under Prof. BILLROTH. While serving as a Prosector to the Copenhagen City Hospital, FENGER wrote his thesis for the degree of Doctor of Medicine, entitled, „On Cancer of the Stomach with Special Reference to its Structural Development and Extension." He was then appointed Privatdozent in pathologic anatomy. When he came to Chicago in 1877, he gave lectures and demonstrations on pathologic anatomy („The science which was unknown to the physicians there.")

Probably because of his Swiss ancestry, the time spent in Germany and Austria early in his career, and the influence exerted by BIRGE, SENN, and FENGER, Dr. A. J. OCHSNER always had close ties with the Germanic countries. Because he realized that their medical training was superior to ours, he arranged for ERWIN SCHMIDT, also a cousin, to serve as an exchange surgical resident under VICTOR SCHMIEDEN in Frankfurt (Main) and under EINAR KEY in Stockholm. He also arranged for me to serve as an exchange surgical resident under PAUL CLAIRMONT in Zürich and for a longer period of time in a similar capacity under SCHMIEDEN in Frankfurt (Main).

* From the Department of Surgery, Ochsner Clinic and Ochsner Foundation Hospital, New Orleans.

I shall always cherish the opportunity I had to work in these two clinics and to come under the influence of two such eminent and stimulating surgical masters. While in Europe, also at Dr. A. J. OCHSNER's suggestion, I visited the clinics of SAUERBRUCH in Munich, BIER in Berlin, PAYR in Leipzig, LEXER in Freiburg, PERTHES in Tübingen, KIRSCHNER in Königsberg, VON EISELBERG and HOCHENEGG in Vienna, HENSCHEN in St. Gallen, DE QUERVAIN in Bern, HOTZ in Basel, KÜMMEL in Hamburg, and ENDERLEN in Heidelberg. I remember vividly, while attending the meeting of the Deutsche Gesellschaft für Chirurgie in 1924, hearing KIRSCHNER's electrifying report of the first successfull pulmonary embolectomy. Some of my most lasting friendships were made during this period.

Before the middle of the nineteenth century, Paris was considered the medical center of the world, but, as White pointed out, "... a change was beginning. Gradually the philosophic German mind, so skeptical and irreverent as to accept no dogma unchallenged, and so patient and industrious in following the suggestions of nature to their source, began to make itself felt. This influence soon became an acknowledged power as the careful observation of devoted students — men who cared for nothing else in life than their studies, who had no higher ambition than their scientific reputation, who knew no other pleasure than was to be found in the laboratory or hospital, and who never aspired to become rich — became known ... 19 of all that is new and important on physiology, pathology, and medical chemistry, is the work of German hands and brains, and is given to the world in their tongue... In Germany the celebrated physician first makes for himself a name of incessant toil and self sacrifice. He cares neither for society, for appearance, for comfort, only for science."

SAUERBRUCH, BIER, PAYR, LEXER, PERTHES, KIRSCHNER, VON EISELSBERG and HOCHENEGG, HENSCHEN, DE QUERVAIN, HOTZ, KÜMMELL, ENDERLEN.

In his scholarly presidential address before the American Surgical Association in 1947, CHURCHILL also recognized the influence of German science on American medicine: "The stream from Germany was a turbulent freshlet of Science, beginning in the middle of the nineteenth century and reaching full flood by 1914... The Germanic influence in American medical education was not apparent until the rise of scientific medicine in Germany in the middle of the 19th century... Philosophical thought was already declining [in Germany] by 1830, but the united and the imperial state fostered a period of industry and achievement in German universities that flowered in research in the natural and medical sciences. The wealth and importance of Germany's intellectual and technical achievements made it a country to which our students turned as a fountainhead and guide of medical science. This was, in all, a brief period, 1850 to 1914, but its impact on medicine and medical education has been enormous... By 1870 the floods of specialized knowledge and technics were bursting forth from German and Austrian universities."

The real advance in medicine in the early 19th century was probably due more to RUDOLPH VIRCHOW than anyone else. Early in life, VIRCHOW was torn between deciding whether to enter the ministry or study medicine. Because he thought that his voice was not strong enough to be an effective minister, he decided to become a physician. What a fortuitous decision this proved to be for medicine. GRAHAM called VIRCHOW LISTER's most distinguished contemporary.

Although VIRCHOW is generally known for his contributions to pathology, he had a much broader interest in medicine. According to QUINCKE, he was interested not only in pathologic physiology and pathologic anatomy but also in clinical medicine, making regular rounds on the wards at the Charité in Berlin. VIRCHOW's concept of cellular pathology was that the cell is the important unit, that cells arise only out of other cells, and that sickness or illness is the reaction of the cell to altered conditions.

STENGEL called VIRCHOW unquestionably "the greatest genius among the medical men of the 19th century." He stated that no man had influenced the workers in any branch of science more than had VIRCHOW on physicians. VIRCHOW advocated accuracy of observation and logical reasoning, and was a strong force in setting aside prevailing empiricism. Yet he took no credit for having discovered the scientific methods of medical research, believing that the world would have found them in time.

VIRCHOW introduced the systematic method of performing postmortem examinations. SMITH, in reminiscing about his experience while working under VIRCHOW, stated that before VIRCHOW's time postmortem examination was performed solely to determine the immediate cause of death and was always terminated the moment this was ascertained. SMITH witnessed for the first time a necropsy performed with the intention of learning all pathologic changes present in that particular cadaver.

WELCH also recognized VIRCHOW as the "chief founder of modern scientific medicine," believing that he would be "for all time to come... one of the greatest figures in medicine." He considered VIRCHOW's establishment of the principles of cellular pathology the greatest scientific advance of all times.

Although it is not commonly known, VIRCHOW also played an eminent rôle in the revolution that resulted in establishment of the United German Commonwealth in 1848 to 1849. While Prosector to ROBERT FRORIEP at the Charité Hospital in Berlin he and BENNO REINHARDT founded the "Archiv für pathologische Anatomie und Physiologie, und für klinische Medizin" in 1847. In 1849 he lost his prosectorship because of his political activities and accepted the Professorship of Pathologic Anatomy at the University of Würzburg. He returned to Berlin, however, in 1856 as Professor of Pathological Anatomy, General Pathology and Therapeutics, and Director of the newly formed Pathological Institute. In 1865 he was challenged to a duel with pistols by BISMARCK, because of a speech which he had made in the Reichstag. At his death, September 5, 1902, when he was almost 81 years old, OSTHEIMER wrote that VIRCHOW "excelled as a scientist, politician, municipal reformer, medical discoverer, thinker and writer of the first order."

OSLER beautifully pointed out the strong influence of Vienna on American Medicine: "As a medical center Vienna has had a remarkable career and her influence, particularly on American Medicine, has been very great. What was known as the first Vienna school in the 18th century was really a transference by VAN SWIETEN of the school of BOERHAAVE from Leyden. The new Vienna school, which we know, dates from ROKITANSKY and SKODA, who really made Vienna the successor of the great Paris school of the early days of the 19th century. But Vienna's influence on American medicine has not been so much through SKODA und ROKITANSKY as through the group of brilliant specialists — HEBRA, SIGMUND and NAUMANN in dermatology; ARLT and JAEGER in ophthalmology; SCHNITZLER and VON SCHRÖTTER in laryngology; GRUBER and POLITZER in otology."

In speaking of Vienna as the Aesculapian center, Osler stated, "Not until she [the Aesculapian center] saw in JOHANNES MÜLLER and in RUDOLPH VIRCHOW true and loyal disciples did she move to Germany, where she stays in spite of tempting offers from France, from Italy, from England and from Austria... I boldly suggested that it was perhaps time to think of crossing the Atlantic and setting up her temple in the new world for a generation or two. I spoke of the many advantages, of the absence of tradition — here she visibly weakened, as she has suffered so much from this poison — the greater freedom, the enthusiasm, and then I spoke of missionary work. At these words she turned on me sharply and said: 'That is not for me. We gods have but one motto — those that honor us we honor. Give me the temples, give me the priests, give me the true worship the old Hippocratic service of the art and of the science of ministering to man, and I will come. By the eternal law under which we Gods live I would have to come. I did not wish to leave Paris, where I was happy and where I was served so faithfully by BICHAT, by LAENNEC and by LOUIS' — and tears filled her eyes; her voice trembled with emotion — 'but where the worshippers are the most devoted, not, mark you, where they are the most numerous; where the clouds of incense rise highest, there must my chief temple be, and to it from all quarters will the faithful flock. As it was in Greece, in Alexandria, in Rome, in northern Italy, in France, so it is now in Germany, and so it *may be* in the new world I long to see.' Doubtless she will come, but not till the present crude organization of our medical clinics is changed, not until there is a fuller realization of internal medicine as a science as well as an art".

BERNHARD VON LANGENBECK, who lived from 1810 to 1887, also exerted a great influence on the development of Germanic surgery. In 1834 he graduated from the University of Göttingen, where he had studied under his famous uncle, KONRAD J. M. VON LANGENBECK. He then studied in Belgium, Paris, and London, where he became a good friend of Sir BENJAMIN BRODIE and Sir ASTLEY COOPER. Returning to Göttingen, he became Professor of Pathological Anatomy at the age of 30, and the next year was appointed Professor of Surgery at Kiel. After serving in the Army, he was appointed Professor of Surgery at Berlin in 1848. Probably because of VIRCHOW's influence, he emphasized the importance of physiology and anatomy in surgery. THEODOR BILLROTH (1924), VON LANGENBECK's pupil, called him the founder of the greatest German School of Surgery. He pointed out that all of VON LANGENBECK's pupils, including himself, had been influenced by the physiologic and anatomic training under him. VON LANGENBECK was the founder of the *Archiv für klinische Chirurgie* (LANGENBECKS), and together with RICHARD VON VOLKMANN and GUSTAV SIMON, in 1874 founded the *Deutsche Gesellschaft für Chirurgie*. In addition to BILLROTH, his assistants were KRÖNLEIN, TRENDELENBURG, ESMARCH, M. MÜLLER, E. GURLT, and A. LÜCKE.

The person who was probably the most direct link between Germanic medicine and development of surgery in the United States is THEODOR BILLROTH, a truly great scientist and teacher, who lived at a time when scientific medicine was developing in the United States. In his monograph "The Medical Sciences in German Universites" BILLROTH (1924) set forth the philosophy of scientific medicine better than probably anywhere else: "A person may have acquired from books a vast amount of medical knowledge, he may even have memorized from books the technic of its application; such a person has much knowledge of medicine, and yet with it all he is no physician. He must see and hear a master's diagnosis, prognosis, and treatment of disease. He must witness the master's skill in action, in order himself to become a practitioner. The more he knows, the more he will be able to accomplish later".

In speaking of a physician's knowledge he pointed out, "... this knowledge is of no value to him if he lacks imagination and the power of synthesis. The student can learn to develop this power, to practise it, to guard against errors, only by observing a master in action."

He emphasized the need for scientific investigation: "Down to the middle of the 19th century teachers contented themselves with showing and explaining to the students finished preparations, their chief concern being to convey to them the results of research in the most condensed and systematized form possible. But since the fourth decade of this century the German professor has been pretty generally required, not only to know the results of the most recent researchs, and to teach these to his students, but himself to be an investigator in the branch of science which he teaches. That combination had been appreciated in the earlier periods also, when happily it chanced to occur; but it is characteristic of the modern spirit of the German universities that they aim to be not only channels for conveying established knowledge, but also centers of research."

He pointed out the need for clinical teaching, "Teachers at the bedside, the 'clinical physician', could only be trained gradually and at the bedside itself, by eminent practising physicians." Concerning surgical training he wrote, "A man who has been assistant in a surgical ward and has not performed the typical operations dozens of times on the cadaver, until he can do them as well in his sleep as when fully awake, will never be an operator. It is much more important to enlighten the students by systematic lectures on surgery in general as to *when* an operation is necessary, and to discuss in these lectures only the simplest operative manipulations, as well as the technic of emergency operations that must be done quickly for the immediate saving of life. All else had better be left to later special study in the surgical wards."

He believed "... that in actual practice it is the *personal influence* of great men that gives rise to schools, and not the special administrative efforts of a government to found them. There is only one way to train capable university teachers — one way that has been practically tested — and that is to secure for the universities the services of the most distinguished men of science, and to furnish them with the necessary equipment for their teaching...

"... I believe that I am justified in saying that the great investigators and physicians have always been of a somewhat visionary, highly imaginative nature, with an urge toward universality; so that the moment they began to speak of their science, they gave their students the impression that they were inspired."

Among the men trained by BILLROTH (1892) were CZERNY, GUSSENBAUER, MIKULICZ, SALZER, WINIWARTER, and WÖLFER. BILLROTH's (1858) pride in his students is evidenced in a letter of February 4, 1881, to Dr. WITTELSHOEFER in which he described the development of gastric resection: "... please forgive me if I have a certain pride in the works of my pupils which makes this progress possible — Numquam retrorsum! was the watchword of my teacher, BERNHARD V. LANGENBECK; it shall be mine and that of my pupils."

The direct link between the Billroth School and American medicine was Johns Hopkins University, and especially HALSTED, who spent a good deal of time in Europe and was greatly influenced by Germanic medicine, particularly the Billroth School. According to BONNER, BILLINGS and WELCH made no secret of their hope to introduce German ideas and methods at the new Johns Hopkins Hospital and Medical

School. BONNER pointed out, "The Johns Hopkins School of Medicine radiated German ideas and practices far beyond Baltimore... HALSTED's influence on American surgery, especially in relating it to basic laboratory research, was tremendous. The Hopkins system of clinical residencies for advanced postgraduate studies, hitherto unknow in this country was widely copied by other medical schools." BONNER noted that in his report to the Carnegie Foundation in 1910 FLEXNER "... said in effect that most of America's medical schools should die or be killed, and the rest rebuilt on German or Johns Hopkins lines. It reflected throughout a strong bias in favor of the German system of training medical men."

HALSTED spent 2 years in Europe working with BILLROTH in Vienna, ERNST VON BERGMANN in Berlin, JOHANNES VON MIKULICZ-RADECKI in Breslau, and KARL THIERSCH in Leipzig (STEUDEL). In a letter to Dr. HENRY BEYER dated February 11, 1915, he wrote, "I should say that the characteristic which stands out in bold relief in German scientific life is of paramount importance of knowledge for its own sake. To know certain things thoroughly, and to contribute to an increase in our knowledge of them seems to satisfy the ambition of many of the best minds. The universities of Germany are her chief glory, and the great boon that she can give to us in the new world is to return our young men infected with the spirit of earnestness and with the love for thoroughness which characterizes the work done in them."

In an address at Yale University on June 27, 1904, in speaking of the opening of Johns Hopkins Medical School in 1893, HALSTED (1924) said, "It was our intention originally to adopt as closely as feasible the German plan, which, in the main, is the same for all the principal clinics of the German universities".

The Hopkins school was also greatly influenced by another great European surgeon, THEODOR KOCHER, a fellow Swiss, who was born in Bern, and who was a pupil of VON LANGENBECK and BILLROTH. He became Professor of Surgery at Bern in 1872 and in 1909 received the Nobel Prize for his work on physiology, pathology, and surgery of the thyroid gland. He revolutionized the surgical treatment of thyroid disease and obtained the unbelieveably low mortality rate at that time of only 4.5% in more than 2,000 thyroidectomies. Although he did total thyroidectomies on many patients, in all of whom myxedema developed, tetany developed in only one. He greatly influenced HALSTED, who worked with him and who was responsible for CUSHING getting surgical training under him. BILLROTH also did a great deal of thyroid surgery, but in contrast to KOCHER, he had a high incidence of tetany. In commenting on this difference HALSTED (1920) said, "I have pondered this question for many years and conclude that the explanation lies in the operative methods of the two illustrious surgeons. KOCHER, neat and precise, operating in a relatively bloodless manner, scrupulously removed the entire gland, doing little damage outside the capsule. BILLROTH, operating more rapidly and, as I recall his manner, with less regard for the tissues and, less concern for hemorrhage, might easily have removed the parathyroids, or at least have interfered with their blood supply, and have left fragments of the thyroid."

Although the United States is now recognized as one of the world centers for the medical sciences, we must not forget our great heritage from the Germanic schools. Those of us who had an opportunity to work in the pioneer institutions of the Germanic countries, and to come under the influence of eminent German surgeons have indeed been fortunate. To have been imbued with the dictum, "Alles für die Wissenschaft" (everything for science) has indeed been a special privilege. Hopefully, we have been able to impart some of this spirit to the immediate past and present generations.

References

BILLROTH, T.: The medical sciences in the German universities. Translated by WILLIAM H. WELCH. New York: Macmillan 1924.

— Open letter to Dr. L. WITTELSHOEFER on Feb. 4, 1881. Wien. med. Wschr. **31**, 162 (1881).

— Milestones in modern surgery, HURWITZ, A., and G. A. DEGENSHEIN. Eds. New York: Paul B. Hoeber 1958.

BONNER, T. N.: American doctors and German universities. A chapter in international intellectual relations. 1870—1914. Lincoln, Neb.: University of Nebraska Press 1963.

CHURCHILL, E. D.: Science and humanism in surgery. Trans. Amer. Surg. Ass. **65**, 1—16 (1947).

GRAHAM, H.: (Pseud. of I. H. FLACK). The story of surgery. Doubleday. Doran and Co. New York: 1939.

HALSTED, W. S.: His letter to Dr. HENRY BEYER, geb. Feb. 11, 1915. HALSTED papers. Welch Med. Library, CUSHING, OSLER, P. 331.

— The operative story of goitre. The author's operation. Johns Hopk. Hosp. Rep. **19**, 71—257 (1920)

— The training of the surgeon. Bull. Johns Hopk. Hosp. **15**, 267—275 (1904).

KRECKE: Feuilleton. THEODORE BILLROTH. Münch. Med. Wschr. **39**, 690—691 (1892).

OSTHEIMER, M.: Death of VIRCHOW. Philad. Med. J. **10**, 358—360 (1902).

OSLER, W.: Vienna after thirty-four years. J. Amer. Med. Ass. **50**, 1523—1525 (1908).

QUINCKE, H.: VIRCHOW's influence on practical medicine. RUDOLPH VIRCHOWS Einfluß auf die praktische Medizin. Med. Klin. **17**, 1254—1256 (1921).

SMITH, A. H.: Reminiscences of VIRCHOW. Postgrad. N. Y. **17**, 469—474 (1902).

STENGEL, A.: The endurance of VIRCHOW's work. Philad. Med. J. **10**, 360—361 (1902).

STEUDEL, J.: Der deutsche Einfluß auf die amerikanische Medizin. Festschrift für WERNER LEIBBRAND zum 70. Geburtstag.

WELCH, W. H.: VIRCHOW: a tribute. Philad. Med. J. **10**, 360 (1902).

WHITE, J. C.: Quoted by Churchill.

American-German Relations in Surgery

F. LINDER

On behalf of my German-speaking colleagues, I have the honor and pleasure to thank the youngest member of our Society, Prof. ALTON OCHSNER, for his kind presentation. As we have heard, the early years of American Surgery were characterised by the simple acceptance of European influences from France, England and — from 1870 onwards — particularly from Germany. There followed a vigorous phase of critical assimilation until in the past 50 years the highest perfection and prime position in world surgery was reached. Our friend the preceding speaker will forgive me for regarding him as the personification of this developement: the Swiss roots of his family, his apprenticeship in Bern and Frankfurt, and then the success of his surgical life culminating in the presidency of the American College of Surgeons and the International Surgical Society — all this is proof enough! Thank you, once more, ALTON OCHSNER.

The evaluation of American Surgery from the German point of view seems more difficult in comparison, since this involves more recent chapters of medical history some of which are by no means completed. It is inevitable therefore that my brief response will be largely based on a personal selection of events and personalities.

At the outset let us not forget, that long before the present culmination, remarkable feats were achieved in North America, which became mile-stones in surgery. One of these was the successful removal of a 22-pound ovarian cyst performed by McDowell in a Kentucky log cabin back in the year 1809. Equally as admirable as the courage and skill of the surgeon — who only took 25 min for the operation — was the pluck and faith of that pioneer lady. Having been fully informed about the risks of this first operation, she appeared willing to undergo the experiment and to ride horseback through wintry forests for 5 days to her surgeon. She preferred a quick decision one way or another to an unproductive invalids life. 5 days after the intervention she made her bed herself, on the 25th day she rode home again for 60miles and lived an active life for another 31 years. McDowell underlined the correctness

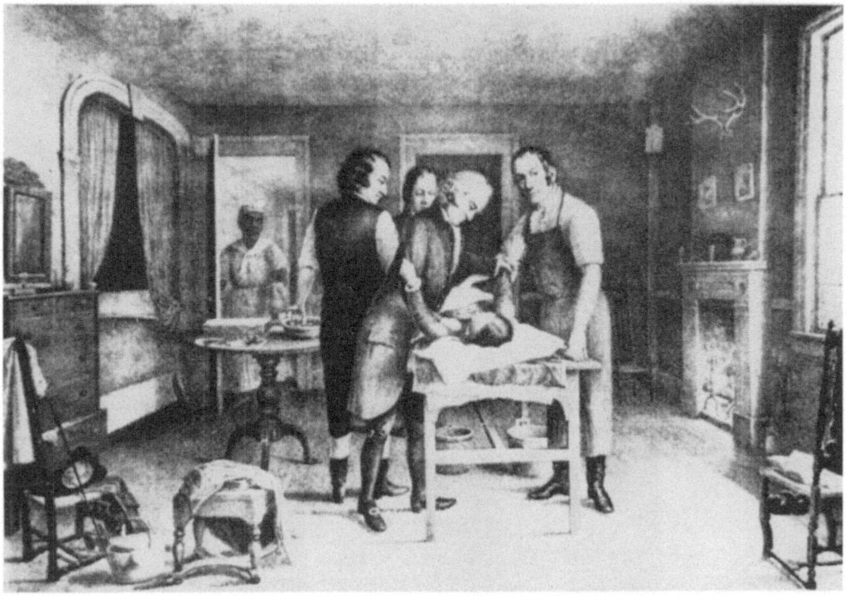

Fig. 1. First successful ovariotomy by Ephraim McDowell in Danville (Kentucky), Dec. 1809

of his decision by publishing a further series of ovariectomies, thus giving the world a first indication for laparotomy — long before the antiseptic era.

Whereas analgesia during McDowell's operations depended largely on the singing of hymns, the delivery from the scourge of pain was a further pioneering American achievement. Popularised by Morton's first public demonstration in the ether dome in Boston, this is one of the two pillars on which, (together with anti- and asepsis) our profession rests.

Oliver Wendell Holmes was the first to use the terms anaesthesia and anaesthetic. The same professor from Harvard, as a predecessor of Lister, realised the contagious nature of puerperal fever and was acclaimed — like Semmelweiss in Europe— as the American saviour of mothers.

Until the turn of the century we note a whole series of American innovations, such as Kimball's removal of a uterine fibroid, Dorsays first splenectomy, Fitz and Albert Ochsner's work on appendicitis, McBurney's point or Murphy's historical button, which have retained their place in German textbooks up to the present. Radical mastectomy according to HALSTED, ROTTER and MEYER — the perfect model of en-bloc cancer surgery — may be regarded as an example of transatlantic teamwork. Whereas HALSTED, with his German system of surgical resident training became the founder of a great American school of surgery (no less than 37 surgical professors in two generations!), the Europeans gratefully received from him the method of nerve blockade and surgical rubber gloves. The latter were originally intended to protect the delicate hands of his operation-nurse, CAROLINE HAMPTON, who subsequently became his wife, from mercuric chloride. Thus Venus and Asclepios cooperated in the introduction of this piece of standard surgical equipment. As a matter of fact, those particular rubber gloves originated in Breslau in COHN-

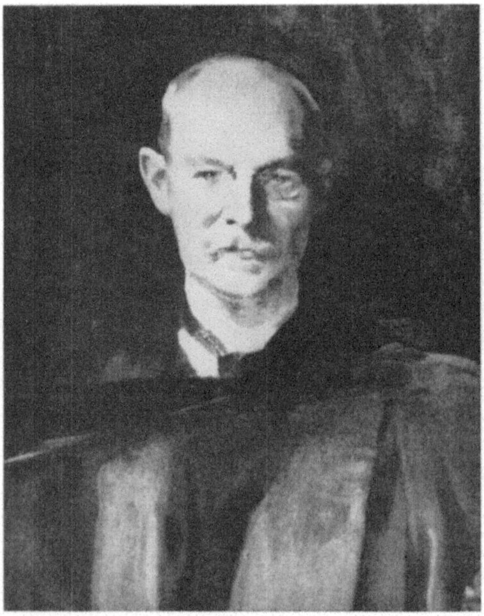

Fig. 2. WILLIAM STEWART HALSTED, 1852—1922

HEIM's laboratory, from where WILLIAM HENRY WELCH, the discoverer of the gas gangrene bacillus took them to America.

HALSTED was regarded so highly by his German colleagues, that he became the first American to be awarded an honorary membership of the German Surgical Society. His acceptance speech — spoken by the way in fluent German — characterised the modesty of this truely great surgeon: the honor was so great, that he could not have deserved it by his own contributions to surgery; he accepted it nonetheless on behalf of his country. This was on April 18th 1914. Soon the lights went out all over Europe and brought the interruption of all the old and fruitful relations between our two countries. They were revived partially and briefly during the Weimar Republic, only to cease completely during the years of isolation following 1933 and the second world war.

In this period, that is to say within the past five decades, the most amazing advances were achieved by American surgery, in part also stimulated by various wars.

Mars — an old Roman proverb reminds us — is the teacher of many things. The reason for this brilliant developement are manifold. In the first place, the intensive study of physiology, biochemistry and biophysics brought a better understanding of pathophysiology and of the metabolic care of the surgical patient. This led to a breakdown of barriers between surgery and other preclinical and clinical fields and stimulated cooperation with other areas of natural sciences such as biophysics and electronics. This analytical spirit was supported by substantial financial aid. Generous grants from federal and private sources facilitated the construction and the work of research laboratories. In addition, new specialities were inaugurated, such as neurosurgery linked to the name of HARVEY CUSHING, which nevertheless did not disrupt

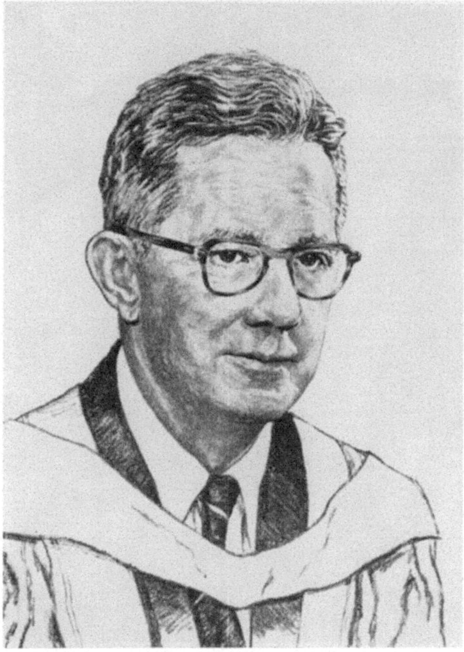

Fig. 3. ALFRED BLALOCK, 1899—1964

the unity of the department as a whole. Thus each specialty benefited from the advances made by the others and, as SIGERIST, the medical historian from LEIPZIG and JOHNS HOPKINS pointed out, remained a wheel within the larger machine. This made American surgical departments more versatile and at the same time more compact than comparable European institutions. "Give me the temples, give me the priests and I will come", the goddess of health had promised WILLIAM OSLER in a vision. There is no doubt — she has moved her chief temple over to the new world!

No wonder that American surgery opened up ever new avenues of therapy, which in spite of their increasing magnitude, retained a reasonable risk. I can mention only a few: 1929 — the first successful exstirpation of an islet cell tumor by ROSCOE GRAHAM in Toronto, where in 1922 BANTING and BEST had discovered insulin.

1933 — the first successful pneumonectomy for bronchial carcinoma in St. Louis by EVARTS GRAHAM, who — after an extra curriculum in chemistry — together with

W. COLE had earlier placed biliary surgery on a sure foundation by the introduction of the cholecystogram.

1940 — the first anastomosis for oesophageal atresia by CAMERON HAIGHT in Ann Arbor and the first duodeno-pancreatectomy for pancreatic carcinoma, performed by WHIPPLE in New York.

In 1943 — again WHIPPLE and his associates carried out the first porto-caval anastomosis at Columbia University and in 1945 — there followed BLALOCK's anastomosis for Fallot's Tetralogy.

In the following years the heart, as the last organ of the human body, became the chief target of surgical therapy. Most of the cardiovascular procedures, which today

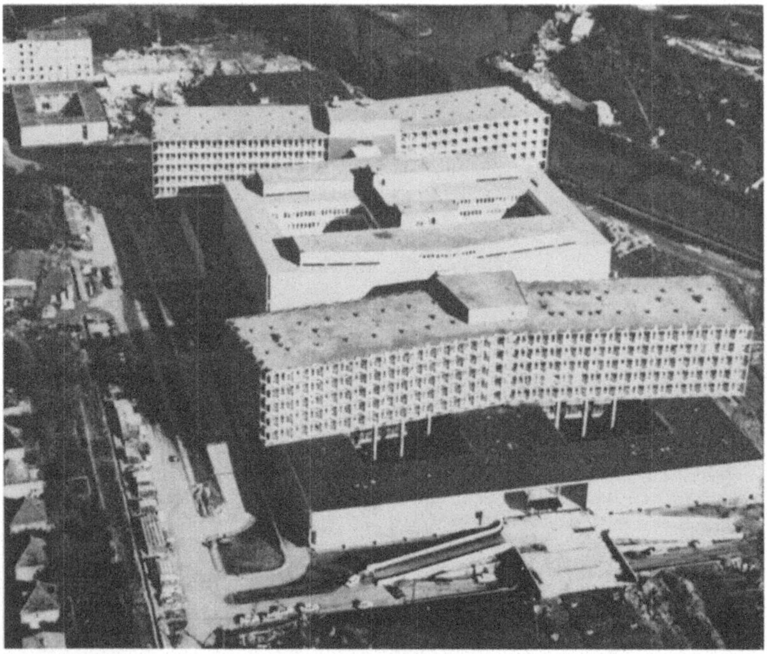

Fig. 4. New medical center of the Free University in West-Berlin under construction

are part of the routine all over the world, originated in the United States or in Canada: in particular the spectacular successes of open heart surgery in hypothermia or extracorporeal circulation and the replacement of cardiac valves and arteries. This was the achievement of many active fellows of the American College of Surgeons with names well-known to all of us.

The gradient between the surgical standards of our two countries was regrettably large after the second world war. The longtime isolation, the destruction of our cities, the loss of man-power through two world wars and the emigration following 1933 as well as a considerable brain-drain in more recent years were the main causes. If today we are once more able to offer our patients an international standard chance of healing, we owe this to the friendly help of many fellows of your college. The exchange of new experiences was begun by men still in uniform whose humanitarian spirit knew of no fraternization ban. Many of my German colleagues still remember the strength that could emanate from an American Surgical Journal received with a pack of cigarettes or candies for the kids. The army surgeons were succeeded by surgical missions with university professors, amongst whom — since the living are excepted — we gratefully recall only the gracious personality of DALLAS PHEMISTER.

Since then uncounted numbers of junior and senior surgeons from this country have had the opportunity to visit and to work in American clinics. The Ventnor Foundation alone, under its presidents I. RAVDIN and H. S. READ have sponsored the exchange of a 1000 young German doctors. Furthermore, untold numbers have crossed the Atlantic River on personal exchange systems and have returned with new knowledge that has been of inestimable value for pre- and postgraduate teaching and surgical practice in Germany. Another institution, the Benjamin Franklin Foundation, has decisively influenced the construction of Germany's most modern hospital for the Free University of Berlin. Like in some other rebuilt faculties its concept of many departments under one roof should give full scope to interdepartmental cooperation.

Reviewing the last century of scientific medicine and surgery an overwhelming radiation from East to West cannot be overlooked in the first half of this period. WILLIAM OSLER at his time gave the credit to German Universities by stating that to their "geist" the entire world stands debtor. During the last decades we can recognize with graditude an enormous feed-back in the opposite direction. From this many patients — not only in the Western world — receive a better care. Therefore it is under the sign of humanity also that this congress is going to meet with all its friendly participants from North America and Europe. With this in mind let's go to work now, but don't forget to have a good time in still rural Munich, our secret German capital. Your patients need a relaxed surgeon. Thank you!

Vascular Disease

Etiology of Arteriosclerosis. Relationships to Systemic Diseases

G. Schettler

"Atherosclerosis is" according to the definition of the WHO [*1*] (1958) "a variable combination of changes of the intima of arteries consisting of the focal accumulation of lipids, complex carbohydrates, blood and blood products, fibrous tissue and calcium deposits, and associated with changes of the media".

The arteries have been altered already considerably for years prior to the first manifestation of circulatory impairment. Time of manifestation and clinical picture are variable and depend upon the location and extension of the occlusion as well as the functional capacity of the collateral circulation. There are often discrepancies between the pathologic-anatomical material and clinical data [*2—4*]. Many anatomical vessel occlusions remain silent clinically as shown by angiographic studies. For example two third of 64 men and 11 women with arterial occlusive disease of the extremities from a pool of 6400 workmen were free of symptoms in the Basle study project of Widmer [*3*]. It has been stated [*3*] that peripheral vascular disease and coronary artery disease have about the same frequency and occur in about the same age. I do not think this conclusion is justified. Hild [*2*], however, found a statistical correlation between peripheral vascular occlusive disease and coronary artery disease in Heidelberg. Arterial occlusive disease in patients with myocardial infarction was demonstrable only in appr. 10% by arteriography. Only half of these patients had symptoms. No definite correlations exist between arteriosclerosis of the aorta and coronary arteries. There is neither in patients with aortic aneurysm nor in patients with aortic occlusive disease a significant increase of coronary artery occlusive disease [*5*, *6*].

One cannot draw conclusions from aortic calcifications as to an increased incidence of coronary artery sclerosis [*7*]. Also there are no definite relations between the incidence of peripheral artery, coronary artery and aortic occlusive disease and cerebral vascular occlusive disease. Even arteriographically demonstrable occlusions of cerebral arteries may remain silent clinically. The occurrence of arteriosclerotic occlusive disease in extracranial or intracerebral arteries which is rather high beyond the 4th decade correlates not always with clinical manifestations [*8*, *9*]. Clinical symptoms in the region of the cerebral vessels are mainly dependent upon the condition of the collateral circulation. The same applies to occlusive disease in the region of the aorta and the peripheral arteries. The renal and coronary arteries are possibly exceptions in this regard. Arteriosclerotic occlusive changes in the renal arteries are rarely isolated findings. They may via liberation of renin and angiotensin lead to hypertension with secondary sequelae. If hypertension is associated with arteriosclerotic renal artery disease, the incidence of symptomatic arteriosclerotic disease in other vascular regions is high. Clinical studies [*10*] revealed a positive correlation between the extent of arteriosclerotic renal artery disease and the frequency of symptomatic coronary, cerebral vascular and peripheral artery disease. These episodes are frequently multiple and shorten the life expectancy.

An indirect proof of the importance of the vessel wall structure is the development of arteriosclerotic lesions in essential hypercholesterolemia. This incompletely dominant transmitted inborn error of metabolism is frequently associated with coronary occlusions, although occlusions of the peripheral arteries, the aorta, the renal or cerebral vessels are not more frequent than in comparative age groups [*11*]. Coronary artery occlusions in this disease are more frequent in men than in women. Striking is the different involvement by arteriosclerosis in hypertriglyceridemias. Comparative studies show that coronary artery occlusions are frequent in carbohydrate-induced hypertriglyceridemia, while occlusions of other arterial areas are not more frequent.

Other factors accelerating arteriosclerosis were examined pathologically and clinically [*12*, *13*]. Excellent results were obtained from prospective epidemiologic studies of coronary artery disease, an example of which is the Framingham-study. The following risk factors were observed since 1949: In the group of metabolic diseases the hypercholesterolemic xanthomatoses, diabetes mellitus, gout and with some reservation hypothyroidism. Elevated blood lipids, obesity, hypertension, abnormal increase of hemoglobin and hematocrit and a decreased vital capacity increase the risk. Disturbances of the general behaviour, physical activity and the so-called stress factor do not correlate with coronary artery disease. A noteworthy result of these studies is the accumulation of the personal risk by the combination of several risk factors. The relative frequent combination of obesity, diabetes mellitus, hyperlipemia or hypercholesterolemia, hypertension and cigaret smoking denotes an unusually high risk of coronary artery disease.

Similar representative results for arteriosclerotic occlusions in other vessel provinces do not exist as yet [*14*]. However, the literature on peripheral and cerebral arterial occlusions allows the cautious assumption that the risk factors of coronary artery occlusions do not correlate with occlusions in other vascular areas. Hypercholesterolemia, obesity and hypertension do not correlate with peripheral arterial occlusions. However, diabetes mellitus and cigaret smoking are definite risk factors in these conditions. It seems that hypertension is no significant factor for cerebral vascular occlusions. The undoubtedly high risk of hypertensive patients to suffer a stroke does not parallel the extent of cerebrovascular occlusive disease. Similarly, the risk factors of coronary artery disease are not or are not at least to the same extent applicable for vascular occlusions of the aorta and renal arteries.

The current theories of atherogenesis are as follows [*15*—*18*]:

1. The lipid infiltration theory claims that lipids derived from plasma diffuse into the inner vessel wall layers.

2. The lipid synthesis theory is based on the proven phospholipid synthesis in the vessel wall tissue itself, although it seems that the massive cholesterol deposits are not synthesized locally but are derived from blood plasma.

3. This theory postulates that the lipids do not simply diffuse into the vessel wall but that reticulo-endothelial cells of the blood plasma are responsible for the appearance of foam cells in the vessel wall.

4. The smooth muscle cells are of great importance for the deposition and conversion of lipids in the vessel wall. Plasma lipids enter the cytoplasma of the smooth

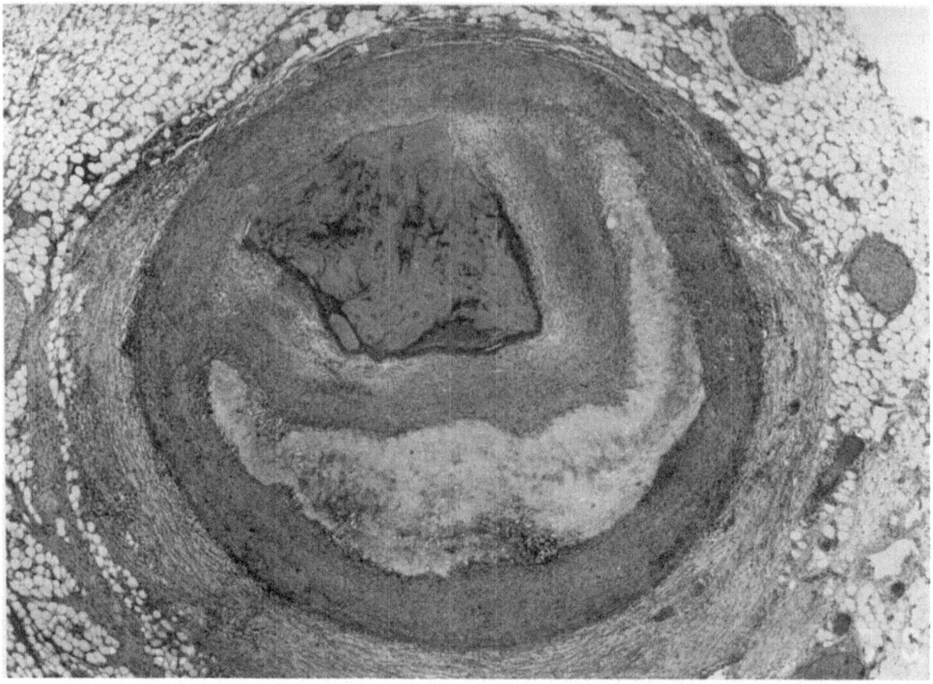

Fig. 1

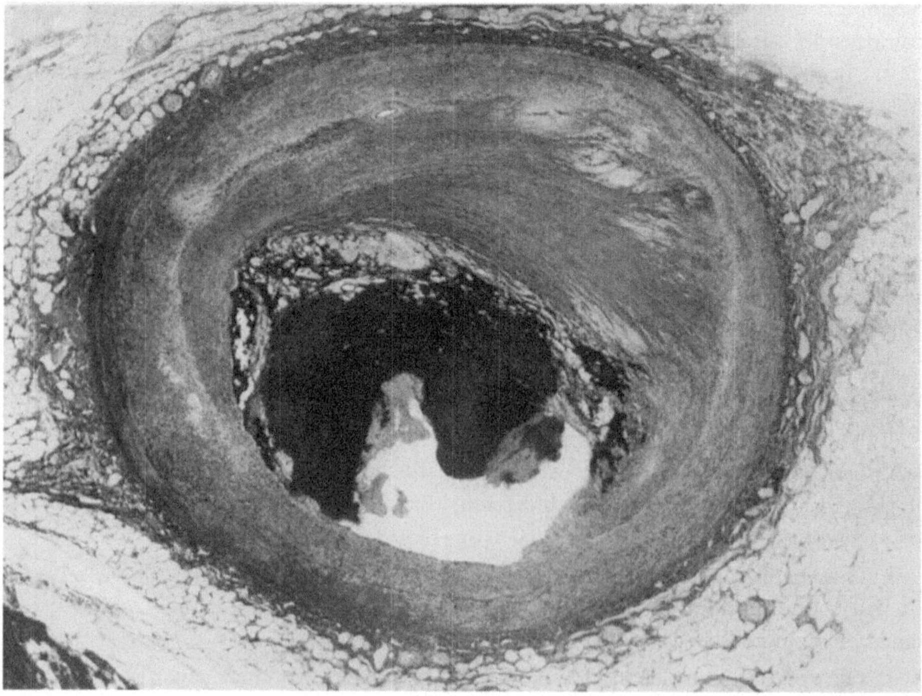

Fig. 2

muscle cells via pinocytosis through the endothelium. Other cell elements like macrophages and lymphocytes participate in these vessel wall changes.

5. Recently particular attention was directed to the ground substance of the vessel wall. The cellular and fibrous elements are located in a gel substance consisting of mucopolysaccharides, hyaluronic acid and chondroitin sulfate C, protein, lipoproteins and lipids. This system contains a considerable amount of enzymatic activity responsible for the transformation into an atherosclerotic process. Arteriosclerosis

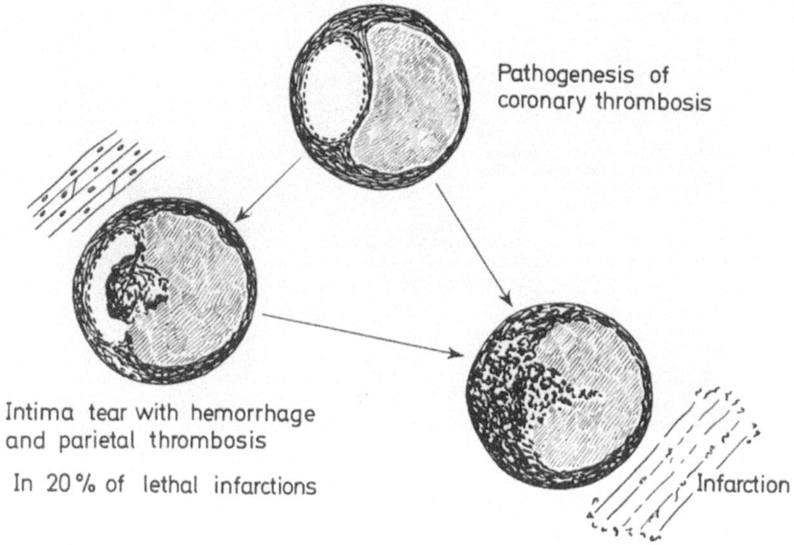

Fig. 3

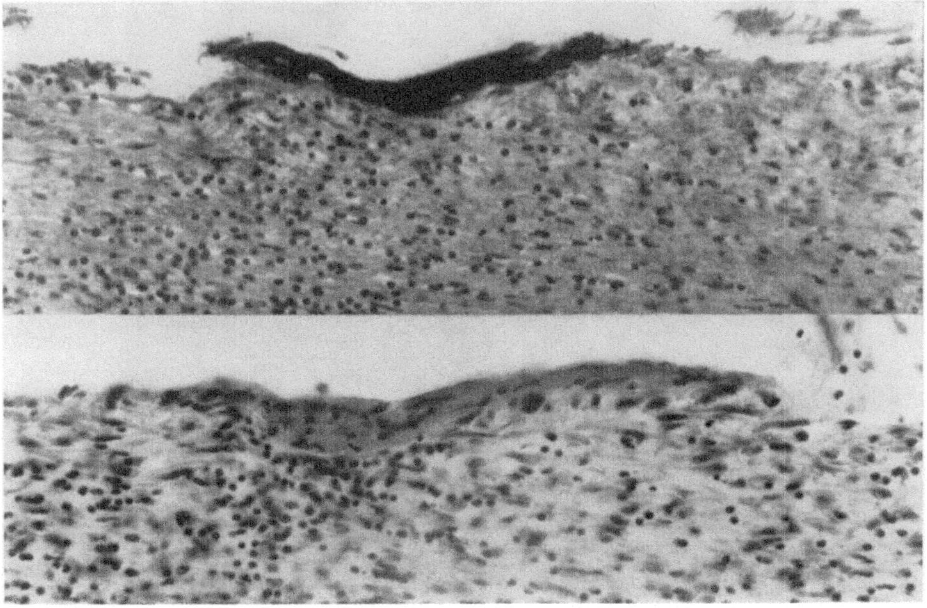

Fig. 4

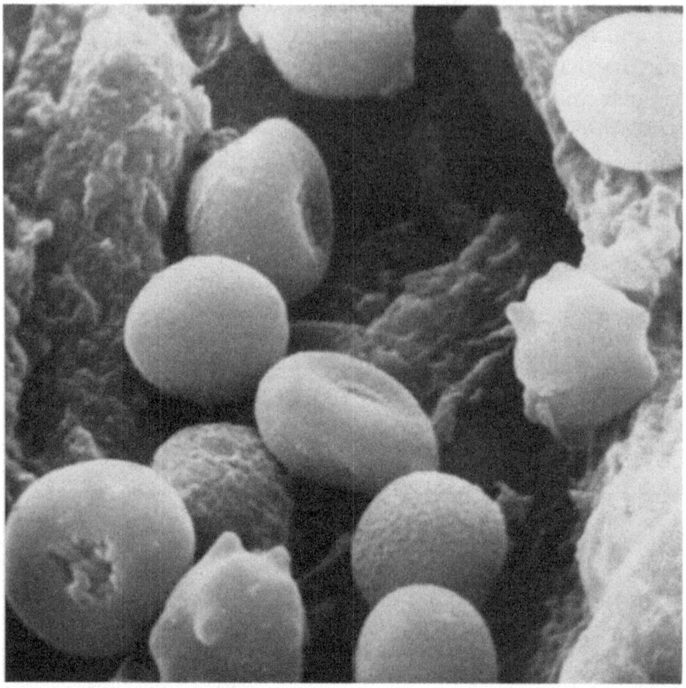

Fig. 5

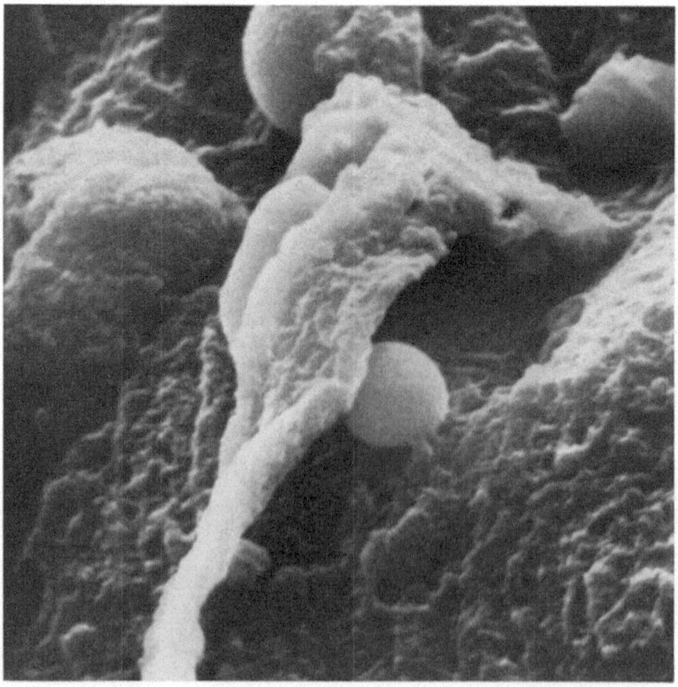

Fig. 6

starts early in life. Fig. 1 demonstrates the extent of changes which might develop even in a young adult of 27 years.

6. Frequently discussed are thrombotic processes in atherosclerotic vessel occlusions. Fig. 2 shows extensive atheromatous intima changes. One necrotic atheromatous plaque has penetrated into the vessel lumen of the coronary artery. Connective tissue has grown through the thrombotic deposits at the point of break-through. Within the vessel lumen one can recognize the remainders of a platelet clot. I am indebted to Prof. KRAULAND [19], the director of the Institute of Forensic Medicine of the Free University of Berlin, for these pictures. A schematic presentation of stenosing coronary thrombi is shown on the next figure (3) following SINAPIUS [20]. At least for the coronary artery system one has to assume that occlusions are caused in the majority of cases by thrombi. The importance of coagulation processes for the early phases of arteriosclerosis has been of a high interest in regard to pathogenesis. The incorporation of fibrinoid into the vessel walls has been demonstrated repeatedly (Fig. 4).

The progress in microscopic diagnostic techniques is demonstrated in the following pictures (Fig. 5, 6) of human aorta (Fraunhofer Institute in Karlsruhe; V. BECKER and coworkers). Coagulation studies and new electronmicroscopic techniques may contribute to the solution of these important problems of atherogenesis. In that case the conditions for prophylactic and therapeutic measures against thrombosis, the most important component of vascular occlusion, would be much improved. The therapy with fibrinolytic and thrombolytic agents together with anticoagulants has augmented the tools of the internists. The achieved results have to remain modest if one considers all the anatomical changes leading to the vascular occlusion. This is the field of the vascular surgeon.

Fig. 1 to 6; legends see text.

References

1. WHO: Classification of atherosclerotic lesions. Report of a study group. Definition of terms. W H O Techn. Rep. Ser. **143**, 4 (1958).
2. HILD, R.: Arteriosklerose der Gliedmaßenarterien. In: Pathophysiological and clinical aspects of lipid metabolism. Ed. SCHETTLER, G., and R. SANWALD. Stuttgart: Thieme 1966.
3. WIDMEX, L. K.: Bibl. cardiol. (Basel) **13**, 67 (1963).
4. —, M. CIKES, P. KOLB, H. LUDIN, M. ELKE und H. E. SCHMITT: Schweiz. med. Wschr. **97**, 102 (1967).
5. GROOM, D., E. E. MCKEE, W. ADKINS, V. PEAN, and E. HUDICOURT: Ann. intern. Med. **61**, 900 (1964).
6. STRONG, J. P., and H. C. MCGILL: Exp. molec. Path. Suppl. **1**, 15 (1963).
7. CHAPMAN, J. M., D. B. LOVELAND, L. S. GOERKE, G. JACOBSON, and W. J. ROTROCK: J. chron. Dis. **12**, No. 5 (1960).
8. DRAKE, JR., W. E., and M. A. L. DRAKE: Circulation **33/34**, Suppl. III, 90 (1966).
9. BERNSMEIER, A., and U. GOTTSTEIN: Internist (Berl.) **5**, 207 (1965).
10. WOLLENWEBER, J., S. G. SHEPS, and G. D. DAVIS: Amer. J. Cardiol. **21**, 60 (1968).
11. HARLAN JR., W. R., J. B. GRAHAM, and E. H. ESTES: Medicine (Baltimore) **45**, 77 (1966).
12. BREST, A. N., and J. H. MOYER (Ed.): Atherosclerotic vascular disease. New York: Appleton-Century 1967.
13. SCHETTLER, E. G., and G. S. DOYD (Ed.): Atherosclerosis. Amsterdam: Elsevier 1969.
14. HEYDEN, S.: Statistics and Epidemiology. In: Atherosclerosis. Ed.: SCHETTLER, F. G., and G. S. BOYD. Amsterdam: Elsevier 1969.

15. Kritchevsky, D.: Current concepts in the genesis of the atherosclerotic plaque. In: Brest, A. N., and J. H. Moyer, Ed. Atherosclerotic vascular disease, p. 1. New York: Appleton-Century-Crotts 1967.
16. Doerr, W.: Perfusionstheorie der Arteriosklerose. Stuttgart: Thieme 1963.
17. — Gangarten der Arteriosklerose. S. Ber. Heidelberger Akademie der Wissenschaften Math. nat. Kl. 1964, Abh. 4. Berlin-Göttingen-Heidelberg-New York: Springer 1964.
18. Bleyl, U.: Habilitationsschrift, Heidelberg 1968.
19. Krauland, W.: Dtsch. med. Wschr. **93**, 807 (1968).
20. Sinapius, D.: Personal communication.

Radiographic Techniques in Diagnosis of Vascular Disease*

W. Wenz

Historical Data

The history of the radiologic evaluation of the blood vessels is as old as x-rays are. 8 weeks after Roentgen's first succesful experiment Haschek and Lindenthal (1896) published the radiography of an amputated hand with the vascular system visualized by a mixture containing calcium and mercury.

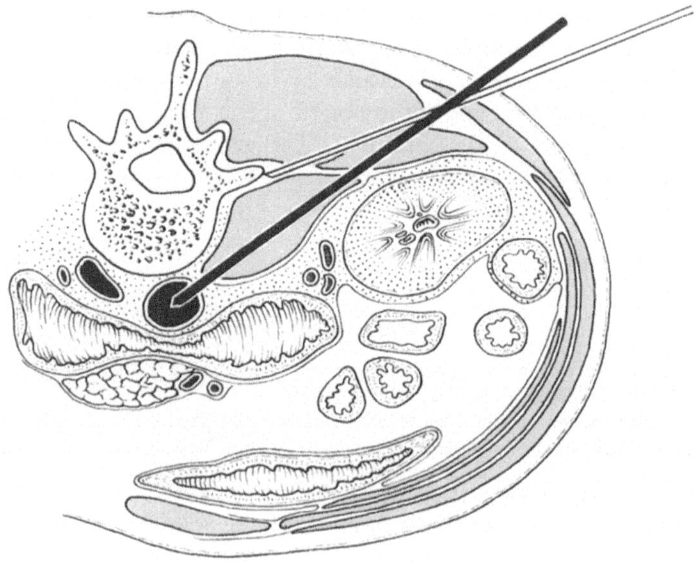

Fig. 1. Dos Santos' technic of direct lumbar aortography

Initially the development of angiography was not so much concerned with techniques of injection as with the problem of toxicity of the contrast material used. With the advent of modern iodine containing contrast media complications are today extremely rare.

Regarding the technique of administration of contrast media there seems to be no vessel in the human body that has not at some time or another been used for this purpose. As an example you see here numerous possible injection sites for the visualization of the thoracic aorta in a somewhat confusing pattern.

* X-ray Department (Head: Dr. W. Wenz) of the Surgical Clinic (Director: Prof. Dr. F. Linder), University of Heidelberg.

We look back on the pioneers of angiography amongst whom there were several surgeons with great respect particularly since they produced excellent radiographs sometimes at great personal risk and under poor working conditions.

I would like to single out two dates as being of particular importance in the development of arteriographic techniques: the direct injection into the lumbar aorta (Fig. 1) by Dos Santos (1929) and the technique of percutaneous catheter replacement of a cannula (Fig. 2) by Seldinger (1953). Both these methods gave tremendous impetus to the further development of angiography.

Practically all of our modern techniques of today derive from these two basic procedures. This paper will be concerned only with aortic and arteriographic techniques.

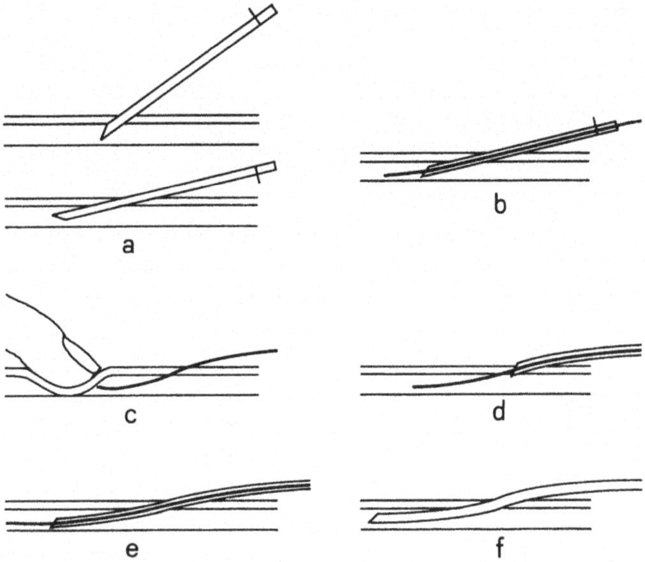

Fig. 2. Catheterization technic according to Seldinger. (a) The artery is punctured; the needle pushed upward. (b) The leader inserted. (c) The needle withdrawn and the artery compressed. (d) The catheter threated onto the leader. (e) The catheter inserted into the artery. (f) The leader withdrawn. (After Abrams, 1961)

General Angiographic Technique

The minimum apparatus required includes a well functioning x-ray unit, a television image intensifier, a rapid serial film changer, tape recording or cinematography.

Primarily there are two ways for the visualization of arteries:

1. the intraarterial injection of the contrast medium,
2. the transvenous injection.

In the first case injection takes place directly into the artery resulting in a selective arteriogram with a low dosage of contrast medium without troublesome superpositions. The injection is performed either by hand or by means of an injection pump.

Following intravenous application the iodine containing substance has to pass the pulmonary circulation before reaching the desired arterial segment after a variable passage time. This method was propagated by Steinberg et al. (1965), who produced

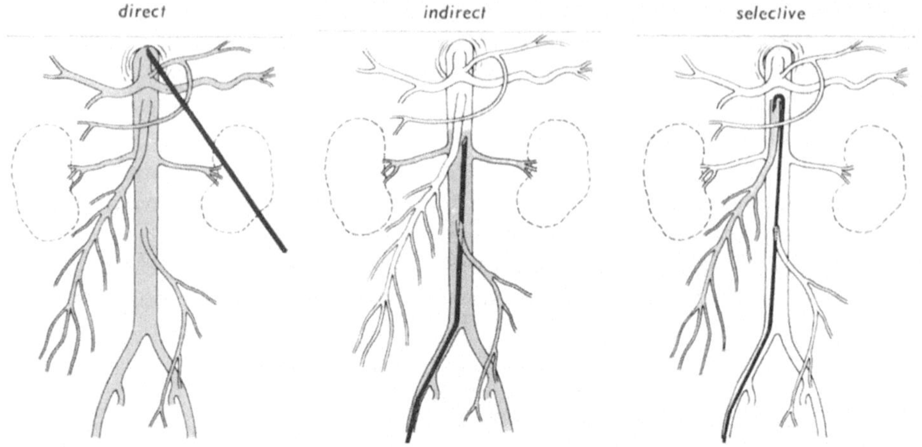

Fig. 3. Technics of abdominal aorto-arteriography. [After WENZ, W.: Langenbecks Arch. klin Chir. Kongr.-Bd. **21,** (1968)]

clear aortographies with doses of around 100 ml of highly concentrated iodine solution. This technique has not become popular in Germany. Exceptions are however pathological changes of the thoracic aorta such as anomalies and posttraumatic aneurysms where a right heart catheter injection seems to be preferable.

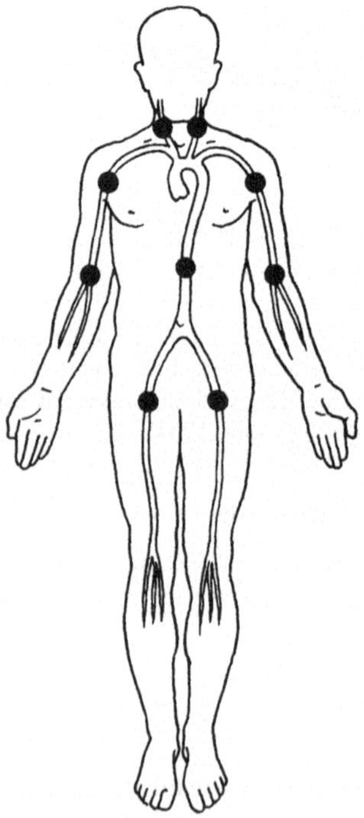

Fig. 4. Injection sites for direct and catheter arterio-aortography as used by the author

For intraarterial contrast injection two techniques are available.

1. direct, percutaneous arteriography,
2. indirect, retrograde arteriography by means of catheter or retrograde contrast injection from the periphery (LUDIN, 1966).

Let me demonstrate this technique for the abdominal aorta and its branches (Fig. 3): This is the original technique of DOS SANTOS (1929) for *direct* visualization of the abdominal aorta, performed in all cases of aortic occlusion or changes of the visceral arteries whenever stenoses or kinking of the iliac arteries prohibits catheterization from below.

In contrast to this SELDINGER's technique of *indirect* catheterization permits a certain selectivity depending on the position of the catheter-tip. Thanks to the curved catheter of ÖDMAN (1956), *selective* angiography of visceral arteries is possible.

It seems unnecessary to discuss the angiography of peripheral arteries in this auditorium. I just want to demonstrate the injection sites that we prefer for direct arteriography (Fig. 4). Combined with the catheter technique they enable us to reach any area of vascular disease.

The indications for direct injection and for catheter technique as used in our department are as follows:

extremities: direct injection; thorax: catheter technique; abdomen: direct injection in occlusive disease, cathetertechnique for selective arteriography and visualization of the retroperitoneal organs; skull: direct injection of the carotid artery, catheterization of the vertebral artery.

In our series the separate techniques were split up as indicated in Table 1:

Table 1. *Localization of arteriographies (X-ray Dept. Surgical Clinic, University of Heidelberg 1. January 1960 to 1. March 1968)*

Arteriography		Number
cerebral	more than	3 000
brachial		111
thoracic		149
abdominal		2 311
femoral		349

During aorto-arteriography a certain amount of vascular damage due to the cannula or catheter is unavoidable. Fortunately most of these cases remain asymptomatic.

In Heidelberg nevertheless we had two fatal cases in a series of more than 6000 angiographies (0,3‰). Apart from that there were several complications such as extravasation, hematoma, thrombosis and one incompletely restored hemiplegia (less than 1%). This complication rate is about the same as in other large series (LANG, 1963; CORMIER et al., 1966; DIEMEL u. SCHMITZ-DRÄGER, 1968).

Special Angiographic Technique

Ladies and gentlemen, undoubtedly you are not only interested in our angiographic technical problems but as surgeons you expect some concrete examples demonstrating our procedure. This excursion into clinical routine shall be followed by the rate of incidence of common arterial disease.

Congenital Anomalies

The most important clinical anomalies affect the aortic root. For the visualization of the left heart we prefer transseptal injection of the contrast medium (Example[1]: Coarctation of the aorta; rt. aortic arch after ligature of a patent ductus, demonstrated via rt. heart catheter).

A further congenital anomaly of the descending aorta was verified in a 30 years old soprano (Fig. 5). Two aortic branches reach an accessory lung within the left thorax while the venous drainage could be followed into the left pulmonary vein.

As a very rare condition we saw a newborn baby with mermaidssyndrome (sirenomelia[1]). There was no sacral bone, two femurs, only one fibula and one talus. The arteries were filled via the umbilical artery. The iliac arteries were missing and we could 'nt find the rt. femoral artery. The fused lower extremities were vascularized by only three arteries. These angiographic findings were later verified at autopsy.

[1] Illustrated in the original lecture.

Acute Arterial Occlusion

There are three possible causes for acute arterial occlusion: trauma, embolism or acute thrombosis. Posttraumatic vascular occlusion may follow stretching of the vessel, dissection of the intima or external compression. The localization of the injury and the site of vascular occlusion are not identical in every patient.

(Example[1]: Occlusion of the axillary artery in the case of a young parachutist who accidentally hung onto the wing of his aeroplane with one arm. He sustained fracture of the humerus and the resulting hematoma prevented direct arterial puncture. The occlusion was visualized by means of femoral catheterization and selective angiography of the lt. subclavian artery).

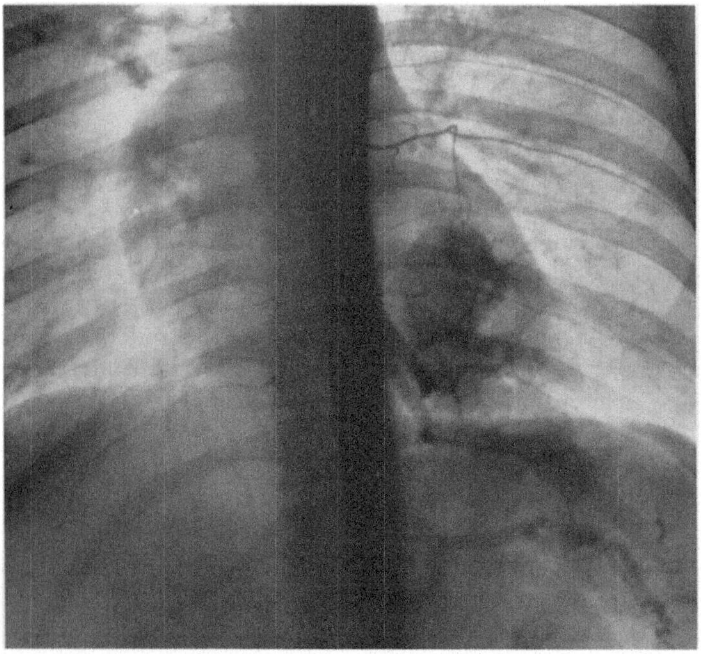

Fig. 5. Catheter aortography: accessory left lung with two aortic branches

Technical difficulties are illustrated in the case of multiple fractures with blunt abdominal trauma. Rupture of the spleen or left kidney — suspected before — could be excluded by selective arteriography, whereas filling of the left femoral artery revealed massive dislocation of the vessels by the bony fragments[1].

As a rule arterial embolism can be localized exactly by simple clinical means. Therefore arteriography is indicated only in rare cases (VOLLMAR, 1967). Exceptions are occlusion of the abdominal aorta and embolic occlusion of important visceral arteries. Fig. 6 demonstrates the typical bifurcation embolism in a patient who had just undergone mitral commissurotomy.

(Example[1]: Mesenteric arterial thrombosis causing acute abdominal symptoms in a 75 years old woman).

As you see we try to diagnose aortic occlusions by means of direct injection and lesions of the aortic branches by selective catheter arteriography.

Apart from the left heart aneurysms are well known sources for peripheral embolism (Example[1]: Embolism of digital arteries due to a poststenotic subclavian aneurysm. Prior to angiography the clinical diagnosis was REYNAUD's disease).

In contrast to this thrombotic occlusions often show arteriosclerotic changes of the vessel wall with collaterals and irregularly pointed ends of the contrast column. This angiographic differentiation between thrombosis and embolism is not always possible but particularly in the case of carotid occlusions it may be of vital importance. The radiologist should rapidly come to a diagnosis by direct puncture or catheter arteriography. (Example[1]: Occlusion of the internal carotid with a pointed irregular stop

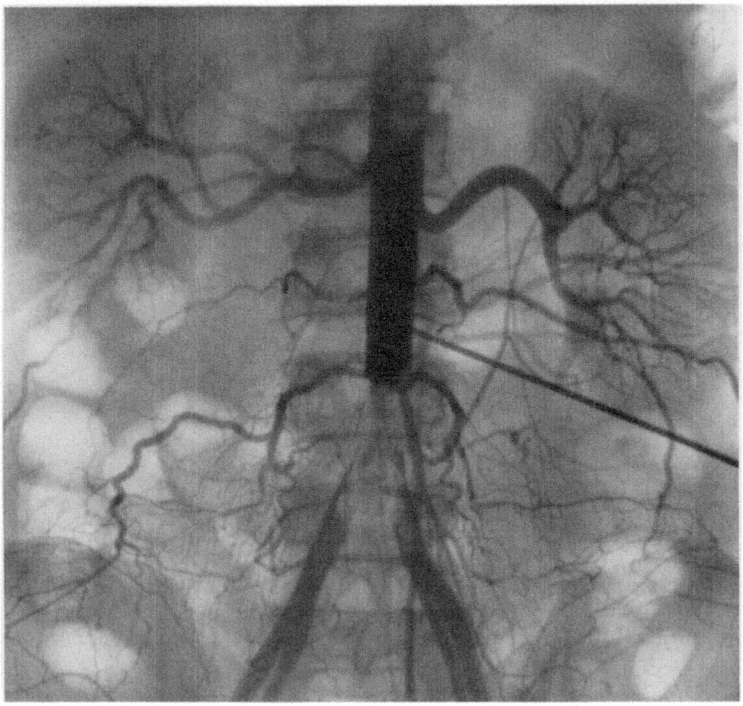

Fig. 6. Lumbar aortography: Bifurcation embolism after mitral commissurotomy

as a sign of thrombosis and a second example reveals embolic occlusion of the middle cerebral artery with a perfectly smooth break of the contrast column.)

Contrast medium entering the external carotid only but not the internal carotid is taken as proof of cessation of cerebral circulation and when repeated within 30 min with identical findings a sign of clinical cerebral death.

Chronic Occlusive Disease

In comparison to the relatively rare acute arterial occlusions in our angiographic series (about 5%) the chronic occlusions are predominant. When localized in the lower extremities the examination was carried out mostly by direct lumbar aortography. We consider it a mistake to attempt catheterization of the iliac arteries in arteriosclerotic disease thus risking loosening of calcified plaques. Our procedure consists of puncture of the lumbar aorta between the 3rd and 4th lumbar vertebra and in cases of high aortic thrombosis the puncture at the level of the 12th thoracic vertebra.

Obviously in the abdominal area the development of collateral circulation is of great importance in chronic occlusion of visceral arteries. We found 68 occlusions or stenoses amongst 398 abdominal aortographies of which only 7 caused clinical symptoms. What is the reason for this discrepancy?

The arteriographic example(1) of multiple occlusions with vascular supply of the upper abdominal organs via the so called Riolan-anastomosis demonstrates the efficiency of those collaterals. It was surprising that this patient weighing 100 kgs had no abdominal complaints.

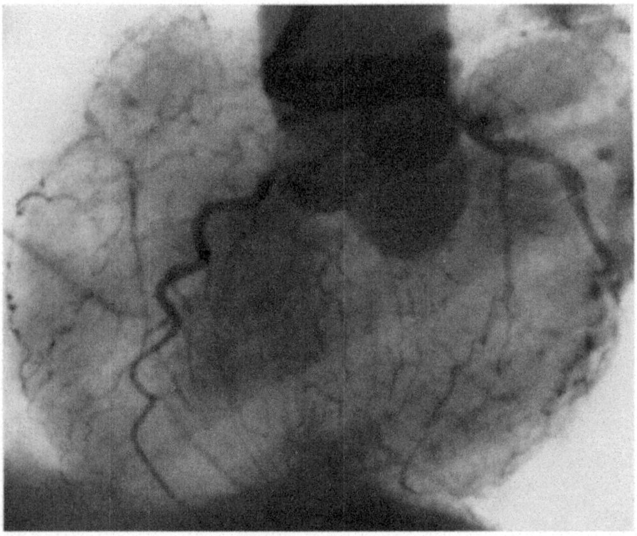

Fig. 7. Coronarography: Typical positioning of the spiral catheter (Paulin) in a case of total occlusion of the rt. coronary artery

Thus angiography supplies objective proof for the importance of the collateral circuit in visceral occlusions. The possible collateral pathways can be demonstrated by aortography or selective arteriography.

The absence of collaterals led to abdominal angina in a patient with stenoses of celiac and superior mesenteric arteries (example[1]). Similar mechanisms apply to occlusive processes of the large supraaortic branches. We know that in particular the vertebral artery can function as a collateral vessel in cases of subclavian occlusion. (Example[1]: Subclavian steal syndrome visualized by retrograde brachial arteriography; injection from the rt. side showing the rt. subclavian, the rt. vertebral artery and filling of the lt. subclavian via the lt. vertebral in which the contrast medium flows in a retrograde direction.)

The method of choice for the visualization of all supraaortic branches is thoracic aortography. For coronary arteriography we prefer the spiral catheter of Paulin (1964) (Fig. 7), whereas Sones (1962) recommends the selective cannulation of the coronary ostia.

Aneurysms

All angiographies in patients with suspected aneurysms require particular care, because some of them show very thin walls. (Example[1]: Posttraumatic aortic aneurysm demonstrated by thoracic catheter aortography).

Fig. 8 shows a historical film of the year 1942 with a brachial aneurysm demonstrated by direct injection-arteriography with THOROTRAST. This technique was abandoned because of the possible complication of bleeding from the injection site.

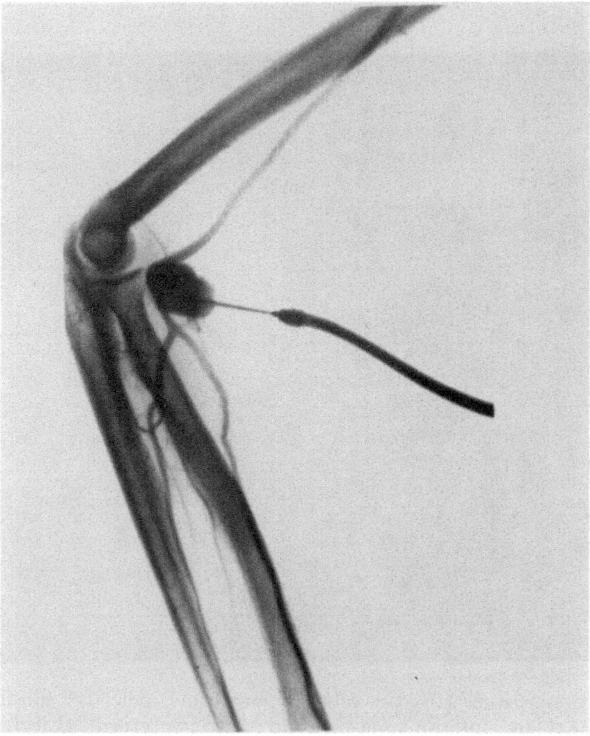

Fig. 8. Direct puncture of a brachial aneurysm: Visualization of the arterial system by THOROTRAST, a thorium containing contrast medium (historical film of the year 1942)

Sometimes the differentiation between aneurysm and angioma can be very difficult as we learned in a case of aneurysmal angioma of the carotid artery confirmed by operation (example[1]).

Arterio-venous Fistula

Aneurysms may be combined with a shunt to the venous system. Mechanisms of the trauma and clinical findings usually permit correct diagnosis. It is the task of angiography to localize the shunt exactly and to provide an estimate of its volume. Technically the contrast medium should be injected as close as possible to the shunt. Registration must be performed by cinematography or by fast serial filming.

(Example[1]: A-v-fistula of the index-finger as a curiosity for which a wall-eyed pike was responsible. The fish apparently mistook the finger for the hook and the subsequent peripheral arteriography presented us with this unusual localization of an arterio-venous shunt.)

Sometimes arterial puncture in arterio-venous aneurysms is very difficult because of the arterialization of the dilated post-shunt veins. Only the direction of flow of the contrast medium under television control will permitt the recognition of the afferent artery.

The case of a-v-fistula 19 years after nephrectomy (Fig. 9) also demonstrates the importance of catheterizing and filling the afferent vessel. The arterial stump, the admixture of arterio-venous blood within the inferior vena cava and the dilatation

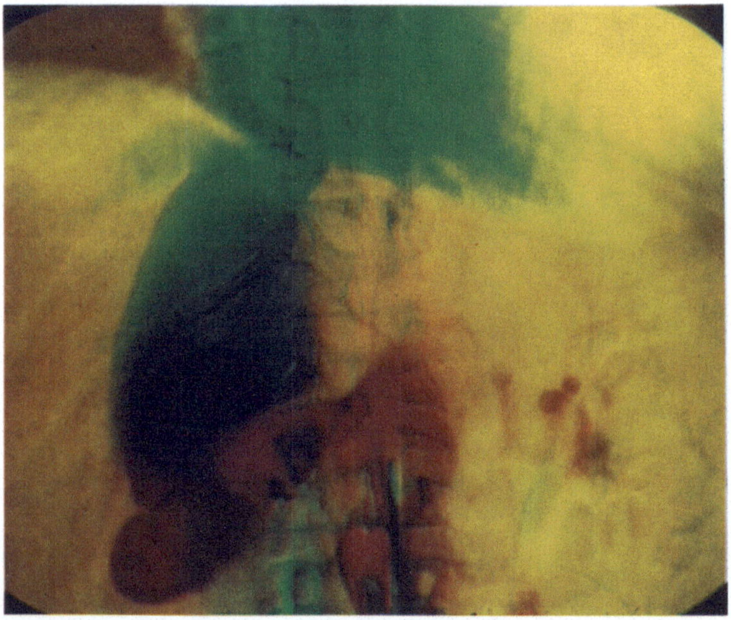

Fig. 9. Arterio-venous fistula 19 years after nephrectomy. Selective filling of the afferent vessel (red) and the dilated inferior vena cava and rt. atrium (green). (Electronic subtraction and color reproduction of the films)

of the cava and right atrium can be clearly outlined by electronic subtraction of the films and color reproduction.

Our excursion into the field of angiographic techniques has shown a great variety of problems. No wonder that radiologists are discussing the next steps in future technical development. Let me offer you one possibility: contrast medium exchange transfusion! Unfortunately this method includes problems that are not purely radiologically, otherwise we would be delighted to inaugurate this method of ideal and total examination here and now.

References

Abrams, H. L.: Angiography. Boston (Mass.): Little, Brown & Co. 1961.

Bücheler, E., L. Beltz, A. Düx und P. Thurn: Radiologe **5**, 217—231 (1965).

Cormier, J. M., C. Hernandez, R. Kieny et J. Natali: Aortographie abdominale (tronc et collatérales). Paris: Masson & Cie. 1966.

Debray, Ch., J. Leymarios und Cl, Hernandez: Cah. Coll. Méd. Hôp. Paris **6**, 739—751 (1965).
Diemel, H., u. H. G. Schmitz-Dräger: Radiologe **8**, 54—65 (1968).
Dos Santos, R., A. Lamas, and J. Pereira-Caldas: Med. contemp. **47**, 93 (1929).
Elke, M.: Röntgenblätter **20**, 412—419 (1967).
Friedenberg, M. J., and T. W. Staple: Surgery **58**, 789—796 (1965).
Heberer, G., G. Rau und H. H. Löhr: Aorta und große Arterien. Berlin-Heidelberg-New York: Springer 1966.
Hernandez, Cl., G. Morin et B. Ecarlat: Presse méd. **73**, 2889 (1965).
Kappert, A.: Leitfaden und Atlas der Angiologie. Bern u. Stuttgart: Hans Huber 1966.
Lang, E. K.: Radiology **81**, 257 (1963).
Ludin, H.: Acta radiol. (Stockh.) Suppl. **256**, 1 (1966).
Nebesar, R. A., and J. J. Pollard: Amer. J. Roentgenol. **97**, 477—487 (1966).
Ödman, P.: Acta radiol. (Stockh.) Suppl. **159**, 1 (1958).
Paulin, S.: Acta radiol. (Stockh.) Suppl. **233**, 1 (1964).
Seldinger, S. I.: Acta radiol. (Stockh.) **39**, 368 (1953).
Sones, F. M.: Selective cine coronary arteriography. Xth International Congress of Radiology, Montreal 1962.
Steinberg, I., and H. L. Stein: Amer. J. Roentgenol. **95**, 684—695 (1965).
Vollmar, J.: Rekonstruktive Chirurgie der Arterien. Stuttgart: Thieme 1967.
Wenz, W.: Die Arteriographie in der chirurgischen Diagnostik der Bauchorgane. 85. Tagung Dtsch. Ges. Chirurgie, München 1968.

Management of Chronic Femoropopliteal Artery Obstruction

J. Vollmar and K. Laubach

Of all the arteries in the body the human femoral artery is most frequently affected by obliterative lesions. Their surgical correction includes many divergent opinions in respect of technic, indication and late results. Alloplastic bypass procedures which were enthusiastically accepted ten years ago lead to a host of failures: on the other hand these failures stimulated many efforts to find new ways for improving the results.

It is evident that the relatively high failure rate of femoro-popliteal reconstructions stands in close correlation with the following patho-physiological facts:

1. The predominance of lengthy occlusions frequently with calcification of the arterial wall (Fig. 1);
2. the relatively small caliber of the vessels with a small minute volume;
3. poor arterial "run-off" caused by concomitant disease of the more distal vessels in 30 to 40% of cases;
4. in the case of vascular prostheses their vulnerability at the level of the knee joint.

The return to autoplastic vascular reconstruction and certain instrumental and technical improvements within recent years have shown the way to overcoming these difficulties. Two autoplastic procedures are in the limelight of discussion today:

1. The femoro-popliteal venous bypass;
2. the open or semi-closed thrombendarterectomy.

We ourselves give preference to the semi-closed disobliteration with ringstrippers as the method of choice for both short and lengthy occlusions (Fig. 1).

Here are some remarks on the technique of the operation: In most cases with segmental lesions it is possible to isolate and remove the occlusive cylinder in retrograde fashion from a single distal arteriotomy (Fig. 2). This simple procedure is based on the assumption that proximal to the diseased vascular segment the intima is normal. The intimal cylinder then tears off in the zone of transition through the normal segment and can be removed in one piece through the distal arteriotomy. On the other hand, short, localized stenoses as seen in this femoral artery with an apparently normal run-in and run-off arteriographically, should not tempt the surgeon to be satisfied with a purely local disobliteration. In actual fact, this 57 year old patient showed severe atheroma of the whole of his femoral artery, necessitating disobliteration right up to the femoral bifurcation. The occlusive cylinder is shown on the right.

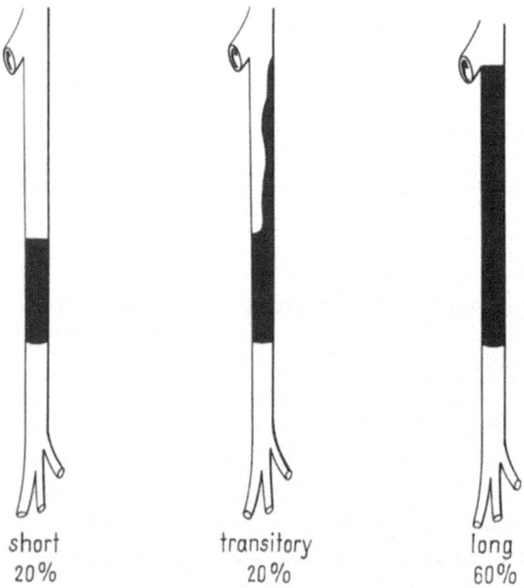

Fig. 1

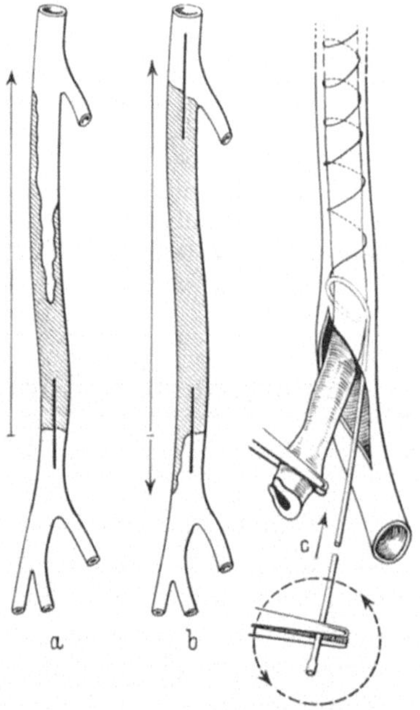

Fig. 2

Fig. 1. Morphological types of femoro-popliteal arterial occlusions

Fig. 2. Principles and technic of semiclosed Thrombendarterectomy by spiraldissection

For all lengthy occlusions we prefer to perform the stripping procedure between a proximal and distal arteriotomy (Fig. 2b).

This also applies when a short stenosis exists at the origin of the deep femoral artery. Reconstruction of the deep femoral run-in will insure survival of the extremity even in those cases where the peripheral vascular procedure may fail.

Additional, intermittent arteriotomies are acquired only rarely if the following technical points are followed:

1. If the media is found to be calcified, the plane of disobliteration should be selected close to the adventitia (Fig. 3). This plane lies close to the external elastic lamina in the zone between media and adventitia.

2. The dissection of the occlusive cylinder should be performed in a spiral fashion, i. e. blunt rings mounted at an angle of 135 ° and advanced within the arterial wall by rotatory movements (Fig. 2c). In this way, areas of intramural calcification can be

Table 1. *3-Point indication for reconstructive arterial procedures*

I. Clinical indication:
Stage I: none
Stage II: relative indication
Stage III and IV: urgent

II. Angiographic indication:
Local operability in relation to localisation and length of occlusion
free "run-in"?
free or sufficient "run-off"?

III. General operability:
No severe concomitant risks
(coronary heart diesease; Diabetes; Hypertension; Carcinoma etc.)

threaded into the ring without much difficulty. In contrast to this the right angled ringstrippers lead to a transverse plane of dissection which meant that the stripping procedure usually failed at the first calcified plaque.

In the last 500 cases of femoro-popliteal occlusion ring disobliteration failed only in 7,4% due to excessive calcification of the media; perforation occurred in 3,4% of cases (Table 2).

The advantages of the semi-closed stripping procedure are evident:

1. Short operating time.

2. The remaining outer vascular cylinder remains practically along its whole length within its natural bed, i.e. it is not separated from its blood supply. This insures a rapid regeneration of the intima which is usually complete within 3 to 4 months.

3. In case of failure, a thrombendarterectomy does not preclude a transplant procedure at a later date.

Table 2. *Complications of semiclosed thrombendarterectomy of the femoro-popliteal arteries (500 operations)*

Technical failure (stripping impossible)	37	7.4%
Perforation of the wall	17	3.4%

In contrast to this open thrombendarterectomy, i.e. splitting of the femoro-popliteal artery from the knee to the inguinal ligament with a long patch, constitutes a lengthy and more extensive procedure. As a result of the extensive dissection of the artery intimal regeneration is slowed. Disturbances of wound healing are also much more common. Apart from optimal visual control, this procedure seems to offer only disadvantages. We prefer to reserve the operation of femoro-popliteal bypass for those cases where the shorter and simpler thrombendarterectomy has failed.

This figure may serve as an example: The segmental occlusion on the left was corrected in 1962 by local thrombendarterectomy with a dacron patch. The vessel remained patent for 2 years. Due to incomplete stripping of the proximal intimal segment a recurrent occlusion occurred. Reoperation with femoral-popliteal vein bypass is shown on the right.

If the venous bypass is performed first, in case of a recurrent occlusion a later return to thrombendarterectomy is usually impossible. The saphenous vein should be preserved as a potential vascular transplant in every patient. This vessel should never be slightly sacrificed, especially in patients with obliterative vascular disease. Vein patches can equally well be taken from one of the branches of the vein.

Table 3. *Survey of 668 reconstructive procedures on 644 patients with chronic femoro-popliteal occlusions* (1. Jan. 1959 to 31. Dec. 1967)

Type of operations		Nr. of ops.	†		Nr. of follow-up	patent		failures	
Thromb-endarterectomy		500	5	(15)	480	377 85%	+ 33 ↑	103	A:4 R:33
Bypass	autoplast. (vein)	70	—	(1)	69	64 95%	+ 2 ↑	5	A:0 R:2
	alloplast. (Dacron)	98	1	(14)	83	21 33%	+ 9 ↑	62	A:15 R:9
Total		668	6	(30)	632	506 = 80%		170 = 27%	

( ) = late deaths; A = amputation; R = successful reoperation.

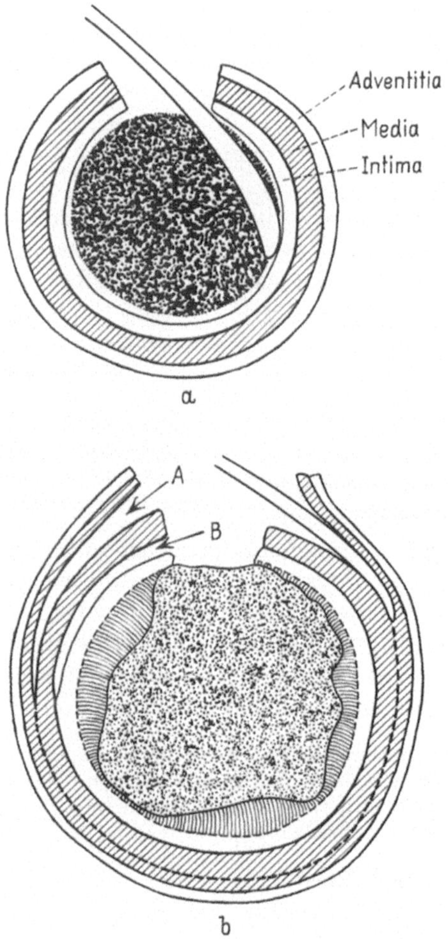

Fig. 3. Principles of disobliteration. a In healthy arteries: removal of clot alone; b In diseased vessels: dissection planes; A inside of external elastic membrane, B along the internal elastic membrane

Table 4. *Early and late results of 668 reconstructive procedures on the femoro-poplit. arteries*

Type of operation				Duration of follow-up															
	Nr.	Nr.	still	1 year		2 year		3 year		4 year		5 year		6 year		7 year		8 year	
	of ops.	of foll.-ups.	pat. tod.	Nr.	pat. %	Nr.	pat. %	Nr.	pat. %	Nr.	pat. %	Nr.	pat. %	Nr.	pat. %	Nr.	pat. %	Nr.	pat. %
Thrombendarterectomy	500	480	377	100	84	112	85	121	75	72	76	52	70	23	70	—	—	—	—
Allopl. bypass or resection and alloplast. interposition	98	83	21	—	—	2	100	3	33	7	43	12	45	23	18	26	23	10	0
Autopl. byp. or resect. and interpos. (vein)	70	69	64	21	81	21	86	26	88	1	100	—	—	—	—	—	—	—	—
Total	668	632	462									(1. Jan. 1959 to 31. Dec. 1967)							

Finally, a survey of our *results*.

Table 3 summarizes early and late results (from 6 months to 8 years) following 668 reconstructive procedures for femoro-popliteal arterial occlusion. Semi-closed thrombendarterectomy and venous bypass show equally favorable results:

85 and 95% of the operated vessels remain open. These figures do, however, include successfully reconstructed recurrent occlusions. All patients were anticoagulated postoperatively.

The further analysis of the follow-up (Table 4) shows that 6 years after semi-closed ringstripping 70% of the arteries remain open (following venous bypass the success rate is nearly the same). The results following alloplastic bypass procedure are far less favorable. Only 16% of these transplants remain patent after 6 years.

The operative mortality for reconstructive procedures on the femoro-popliteal segment is extremely low — it amounts to 0,9% in our clinic.

78% of the patients belonged to stage II, 22% to stage III or IV. 19 extremities had to be amputated in the course of the disease, 16 times following reocclusion of a dacron bypass.

Finally, it must be noted that even today the discussion as to the most suitable procedure for femoro-popliteal arterial occlusions is in no way settled. Strippers, grafters and patchers have taken up more or less reconcilable positions. In our point of view, these are not competitive but rather complimentary methods. It seems most important, however, that the first operation is selected in such a way that in case of recurrent occlusion a further operation remains possible. For this reason, the best solution today appears to be thrombendarterectomy first, followed, if necessary, by a venous bypass.

References

de Bakey, M. E., E. S. Crawford, G. C. Morris, D. A. Cooley, and H. E. Garret: J. cardiovasc. Surg. (Torino) **5**, 473 (1964).

de Weese, J. A., H. B. Barner, E. B. Mahoney, and C. G. Rob: Ann Surg. **163**, 205 (1966).

Vogt, B.: Die rekonstruktive Gefäßchirurgie. Stuttgart: Thieme 1965.

Vollmar, J.: Akt. Chir. **1**, 91 (1966).

— Rekonstruktive Chirurgie der Arterien. Stuttgart: Thieme 1967.

—, M. Trede, K. Laubach, and H. Forrest: Ann. Surg. **168**, 215 (1968).

Wylie, E. J., F. M. Binkley, and R. J. Aldo: Amer. J. Surg. **108**, 215 (1964).

Indications for and Techniques of Surgical Treatment for Carotid Artery Stenosis

Charles Rob

In 1954 Eastcott, Pickering, and Rob reported that a patient suffering from recurrent transient strokes had been cured by reconstruction of a stenosed internal carotid artery. Before that a number of surgeons including Strully, Hurwitt, and Blankenberg (1953) had attempted unsuccessfully to restore the flow through a completely thrombosed internal carotid artery. Today most surgeons prefer to operate upon the carotid artery at the stage of arterial stenosis, because the results of surgery at this stage are so much better. Table 1 illustrates this point, a good flow having been established in 98 per cent of our patients with stenosis of the internal carotid artery and only 36% with a thrombosis of this artery.

Table 1. *Results of arterial reconstruction in 609 patients with stenosis or thrombosis of the internal carotid artery*

Type of occlusion	Number of patients	Good flow established
Arterial stenosis	468	459 (98.36%)
Arterial Thrombosis	141	51 (36.12%)

Indications for Operations

The indications for reconstruction of a stenosed carotid artery include transient strokes or transient ischaemic attacks; an asymptomatic stenosis if major surgery is planned for another lesion, such as an abdominal aortic aneurysm; senile mental changes if associated with stenosis of the carotid arteries; completed strokes when either carotid artery is stenotic and stenosis of the common carotid arteries including those patients in whom this is part of the aortic arch syndrome.

Transient ischaemic attacks are frequently associated with arteriosclerosis of the cervical position of the carotid arteries. In some patients the cause is an alteration of the blood flow due to stenosis of the carotid arteries. In our view a more frequent cause is microembolization, the microemboli arising from a plaque of atheroma at the bifurcation of the common carotid artery. As Table 2 shows, transient ischaemic attacks have been the major reason why we have reconstructed the carotid artery. But it must be stressed that operations in these patients is essentially a prophylactic procedure designed to prevent further attacks and possibly a major hemiplegia.

Table 2. *Results of reconstruction of the carotid arteries in 609 patients*

Type of stroke	Number of patients	Good flow established	Asymptomatic	Objectively better	No change	Died
Transient or incipient	444	429	298	92	47	7
Progressing	74	35	15	15	32	12
Completed	91	46	21	36	29	5

Asymptomatic Stenosis

These are patients with a bruit over the carotid bifurcation and in whom the diagnosis of stenosis of the carotid artery has been confirmed by arteriography. We recommend surgical correction here if major surgery is planned for another lesion. The reason for this is that a fall of blood pressure may precipitate a major stroke in these patients and it is, therefore, better to correct the carotid lesion before undertaking a major elective surgical procedure.

Early Senile Mental Changes

Some patients notice a considerable restoration of their memory and mental capacity after reconstruction of the carotid arteries. This is especially so if there has been only a short history of mental deterioration or if the common carotid or innominate arteries are occluded. It is possible that in the future the restoration of a normal or nearly normal flow through the carotid and other extracranial cerebral arteries may become for some of our middle aged and elderly citizens a useful method of preventing the premature development of senile mental changes and mental deterioration.

Completed Strokes

At one time we recommended early surgery on patients with acute completed strokes due to the thrombosis of the internal carotid arteries. But as early at 1957 (Rob and Wheeler, 1957) we were beginning to doubt the wisdom of this procedure. And we now believe that such surgery is mistaken and that with the possible exception of patients who are operated upon 2 or 3 hours after such an arterial occlusion, surgery is best deferred until the acute situation has passed.

Our management today of a patient with an acute completed stroke due to thrombosis of the internal carotid artery is to admit the patient to the hospital and commence medical treatment. The diagnosis may be confirmed by ophthalmodynamometry. Later after about a week and after the patient has commenced to improve, we perform an arteriogram of the extracranial cerebral arteries. By this time any surgery is unlikely to influence the outcome of this particular stroke and it will be technically impossible to restore a flow through a completely thrombosed internal carotid artery. However, carotid arterial surgery may still have a place in the treatment of such a patient; if the arteriogram shows a stenosis of either carotid artery. Then correction of this lesion will improve the whole cerebral blood flow, with the result that recovery may be accelerated and future strokes prevented. In many such patients the arteriogram shows thrombosis of one internal carotid artery and stenosis of the other; here reconstruction of the stenotic artery may be worthwhile.

Lesions of the common carotid arteries are not common if one excludes the distal vessel in the region of the carotid bifurcation. The aortic arch syndrome consists of occlusions of the three main branches of the aortic arch: the innominate, left common carotid and left subclavian arteries, diseases of the main stem of the common carotid arteries is part of this syndrome. This syndrome although not common, is very favorable for surgery and the results of arterial reconstruction have been good (Rob, 1966).

Special Problems

Recently we have been interested in two problems. The association of stenosis of the carotid arteries with stenosis of the renal arteries and the association of stenosis of the carotid arteries with cerebral tumors.

In our series 64% of patients with occlusive diesases of the extracranial cerebral arteries also have arterial hypertension. We now perform our arteriogram of the renal arteries as well as of the extracranial cerebral arteries in many of these patients. This has demonstrated a significant stenosis of the renal arteries in 7.8% of these patients or 5% of the whole group (Fig. 1 and 2 illustrate this problem). We believe that the best procedure in such patients is to correct the carotid stenosis first, whilst the blood pressure is still elevated, and to operate upon the renal artery stenosis 4 or 5 days later.

In the case of an association between stenosis of the carotid arteries and cerebral tumors two points will be stressed. First some cerebral tumors may cause symptoms similar to transient strokes or transient ischaemic attacks, and here a correct preoperative diagnosis is important. Second, some patients may have both a stenosis of an extracranial cerebral artery and a cerebral tumor. If the tumor is considered to be

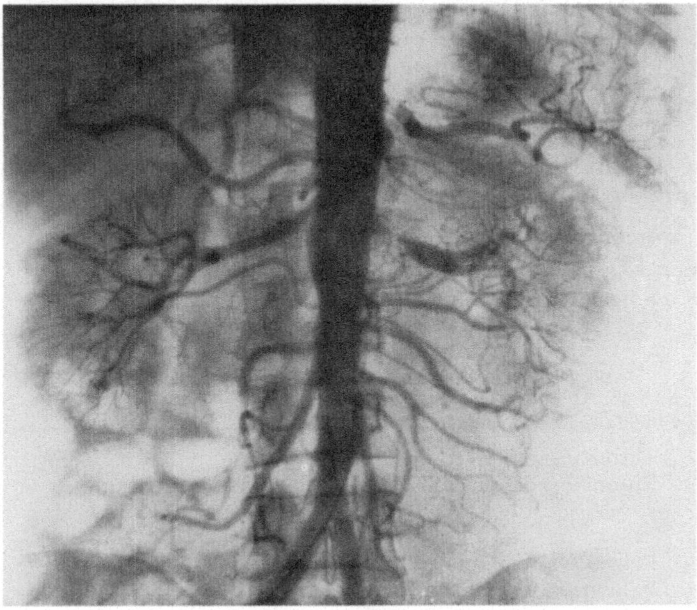

Fig. 1. Stenosis of the left renal artery in a 47 year old patient with transient attacks of cerebral vascular insufficiency and arterial hypertension

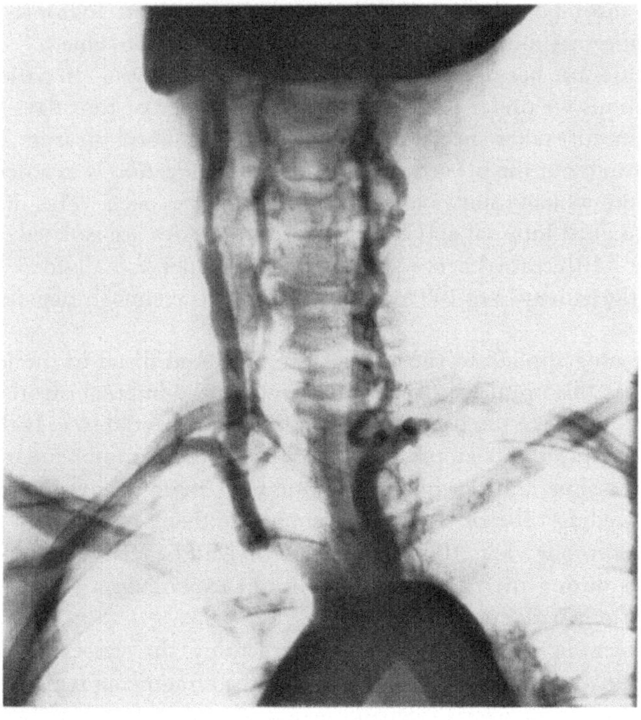

Fig. 2. The patient shown in Fig. 1 also has a stenosis of the first part of the left internal carotid artery. Correction of the carotid lesion followed 4 days later by thromboendarterectomy of the left renal artery has been successful in reducing this patient's blood pressure to normal and preventing further transient ischaemic attacks or transient strokes

benign and resectable it is best to restore a normal carotid flow before the tumor is resected. The reason for this is that the neurosurgeon can control hemorrhage but he cannot control arterial thrombosis if there is a low pressure and slow flow in the carotid arterial system.

The Technique of Operations for Carotid Arterial Stenosis

As stated in Table 1 we now have experience of operations in 609 patients with stenosis or thrombosis of the carotid arteries. In 105 of these patients the operation was bilateral making a total of 714 operations in 609 patients. Table 3 lists the procedures which we have used.

Table 3. *Technique of operation for carotid arterial stenosis and thrombosis*

Thromboendarterectomy	685
Thromboendarterectomy and patch graft angioplasty	
Venous patch	11
Prosthetic patch	6
Resection and end to end anastomosis	7
Vein graft replacement of by pass	5

Table 3 shows that the technique which we have employed most frequently has been a simple thromboendarterectomy without a patch graft angioplasty. The other procedures being used only when this technique was not possible.

The procedure has been performed under general anesthesia. In patients requiring bilateral operations we prefer to leave an interval of three or four days between each side. The anesthestist takes special care to maintain the blood pressure at the preoperative level throughout the procedure. The carotid bifurcation is exposed through an cervical incision which follows the skin folds of the neck. The distal common carotid and proximal internal and external carotid arteries are isolated. Care is taken to preserve the XIIth cranial nerve. The carotid sinus nerve is divided. The anesthetist now gives the patient 75 to 100 mgms of heparin intravenously depending upon the body weight.

Clamps are now applied to the arteries proximal and distal to the lesion and the vessel incised. At this point we release the clamp on the internal carotid artery distal to the lesion and observe the back flow from the distal arterial tree. If this is fast and red, then we reapply this clamp and proceed with the thromboendarterectomy. If this back flow is slow and the blood cyanotic or if there is any doubt, we insert a temporary indwelling tube of silastic as a shunt and then proceed with the thromboendarterectomy. In our view, this is an inexpensive and effective way of monitoring the blood gases during the procedure, and in our experience a shunt is required in less than 5% of our patients.

After completion of the thromboendarterectomy the vessel is very carefully flushed with saline and inspected to confirm that no fragments remain in the lumen as potential emboli. The arterial incision is now closed with a continuous suture of silk and the shunt removed, if present, just before completion of this suture line. The heparin effect is now reversed with protamine sulfate and the arterial clamps are removed.

Occasionally a patch graft is required if it appears that a simple closure will produce a stenosis and we prefer a venous segment for this. Sometimes the lesion is not true arteriosclerosis but another form of arterial disease and then a thromboendarterectomy is often not possible. In these patients continuity is restored either by an end to end anastomosis or by the insertion of a venous graft.

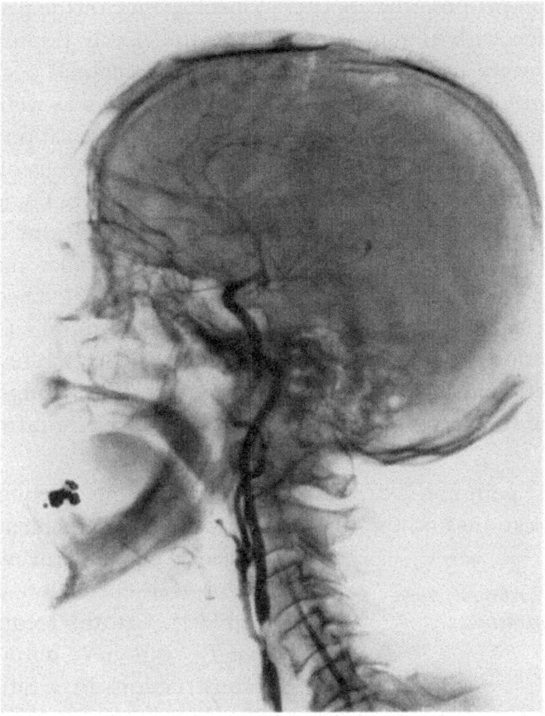

Fig. 3. This arteriogram demonstrates the occasional association of stenosis of the arterial carotid artery with a cerebral tumor

Recurrent Stenosis

This appears to be an uncommon event. We have only operated upon seven such patients and our follow up now extends to over 14 years in our longest surviving patient. The reasons for this may include the localised nature of the disease, the fact that the internal carotid artery distal to the operation site is usually normal and this provides a satisfactory out flow unlikely to be constricted by flexion of joint.

References

EASTCOTT, H. H. G., G. W. PICKERING, and C. G. ROB: Lancet **1954**, 994.

ROB, C. G.: Obliterative diseases of the extracranial cerebral arteries. Thule International Symposium, p. 267. Stockholm: Nord Bokhandelns Forlag. 1966.

—, and E. B. WHEELER: Brit. med. J. **2**, 264 (1957).

STRULLY, K. J., E. S. HURWITT, and H. W. BLANKENBERG: J. Neurosurg. **10**, 474 (1953).

The Vertebral Artery in Cerebral Anoxia*

George C. Morris Jr., E. Stanley Crawford, and
Michael E. de Bakey

Transient symptoms pointing to arterial insufficiency in the posterior circulation of the brain are seen with extreme frequency in the elderly population. These symptoms may be the only manifestations of serious extracranial occlusive lesions not only of the vertebro-basilar system but the carotid pathways as well. Proper management of problems in the vertebral arteries requires full appreciation of the entire cerebral circulation both intracranial and extracranial. Combinations of occlusive lesions involving both the anterior and posterior circulations to the brain, intracranial as well as extracranial, are very common. To compound these variations with their protean neurological manifestations is the great frequency of natural anatomical variations and resulting variability in collateral blood supply to the brain [*2*]. The usual locations of arteriosclerotic occlusive lesions are well recognized and quite characteristic. These usual sites of occlusion are the great branches of the aortic arch near their orifices of origin, the bifurcation of the innominate artery, the bifurcations of the common carotid arteries, and the vertebral arteries adjacent to their origin from the subclavian arteries.

By far the most common extracranial occlusive lesions encountered are located in the carotid bifurcations and the vertebrals at origin. The incidence of these lesions is nearly equal. However, the incidence of surgical correction is quite unequal (Table 1). Carotid reconstructions in the past 15 years have outnumbered vertebral reconstructions by a ratio of nearly six to one. The basis for this more aggressive surgical attack on the carotid bifurcation is the result of firm clinical experience. Permanent and disabling neurologic disability or even death is the usual end when carotid stenosis leads to complete occlusion of the internal carotid artery with thrombus. On the other hand extracranial vertebral stenosis rarely leads to catastrophic basilar artery thrombosis. Basilar artery thrombosis is usually the direct result of basilar artery arteriosclerotic disease. Therefore, surgical correction of a carotid lesion is given priority when associated with vertebral stenosis even if symptoms are primarily or even exclusively vertebro-basilar in character [*3*]. Furthermore, our experience indicates that vertebro-basilar symptoms will disappear in over 80% of cases with combined lesions when the carotid stenosis is corrected. A further factor in this disproportion is related to microembolic phenomena. Carotid plaques are often ulcerated in character and prone to embolic dissemination of debris. On the other hand, vertebral stenosis is usually produced by a smooth, fully endotheliazed sclerosis in ring-like fashion at the junction of the subclavian artery and not prone to produce microembolism.

Table 1. *Cerebrovaslucar reconstruction*

Carotid	2100
Vertebral	365
Arch	299

* From the Cora and Webb Mading Department of Surgery, Baylor University College of Medicine and The Methodist Hospital, Houston, Texas.

Clinical Picture

Characteristic and usual presenting symptoms of vertebro-basilar arterial insufficiency are vertigo, visual disturbances (most commonly diplopia) and variable parasthesias of the body and extremities such as numbness and tingling. However, because of the frequency of multiple lesions, variations in arterial anatomy and the passage of motor pathways through the area of posterior blood supply, symptoms can be extremely variable and misleading. Pertinent points of physical examination should include auscultation for supraclavicular and carotid murmurs and their separation from transmitted cardiac murmurs. Bilateral comparison of carotid, subclavian, and brachial pulses should be made together with comparative blood pressures in the upper extremities. However, if symptoms, even through transient and infrequent, suggest the possibility of cerebrovascular disease, complete four-vessel arteriography is indicated despite the absence of any positive physical findings.

Arteriography

Several techniques with many variations have evolved in the past 15 years, each of which has the potential for high quality delineation of the carotid and vertebro-basilar systems. Selection of specific techniques is a matter of individual adaptation and choice provided the method results in high quality visualization of the entire circulation both intracranial and extracranial. Catheter injection of the aortic arch, while giving high quality visualization of extracranial vessels, has deficiencies in quality of intracranial visualization. The Seldinger technique and modifications will provide excellent X-rays of both intracranial and extracranial areas but does require ordinary needle puncture and injection of the left carotid artery. We employ all of the accepted techniques to meet individual requirements, but for speed, simplicity and safety we prefer direct Cournand needle injection for most four-vessel studies. We believe general anesthesia makes the study more pleasant for patient and doctor, and adds a significant factor in safety.

Occlusive Lesions and Surgical Correction

Aortic Arch

Stenotic and occlusive lesions of the great vessels arising from the aortic arch are pertinent to discussion of vertebral artery disease since decreased perfusion of the subclavian artery must effect vertebral artery blood flow. Furthermore, occlusive

Table 2. *Location and extent of 412 lesions in 299 patients*

	Extent of obstruction		Totals
	Incomplete	Complete	
Innominate artery	40	26	66
Right common carotid artery	5	19	24
Right subclavian artery	30	29	59
Left common carotid artery	24	37	61
Left subclavian artery	69	133	202
Total	168	244	412

disease of the left subclavian artery is the most common type of arteriosclerotic disease of the aortic arch vessels (Table 2). Left subclavian occlusion is the pathologic basis for the physiologic disorder known as the left subclavian steal syndrome. In this condition, flow is reversed in the vertebral artery which acts as a prime source of collateral blood supply to the arm and proportionately decreasing arterial perfusion in the posterior circulation (Fig. 1). This disorder may occur on the right also and the anterior circulation also may be depressed according to the anatomy of the posterior communication arteries.

Specific surgical techniques for correction of occlusive lesions of the great vessels arising from the aortic arch must be individualized to meet specific case requirements. The bypass method of revascularization was the first used in treating this condition

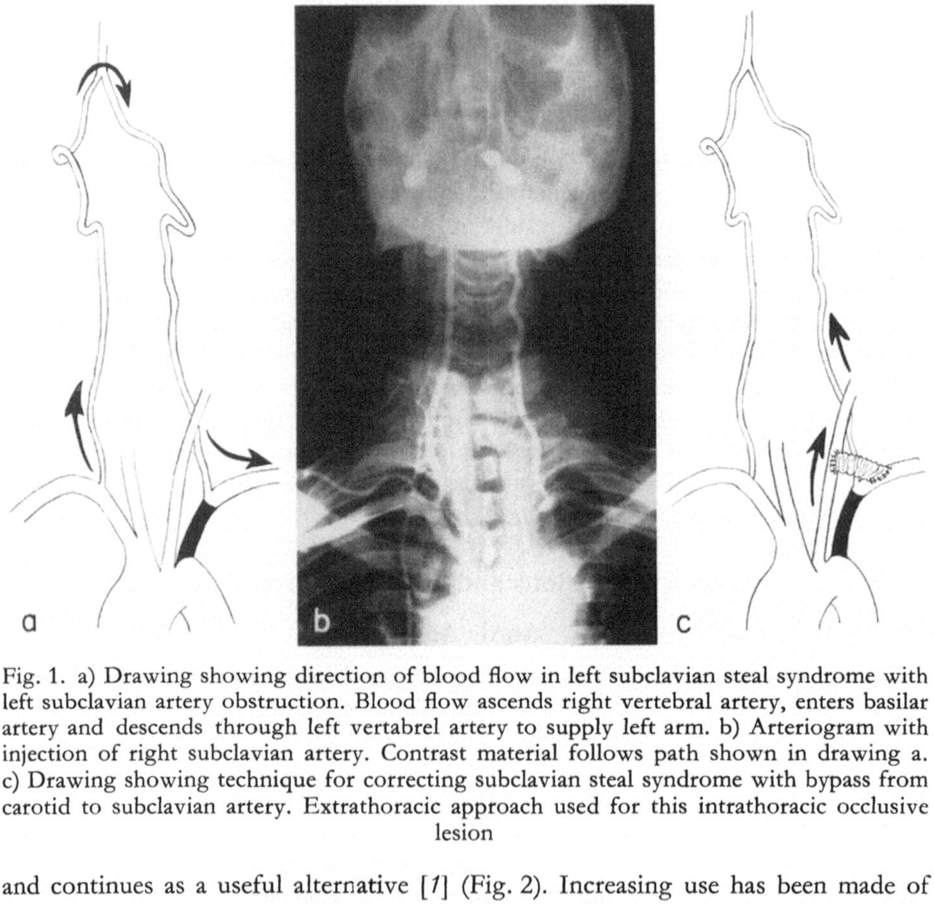

Fig. 1. a) Drawing showing direction of blood flow in left subclavian steal syndrome with left subclavian artery obstruction. Blood flow ascends right vertebral artery, enters basilar artery and descends through left vertabrel artery to supply left arm. b) Arteriogram with injection of right subclavian artery. Contrast material follows path shown in drawing a. c) Drawing showing technique for correcting subclavian steal syndrome with bypass from carotid to subclavian artery. Extrathoracic approach used for this intrathoracic occlusive lesion

and continues as a useful alternative [*1*] (Fig. 2). Increasing use has been made of direct attack with endarterectomy and patch graft angioplasty through a midsternotomy incision. However, the most important trend through the years has been the extrathoracic approach to intrathoracic occlusion usually by means of bypass (Fig. 3). Particularly cogent to this consideration has been the great frequency of isolated left subclavian occlusion and the excellent results obtained in 162 cases treated by common carotid to left subclavian bypass performed through a small supraclavicular incision (Fig. 4). The procedure has been tolerated very well by the elderly and in no instance have symptoms of iatrogenic left carotid steal been observed.

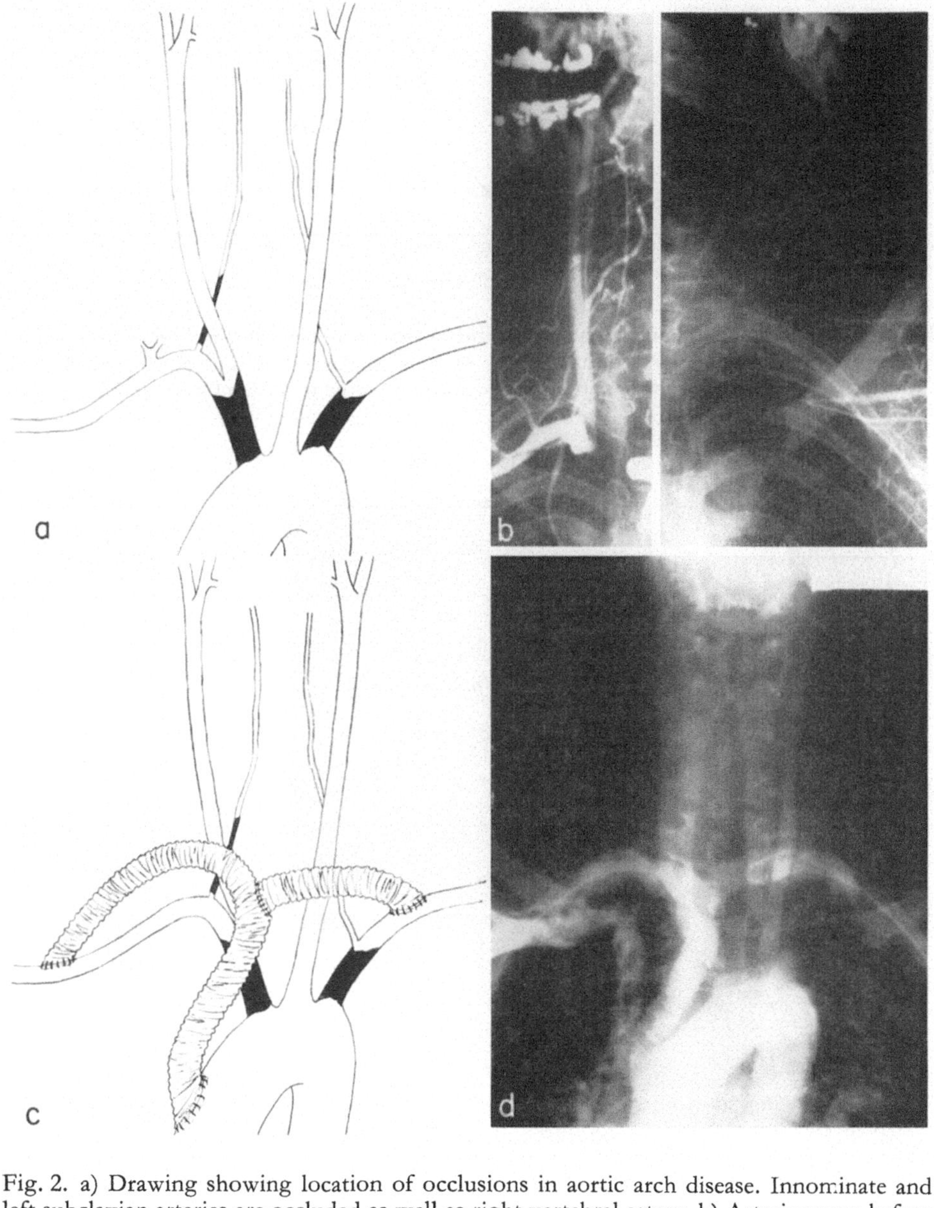

Fig. 2. a) Drawing showing location of occlusions in aortic arch disease. Innominate and left subclavian arteries are occluded as well as right vertebral artery. b) Arteriograms before operation showing locations of occlusive lesions. c) Drawing showing technique of aorta to subclavian artery bypass bilaterally. Proximal graft attachment to aorta is made through right anterior second interspace incision. Distal attachments to subclavian arteries are made through supraclavicular incision. d) Arteriogram made after operation showing functioning bypass graft correcting this form of aortic arch occlusive disease

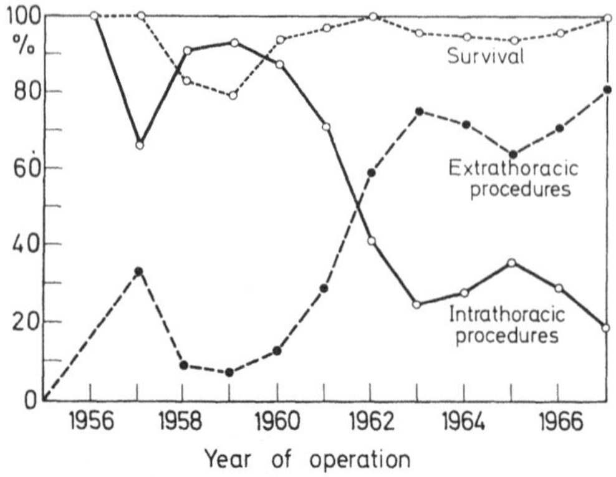

Fig. 3. Line graph contrasting frequency of intrathoracic and extrathoracic procedures used during past 11 years for correction of aortic arch occlusive lesions and operative survival. Note striking trend toward extrathoracic procedures and low mortality figures in recent years

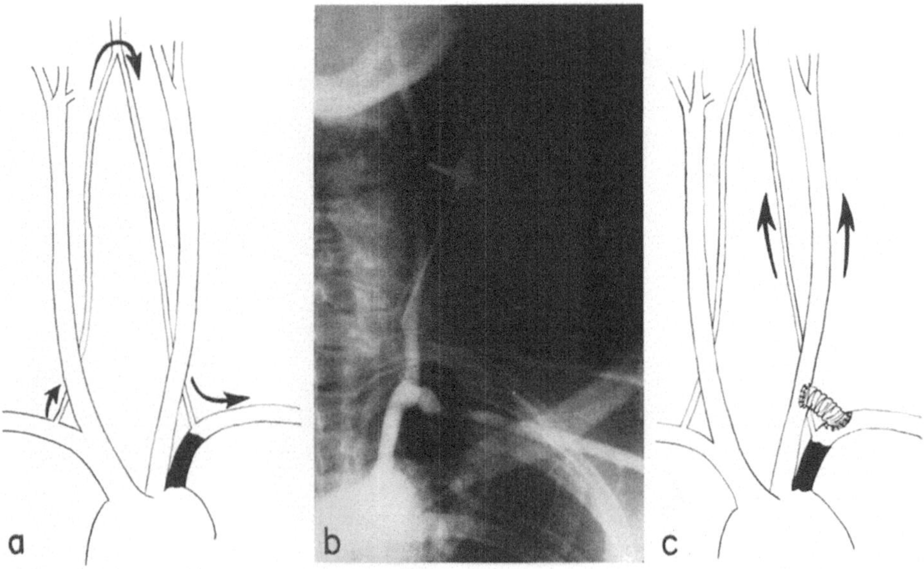

Fig. 4. a) Drawing showing direction of blood flow before operation in patient with left subclavian steal syndrome. b) Arteriogram made after operation showing functioning bypass graft from left carotid artery to left subclavian artery. c) Drawing showing technique of left carotid artery to left subclavian artery bypass with graft

Vertebral Stenosis

The most frequent form of vertebro-basilar arterial insufficiency is produced by circumferential sclerosis of the vertebral orifice and is in part a product of subclavian arteriosclerotic disease. When there is disproportion in vertebral size, the left is usually the larger and hence the more commonly repaired artery (Table 3).

Early in our experience attacks on this lesion included trans-subclavian endarterectomy, simple trans-subclavian dilatation and later endarterectomy with dacron patch extending out the vertebral artery. Long-term evaluation has shown these methods to be not uniformly reliable. Because the intima is smooth with these sclerotic lesions, simple angioplastic widening of the subclavian-vertebral junction with saphenous vein patch and without endarterectomy has been the usual technique by the senior author. Long-term evaluation with critical evaluation of late arteriographic study has shown good results (Tables 4 and 5). However, the method does require fine and meticulous surgical technique. Occasional lesions may lend themselves to other autoplastic methods of reconstruction such as side-to-side anastomosis between redundant post-stenotic vertebral artery and subclavian artery.

Table 3. *Vertebral reconstruction (74 patients) type angioplastic reconstruction*

Type angioplastic reconstruction		Number of procedures Number	%
Patch graft with vein		52	64
Patch graft with dacron		8	10
Reimplantation		8	10
Side-to-side anastomosis		7	8
Endarterectomy		7	8
	Total	82	100
	Left	51	69
Carotid reconstruction		29	39

Table 4. *Vertebral reconstructions (74 patients) results — 6 months to 10 years*

		Number	%
Asymptomatic		47	64
Improved		13	17
Unchanged		5	7
Dead		5	7
Unknown		4	5
	Total	74	100

Table 5. *Vertebral reconstruction (74 patients) follow-up arteriography*

		Number	%
Widely patent		13	82
Stenosis		2	12
Occluded		1	6
	Total	16	100

Other Vertebral Lesions

The most common non-arteriosclerotic occlusive lesion of the vertebral artery in the transient type associated with head turning [*5*]. Impingement of the artery owing to its course through the transverse processes of the cervical spine may reach such a degree with the head in certain positions as to produce temporary complete occlusion (Fig. 5). Aging and osteoarthritis contribute to this problem. Usually surgical intervention is unwarranted and instruction is given to the patient about avoidance of certain forms of cervical rotation. Another form of non-arteriosclerotic

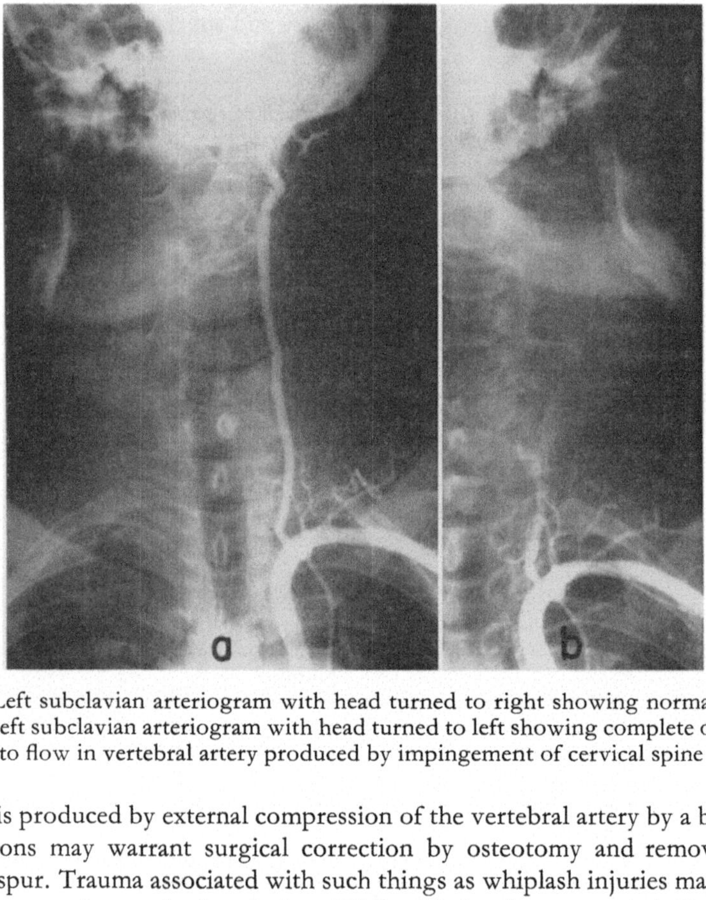

Fig. 5. a) Left subclavian arteriogram with head turned to right showing normal vertebral artery. b) Left subclavian arteriogram with head turned to left showing complete obstruction to flow in vertebral artery produced by impingement of cervical spine

occlusion is produced by external compression of the vertebral artery by a bony spur. These lesions may warrant surgical correction by osteotomy and removal of the offending spur. Trauma associated with such things as whiplash injuries may produce acute, symptomatic vertebral occlusion. While this has been a statistically insignificant lesion in our surgical experience, it is suspected that it is a more common lesion and usually unrecognized. Fibromuscular, intimal and medial hyperplasia has been recognized but as yet has not assumed surgical importance [*3*, *4*].

Discussion and Results

Current autogenous techniques for correcting extracranial vertebral artery occlusive disease have proven most gratifying in long-term results. While occlusive disease of the vertebro-basilar system takes lower priority than that of the carotid system in respect to surgical reconstruction, symptoms of this disorder are so ubiquitous in the elderly population as to magnify the problem in any consideration of cerebrovascular disease. Furthermore, little can be more satisfying to the surgeon than bringing back the sweetness of life to a patient totally disabled by vertigo and/or severe visual impairment; and doing this with an operation seeming relatively trivial to the patient and requiring only a few days of hospitalization. Patients exhibiting infrequent and less severe symptoms can be managed conservatively provided significant carotid disease has been ruled out by arteriography. Nicotinly alcohol tartrate appears to bring decided symptomatic improvement to many such patients.

For purposes of this report, 82 consecutive vertebral artery reconstructions in 74 private patients of the senior author (GCM) were reappraised. Adequate follow-up information was obtained from all but four patients 6 months to 10 years after operation. Age averaged 61 years and 65% of the patients were male. Associated occlusive disease of the carotid system was present in 62% and when surgically correctible was given priority. Bilateral vertebral disease or stenosis in the only vertebral artery communicating with the basilar artery was observed in 74% of cases. Patch graf angioplasty of the subclavian-vertebral junction using saphenous vein without endarterectomy was used in 64% of patients and exclusively during the past 6 years (Table 3). Operative mortality occurred in only one patient and 93% of patients arc still living (Table 4). Of the original 74 patients, 64% are neurologically asymptomatie and 17% are significantly improved. Five patients were unimproved and all but one of these had received obsolete surgical techniques of repair. Follow-up arteriography was possible in 16 patients. In this group the reconstruction appeared widely patent in 13 or 82%. Two were patent but showed some degree of narrowing at the site of reconstruction. One of these followed side-to-side anastomosis between redundant post-stenotic vertebral and subclavian artery. One reconstruction had occluded and this one followed endarterectomy and dacron patch.

References

1. DE BAKEY, M. E., G. C. MORRIS JR., G. L. JORDAN JR., and D. A. COOLEY: J. Amer. med. Ass. **166** (9), 998—1003 (1958).
2. FIELDS, W. S., M. E. BRUETMAN, and J. WIEBEL: Monogr. surg. Sci. **2**, 183—259 (1965).
3. MORRIS, G. C., JR., and M. E. DE BAKEY: Surgical therapy of carotid and vertebral insufficiency. Stuttgart: Thieme 1966.
4. —, A. LECHTER, and M. E. DE BAKEY: Arch. Surg. **96**, 636—643 (1968).
5. WEIBEL, J.: Acta radiol. (Stockh.) **5**, 570—580 (1966).

The Superior Mesenteric Artery Syndrome

GEORGE D. ZUIDEMA

Occlusive disease of the mesenteric arteries has been recognized as a clinical entity for many years. TIEDEMANN reported the first case of superior mesenteric artery occlusion in 1843 [*21*]. Other reports soon followed, and by 1904, JACKSON et al. [*11*] presented an article summarizing the cases studied up to that time. TROTTER [*22*], in 1913, compiled the clinical and experimental work on the subject in an authoritative monograph. The subject has continued to be of interest, and as vascular surgery developed the emphasis has shifted from a review of autopsy studies to the surgical considerations involved in the diagnosis and treatment of the syndromes seen in acute and chronic mesenteric artery occlusion. This transition is well shown by the review article by LAUFMAN et al. [*13*] published in 1964.

Although sudden, complete occlusion of the superior mesenteric artery usually results in extensive intestinal infarction, partial occlusion may present a much different picture. The intestine, when gradually deprived of its blood supply, may show altered function rather than necrosis. The syndrome of mesenteric arterial insufficiency was described by GILBRIDE [*10*] in 1909 and DAVIS [*4*] in 1921 noted the similarity to intermittent claudication in the extremities and angina pectoris, where blood supply is sufficient to maintain life, but inadequate to maintain normal function. It was not until 1958 that SHAW and MAYNARD [*19*] reported the first successful operative correction of superior mesenteric arterial occlusion.

In exceptional circumstances, gradual complete occlusion may occur without intestinal necrosis. CHIENE [*3*], in 1868, reported an autopsy case of a 65 year old woman dying of other causes, who had complete occlusion of the aorta and the superior mesenteric artery. This is atypical, however, and more often chronic symptoms will appear. If unheeded, the condition may progress to complete occlusion with massive intestinal infarction.

Clinical Picture

The most common symptom of chronic mesenteric arterial insufficiency is pain. This tends to be post-prandial, coming on within 30 min after meals and lasting 1 to 3 h. It may become almost constant. The pain is poorly localized so that patients will often note generalized or lower abdominal discomfort. If severe, nausea and vomiting may also occur. Associated with the onset of pain, the patients experience distention, flatulence, and diarrhea. Loose stools may be passed following meals, although this is inconstant, and constipation has also been reported in some instances.

A second common manifestation of the syndrome is weight-loss and emaciation. This is usually severe and may be rapidly progressive. Most of the weight loss can be explained by decreased food intake. Patients find that pain can be avoided by voluntary restriction of meals, and this soon results in marked weight loss. As an alternative, some change their dietary habits and find that frequent feedings of small amounts are tolerated. This pattern has been termed the "small meal syndrome".

The tendency to weight loss may be enhanced by a chronic malabsorption syndrome which has been described in some patients. This aspect of the syndrome is characterized by the passage of bulky, foamy stools. Fat and protein absorption is impaired [*5*], although carbohydrate absorption remains relatively unchanged [*16*].

Many patients will have histories reflecting systemic arteriosclerosis such as cerebral ischemic attacks, carotid artery occlusion, angina pectoris, myocardial infarction, aneurysm or occlusive disease of the distal aorta, iliac arteries or femoral arteries. In some instances, symptoms have appeared following resection of abdominal aortic aneurysms, with ligation of the inferior mesenteric artery. Patients with evidence of peripheral arterial occlusive disease should be questioned closely for the symptoms of mesenteric arterial involvement.

Most patients are in the fifth, sixth or seventh decades of life, although infrequently the syndrome may be seen in younger individuals. Males are affected about four times as often as females.

On physical examination the patient appears to be chronically ill with evidence of marked weight loss. His emaciation is prominent, and his physiological age will often appear to be advanced in excess of his chronological age. Vital signs are usually unremarkable. A systolic bruit may be heard over the mid-portion of the abdomen but this is nonspecific, and this finding alone is not of precise diagnostic significance. These patients usually have extensive arteriosclerosis, and involvement of any of the peripheral arteries in this region may give rise to a bruit. Other peripheral pulses may be absent or decreased.

Approximately 80% of patients with superior mesenteric arterial insufficiency will show evidence of the typical triad of abdominal pain, weight loss and intestinal dysfunction.

Laboratory Studies

The routine laboratory studies are likely to be of little diagnostic help. Perhaps one third of the patients may have occult blood detectable in the stool, but this is inconstant. Barium enema and upper gastrointestinal X-rays are usually within normal limits. Patients in this age group may have colonic diverticula or other incidental lesions which may serve to obscure the diagnosis.

Aortography is the single most important diagnostic study which can be used to establish the diagnosis. The decision to perform this study must be made on clinical grounds on the basis of a high index of suspicion. Mesenteric arteriography can be carried out by either the retrograde brachial or translumbar route. The former is probably the method of choice because of its greater flexibility and safety. Retrograde femoral studies are less reliable because of the frequency with which arterial occlusive disease of the distal aorta and its major branches will coincide with mesenteric artery involvement. It is important to visualize the celiac axis as well as the superior and anterior mesenteric arteries in the study; and lateral views are particularly heplful in bringing out precise definition of the occlusive lesions.

In some patients it is possible to demonstrate fat or protein malabsorption. This, however, is non-specific and inconstant. Experimental studies using ^{131}I tagged polyvinylpyrolidone to show loss of integrity of the intestinal mucosa have also been disappointing [*23*].

Surgical Treatment

Shaw and Maynard's [*19*] report in 1958 of successful reconstruction of superior mesenteric artery occlusion awakened interest in direct surgical attack upon the lesion. Several other reports have followed, but the number of patients treated operatively remains small.

Three methods of arterial reconstruction are available; bypass grafting from the distal aorta, employing a vein graft or prosthetic material; thrombendarterectomy; and reimplantation of the superior mesenteric artery into the distal aorta. In most instances, the stenotic portion of the superior mesenteric artery lies at its origin from the aorta. Exposure of this area may be difficult; and the approach may be made retroperitoneally by thoracoabdominal incision [*9*], or transperitoneally either from below the transverse mesocolon [*1*] or through the gastrocolic ligament with reflection of the stomach superiorly [*13*].

Bypass grafting is technically easier than endarterectomy, and is probably a safer procedure if the quality of the distal aorta will permit its use. It avoids the necessity of cross clamping major aortic branches; and endarterectomy of the celiac axis or superior mesenteric artery is often less than satisfactory because of poor quality of these vessels, initial dissection and thrombosis. A patch graft may be necessary to avoid narrowing the vessel after endarterectomy. In females, the ovarian vein may be used as a vein graft. In other instances it may be possible to revascularize the superior mesenteric artery via the splenic artery, providing the celiac axis is free of disease.

Reimplantation of the superior mesenteric artery is a third alternative when the condition of the distal aorta is satisfactory.

Discussion

The clinical significance of the syndrome of intestinal angina has been well documented. DUNPHY [*8*], in 1936, noted that the syndrome preceded mesenteric infarction. FRY and KRAFT, in 1963 [*9*], studied the records of 20 patients who had succumbed from mesenteric infarction. In this review they noted that symptoms were present for periods ranging from 3 weeks to 24 months before infarction occurred.

Anatomical studies have shown that the atherosclerotic plaques in the mesenteric arteries usually lie at the origin of these vessels. This makes bypass grafting or limited endarterectomy feasible in most instances. KUMMEL, in 1906 [*12*] demonstrated that 17 of 42 patients (40.5%) coming to autopsy had stenosis of the proximal superior mesenteric artery. A similar study by DERRICK, in 1958 [*6*], confirmed this finding in 37% of the patients autopsied in his series. With this frequency, it is puzzling that the syndrome is not more common. A partial explanation probably lies in the fact that patients are usually asymptomatic unless occlusive disease involves at least two of the three visceral arteries. This observation has been made by MIKKELSON [*16*], MORRIS et al. [*17*] and FRY and KRAFT [*9*]. This point underlines the importance of visualizing all three vessels by aortography preoperatively.

Initial results of reconstructive arterial surgery have been good. Patients are relieved of pain, have regained weight, and intestinal dysfunction is improved. The evaluation of long term results, always significant in interpreting results of vascular surgery, awaits a wider operative experience and longer periods of follow-up.

Although most attention has been directed towards patients with arteriosclerotic occlusive disease, other conditions may also be responsible for the production of intestinal ischemia. RIPLEY [*18*] has reported the occurrence of abdominal angina secondary to fibromuscular hyperplasia of the celiac and superior mesenteric arteries

In 1917, LIPSCHUTZ [*14*] pointed out that in some patients the celiac axis arises from the thoracic aorta and may be compressed by the diaphragm. This has been confirmed by others [*2, 15*] and noted to be present in about 20% of patients studied. DUNBAR et al. [*7*] reported a series of patients with abdominal pain resulting from compression of the celiac axis by the arcuate ligament of the diaphragm. They found this disorder to be prevalent in females. STONEY and WYLIE [*20*] studied eight patients in whom visceral ischemic symptoms were thought to be on this basis. These authors confirmed the prevalence in females, but noted wide variation in the pattern of epigastric pain, its duration und severity. There was no apparent relationship with the ingestion of food. Operation may consist of simple division of the crural fibers compressing the celiac axis. In some patients, however, the vessel may show residual narrowing, and resection of the stricture may be necessary to relieve the pressure gradient within the artery. In most instances symptomatic relief will be obtained. Inasmuch as celiac axis compression is frequently present in absence of symptoms, caution must be urged in attributing abdominal pain to this cause. Additional experience is necessary in the evaluation of patients with celiac axis compression. The wider application of aortography in the diagnosis of abdominal pain of obscure origin will be of help in further defining this syndrome.

Despite efforts to identify patients with abdominal angina and carry out elective reconstructive surgery, inevitably some will present with acute mesenteric occlusion and require emergency surgery. It is important to distinguish patients with embolic disease from those with acute mesenteric artery thrombosis. Patients with arterial obstruction on an embolic basis will usually have a source for emboli, and will therefore present with either myocardial infarction or atrial fibrillation. In absence of either of these cardiac conditions one should suspect arteriosclerotic occlusion and carry out thrombendarterectomy or bypass grafting. The cases reported by SHAW and MAYNARD [*19*] and by BRITTAIN and EARLEY [*1*] illustrate this point.

References

1. BRITTAIN, R. S., and T. K. EARLEY: Ann. Surg. **158**, 138—143 (1963).
2. CAULDWELL, E. W., and B. J. ANDSON: Amer. J. Anat. **73**, 27 (1943).
3. CHIENE, J.: J. Anat. Physiol. (Lond.) **3**, (second series) 65—72 (1868—1869).
4. DAVIS, B. B.: Neb. St. med. J. **6**, 101 (1921).
5. DELANGEN, C. D.: Acta med. scand. **146**, 719 (1953).
6. DERRICK, J. R., and W. D. LOGAN: Surgery **44**, 823—827 (1958).
7. DUNBAR, J. D., W. MOLNAR, F. F. BEMAN, and S. A. MARABLE: Amer. J. Roentgenol. **95**, 731 (1965).
8. DUNPHY, J. E.: Amer. J. med. Sci. **192**, 109—113 (1936).
9. FRY, W. J., and R. O. KRAFT: Surg. Gynec. Obstet. **117**, 417—424 (1963).
10. GILBRIDE, J. J.: J. Amer. med. Ass. **52**, 955—957 (1909).
11. JACKSON, J. M., C. A. PORTER, and W. C. QUINBY: J. Amer. med. Ass. **42**, 1469; **43**, 25, 110, 183 (1904).
12. KUMMEL, R.: Zbl. allg. Path. **17**, 129 (1906).
13. LAUFMAN, H., F. P. NORA, and A. I. MITTELPUNKT: Arch. Surg. **88**, 1021—1044 (1964).
14. LIPSCHUTZ, B.: Ann. Surg. **65**, 159 (1917).
15. MICHELS, N. A.: Blood supply and anatomy of the upper abdominal organs, p. 140. Philadelphia: J. B. Lippincott Co. 1955.
16. MIKKELSEN, W. P., and C. J. BERNE: Surg. Clin. N. Amer. **42**, 1312—1328 (1962).
17. MORRIS, G. C.: Arch. Surg. **84**, 95—107 (1962).
18. RIPLEY, H. R.: Angiology **17**, 297—310 (1966).
19. SHAW, R. S., and E. P. MAYNARD: III: New Engl. J. Med. **258**, 874—878 (1958).
20. STONEY, R. J., and E. J. WYLIE: Ann. Surg. **164**, 714—722 (1966).
21. TIEDEMANN, F.: Von der Verengung und Schließung der Pulsadern in Krankheiten. Heidelberg und Leipzig: K. Groos 1843.
22. TROTTER, L. B. C.: Embolism and thrombosis of mesenteric vessels. New York: Cambridge University Press 1913.
23. ZUIDEMA, G. D., J. G. TURCOTTE, E. F. WOLFMAN JR., and C. G. CHILD III.: Arch. Surg. **85**, 146—151 (1962).

Renal Artery Stenosis*

EDWIN J. WYLIE, WILLIAM K. EHRENFELD and RONALD J. STONEY

This paper presents the surgical experience at the University of California Medical Center, San Francisco, in attempts to alleviate or cure hypertension caused by renal

* From the Department of Surgery, University of California, School of Medicine, San Francisco, California.

Table 1. *Renovascular hypertension*
University of California 1952 to 1968
Hypertensive patients studied with arteriography
Total — 850

Major renal artery defects		Operated 307	(36%)
Atherosclerosis	152	102	
Fibromuscular hyperplasia	105	67	
Other	50	25	
Minor abnormalities			90
Normal renal arteries			453

artery occlusive disease. Table 1 tabulates the incidence of renal artery lesions in a series of 850 hypertensive patients who were studied by arteriography in the period from 1953 to 1968. Many of these patients were selected for arteriography because of other presumptive evidence of renovascular disease. Hence a 36% yield does not represent the true incidence of renal artery disease in the hypertensive population. This report is primarily concerned with the results of operation in the patients with atherosclerosis (102) and fibromuscular hyperplasia (67) of the renal arteries. The experience with each group will be described separately. In both groups the indications for operation and the surgical techniques employed progressed through a period of evolution as experience was developed and the results were analyzed.

Atherosclerosis

Table 2 indicates the surgical experience with renal artery atherosclerosis. In the 10 years preceding 1963 the most commonly used criterion for undertaking operation was the radiologic demonstration of a seemingly operable lesion in one or both renal arteries. Many elderly patients with associated degenerative or obstructive disease in other major abdominal arteries were included. Local endarterectomy through a

Table 2. *Atherosclerosis*

	1953—1962	1963—1968
Total patients	60	78
Operated	52	46
Technique		
Nephrectomy	8	9
Endarterectomy		
transrenal	22	
transaortic	18	35
Spleno-renal	3	
Dacron bypass	1	
Autograft bypass		2
Results—1 year postop.		
Cured	6 } 40%*	16 } 57%**
Improved	15 } 40%*	11 } 57%**
No change	9	18
Died	11 (8 p. o.)	1 (p. o.)

* 51% of survivors. — ** 60% of survivors.

transverse renal arteriotomy was the most common method for removal of the obstructing lesions. Associated aorto-iliac and mesenteric artery lesions, if present, were operated on at the same procedure. An unanticipated high operative mortality rate of 16% was encountered. Another 6% died within the first year from problems related to extra-renal atherosclerotic disease. Except for the reversal of uremia, which occurred in three patients, the advantages of surgical over medical management of hypertension were, at that time, highly questionable. Accordingly in 1963 the criteria for selection of patients for surgery and the operative techniques employed were changed. The indications for operation were restricted to patients who presented less of an operative risk and in whom longevity was not already threatened by concurrent disease. Hence, patients with generalized atherosclerosis, especially those with advanced coronary artery disease, were treated medically. Patients over the age of 65 were operated on only if uremia had developed from bilateral operable renal artery lesions.

It had also been observed in that 10 year period that the simplest and most enduring surgical technique was endarterectomy through the opened abdominal aorta. Endarterectomy is particularly suited for renal artery stenosis caused by atherosclerosis. The lesion begins almost invariably at the renal artery orifice and is sharply limited in its extent, i.e., there is an abrupt demarcation between diseased and normal intima. The transaortic approach has several advantages. The period of renal ischemia from cross-clamping the aorta need be no longer than 15 minutes, well within renal tolerance. Removal of thickened intima from the contralateral or accessory renal arteries may be accomplished almost simultaneously without increasing the time of aortic occlusion. Only rarely is it necessary to perform an additional renal arteriotomy to establish an adequate end point. The new arterial lumen has an even greater than normal diameter. The need for additional patch or by-pass grafting by synthetic or other materials is avoided. The only disadvantage is the lengthy period of meticulous dissection required to free the abdominal aorta proximal to the renal arteries.

Operative Technique (Fig. 1)

Access to the aorta at and proximal to the renal arteries is greatly facilitated by division of the ligamentous portions of the crura of the diaphragm which encase the aorta on each side. The aorta between the celiac axis and superior mesenteric artery is then free of its investing tissue. Following temporary clamp occlusion of the aorta at this level and below the renal arteries, of the lumbar arteries posteriorly, the renal arteries laterally, and the superior mesenteric arteries anteriorly, the aorta is incised in the midline. It is usually necessary to extend the aortotomy superiorly lateral to the superior mesenteric artery to gain sufficient exposure of the renal orifices. If only one renal artery is involved and the aorta and opposite renal artery have intima of normal thickness, a circular incision twice the external diameter of the renal artery is made in the aortic intima around the renal orifice. Centripetal dissection in the customary endarterectomy plane raises a disc of aortic intima and establishes the plane for endarterectomy of the renal artery. The renal artery media is gently displaced from the intima using a blunt dissecting instrument, i.e., a Halle dural elevator. As the surgeon continues to develop this plane all the while exerting mild traction on the central intimal core, his assistant gently pushes the distal renal clamp toward the midline. This causes the renal artery to prolapse into the lumen of the aorta and the final dissection to be performed under direct vision. The specimen generally breaks free at the point where the atherosclerotic involvement ends. If not it may be cut away at the media-intima interface. It is important that the dissecting instrument is not allowed to extend the plane beyond the point of eventual separation. In three of the early operations this occurred inadvertently and required a distal renal arteriotomy to remove the intima flap. Although the endarterectomy is performed almost entirely under direct vision in the aortic lumen it is relatively simple to prolapse the entire length of the renal artery to remove unusually lengthy lesions.

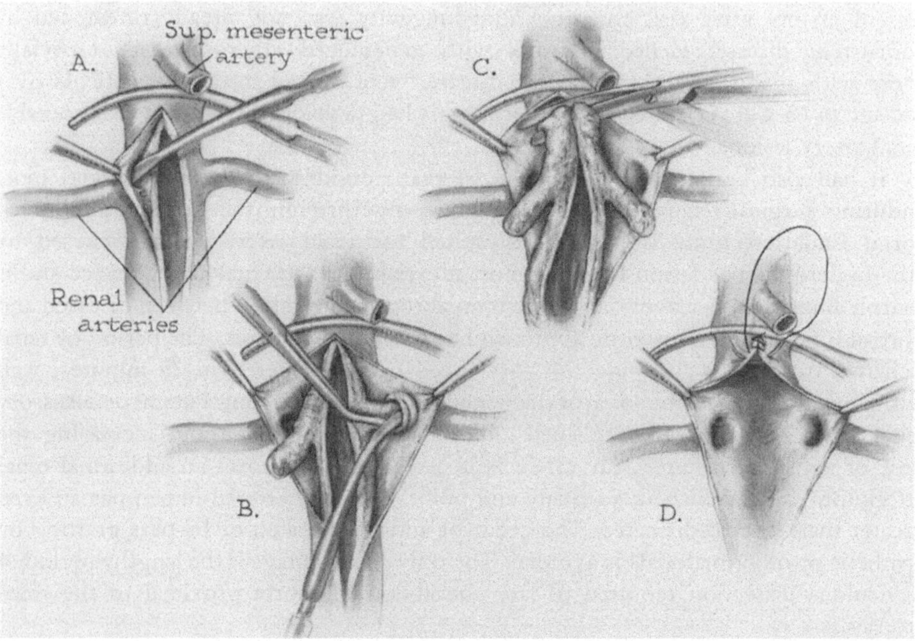

Fig. 1. Steps in the operative technique of "sleeve" endarterectomy of the aorta and renal arteries. When atherosclerosis is limited to the renal arteries only the aortic intima adjacent to the renal orifice is removed.

Whenever there is multiple renal artery involvement, or if the entire aortic intima is unusually thickened, a sleeve aortic endarterectomy is performed. Care is taken to avoid raising a distal intimal cuff in the aorta. The lesion in each renal artery is removed with the aortic intima in the manner described above.

If there is aorto-iliac occlusive disease requiring distal extension of the endarterectomy the upper portion of the aortotomy is first closed and the aortic occluding clamp moved to a infra-renal position.

Unilateral disc endarterectomy was performed in 10 patients; bilateral in 13.

In the 20 patients in whom sleeve endarterectomy was performed, 11 had one or more partially occluded accessory renal arteries that were satisfactorily re-opened at the time of operation. Of the 53 patients operated on by this method, thrombosis of the endarterectomized segment requiring subsequent nephrectomy occurred in only two. The one postoperative death in the 46 patients operated on since 1963 was caused by coronary thrombosis. Normal blood urea nitrogen (BUN) and creatinine levels were restored in four of five patients with uremia.

All patients have been re-examined at 3-month-intervals to assess the influence of operation on the relief of hypertension. Patients were classified as cured if blood pressures were consistently below 150/90. Patients whose diastolic pressures dropped to 90 mm or lower but whose systolic pressures remained over 150 mm were classified as improved. In most of these patients systolic pressures could be lowered to normal levels by the milder antihypertensive agents, reserpine or diuril. Fig. 2 illustrates the pre- and post-operative appearance of the renal arteries following transaortic endarterectomy.

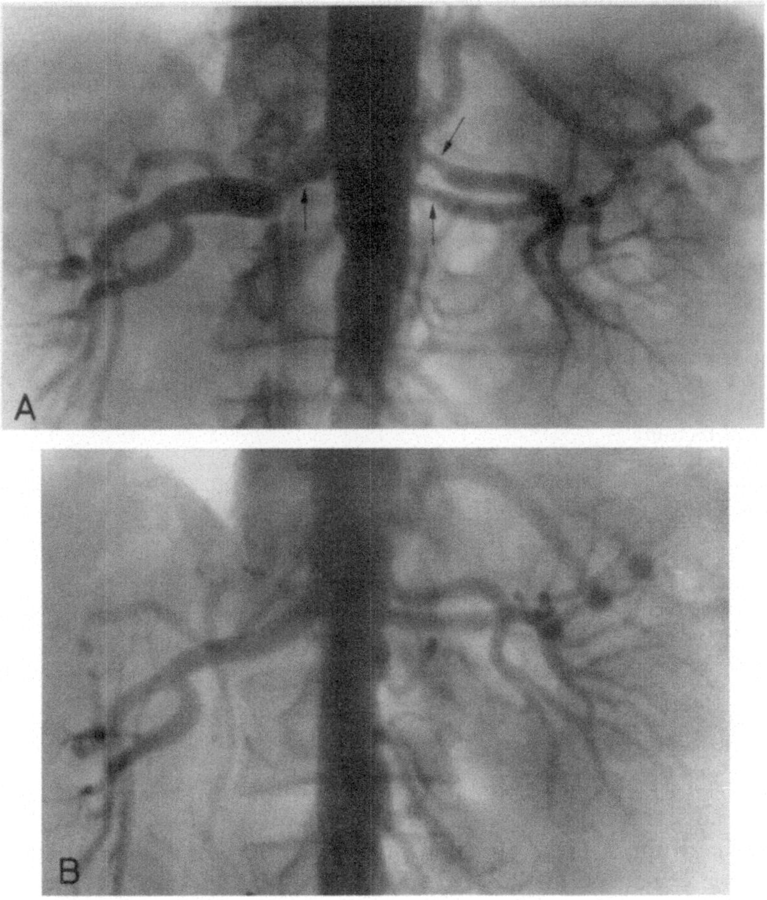

Fig. 2. Pre- and post-operative renal arteriograms in a 55 year old hypertensive man. (A) Atherosclerotic stenosis is demonstrated in the orifices of the right and the paired left renal arteries. (B) A normal lumen in all three arteries has been restored after sleeve endarterectomy of the aorta and the renal orifices.

Complete postoperative studies have not as yet been accomplished on all of the patients who failed to respond to operation. Residual peripheral arterial defects thus far appear to account for only a small number. The significance of parenchymal nephrosclerosis, shown by renal biopsy to be present in a few patients, is difficult to assess since similar changes were found in some patients who responded to operation. Although the reasons for the current failure rate of 40% are obscure, it is apparent that in many patients renal ischemia from disease in the renal artery orifice was not the sole cause of hypertension.

Fibromuscular Hyperplasia

The results of operations for hypertensive patients with fibromuscular hyperplasia of the renal arteries are more encouraging (Table 3). In a previous publication the pathologic characteristics and the results of operation in the first 22 patients in this series were reported (WYLIE, et al., 1962). Simple resection of the diseased segment and reanastomosis continued to be employed until 1964 at which time a total of 33 patients had undergone operation. During the first year after operation 69% were cured or improved. Late recurrence of hypertension subsequently appeared in 3

Table 3. *Fibromuscular hyperplasia*

	1958—1963		1964—1968	
Total patients	56		47	
Operated	33		34	
Technique	Total cases	B. P. Unchanged	Total cases	B. P. Unchanged
Segmental resection	28	8*		
Autograft			22	2
Autograft + contralateral nephrectomy			3	
Nephrectomy	3		7	
Patch	1	1	2	
Spleno-renal	1**			
Results — 1 year postop.				
Cured	19 } 69%		18 } 91%	
Improved	4 }		13 }	
No change	9		2	
Dead	1 (c. v. a.)		1 (c. v. a.)	

* hypertension recurred after the first year in three additional patients.
** hypertension recurred 2 years post-op.

of these patients, lowering the success figure to 60%. Postoperative renal arteriograms were performed on all patients who failed to respond to operation. Contralateral chronic pyelonephritis in 3 patients, progressive renal atrophy of unknown cause in 1, and residual fibromuscular lesions in an accessory artery account for 5 patients in whom failure of operation could have been anticipated. In the remaining 8 patients, immediate failure or late recurrence appeared to be related to the operation itself. Occlusion of branch arteries not present before operation was found in 4. 4 additional patients developed stenosis at the site of the arterial anastomosis. These 4 had undergone segmental resection with simple reanastomosis in 3 and a splenorenal shunt in the 4th. It seemed possible that anastomosis under tension, as was frequently the case, could produce late arterial narrowing at the site of anastomosis or stretch attentuation of the distal branches.

Beginning in 1964 a new operative technique was designed to provide an autogenous replacement of the renal artery which could be anastomosed without tension.

This technique was a renal artery by-passing operation using one of the patient's own hypogastric arteries as a free autogenous arterial graft. Previous clinical experiences had demonstrated the value of arterial autograft for arterial replacement (WYLIE, 1965). The hypogastric artery is particularly suitable for renal artery repair. It is of sufficient length that, when substituted for a renal artery, the anastomoses can be made without tension. Its diameter is only slightly greater than the renal artery. It is technically more simple to create a perfect union at the site of anastomosis with an arterial autograft than with other grafting materials, either venous or synthetic. No significant dysfunction follows removal of one hypogastric artery.

Technique

Through a trans-abdominal approach the segment of the renal artery distal to the lesion demonstrated at arteriography is freed. The kidney generally is unusually mobile and lying in a low position. The range of its mobility is estimated by moving it cephalad and caudad to its full extent. The mid-point of this range determines the level for the aortic anastomosis of the autograft. This site is usually 4 to 6 cm caudad to the normal origin of the renal artery. After the external diameter of the hypogastric artery is measured it is removed.

The aorta is then flattened between two totally occluding clamps so that the edge of the flattened aorta is slightly posterior to a true lateral position. A circular opening is cut in the aortic edge with a bone rongeur to approximate in size the previously deternimed external diameter of the hypogastric artery. The proximal anastomosis is completed using 5-0 arterial silk and the aortic clamps removed. If it is preferred to make the distal anastomosis in an end to end fashion (as in 82% of the operations) the renal artery is transected distal to the zone of stenosis. The distal renal artery is dilated with a clamp and its lumen inspected to make certain that the arterial wall is free of disease. The autograft-to-renal artery anastomosis is made with 6-0 interrupted arterial silk sutures. Grafts to the right renal artery are placed posterior to the vena cava.

Bilateral autograft replacement was used in one patient with bilateral operable renal artery lesions. In three additional patients with bilateral involvement, only one side was considered operable. In these an autograft bypass operation was performed on the operable side. Contralateral nephrectomy was performed 1 year later following radiologic demonstration of normal excretory function of the kidney on the operated side and a normal appearance of the graft. Return of blood pressure to normal levels followed the second operation in each. Fig. 3 illustrates the pre- and post-operative appearance of the renal artery in a patient with fibromuscular hyperplasia treated by an arterial autograft.

The results from the autograft technique have thus far been superior to previous methods. Graft thrombosis occurred in only one patient. In this patient, who has refused nephrectomy, hypertension persists. The presence of distal partially occlusive lesions may have contributed to graft occlusion. The only other failure to improve hypertension since 1964 occurred in the autograft group. Adequate function of the graft was demonstrated by X-ray. Renal biopsy had shown advanced bilateral nephrosclerosis.

The two operative deaths that occurred in combined series of patients with fibromuscular hyperplasia represent a problem unique to the disease rather than to the operation. Both deaths were caused by rupture of intracranial aneurysms. One additional patient has subsequently died from the same cause and two others have developed hemiparesis. All five were females under the age of 47. In a previous publication we called attention to the similarity of the pathology of some intracranial aneurysms to the pathology of renal artery aneurysms which are frequently found in association with the obstructive lesions of fibromuscular hyperplasia (WYLIE, et al., 1966).

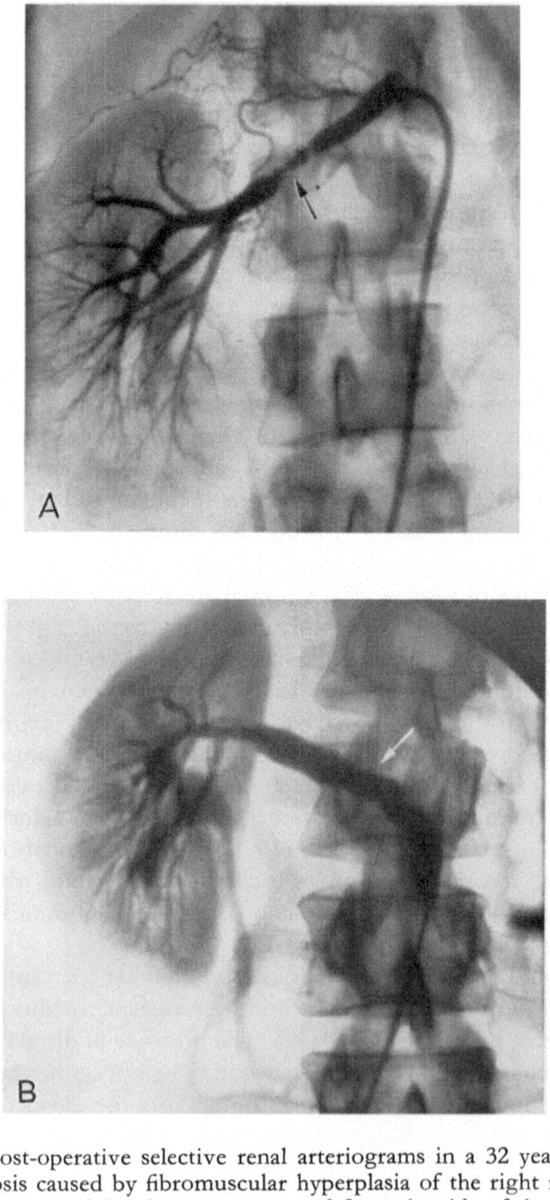

Fig. 3. Pre- and post-operative selective renal arteriograms in a 32 year old hypertensive woman. (A) Stenosis caused by fibromuscular hyperplasia of the right renal artery. (B) A hypogastric artery autograft has been anastomosed from the side of the infrarenal aorta to end of the transected renal artery

References

WYLIE, E. J.: Surgery **57**, 14—21 (1965).
—, F. M. BINKLEY, and A. J. PALUBINSKAS: Amer. J. Surg. **112**, 149—155 (1966).
—, D. PERLOFF, and J. S. WELLINGTON: Ann. Surg. **156**, 592—609 (1962).

The Treatment of Abdominal Aortic Aneurysms*

G. HEBERER and R. GIESSLER

Since OUDOT in 1949 and DUBOST in 1951 initiated the treatment of aneurysms of the abdominal aorta by resection in Europe, American surgeons, especially DEBAKEY and his associates, have standardized this operation as a routine procedure with relatively low mortality. For several reasons it seems worthwhile to discuss the

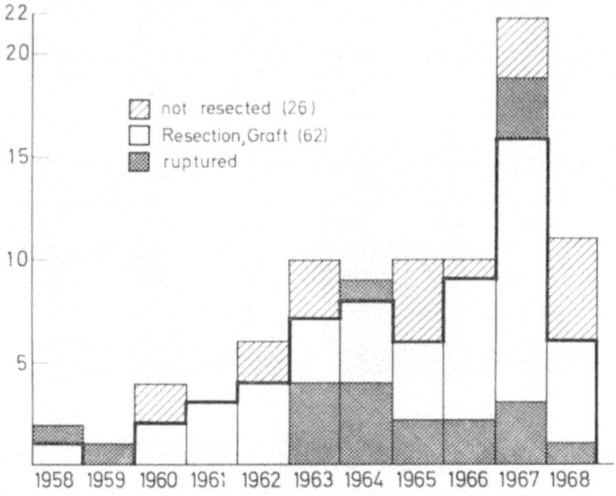

Fig. 1. Abdominal aortic aneurysms in our observation during the last 10 years (88 patients)

treatment of abdominal aortic aneurysms from the present point of view. According to our own experience in 92 cases since 1955 or respectively 88 cases during the last 10 years (Fig. 1) the most important factor is the fact that the abdominal aortic aneurysm is either still recognized too late or not diagnosed at all. Therefore, it can be assumed that the incidence of aneurysms is virtually higher in Europe. On the other hand, 17 years after the first successful resection late results as well as newer statistical analyses in regard to prognosis of the untreated abdominal aortic aneurysm allow a critical evaluation of the operative indication. Last not least, the improved follow-up treatment has to be discussed.

In former years, the diagnosis of an abdominal aortic aneurysm was usually made by obvious symptoms like the finding of a pulsating mass in the abdomen as is demonstrated by this 60 year old male patient with an aneurysm penetrating into the transverse colon. Incidentally, this patient upon whom we operated almost 10 years

* From the Department of Surgery of the University of Cologne School of Medicine (Chairman: Prof. Dr. G. HEBERER)

ago, celebrated recently his 70th birthday. 5 years later his 52 year old brother was also operated upon because of an abdominal aortic aneurysm. Furthermore, it is definitely a great diagnostical improvement that most of the aneurysms are now being diagnosed by means of angiological examination. Unfortunately, 10 to 50% of the patients still arrive at the hospital with a ruptured aneurysm, imposing a rather poor prognosis. Since most of the expanding aneurysms are not instantly lethal, the time intervall can be used for an emergency procedure. Thus, the main interest is concerned with symptoms which indicate *impending rupture*. Besides exacerbation of already existing pain, there are particularly signs of compression of surrounding structures and thrombotic occlusion of vessels. The predilective site of rupture of an aneurysm into surrounding structures is well known. Yet almost unknown is the fact that in more than 50% abdominal aortic aneurysms are associated with gastro-intestinal symptoms (SONDHEIMER and STEINBERG, 1964). The clinical picture of

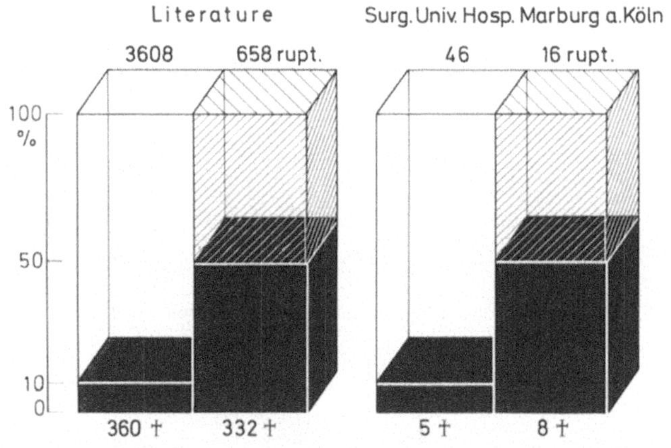

Fig. 2. Operative letality of abdominal aortic aneurysms in elective operations and in the ruptured state (June 1968)

gastric dilatation or high gastro-intestinal obstruction due to compression of the ascending portion of the duodenum near the ligament of Treitz was already described by OSLER in 1905 and SPISHARNY in 1907. We observed this rare complication in a 51 year old patient 8 days after peripheral embolectomy. Postmortem examination revealed a formerly asymptomatic aneurysm.

According to CULP and BERNATZ (1961) *urological symptoms* can also be caused in 10% of the cases by an aortoiliac aneurysm such as colicky pain attacks radiating to the left scrotal region, partial obstruction of the crossing ureter and oliguria or anuria due to shock.

An interesting manifestation of an already perforated aneurysm should be specially emphasized: the perforation into the inferior vena cava, since this complication is not necessarily followed by exsanguination. It rather leads to cardiac decompensation, to anuria or even liver insufficiency, usually within a period up to 6 weeks. In a clinical history of increasing abdominal pain, increasing cardiac insufficiency, pedal edema and a loud bruit over the expanding pulsating mass, as in this 60 year old male physician, surgical intervention with resection and transaortal closure of the vena cava is mandatory. DEBAKEY and associates (BEALL et al.) 10 years ago described an incidence of this complication in less than 1%. We observed this complication four times in 62 operated cases (6.5%). In one of these cases the perforation spontaneously closed by thrombi at the site of the compressed inferior vena cava, thus leading to spontaneous healing.

Acute as well as chronic arteriosclerotic *obstructive disease* of the legs quite often predominate the clinical picture and may be misleading. These symptoms, however, can be caused by emboli originating from the aneurysm as well as by thrombosis. 40% of our operated patients also had symptoms of chronic arteriosclerotic obstructive disease. Very often a similar symptomatology can be seen in cases with aneurysms in the popliteal-femoral region which is not rarely associated with abdominal aortic aneurysms. Having these more or less rare symptoms in mind, a thorough clinical and angiologic examination should be undertaken for the diagnosis of an abdominal aortic aneurysm. The case of this 49 year old patient, who was amputated on the left side, is interesting for several reasons. The aortogram shows an infrarenal occlusion of the aorta with a moderate degree of left renal artery stenosis. Some weeks later there is a severe stenosis of this left renal artery. During the operation a fusiform thrombosed aneurysm of the abdominal aorta was found. The hemodynamic interpretation is: The left sided amputation and the right sided arteriosclerotic obstructive disease lead to stagnation and thrombosis due to increased peripheral flow resistance. An aorto-iliac prosthesis with connection to the left renal artery was inserted in this case. Whenever a high aortic occlusion is suspected clinically, an aortic aneurysm should be thought of as underlying cause. Aortography should be carried out in such cases only suprarenally. Aortography, however, has not been recommended for the diagnosis of abdominal aortic aneurysms by most vascular surgeons.

Should all abdominal aortic aneurysms be operated upon? This question is answered in part by the grave prognosis of the untreated aneurysm on one hand and the relatively good early results on the other. During the first 10 years of the resection era it was felt that the indication for the operation is given with the diagnosis of an aneurysm. Yet, a more critical view has to be put upon the question of the operative risk. Besides substitution of homografts by synthetic prostheses the technique of resection has not significantly changed since DUBOST. However, the improved technique and the thorough prophylaxis and prevention of complications has led to a considerable decrease of the operative risk in elective surgery from 20% in the early days to nearly less than 10% (Fig. 2). In particular, the technical variation of the resection which leaves the outer layers of the aneurysm in situ being closely attached to surrounding structures avoids injuries to veins or the ureter (Fig. 3). Further important points to be considered are the following (Fig. 4): The prevention of kidney complications by careful clamping at the neck of the aneurysm below the renal arteries, and if necessary the revascularization of a narrowed renal artery or reimplantation of an aberrant vessel originating from the aneurysm; the prevention of ischemic injury of the descending and sigmoid colon by ligation of the inferior mesenteric artery, by protecting collaterals, or by leaving at least one internal iliac artery intact; the prevention of embolisation from the aneurysm by careful dissection, specially in the vicinity of renal arteries and early clamping of the large vessels; the protection of the proximal anastomosis with additional viable tissue for prevention of aorto-duodenal fistulas should be emphasized especially (DE BAKEY and associates). The resection of a small saccular aneurysm leaving the main vessel intact by either

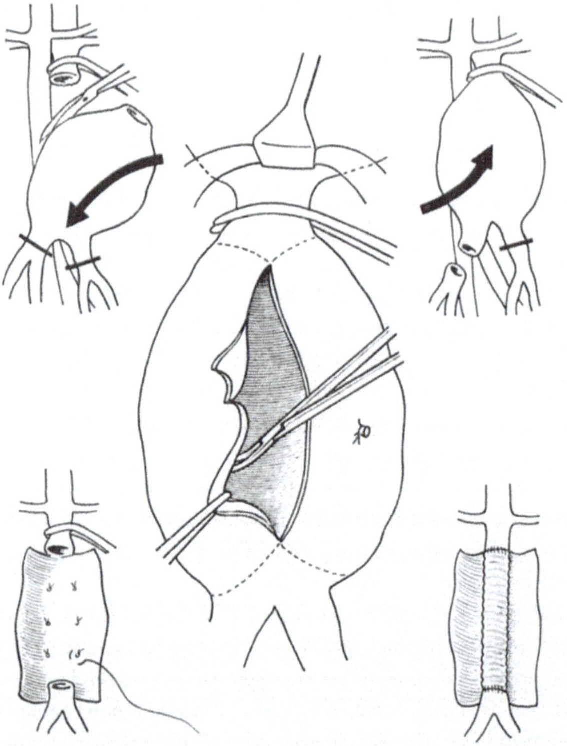

Fig. 3. Resectional techniques of the abdominal aortic aneurysm, dissecting method. Suture ligation of the lumbar arteries (below left) and covering of the anastomoses with periaortic tissue (below right). Small aneurysms which are free of adhesions can be totally removed (upper inserts)

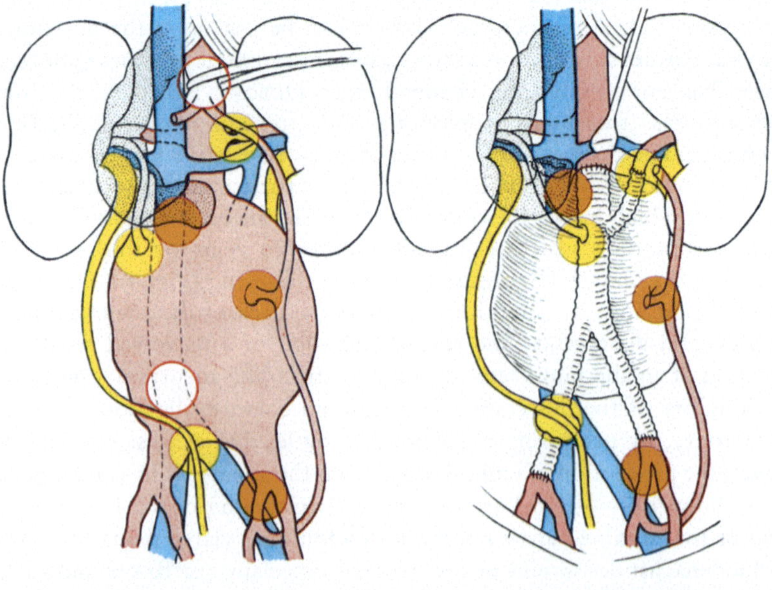

Fig. 4. Technique of resection: Prevention of intraoperative complications (s. text).

reconstructive aneurysmorrhaphy or by patching can be used probably in only rare instances. In the case of a 65 year old woman, who is doing well now 13 years after the operation, a small saccular aneurysm had penetrated into the duodenum leading to melena and chronic anemia.

The improvement of the *postoperative intensive care* is mainly due to therapy of respiratory insufficiency. Even though pulmonary complications do not represent the main cause of postoperative deaths, probably the improvement of O_2-saturation of the blood will lead to a decrease of ischemic cardiac and cerebral complications. The prophylactic intra- and postoperative application of mannitol and the maintenance of a constant blood pressure have led to a considerable decrease of kidney complications following aneurysmal resections. Intensive shock treatment however was not able to improve the survival rate of patients with ruptured aneurysms. Furthermore, additional risk is put on patients with expanding aneurysms by serum-hepatitis due to multiple blood transfusions. In our experience during elective procedures blood transfusions can be reduced by careful technique and application of blood substitutes.

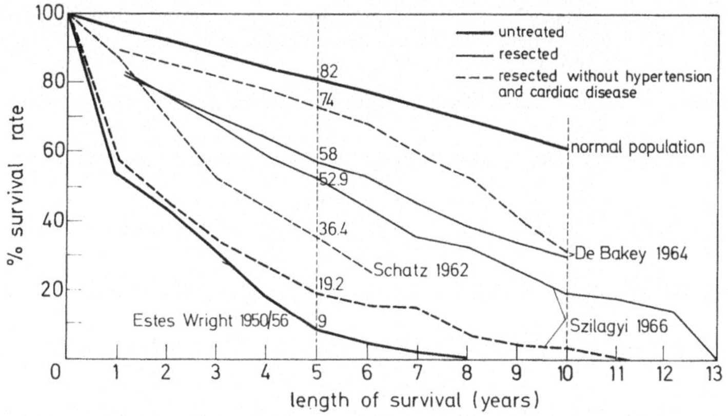

Fig. 5. Prognosis of patients with abdominal aortic aneurysm

Late complications add to the risk of operative treatment. A typical late complication of the implanted prosthesis is the dehiscence at the suture line, because of the progressive nature of the underlying disease. We have seen false aneurysms at the distal anastomosis of the prosthesis in 15% of 199 patients, who were operated upon more than 5 years ago because of occlusions, aneurysms or arterio-venous fistulas in the aorto-iliac-femoral region (GIESSLER, GEHL, and HEBERER, 1968). Therefore, special attention has to be placed upon the suture, the double-layer-coverage with additional viable tissues at the site of the anastomosis and, if possible, the use of the iliac bifurcation for the distal anastomosis rather than the groin.

The *operative results* do not depend mainly on the outcome of the operation, but rather on the cardiac and cerebral complications of the underlying arteriosclerotic disease. Even though DEBAKEY has shown survival curves parallel to the natural death rate of a comparative healthy group (Fig. 5), SZILAGYI as well as other authors have demonstrated a significantly shorter life expectancy in these patients. Obviously patients without hypertension and coronary disease have a better chance during and after operation.

Recent publications by SCHATZ of the Mayo Clinic and SZILAGYI (1966) in regard to the prognosis of the untreated abdominal aortic aneurysm revealed a somewhat better life expectancy as results reported by ESTES in 1950 and WRIGHT in 1957. This discrepancy can be explained by earlier recognition even of small aneurysms which have a lower wall tension according to the law of LA PLACE with less tendency to rupture. Therefore, several authors (BERNSTEIN et al., 1967; KLIPPEL and BUTCHER, 1966; SCHATZ et al., 1962; STEINBERG and STEIN, 1966; SZILAGYI et al., 1966; WOLFFE and COLCHER, 1966) have stressed the fact that the risk of rupture of a small aneurysm is less than the operative risk of arteriosclerotic patients in advanced age.

However, reliable criterias for the recognition of a small but expanding aneurysm are not yet established in view of the poor symptoms. This is proven by a thorough comparative statistical analysis by SZILAGYI (Fig. 6) of 44 not operated and 47 operated patients having a small aneurysm. The following *conclusions* can be drawn:

1. In selecting patients for operation the overall risk of cardiovascular complications of the underlying arteriosclerotic disease should individually be compared

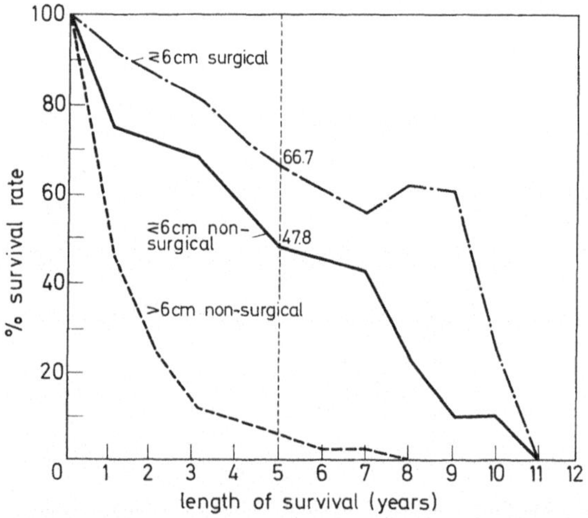

Fig. 6. Prognosis of patients with a small abdominal aortic aneurysm compared with the survival curve of untreated patients with large aneurysm (SZILAGYI et al., 1966)

with the risk involved in the presence of an aneurysm (rupture, compression, thrombosis).

a) Symptomatic aneurysms of any size as well as asymptomatic aneurysms without associated cardiovascular disease should be operated upon.

b) Small asymptomatic aneurysms with associated cardiovascular arteriosclerotic disease should be carefully followed until symptoms of ruptur occur. The risk of rupture must be accepted as a fate.

c) Large aneurysms with associated arteriosclerotic disease and age over 70 years impose a difficult decision. Personal experience will often be the decisive factor.

2. Special attention should be placed upon the thorough preoperative treatment in elective procedures. (Weight reduction, breathing exercises, specific therapy of bronchitis and emphysema, cardiac treatment).

3. Postoperative treatment has to be intensified in patients with hypertension and coronary disease in the light of modern antihypertensive drugs and coronary dilators. To improve the life expectancy of the patients with aneurysms one should call for a combined effort of general practicians, internists and surgeons alike.

References

BEALL, A. C., JR., D. A. COOLEY, G. C. MORRIS JR., and M. E. DEBAKEY: Arch. Surg. **86**, 809—818 (1963).

BERNSTEIN, E. F., J. C. FISHER, and R. L. VARCO: Surgery **61**, 83—93 (1967).

CULP, O. S., and P. E. BERNATZ: J. Urol. (Baltimore) **86**, 189—195 (1961).

DEBAKEY, M. E., E. S. CRAWFORD, D. A. COOLEY, G. C. MORRIS JR., T. S. ROYSTER, and W. P. ABBOTT: Ann. Surg. **160**, 622—639 (1964).

GIESSLER, R., u. G. HEBERER: Chirurg **38**, 514—520 (1967).

—, H. GEHL und G. HEBERER: Nahtaneurysma nach alloplastischem Gefäßersatz. 85. Verh. dtsch. Ges. Chir., München 1968.

HEBERER, G., G. RAU und H. H. LÖHR: Aorta und große Arterien. Berlin-Heidelberg-New York: Springer 1966.

KLIPPEL, A. P., and H. R. BUTCHER JR.: Amer. J. Surg. **111**, 629—722 (1966).

OSLER, W.: Lancet **1905 II**, 1089—1096.

SCHATZ, I. J., J. F. FAIRBAIRN II, and J. L. JUERGENS: Circulation **26**, 200—205 (1962).

SONDHEIMER, F. K., and I. STEINBERG: Amer. J. Roentgenol. **92**, 1110—1122 (1964).

SPISHARNY, J. K.: Zbl. Chir. **34**, 574 (1907).

STEINBERG, I., and H. L. STEIN: J. Amer. med. Ass. **195**, 1025—1029 (1966).

SZILAGYI, D. E., R. F. SMITH, F. J. DERUSSO, J. P. ELLIOTT, and F. W. SHERRIN: Ann. Surg. **164**, 678—699 (1966).

WOLFFE, J. B., and R. E. COLCHER: Vasc. Surg. **3**, 49—57 (1966).

Management of Thoracic Aortic Aneurysms*

W. GERALD AUSTEN

In recent years, there have been major advances in the therapy of thoracic aneurysms, both dissecting aneurysms (DEBAKEY et al., 1965; WHEAT et al.; BAHNSON) and non-dissecting aneurysms (DEBAKEY et al., 1958, 1962). Both medical and surgical therapy have been extensively investigated.

It is the purpose of this report to review recent experience at the Massachusetts General Hospital with 55 proven cases of dissecting thoracic aneurysms and 35 cases of non-dissecting thoracic aneurysms.

Dissecting Aneurysms

The proper therapy for this life-threatening disease currently remains a matter of some controversy. The development of extracorporeal circulation has made a definitive surgical approach possible (DEBAKEY et al., 1965; AUSTEN and DESANCTIS), but reported results are variable and marked by relatively high mortality and morbidity (LINDSAY and HURST). Poor surgical results in some centers have led to the espousement of a vigorous medical attack on dissecting aneurysm, using drugs which both lower the systemic blood pressure and protect the aorta from further dissection by diminishing the velocity of ventricular contraction (WHEAT et al., PALMER and WHEAT).

Case Material

Surgical Resection: Surgical resection was carried out in 35 patients with proven dissecting thoracic aneurysms. The diagnosis was confirmed preoperatively with

* From the Department of Surgery, Harvard Medical School and the General Surgical Services, Massachusetts General Hospital. — Supported in part by U.S.P.H.S. Grants HE-06664 (HEPP) and HE-08043.

angiography in all instances. All patients were operated on within two weeks of the onset of their symptoms, except for four who underwent surgery between 3 weeks and 5 months after onset of their original symptoms because of either severe aortic insufficiency or progression of their dissection. The majority of resections was carried out within 48 h of the onset of the symptoms.

Ten of the patients had dissections which began in the proximal ascending aorta and these were handled by the following technique. A median sternotomy was used.

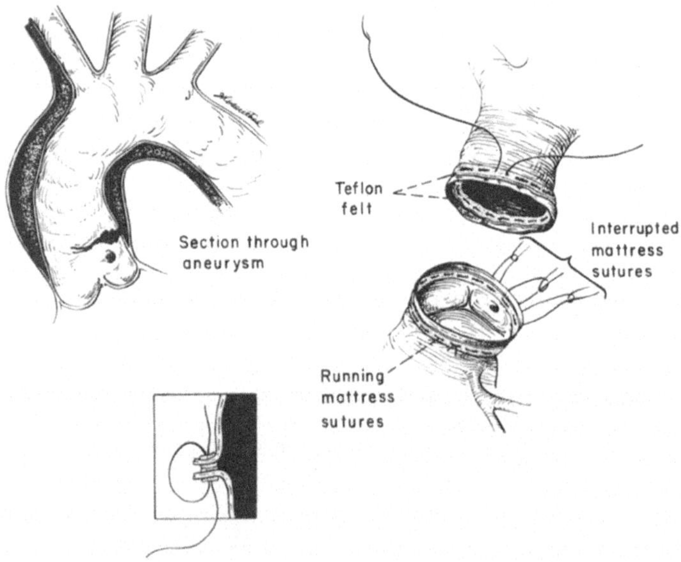

Fig. 1. Schematic representation of the pathology and surgical treatment of a dissection originating in the ascending aorta. The use of Teflon felt reinforcement and end-to-end anastomosis is illustrated

The patients were placed on total cardiopulmonary bypass and the ascending aorta was clamped proximal to the right innominate artery. The aorta was transected just above the coronary ostia and the heart maintained with coronary perfusion. The point of intimal tear was excised. The distal dissection was obliterated by reapproximating the aortic layers either with running mattress sutures or, in friable areas, with interrupted mattress sutures and Teflon felt reinforcement. The proximal dissection was similarly handled. Interrupted mattress sutures were added in some cases to further anchor the valve commissures in order to correct aortic valvular insufficiency. In two instances, prosthetic aortic valve replacement was required. A ring of Teflon felt was wrapped around both aortic ends in order to avoid tearing of the disseased aortic wall (Fig. 1). In the severely diseased aorta, Teflon felt reinforcement was also on the intimal side. Reconstitution of the aorta was then accomplished either by used direct end-to-end anastomosis or with an interposed prosthetic graft.

In the remaining 25 patients, the dissection began at or just distal to the left subclavian artery and these cases were managed in a similar manner (Fig. 2). Left thoracotomy and partial left heart bypass from the left atrium to the femoral artery were utilized. The proximal aorta was clamped, usually just proximal to the left subclavian artery and the distal descending aorty was clamped at an appropriate level.

The aorta was transected and the intimal tear and adjacent area of dissected aorta were resected. The disrupted layers at both ends of the aorta were reapproximated with a running mattress suture and Teflon felt reinforcement. In all cases, a prosthetic graft was then inserted between the transected ends of the aorta.

In these 35 cases, proximal resection has been attended with a hospital mortality of 30% and distal resection has been associated with a mortality of 20%. In the proximal resection group, two of the deaths occurred early in the series and were due

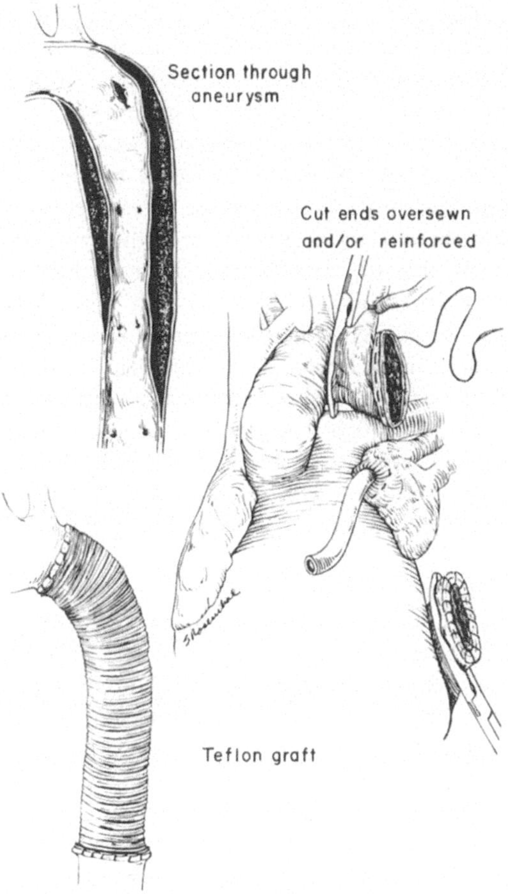

Fig. 2. Schematic representation of the pathology and surgical treatment of a dissection originating in the aorta distal to the left subclavian artery

to disruption of the aortic suture line at the time of surgery. The use of interrupted sutures and Teflon felt reinforcement has recently prevented this complication. The third death resulted from cerebral injury occurring at the time of the acute dissection. In the distal resection group, two patients died at the time of operation, one from disruption of the suture line and the other from a bleeding diathesis. Two patients died from postoperative dissection and the fifth death was due to renal failure. The 27 surviving patients are all doing well, 6 months to 4 and $^{1}/_{2}$ years postoperatively. There have been no late postoperative deaths in any of the patients who have undergone surgical resection of their dissection.

Medical Therapy: 20 patients with dissecting aneurysms have been treated medically. Dissection was confirmed by angiography in all but one case, in whom angiography was not performed because of known hypersensitivity to contrast substances. Of these 20 dissections, 16 were acute (arbitrarily defined as 14 days or less from onset of symptoms to onset of treatment) and four were subacute or chronic (onset of treatment more than 14 days after onset of symptoms). Sex and age distribution were not statistically different from the surgically treated patients and are similar to those of other reported series (LINDSAY and HURST).

Acute medical management was instituted similar to that reported by (WHEAT et al.) except for the use of methyldopa (Aldomet) in place of guanethidine (Ismelin) in most instances. Prior to and following angiography, close monitoring of vital signs, venous pressure, urine output, cerebral function, and the status of the peripheral pulses was carried out. If the blood pressure was elevated, acute lowering to levels of 100 to 110 mm. Hg systolic was affected by the use of an intravenous drip of Trimethaphan (Arfonad), 2 mg per cc. Pressures were kept at that level or as close as possible thereto, as long as urine output and other monitored signs remained satisfactory. Within the first 24 to 36 h, methyldopa was started, usually given intravenoulsy in doses of 250 mg every 4 h with dosage being increased according to the response elicited. The blood pressure could usually be controlled with methyldopa by the time tachyphlaxis to trimethaphan developed. The patients were maintained on bed rest until their condition appeared completely stable, usually a period of 2 to 3 weeks, at which time gradual increase in activity was permitted. As soon as feasible, usually at the end of the first week of therapy, patients were changed to oral therapy as intravenous drugs were discontinued. A combination of methyldopa with chlorothiazide (Diuril) or hydrochlorothiazide (Hydro-Diuril) was generally used.

The patients in the medically treated subacute group all had a period of 24 or more days and usually a number of months from the onset of symptoms to the time therapy was initiated. In these patients, all of whom were obviously stable on admission, the blood pressure was controlled with methyldopa administered orally only. The use of trimethaphan acutely was not considered necessary. All were continued on long-term antihypertensive agents.

In nine of the patients with acute dissection, the site of origin could not be determined with certainly (eight of these had angiograms, one did not due to sensitivity to contrast material). This played a large role in the decision to treat these patients medically. Four of this group died in the hospital, and at postmortem examination, two had origin of the dissection distal to the left subclavian artery, one originated in the abdominal aorta and one originated in the ascending aorta. There was one late death at 8 months without postmortem. In the other seven patients with acute dissection, medical therapy was undertaken usually because the patient was considered a poor surgical risk. In this group, six had sights of origin demonstrated just distal to the left subclavian artery and two of these were late deaths occurring at 1 month and 12 months. The one patient with a demonstrated ascending aortic dissection died in the hospital under treatment.

Of the eight deaths in the medically treated group, five occurred acutely in the hospital. Three of these were due to further dissection and rupture and one was associated with acute tubular necrosis, most likely related to the hypotensive therapy. One patient died of complications following massive gastrointestinal bleeding. Of the three late deaths, one died from aneurysm rupture at approximately 1 year. A second died 1 month after discharge in uremia; terminally, he had abdominal pain which was consistent with further dissection but no postmortem examination was done. The final patient died at 8 months of femoral artery occlusion and a cerebrovascular accident, again possibly related to the previous dissection. Thus, of the eight deaths in the 16 acute dissections, probably six were due to progression of the dissection despite apparently adequate antihypertensive treatment. One death was probably the result of hypotensive therapy.

The eight surviving patients with acute dissections have been followed for 6 to 35 months; they are all doing well. All four patients of the subacute group have survived well with follow-up of 21 to 36 months.

Comment

Although dissecting thoracic aneurysm remains a highly lethal disease, there seems to be little question that the development of an aggressive surgical and medical attack on this condition has improved survival. Thus, in 50 cases of untreated dissecting aneurysms seen at this hospital during the period of 1950 to 1960, only 14% survived at the end of 1 year, (AUSTEN and DESANCTIS) a figure similar to that reported by others (HIRST et al.) In contrast, in the present series, 70% of patients with dissection arising in the ascending thoracic aorta and 80% with dissection arising in the descending thoracic aorta survived surgical resection and are doing well to the present — 6 months to 4 and $^1/_2$ years following operation. Furthermore, it is likely that improved surgical techniques will further increase operative survival in the future. Perhaps the overriding surgical problem technically lies in the friability of the diseased aortic tissue. Surgery must be performed meticulously in order to avoid tearing the aortic suture line. We have found Teflon felt reinforcement of the aortic closure to be of inestimable value in this regard.

Surgical therapy requires accurate identification of the site of the intimal tear. This can usually, but not always, be delineated by angiography which we consider mandatory in all cases of suspected dissection. We prefer to opacify the aorta from an injection of contrast material into the main pulmonary artery, but we will proceed to direct aortic angiography if the results of venous angiography are equivocal (DINSMORE et al.).

Discouraging results with surgical therapy in some centers has led to a vigorous medical approach with remarkably good results. The objective of medical therapy is to use drugs which not only lower the arterial pressure but also diminish the velocity of ventricular contraction so as to protect the dissected aorta from the percussion impact of ventricular systole. This can be accomplished with a variety of agents, inclusing trimethaphan, reserpine, guanethidine, and methyldopa. Our experience with medical therapy in acute dissecting aneurysm has been less satisfactory than that of others, with a survival rate of 50%. Nevertheless, there have been some good results, and, furthermore, our mortality in medically treated patients will be increased by virtue to the fact that patients who pose a poor risk for surgery are more likely to be treated medically. Medical therapy itself is not without hazard as evidenced by the precipitation of fatal renal failure in one of our patients by overly enthusiastic hypotensive therapy. Medically treated patients must be watched very carefully in order to assure that perfusion of the vital organs, particularly the heart, kidneys and brain, is not compromised by the treatment.

The long term survival of our surgically treated patients has been surprisingly good in that there have been no "late" deaths. There have been a few late deaths in the medically treated group.

In the light of the experience presented in this series, we prefer to individualize the therapy of dissecting aneurysms. Our approach to acute dissecting aneurysms is as follows. In all patients suspected of having an aortic dissection, confirmatory angiography is performed. If, on the basis of angiographic and clinical findings, there is reasonable certainty as to the site of origin of the dissection and if the patient is a reasonable operative risk, surgical repair is undertaken. In each patient, the blood pressure is lowered with trimethaphan while preparation for surgery is underway. If the site of origin cannot be identified either angiographically or at thoracotomy, if the origin of the dissection appears to be in the aortic arch, or if the patient is a poor operative risk, resection is not done and vigorous medical treatment is continued. In patients with stable subacute or chronic dissection, medical therapy is usually employed. Medically treated patients must be followed closely for any evidence of progression of the dissection, expansion of localized aneurysms, or aortic insufficiency that might necessitate early or late surgical intervention.

Non-dissecting Thoracic Aneurysms

Fusiform and saccular aneurysms of the thoracic aorta represent a difficult and interesting surgical problem. While usually lacking the dramatic onset and obvious need for immediate treatment of dissecting aneurysms, they carry a high mortality rate from rupture or obstruction of adjacent vital organs if treated conservatively (CRANLEY et al.).

Case Material

Of the 35 patients to be presented there were 15 aneurysms of the ascending thoracic aorta and 20 of the descending thoracic aorta. Only non-ruptured aneurysms are included in this discussion. No aneurysms primarily involving the arch are included; the author feels resection of this lesion is so hazardous that we usually do not undertake elective resection.

16 of the 20 aneurysms of the descending aorta were arteriosclerotic and 12 of these patients were hypertensive. Syphilis was the etiologic agent in two patients and trauma was the cause in the other two. Of the 15 ascending aortic aneurysms, there was one case of giant cell aortitis, one instance of non-specific aortis, five cases of tertiary syphilis, three cases of arteriosclerosis, and five cases of medial cystic necrosis.

Unquestionably, the most valuable aid in diagnosis was a PA and lateral chest X-ray. This usually proved the presence and general location of the aneurysm. Aortic angiography may be necessary for diagnosis and was frequently helpful in determining the extent of the aneurysm and, therefore, the ease of resectability.

Aneurysms of the ascending aorta require a median sternotomy incision and total cardiopulmonary bypass for operative treatment (DEBAKEY et al., 1958). Ideally, aneurysms should be completely resected and replaced with a graft. In this series, five patients had complete resection of the ascending aorta (Fig. 3a and 3b). The remaining ten patients had either a true saccular aneurysm or at least a thick, substantial posterior wall and they underwent aneurysmorrhaphy (Fig. 3c and 3d) with primary closure of the aorta while on cardiopulmonary bypass; usually there were reasons for expediting the procedure such as a poor risk patient or inability to accomplish satisfactory coronary perfusion during aortic clamping. Eleven of the patients had significant aortic regurgitation and underwent, in addition, STARR-EDWARDS aortic valve replacement.

Aneurysms of the descending thoracic aorta require a left thoracotomy incision and left heart bypass for operative treatment (DEBAKEY et al., 1958). 18 of the 20

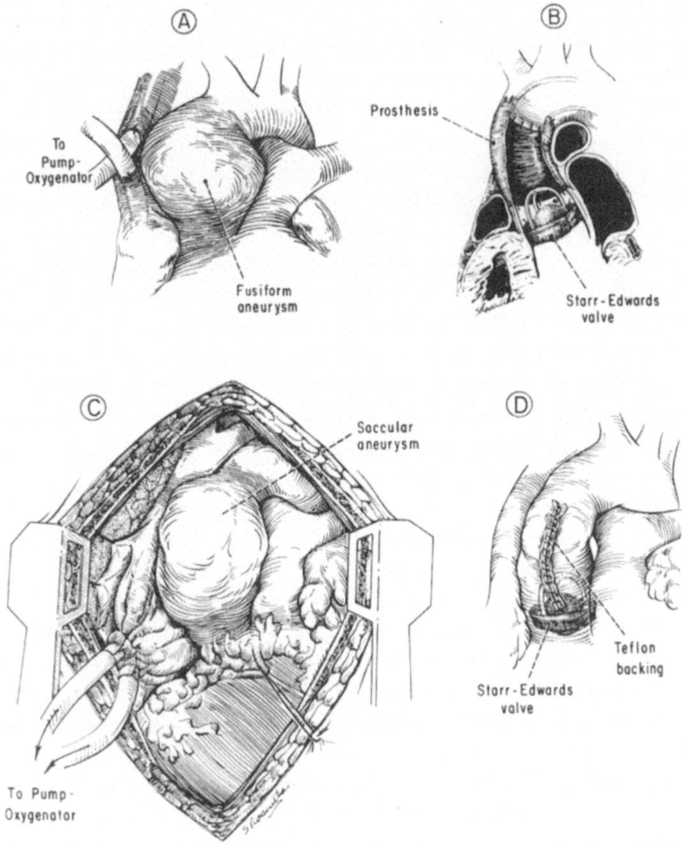

Fig. 3. Fusiform aneurysm of ascending thoracic aorta with associated aortic regurgitation (A) is treated by (B) resection of the ascending aorta, insertion of prosthetic graft and replacement of the aortic valve employed total cardiopulmonary bypass. Saccular aneurysm of ascending aorta with associated aortic regurgitation (C) may be treated by (D) resection of the aneurysmal sac with primary closure of the aorta and aortic valve replacement

aneurysms involving the descending aorta were fusiform. These were all treated with resection of the aneurysm and prosthetic graft replacement (Fig. 4a and 4b). Two aneurysms were saccular and were treated with aneurysmorrhaphy (BANHSON) with primary closure of the aorta with the patient maintained on left heart bypass (Fig. 4c and 4d); one of these aneurysms was secondary to trauma from many years previously and the surrounding aorta was clearly of good quality and the other case was a very poor risk patient with severe angina where an abbreviated procedure was thought advisable.

There were a total of nine hospital deaths (26%), three of 15 ascending aortic aneurysms and six of 20 descending aortic aneurysms. All three deaths in the ascending thoracic group were due to postoperative cardiac arrhythmias and/or cardiac failure. Three of the six deaths in the descending thoracic group were due to cardiac arrhythmias and cardiac failure during the surgery; one death was due to a central nervous system problem and two deaths were due to postoperative renal failure.

The surviving patients have been followed from 6 months to 4 and $^1/_2$ years. One patient died approximately 2 years following surgery, presumably from a myocardial infarction. All other patients are doing well.

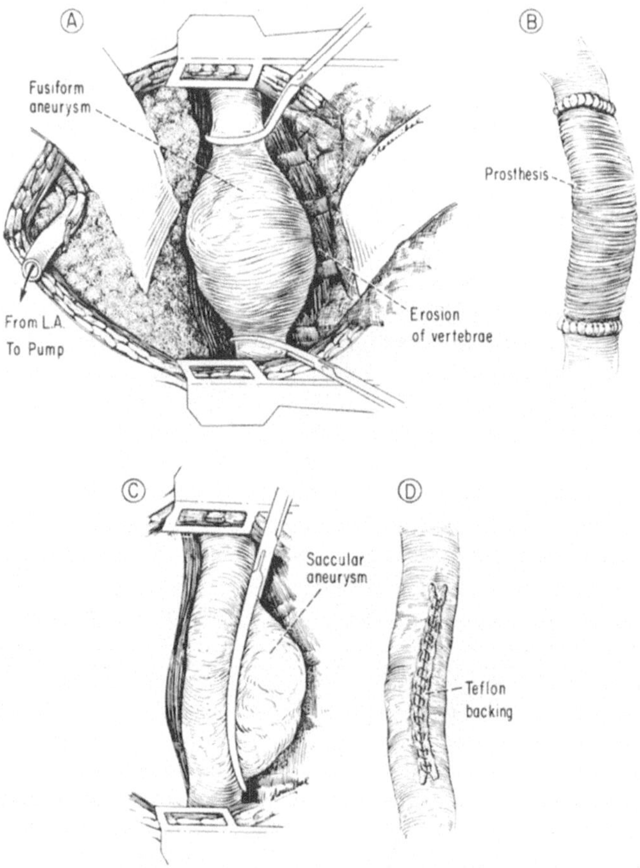

Fig. 4. Fusiform aneurysm of the descending thoracic aorta (A) is treated by (B) resection and graft employing left heart bypass. Saccular aneurysm of the descending thoracic aorta (C) may be treated by resection of the aneurysmal sac with primary closure of the aorta (D)

References

AUSTEN, W. G., and R. W. DESANCTIS: Clin. N. Amer. **46**, 573—586 (1966).

BAHNSON, H. T.: Surg. Gynec. Obstet. **96**, 383—402 (1953).

CRANLEY, J. J., L. G. HERRMANN, and R. M. PREUNINGER: Arch. Surg. **69**, 185—197 (1954).

DEBAKEY, M. E., D. A. COOLEY, E. S. CRAWFORD, and G. C. MORRIS JR.: J. thorac. cardiovasc. Surg. **36**, 393—420 (1958).

DeBakey, M. E., W. S. Henly, D. A. Cooley, G. C. Morris Jr., E. S. Crawford, and A. C. Beall Jr.: J. thorac. cardiovasc. Surg. **49**, 130—149 (1965).
— — —, E. S. Crawford, G. Morrow C. Jr., and A. C. Beall Jr.: Surg. Clin. N. Amer. **42**, 1543—1554 (1962).
Dinsmore, R. E., J. A. Rourke, and R. W. Desanctis: New. Engl. J. Med. **275**, 1152—1157 (1966).
Hirst, A. E., Jr., V. J. Johns Jr., and S. W. Kime Jr.: Medicine (Baltimore) **37**, 217—279 (1958).
Lindsay, J., Jr., and J. W. Hurst: Circulation **35**, 880—888 (1967).
Palmer, R. F., and M. W. Wheat Jr.: Ann. thorac. Surg. (To be published.)
Wheat, M. W., Jr., R. F. Palmer, T. D. Bartley, and R. C. Seelman: J. thorac. cardiovasc. Surg. **50**, 364—373 (1965).

Cardiac Surgery

Plastic Homologous and Heterologous Valves

D. N. Ross

Mr. Chairman, Ladies and Gentlemen I should make it clear to you from the start that I have no personal experience in the use of heterograft heart valves. Therefore I have to confine my observations largely to homologous and autogenous valves, but what I have to say about these applies largely to heterografts also, provided we are dealing with non-living transplants.

Once we consider living heterograft valves, and it seems likely that we have to take viability into consideration if we are to get long term durability, then I believe we are up against a very important *species incompatibility barrier* which has not been satisfactorily surmounted with the immunosuppression therapy at present available. Certainly it is clear particulary from the work of Paton of Denver immunosuppressives are necessary in using living heterograft aortic valves in dogs.

Table 1. *Table of comparison of mortality in 100 consecutive cases of biological and mechanical valves. Last 100 Aortic valve replacements including multivalve disease*

			Deaths
Homografts	23	47	2
Autografts	24		3
Starr valves	53		5
	100		10

My attitude to the use of plastic and homologous valves, (particularly in the aortic area) has crystallised somewhat over the past 5 years. My surgical inclination has always been towards the use of biological tissue wherever possible but like most surgeons I have been aware of the convenience of a readily available easily inserted mechanical prosthesis.

I am satisfied that both mechanical valves and homograft aortic valves can be inserted with similar mortality in my hands (Table 1) and both types of implant can work effectively as valve substitutes for at least 5 years. However the over-riding consideration which has made me persevere with homografts has been the total free dom from embolic complications and the need for anticoagulants. This latter feature is perhaps not so important in highly developed countries but is of very great importance in many underdeveloped and remote countries.

However I have come to recognise that, like plastic valves, non-living homografts have durability problems of their own particulary late calcification which I have seen on a number of occasions. This problem of calcification is one which I believe we may well be able to overcome by the use of young valves suitably pre-treated and by a better understanding of the physiochemical factors which determine the laying down of calcium in the aortic area.

Nevertheless the feature of the dead homograft valve which has been the greatest disappointment to me has been the lack of any living cellular repopulation of the transplant (Fig. 1).

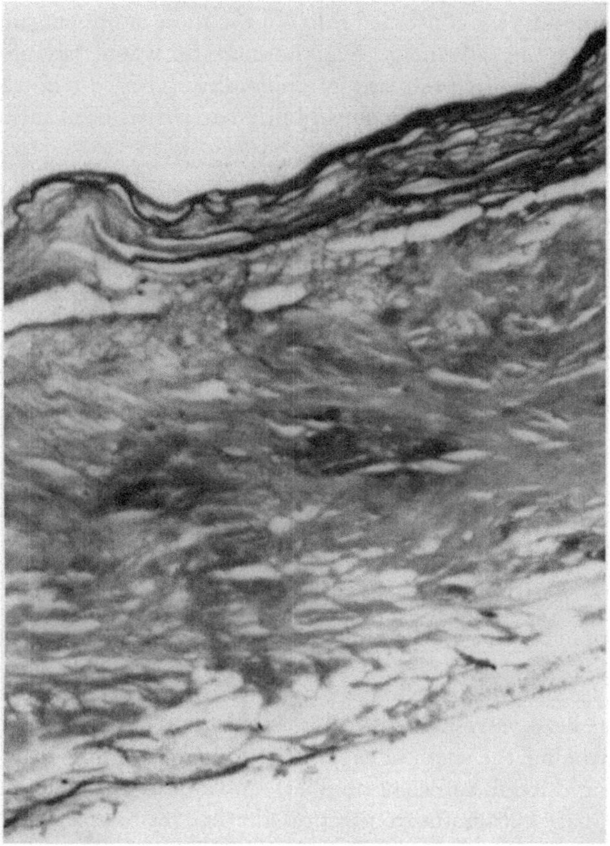

Fig. 1. The acellular structure of a homograft cusp 2 years after insertion

Any non-living structure within the body, particularly a moving one, will I believe ultimately fail unless it has living tissue incorporated, since only living tissue has the unique ability to replace its structure and make good the effects of wear and tear.

Therefore I, like others, forsee the need for living homograft valves in the future just as with a corneal, kidney, liver or heart transplant. This poses an enormous problem since it is almost impossible to provide enough living valves to meet the present surgical needs.

The alternatives, apart from the use of mechanical prosthesis, are to use heterografts and I have already mentioned immunological problems involved here, or pulmonary autografts, that is to borrow the patient's own pulmonary valve for reimplantation in the aortic or mitral valve position (Fig. 2).

I have used the patient's own living autogenous pulmonary valve now on 28 occasions in the aortic area and twice in the mitral area and although the follow-up is now only 18 months the result is in every way comparable with homograft valves and offers the prospect of a really long term implant which being in its natural environment should continue to live and renew its structure.

Consequently I shall try to summarise my views and policies with regard to my present selection of valve replacements.

As far as heterografts are concerned I do not use these at present since they do not seem to me to have any advantage over homografts when they are dead and as living structures they raise problems of immunity. They do however hold out future prospects once the species incompatibility barrier has been surmounted.

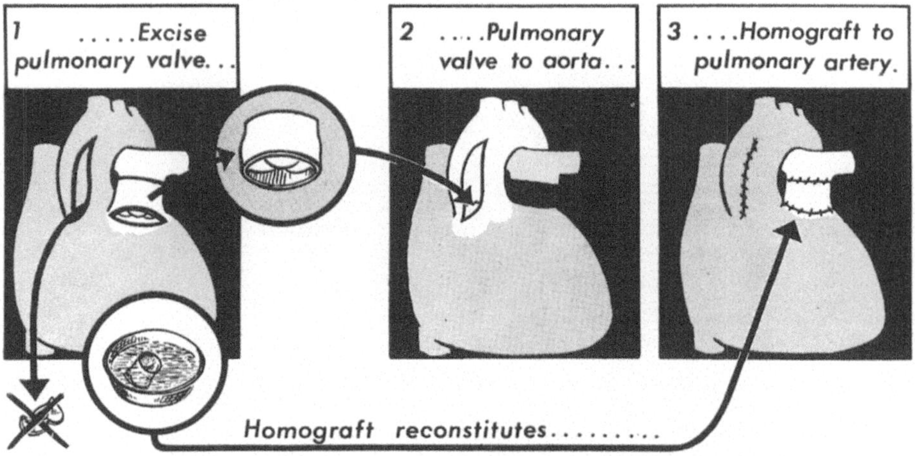

Fig. 2. Steps in the replacement of the aortic valve with a pulmonary autograft

Homografts are still my first choice particulary for aortic valve replacement but I recognise that the dead valve must have a limited outlook. This may be overcome or improved by changing the method of preparation or by using truly living valves if these can be harvested in sufficient numbers, and stored in a viable state.

Living pulmonary autografts are practical alternatives for aortic replacement and possibly for mitral replacement also but they involve a longer period on bypass. However in the young patient under 40 years of age this is my operation of election at present.

In patients over 60 years of age and particularly those with associated coronary artery disease I use a plastic valve, usually a Starr-Edwards unless there is a contraindication to the use of anticoagulants. These older patients I believe benefit from the shorter bypass involved and the operative risk is correspondingly low. More recently in some of them we have combined a Starr replacement with a bilateral Vineberg procedure.

In other words, at present I am using a combination of a number of available methods of valve replacement including homografts, autografts and mechanical prosthesis believing them to be complementary rather than competitive in covering the various clinical indications and age groups.

With regard to our recent transplant experience we have little to add to the admittedly scanty clinical knowledge available to the world. From the surgeons, point of view the surgical details are uncomplicated but the organisation and post-operative management are the important features which distinguish this type of work from our more day-to-day surgery.

In the first place we decided that we as surgeons should not concern ourselves primarily with the selection of cases. Consequently we organised a selection panel of cardiologists within our hospital to assess the clinical suitability of about four to five potential recipients. Also these patients were tissue-typed and it was explained to them that a transplant would be considered in their cases. In general we believe that the severely incapacitated coronary patient with gross myocardial damage

Table 2. *Summary of the clinical details of the recipient*
Investigation of F.W. age 45
At kings college Dr. RAFTERY

L.V. 100/10	Aorta 100/80
R. cor. art.	total block $1^1/_2$" from origin
L. cor. art.	Large circumflex
	total block anterior descending
L.V. angio.	dilated. poor contraction.
	no contraction anterior.

Table 3. *The donor picture*
Clinical details donor P.R. age 24 male

Fell 20 ft Laying concrete blocks
Depressed compound skull fracture
Multiple fractures and contusions
Unconscious
Burr holes — elevated fracture — I.P.P.R.
Flat EEG. — 24 hours
3 cardiac arrests

represents the most deserving recipient and the young patient with a progressive cardiomyopathy is also a likely candidate.

At the same time we organised our potential donor hospitals and a service for collecting the donor and getting his tissue type as quickly as possible. In addition we went to the dog lab. as a team to practice the technical details of the transplant.

Our recipient was a comparatively young man of 45 years who had had four to five major coronary attacks and about 20 hospital admissions. Coronary angiography confirmed major disease of all three coronary arteries plus an area of nonfunctioning myocardium in the left ventricular angiogram (Table 2). At the time of the hospital admission he was stable and not in left ventricular failure. At this stage of cardiac transplantation work we believe there should be a reasonable prospect of clinical success. This excludes cases in terminal congestive cardiac failure.

The donor was a young man of 28 years who had fallen on his head and had been admitted to another hospital about 24 h earlier (Table 3). There the traumatic service considered him moribund but referred him to the neuro-surgeons who performed burr holes but without relief and his condition was considered irrecoverable. He was maintained on a respirator but no electrical activity could be recorded from the brain.

On the following day after being resuscitated from two episodes of cardiac arrest he was referred to us and we transferred him to our hospital and at the same time sent his blood for tissue typing — the blood groups being compatible.

On arrival in the hospital he had a further cardiac arrest and was resuscitated and he was kept in the operating room with a heart-lung machine standing by in order to perfuse him via the femoral vessels if necessary. This did not prove necessary but we think it is important to bring the donor to the recipient's hospital and not to remove the heart prematurely or try to perfuse it or store it. I don't believe our methods of preserving hearts in a fully viable state have advanced to this stage yet.

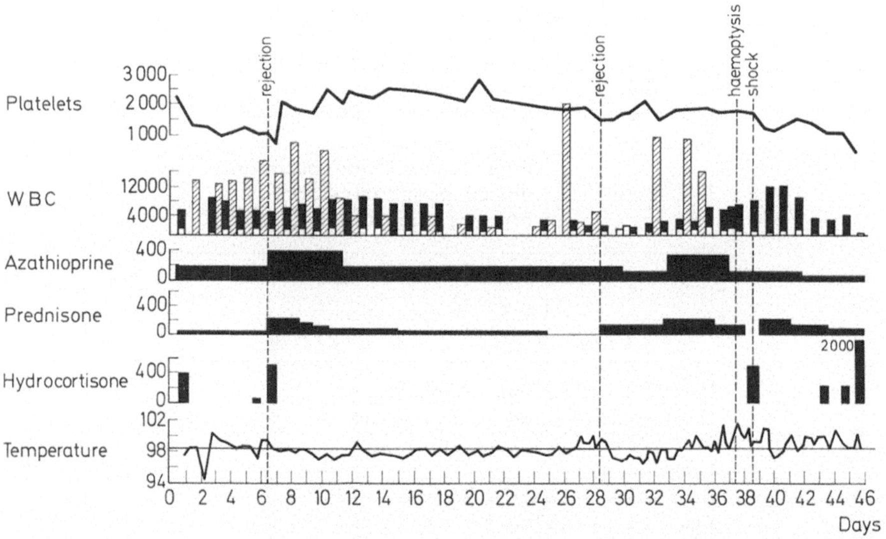

Fig. 3. Summary of the immunosuppressive details and course of the recipient from time of transplantation to death

As soon as our tissue typing indicated an acceptable match, the recipient was brought to the adjacent operating room — that was about 2 h after the arrival of the donor and his chest was opened and prepared for bypass. The donor's respirator was then turned off electively and heart function ceased in order to satisfy all possible criteria of death i.e. cerebral, respiratory and cardiac.

The donor heart was then rapidly excised together with its atria and at the same time I in another room excised the recipient's heart just above the atrioventricular groove and the cut edges were oversewn for added haemostasis. The subsequent course of events has shown that I probably left too much of the recipient atria behind since these will be poorly perfused and are likely to be a source of disturbed function from early paradoxical pulsation and later arrhythmias as the remnant fibroses.

The donor heart was brought in and sutured immediately in position without any attempt being made to cool or perfuse it.

After completion of the atrial suture lines, the aortic anastomosis was completed and after eliminating air the heart started promptly in sinus rhythm — the period of ischaemia being about 48 min. About 5 min later the aorta was again clamped and the pulmonary artery anastomosis was carried out.

Again the heart started without difficulty but the double poradoxically contracting atria tended to distend and we had a further short period of bypass in order to stabilize. Subsequently an isoprenalin drip was set up and pacemaker wires were inserted, after which the rest of the procedure was routine.

The patient was taken off the respirator the following morning and kept on antibiotics for 3 days. Altogether he remained in a bed in the operating room for 14 days while an air conditioned room was prepared in the recovery ward area.

Immunosuppression has been based on azothioprine and prednisone under the direction of Dr. Mowbray, London, and anti-lymphocytic serum has not been used although we had generous offers of this serum both from Munich and France. We had preferred to reserve its use until we had more clinical information.

The subsequent course of the patient is summarised as follows (Fig. 3). At 6 days post-operatively the patient felt weak and out of sorts. Also the cardiac output was clearly inadequate and the pulse rate was slow at about 70 to 80 and unvarying.

There was some improvement on isoprenalin but he developed some fever and his platelets, which had fallen as a result of the bypass, failed to rise. The combination of fever, low platelets, reduced cardiac function added up to rejection, and increasing his steroids and azothioprine produced a dramatic response in circulation and wellbeing within 6 h.

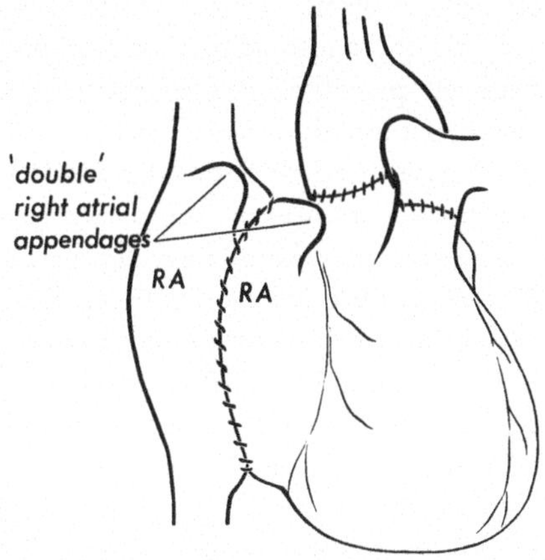

Fig. 4. Diagram illustrating the residual recipient atrial appendage which was a source of emboli

There after his case was uneventful until 4 weeks post-operatively when he again felt out of sorts, had a fever and platelet drop. Again he was treated, we believe correctly, for a second and minor rejection episode.

However from this stage on we mismanaged his post-operative course, for between the 4th and 5th post-operative weeks he developed a cough and blood-stained sputum plus signs at the right base, together with atrial fibrillation. This was thought initially to be a pulmonary embolus but the sputum became purulent and he was considered to have a lung infection.

The following day he collapsed acutely with hypotension and again we considered this to be infective, probably a gram-negative septicaemia.

Anuria followed and progressive deterioration until his death on the 45th day just over 6 weeks post-operatively.

The autopsy confirmed a terminal pyocyneus septicaemia, and no evidence of rejection macroscopically at the suture lines. However the lungs showed multiple pulmonary emboli and a source in the recipient right atrial appendage which contained a clot. There was no clot elsewhere in the venous system.

We conclude that death in this case was due to multiple pulmonary emboli arising in the patient's right atrial appendage and this should have been preventable if the recipient atria had been amputated closer to the great veins (Fig. 4). We believe that this death was unrelated to rejection and feel encouraged to continue with the work.

Reconstruction and Replacement of the Mitral Valve*

FRANK GERBODE[1], WILLIAM J. KERTH[2], PEDRO A. SANCHEZ[3], and GORDON H. PURYEAR[4]

A rather large number of congenital defects and acquired diseases produce lesions of the mitral valve which are sufficiently severe to require surgical correction. Various procedures other than replacement of the valve are now available for the treatment of some of them. Our basic philosophy with respect to surgical therapy for mitral valve lesions may be summarized as a definite preference for reconstruction whenever possible. Replacement is reserved only for those lesions which we consider irreparable.

We have used the Starr-Edwards prosthesis almost exclusively for mitral valve replacements. However, the disadvantages and uncertainties attendant with the use of ball valve prostheses have led us to investigate the use of aortic heterografts for this purpose. We have used these in a modest number of cases and the results thus far have been sufficiently encouraging to warrant continuing their use.

We have devised a rather complete classification of mitral valve lesions producing essentially pure incompetence, which is in press elsewhere [*1*]. A suitable classification with respect to the larger categories of mitral valve disease, including stenosis, with which we shall be dealing in this communication is set forth in Table 1.

The diagnostic categories of mitral valve lesions into which the largest numbers of our patients fall are rheumatic heart disease, congenital mitral insufficiency and ruptured chordae tendineae.

Congenital Mitral Insufficiency

Our experience with congenital mitral insufficiency consists of 66 cases [*2*]. Three of these were cases of isolated cleft of the mitral valve, two were of mitral insufficiency associated with corrected transposition of the great vessels and 61 were cases of mitral incompetence associated with endocardial cushion defects. An outline of this experience complete with early and late mortality figures is given in Table 2.

Extracorporeal circulation and moderate (31 to 33 °C) hypothermia were employed for essentially all of the repairs. Wherever feasible, the mitral valve was exposed through a right anterolateral thoracotomy. In the cases of endocardial cushion defect,

---

* From the Department of Cardiovascular Surgery, Presbyterian Hospital and the Institute of Medical Sciences of the Pacific Medical Center, San Francisco, California. Aided in part by U.S.P.H.S. grants HE 06311 and HTS 5349.

[1] Chief, Department of Cardiovascular Surgery, Pacific Medical Center; Clinical Professor of Surgery at Stanford University Medical School, Palo Alto, and University of California Medical School, San Francisco.

[2] Associate, Department of Cardiovascular Surgery Pacific Medical Center; Director, Cardiovascular Surgical Laboratory, Institute of Medical Sciences; Clinical Instructor in Surgery, University of California Medical School, San Francisco.

[3, 4] Fellows in Cardiovascular Surgery, Pacific Medical Center, San Francisco, and Stanford University Medical School, Palo Alto.

a right atriotomy was used. A complimentary right ventriculotomy was also employed in those cases having a fairly large ventricular septal defect as part of the endocardial cushion lesion.

Our technic of repair of the cleft mitral valve associated with endocardial cushion defects has been reported [3 to 7]. In short, the cleft is closed with interrupted silk sutures starting with one placed precisely through the thickened nodules which are almost always present on the leading edges of the affected leaflet at the margins of the cleft. In the cases of isolated congenital cleft of the mitral valve, simple suture closure was found to be sufficient in all. This was a most gratifying lesion to treat because of its simplicity and there was no mortality in the three cases.

Table 1. *An abridged classification of lesions of the mitral valve*

I. Lesions producing mitral insufficiency
   A. Congenital mitral insufficiency
   B. Ruptured chordae tendineae
   C. Rheumatic mitral valvulitis
   D. Ischemic lesions
      1. Ruptured papillary muscle
      2. Papillary muscle dysfunction
      3. Myocardial fibrosis with left ventricular failure and dilatation of the mitral annulus
   E. Heritable diseases of connective tissue (Marfan's syndrome, floppy valve syndrome)
   F. Bacterial endocarditis
   G. Miscellaneous (tumors of left atrium, idiopathic hypertrophic subaortic stenosis, aortic valvular disease, trauma)

II. Lesions producing mitral stenosis
   A. Rheumatic mitral valvulitis
   B. Tumors of left atrium
   C. Miscellaneous (congenital mitral stenosis, thrombi)

Table 2. *Congenital mitral insufficiency cases*

	Number	Mortality	
		Early	Late
Isolated cleft mitral valve	3	0	0
Mitral insufficiency as part of endocardial cushion defects:			
Partial A-V canal	38	8	3
Complete A-V canal	23	4	0
Mitral insufficiency and corrected transposition of the great vessels	2	1	1
	66	13	4

There were twelve early deaths among the endocardial cushion defect cases which amounted to a 21% mortality in the partial A-V canal group and a 17.4% mortality in the complete A-V canal group. For the complexity and serious nature of this group of lesions, these mortality rates are considered acceptable by most workers in the field and we have found no reason thus far to implicate the mitral repair as a significant source of mortality [7].

Only four patients required reoperation to correct residual mitral insufficiency, and two of these, both adults, required replacement of the valve. The pathology of the mitral valve in these cases was similar; specifically, dilatation of the annulus and elongation of chordae tendineae, and not a congenital deficiency of valve substance. This had occurred after heart failure from septum primum defects. An early postoperative death occurred in a 15 year old boy who had corrected transposition and mitral insufficiency. A repair of his mitral valve subsequently proved to be inadequate as severe mitral insufficiency prevailed and congestive heart failure progressively worsened. Three weeks after the first procedure, reoperation revealed that the valve tissue had originally been inadequate and the valve was replaced with a Starr-Edwards prosthesis. Death occurred on the seventh postoperative day due to bronchopneumonia and pulmonary edema.

A 6 month to 8 year follow-up on the surviving patients revealed an improvement in symptoms and exercise tolerance in 90%. There was a decrease in the size of the heart on chest roentgenogram in 85% of the patients and a decrease in pulmonary hypervascularity in 90%. A soft systolic murmur remained in 70% of the patients but in no instance was it thought to be significant.

Several authors have advocated the use of prosthetic valves in children with A-V canal defects associated with severe mitral insufficiency [*8*, *9*]. We have avoided this as we think that in the long run, it is not a satisfactory answer. We feel that a repair should always be attempted first and our results thus far would seem to substantiate this policy.

Ruptured Chordae Tendineae

Rupture of the chordae tendineae was once thought to result in sudden mitral insufficiency of such proportions as to categorically produce fulminating and rapidly fatal heart failure. The continued experience with this lesion afforded by open heart surgery has allowed modification of this concept to a substantial degree. Some authors continue to report death from this lesion within a year of its first manifestation but the experience of others has been that ruptured chordae seem to provoke a spectrum of physiological responses from very severe heart failure and disability on the one hand to very mild symptoms on the other [*10*, *11*]. The severity of symptoms and disability seems to be fairly well correlated with the number of chordae ruptured.

There has been a changing etiology noted in this disease as well. Prior to the availability of antibiotics, bacterial endocarditis was the most prevalent cause of ruptured chordae. Now, sequelae of rheumatic carditis produce the majority of ruptured chordae. Lately, however, there have been more and more cases of ruptured chordae reported for which no etiology can be found. These cases have been grouped into a classification termed "spontaneous" or "idiopathic" rupture of chordae tendineae. Between 20 and 46% of many series of cases reported over the past 8 years belong to this group [*10* to *14*].

We have treated surgically a total of 26 patients. Our experience has indicated that chordae to the posterior leaflet are the most likely to be ruptured in the spontaneous group whereas chordae to the anterior leaflet or to both leaflets are more frequently involved in cases due to bacterial endocarditis or rheumatic valvulitis.

A syndrome has been defined with respect to isolated rupture of chordae tendineae which support the posterior leaflet [*11*, *15*] (Figs. 1, 2). When a segment of this leaflet becomes flail, the regurgitant jet is directed against the atrial septum above the aortic root. In addition to the apical pansystolic murmur usually heard in mitral incompetence, such patients have a murmur at the base of the heart which is "diamond

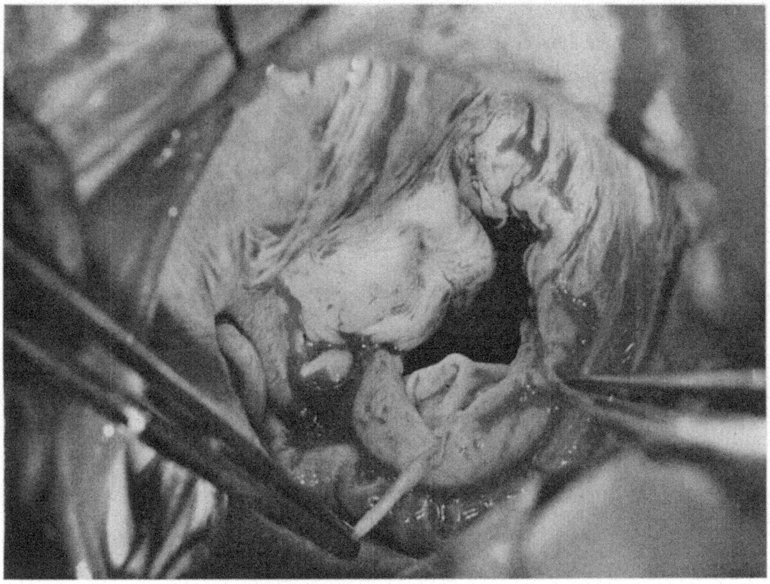

Fig. 1. Operative photograph of ruptured chordae tendineae — posterior leaflet of the mitral valve

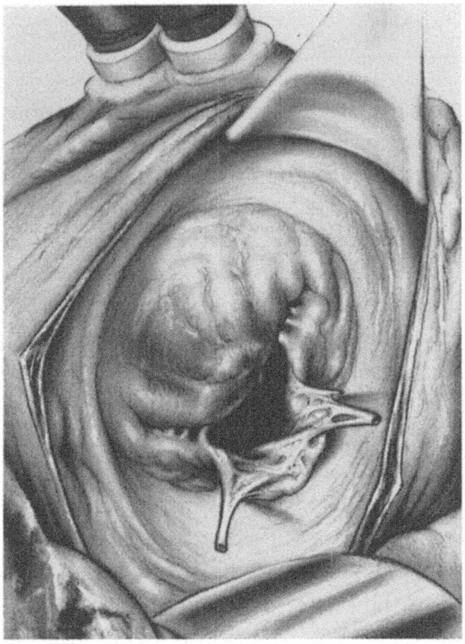

Fig. 2. Artists' illustration of ruptured chordae tendineae — posterior leaflet of the mitral valve (from Gerbode et al.: Circulation Suppl. 37—38, II, 119 (1968)

shaped" and frequently simulates aortic stenosis. This murmur quite often is transmitted to the carotids and these patients may not have transmission of the apical systolic murmur to the posterior axilla and to the back. In addition to the murmur simulating aortic stenosis, the diagnostic features of this syndrome which serve to distinguish such patients from those that have ruptured chordae to the anterior leaflet or both leaflets are listed in Table 3 [*11*]. The numbers of patients which had each feature in a series of 20 cases are also listed.

The diagnostic features of ruptured chordae to the anterior leaflet are usually quite different.

Cardiopulmonary bypass and moderate (31 to 33 °C) hypothermia were employed in all 26 operations. A right anterolateral thoracotomy was used to expose the mitral valve wherever possible. Separate cannulation of the cavae through stab wounds in the right atrium was employed to allow for a transseptal approach should it become necessary. The heart beat was maintained in all cases to permit assessment of the results of repair.

Table 3. *Clinical features in a series of 20 cases of isolated rupture of the chordae tendineae*

Clinical features	Cases
Absence of valvular calcifications	20
Absence of history of rheumatic fever or bacterial endocarditis	19
Male sex	18
Age 40 to 60 years	18
Sinus rhythm	18
Murmur simulating aortic stenosis	18
Normal or middly enlarged heart in roentgenogram	14
Absence of left ventricular hypertrophy pattern in ECC	11
Abrupt onset of symptoms and heart failure	8
Sudden Appearance of a murmur	5

Our first two operations for ruptured chordae tendineae consisted of reattachment of the torn chordae in both cases and repair of a co-existing cleft in the posterior leaflet in one [*16*]. The results are shown in Table 6. Our relative dissatisfaction with the reattachment procedure led to the development of our present technic. In the subsequent cases, the edges of the posterior leaflet on each side of the defect, which were still supported by chordae, were plicated in such a fashion as to invert the flail segment and result in restitution of chordal support for the entire free margin of the leaflet. Tension on the repaired leaflet was relieved by carrying the plication beyond the annulus at the same site (Fig. 3). Usually five or six interrupted silk sutures were sufficient for the entire procedure. The fairly abundant leaflet tissue often present in this type of lesion usually allowed a rather generous plication of the posterior leaflet without producing stenosis (Fig 3 and 4). Ordinarily the leaflet tissue was sufficiently strong to hold sutures quite well. When it was not, the sutures were first passed through small pledgets of teflon felt to act as bolsters.

Subsequent to our first two cases, we have operated upon 16 patients with ruptured chordae limited to the posterior leaflet and whose clinical findings in most instances fit the syndrome mentioned previously. The plication procedure was used in all of these patients. Results in 13 patients may be described as excellent and as good in two. The experience in all 26 cases is tabulated in Tables 4, 5, and 6.

The one patient that died following a plication procedure had a flail segment of the posterior leaflet due to ruptured chordae as well as fenestrations of both leaflets. The initial result of repair of the fenestrations and plication of the posterior leaflet was satisfactory but within 3 weeks, the complicated repair broke down and the patient succumbed.

All of the cases in which the valve was replaced with a prosthesis had either ruptured chordae to the anterior leaflet or to both leaflets. We, unlike McGoon, have never been able to repair an anterior leaflet made flail by rupture of chordae tendineae [*17*].

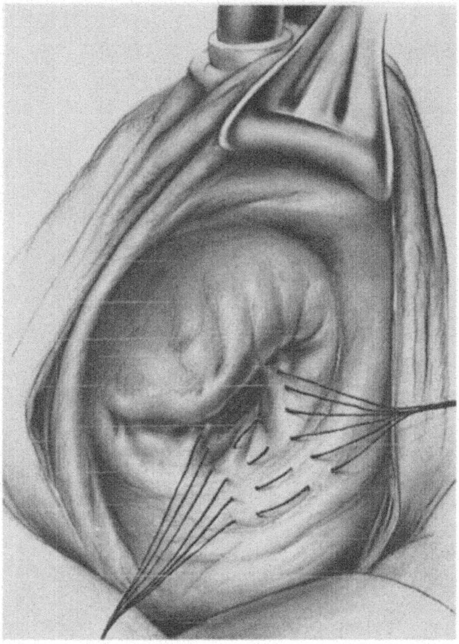

Fig. 3. Artist's illustration of the technic of plication of the flail segment of the posterior leaflet with extension of the plication across the annulus at the same site

Our experience has led us to believe that valve repair is superior to replacement with a prosthesis in those cases in which there is isolated rupture of chordae supporting the posterior mitral leaflet only.

Within the two large categories of mitral valve disease, insufficiency is the lesion that most frequently permits reconstruction of the valve. We have indicated a number of other types of insufficiency in our classification which are of major importance. However, we happen to have very few cases of any of these categories from which to draw conclusions. For instance, we have treated only one case of isolated mitral incompetence in a patient with Marfan's syndrome. A reconstruction was performed which restored competence initially but within 20 months, mitral insufficiency had obviously recurred. A recent publication indicated that two patients which the authors had treated by reconstruction of the valve had had results similar to ours [*18*]. It might seem from this very small cumulative experience that perhaps valve replacement should be the treatment of choice in this lesion.

The mitral insufficiency produced by rheumatic valvulitis is usually on the basis of ruptured chordae tendineae or scarring, with attendant fixation of the leaflets, prohibiting complete valve closure. Therapy for ruptured chordae tendineae has been discussed above. Cardiovascular surgeons are quite familiar with the fact that an adequate, careful and complete commissurotomy, with adequate debridement as indicated, under direct vision, may be expected to restore competence of the valve in a large number of cases of rheumatic mitral insufficiency. Replacement of the valve is the usual alternative to this.

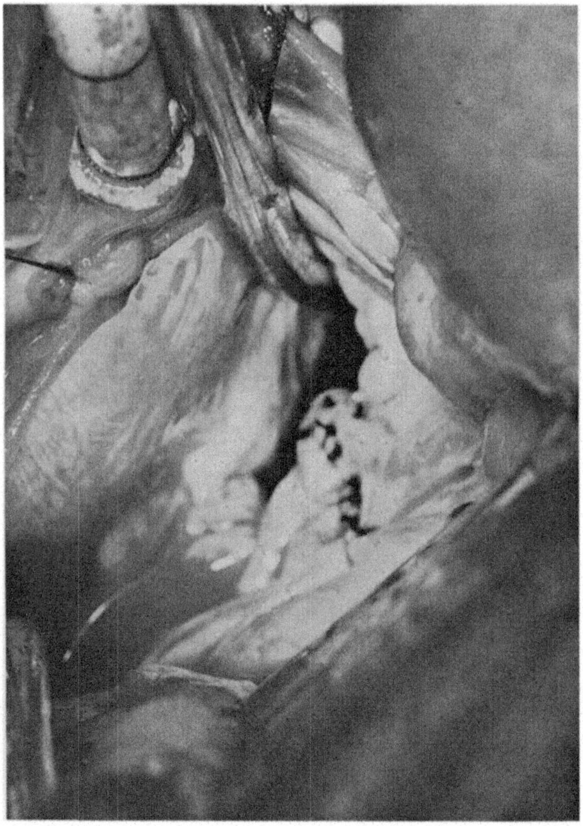

Fig. 4. Operative photograph, completed plication of posterior leaflet for ruptured chordae tendineae

Table 4. *Site of ruptured chordae — 26 patients*

Site	Cases
Posterior leaflet only	16
Anterior leaflet only; or to both leaflets	9
Posterior leaflet plus fenestration both leaflets	1
Total	26

Table 5. *Surgical procedures performed on 26 patients with ruptured chordae tendineae*

Surgical procedure	cases
Plication, posterior leaflet with associated annuloplasty	15
Reattachment of chordae	2
Plication, posterior leaflet plus repair of fenestration both leaflets	1
Valve replacement, starr-Edwards protheses S	8
Total	26

Table 6. *Results of operation in 26 cases of ruptured chordae tendineae*

1. Plications	
Excellent — Returned to normal heart size, asymptomatic, no murmur	13
Good — Returned to normal heart size, virtually asymptomatic, Grade II/VI systolic murmur	2
Death — 3 weeks — breakdown of complicated repair	1
2. Reattachment	
Death — 44 months; 7 months	2
3. Replacements	
Excellent results	2
Deaths — 4 early operative; 2 late	6
Total	26

Prosthetic Replacements of the Mitral Valve

The need for accurate statistical analyses of the results obtained from replacement of any of the heart valves is obvious to all physicians. That providing such statistics in a valid and meaningful manner is extremely difficult, if perhaps not impossible, is a fact well known to all who work objectively with these facets of the cardiovascular field. The factors of age, genetic background, type of primary illness and the possible side effects of the cardiac valvular lesion on other organs such as lungs, liver, and the myocardium itself are so intimately interrelated with respect to the eventual result of valve replacement in any single patient that they are virtually unique for the individual. In view of this concept, which is unquestionably valid, attempts to make comparisons of results based on isolation of any one or perhaps even several of these factors would seem to be doomed to failure. Yet, some attempt must be made. Fortunately, many investigators have risen admirably to the challenge. Our total experience with mitral valve replacements shows an early and late mortality of 48%.

In our search for methods of evaluating results of mitral valve replacement, we have found that if we limit the comparison to isolated replacements of the mitral valve and relate the mortality figures to the presence or absence of pulmonary hypertension, that there appears to be a fairly significant point of differentiation. Table 7 shows our experience with a group of 93 patients when early mortality is related to pulmonary hypertension defined as a pulmonary vascular resistance exceeding 250 dynes sec cm^{-5}. The difference between a 10% and a 33% mortality is obviously striking and the numbers of patients in each group appear to be sufficiently large to consider the difference valid. The presence or absence of pulmonary hypertension would, therefore, seem to be one of the most important parameters to consider when attempting an evaluation of the results of such procedures .

We have been fortunate to have a very low incidence of embolic phenomena following prosthetic replacement of the mitral valve. The total incidence has been 6%. As we have stated, we have almost exclusively employed the Starr-Edwards prothesis for mitral valve replacement. We attribute the low incidence of emboli to an effective anticoagulant program.

Our gross early and late mortality figures, however, have continued to be a matter of considerable concern to us. As we have cared for these patients over the years, we have gotten a distinct impression, which we are not yet able to corroborate by

Table 7. *Single mitral valve replacements related to pulmonary hypertension (PVR > 250) 1/1/63 to 5/31/68* (93 patients)

Pulm. hypertension (PVR > 250) — 63 patients		
Living	42	(67%)
Hospital deaths	21	(33%)
	63	(100%)
No pulm. hypertension (PVR < 250) — 30 patients		
Living	27	(90%)
Hospital deaths	3	(10%)
	30	(100%)

measurement, that many of them would benefit significantly from a larger flow area than the existing prostheses allow. For this reason, plus the desirability of eliminating an anticoagulant program from the care of these patients, in increasing frequency we have been using preserved heterograft aortic valves to replace the mitral valve. The results so far have been very encouraging.

References

1. Gerbode, F., W. J. Kerth, and G. H. Puryear: Progr. cardiovasc. Dis. (In press). —
2. — —, J. D. Hill, P. A. Sanchez, and G. H. Puryear: Surgical treatment of non-rheumatic mitral insufficiency. To be presented at the European Society of Cardiovascular Surgery, XVIIth International Congress, London, July 1968. (To be published).
3. — Ann. Chir. thorac. cardiovasc. **1**, 753 (1962).
4. —, J. B. Johnston, J. S. Robinson, G. A. Harkins, and J. J. Osborn: Surgery **49**, 69 (1961).
5. —, and E. F. Sabar: J. cardiovasc. Surg. (Torino) **5**, 223 (1964).
6. — —, and F. B. Main: Bull. Soc. int. Chir. **23**, 446 (1964).
7. —, P. A. Sanchez, R. Arguero, W. J. Kerth, J. D. Hill, P. A. deVries, A. Selzer, and S. J. Robinson: Ann. Surg. **166**, 486 (1967).
8. Rastelli, G., R. B. Wallace, P. A. Ongley, and D. C. McGoon: Mayo Clin. Proc. **42**, 417 (1967).

9. COOLEY, D. A., R. D. BLOODWELL, and G. L. HALLMAN: Surgical treatment of endocardial cushion defects in 132 patients including results of radical repair of atrioventricularis communis. Presented at 40th Scientific Session, American Heart Association, San Francisco, 1967.
10. SANDERS, C. A., W. G. AUSTEN, J. W. HAWTHORNE, R. E. DINSMORE, and J. G. SCANNELL: New Engl. J. Med. **276**, 943 (1967).
11. SELZER, A., J. J. KELLY JR., M. VANNITAMBY, P. WALKER, F. GERBODE, and W. J. KERTH: Amer. J. Med. **43**, 822 (1967).
12. ELLIS, F. H., JR., R. L. FRYE, and D. C. MCGOON: Surgery **59**, 165 (1966).
13. MORRIS, J. D., D. A. PENNER, and R. L. BRANDT: J. thorac. cardiovasc. Surg. **48**, 772 (1964).
14. MENGES, H., JR., J. L. ANKENEY, and H. K. HELLERSTEIN: Circulation **30**, 8 (1964).
15. GERBODE, F., J. D. HILL, J. J. KELLY JR., A. SELZER, and W. J. KERTH: Circulation Suppl. 37—38, II, 119 (1968).
16. —, W. J. KERTH, J. J. KELLY JR., and A. SELZER: Bull. Soc. int. Chir. **5**, 483 (1966).
17. MCGOON, D. C.: J. thorac. cardiovasc. Surg. **39**, 357 (1960).
18. SIRAK, H. D., and M. M. RESSALAT: J. thorac. cardiovasc. Surg. **55**, 493 (1968).

Multiple Valve Replacement

Review of 5 Years Experience

JOHN C. BIGELOW and ALBERT STARR

Introduction

The management of patients whose advanced valvular heart disease requires the replacement of more than one valve has improved greatly during the past 5 years. The most significant changes have been the development of more suitable prostheses, a more complete diagnosis of associated pathological valves, and an improved aggressive operative approach. It is now possible to operate upon these patients with a risk nearly identical to isolated valve disease patients. This report reviews 152 patients who have undergone multiple valve replacement at the University of Oregon Medical School between June, 1962 and January, 1968.

The Prosthesis

This experience with replacement procedures has utilized only the mitral and aortic ball-valve prostheses developed in this laboratory. Both prostheses have undergone gradual improvement in design and these changes have been detailed in previous reports (STARR et al., 1960, 1963, 1967; HERR et al., 1967, 1968). The current prostheses are illustrated in Fig. 1. The ball-valve prostheses (Mitral no 6300, and Aortic no 2300) promote more complete encapsulation with neointima because the metallic areas are entirely cloth-covered. Thromboembolism data for all models is compared in Tables 7 and 8. The use of hollow Stellite spheres diminishes the risk of ball variance which has been noted with the silastic rubber poppets. The low profile mitral prosthesis (no 6500) with a hollow Stellite lenticular poppet is now being evaluated clinically in the mitral and tricuspid areas in specific cases of small ventricle. Laboratory testing is also in progress to evaluate two new polymer poppets.

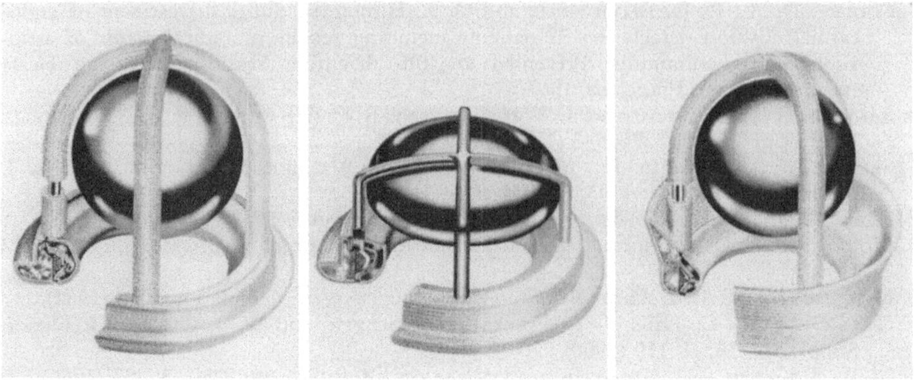

Fig. 1. This is a cut-away diagram of the current experimental prostheses. a) Hollow Stellite ball, completely cloth covered, mitral prostheses (model 6300). b) Hollow Stellite lenticular poppet, naked struts, low-profile, mitral prosthesis (model 6500). c) Hollow Stellite ball, completely cloth covered, aortic prosthesis (model 2300)

Clinical Material

There were 152 patients in this series. Aortic and mitral valve replacement was performed in 103, mitral and tricuspid replacement in 16, and aortic, mitral and tricuspid replacement in 33. Two patients with previous aortic valve replacement subsequently had a mitral valve replacement. One patient with an isolated mitral valve replacement subsequently had an aortic valve implanted, and three subsequently had a tricuspid valve implanted.

The age distribution of the patients is indicated in Fig. 2, with a range from 20 to 66 years and a mean of 47 years. An additional 31 patients have undergone isolated valve replacement and concomitant valvulotomy or valvuloplasty of one or more of the remaining valves. They are not included in the above total. 15% of the patients had previous closed mitral commissurotomy. Three patients had tricuspid valve repair with an unsatisfactory late result requiring subsequent replacement.

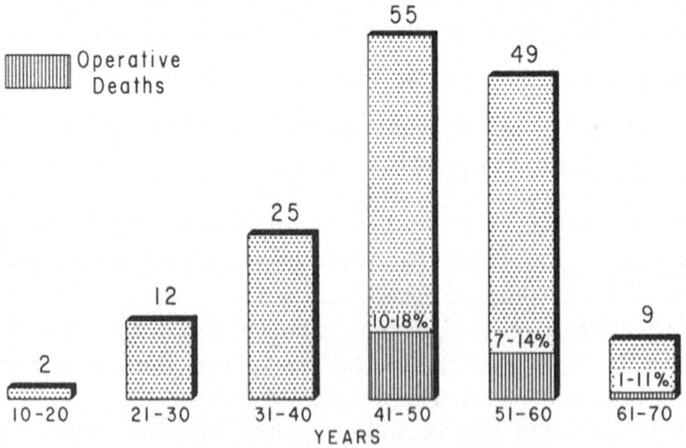

Fig. 2. The age distribution of 152 patients undergoing multiple valve replacement, and the operative mortality for the age groups is shown graphically. June 1962 to Jan. 1968

All patients selected for operation were Functional Class III or IV by the New York Heart Association Classification System. Their clinical appearance was dominated by the symptoms and physical signs of either long standing mitral or aortic valve disease. These signs are often misleading in the presence of multiple valve lesions. Accurate diagnosis can only be made during surgical exploration of the pathological anatomy. Tricuspid valve disease is frequently accompanied by obvious diagnostic signs but it was not suspected preoperatively in 10 of the 49 tricuspid valve replacement patients. Although a complete catheterization study is useful in discovering unsuspected multiple valve disease, six of the ten had complete right heart catheterization.

The catheterization pressures may suggest only mild multiple valve disease, but the combined valvular abnormalities may result in marked restriction of performance as determined by cardiac output and arteriovenous oxygen difference with rest and exercise. Supravalvular cineaortography is of value in uncovering subclinical aortic valve disease. Left ventriculography often demonstrates the anatomy and severity of concomitant mitral valve disease. Coronary angiography in patients over 40 years of age helps identify severe coronary atherosclerosis. A careful preoperative study of hepatic, renal, and pulmonary function is important.

If the patient is precarious it may be risky to undertake extensive diagnostic studies and the clinical evaluation may be sufficient to define the need for operation. Complete surgical exploration provides the necessary information to determine the nature and the extent of the pathology.

No patient has been denied surgery because of the severity of cardiac disability as determined either clinically or by hemodynamic studies. Surgery has been denied to some patients with serious associated disease such as alcoholic cirrhosis, chronic renal failure, and pulmonary fibrosis and emphysema. Ten patients beyond the age of 60 have undergone multiple valve replacement and nine are surviving. It does not appear that age alone contraindicates an operation.

Patients are admitted to the hospital at least 1 week prior to operation to gain the maximum benefit of medical therapy. This allows the patient's staphylococcal flora to be controlled and any occult foci of infection to be identified and treated. Dental examination is an important part of the initial workup and abscessed teeth should be treated prior to the operation. Cultures of the urine and external nares are obtained. The patients undergo a rigid program of antibacterial prophylaxis with instillation of a broad spectrum antibiotic ointment into the nasal vestibule, showers or bed baths with surgical soap twice daily, and a shampoo every other day. Parenteral Penicillin, Methicillin and Streptomycin are given the day before operation and for 1 week postoperatively. Penicillin sensitive patients are treated with Cephalothin. Long acting digitalis preparations are withheld 24 to 48 h prior to operation. Fluid restriction is employed if a rapid weight gain occurs during the preoperative period; diuretics are withheld except in patients with overwhelming congestive heart failure. Occasionally peritoneal dialysis is required to reverse the failure. Many of these patients are receiving an anticoagulant at the time of admission. The drug is discontinued early enough to assure normal prothrombin function. In the presence of congestive hepatomegaly this may require 5 to 6 days and supplemental vitamin K. Temporary pervenous atrial or ventricular electrical pacing is sometimes indicated to support the patient during the induction of anesthesia.

Operative Findings

The 152 patients in this series had rheumatic heart disease except one with cystic medial necrosis, aneurysmal dilatation of the sinuses of VALSALVA, and aortic regurgitation. Mitral regurgitation in this case was secondary to ruptured chordae tendineae.

The usual aortic valve pathology included commissural fusion, loss of leaflet substance, and thickening of the leaflets at their attached margins. Massive calcification is common with congenital stenosis, but is uncommon in this group. When calcification occurs it may involve the aortic and mitral valves as a single unit suggesting the rheumatic process extends into the tissue between the valves. A failure to consider this point during mitral valve resection may cause an obstructing cuff of tissue to be left in-situ.

Most of the resected mitral valves had either a combined stenotic and regurgitant lesion or a stenosis with massive calcification. Adequate repair of the mitral valve was possible in only 24 patients with multiple valve disease not included in this series. The decision between repair and resection is determined solely by the operative findings. The mitral valve is not resected for simple dilatation of the annulus as the result of left ventricular failure secondary to aortic valve disease. Many such valves have been encountered in this clinic during isolated aortic valve replacement, but none has required mitral valve replacement. The functional mitral regurgitation and the elevated left atrial pressure usually disappear immediately after the bypass.

49 patients had sufficiently severe tricuspid valve disease to warrant replacement of the valve. Combined tricuspid stenosis and regurgitation with thickening of the leaflets and the subvalvular mechanism occurred in 25 of the 49 patients. Although functional tricuspid regurgitation may frequently occur, all of the 22 valves resected for pure regurgitation showed gross evidence of thickening of the leaflets and shortening of the chordae tendineae. Two resected specimens showed pure tricuspid stenosis. None of the 49 specimens had gross calcification.

4 patients had tricuspid replacement after an annuloplasty had failed to correct the regurgitation. An additional 27 patients with thin, delicate tricuspid valve leaflets had significant regurgitation palpated immediately prior to bypass; 20 had decreased their regurgitation following corrective mitral surgery and did not require tricuspid surgery. The remaining seven patients had unchanged persisting regurgitation; however, a replacement was not performed because of their favorable early clinical course. Three have subsequently required tricuspid replacement to correct persisting right heart failure.

Operative Technique

The techniques of isolated mitral and aortic valve surgery, and simultaneous multiple valve replacement have been described in previous reports (STARR et al., 1960, 1963, 1964, 1966, 1967; HERR et al., 1967, 1968). Several technical features are important in multiple valve replacement: 1. flexible exposure, 2. prolonged cardiopulmonary bypass, 3. myocardial protection during aortic cross-clamping and 4. sequence of implantation.

All patients are operated upon through a midline sternotomy incision. Pressures are routinely measured in the right ventricle and both atria. The tricuspid valve is routinely palpated prior to bypass.

The pump prime for prolonged cardiopulmonary bypass consists of citrated blood stored for 1 to 5 days and 20% Mannitol solution to a total dose of 2 gm/kg of body weight. The osmotic effect of the Mannitol shifts excess extracellular fluid into the intravascular space causing mild hemodilution (PORTER et al.). No other exogenous diluents are used. Initially the patient is heparinized with 3 mg of heparin per kg of body weight. An additional 1 mg/kg/h of bypass is given if the bypass exceeds 2.5 h. The patient is cooled to 30 °C and the pump flow is reduced. The mean arterial pressure is maintained at approximately 65 mmHg.

The mitral valve is exposed first. The pericardial reflection between the inferior vena cava and the right inferior pulmonary vein is divided and the posterior interatrial groove is recreated. The ascending aorta is cross-clamped. A small stab incision is made in the exposed anterior wall of the left atrium. The mitral valve is palpated in the partially decompressed, beating heart to differentiate functional insufficiency from organic disease. If the valve requires repair or replacement, the left atrial incision is extended downward between the inferior vena cava and the right inferior pulmonary vein to reach the back of the heart. When exposure is difficult the incision is extended posteriorly toward the left inferior pulmonary vein. Visualization of the mitral valve is facilitated by anoxic relaxation of the myocardium and decompression of the aortic root. Both are achieved by intermittent cross-clamping of the ascending aorta in the absence of significant aortic regurgitation. Air is aspirated from the proximal aortic sement prior to each declamping to prevent coronary air embolus.

Many patients with multiple valve disease have aortic insufficiency and require continuous aortic cross-clamping during aortic and mitral replacement. A transverse aortotomy is made. The coronary arteries are perfused with blood which is obtained from the oxygenating chamber, and delivered to the hand-held coronary cannulae at a combined flow of 350 to 400 cc/min. 3 min periods of coronary perfusion are repeated every 15 to 20 min until the cross clamp is removed. No intra-pericardial coolant is employed.

Intermittent coronary perfusion allows sufficient myocardial relaxation to expose the mitral valve without injuring the heart by retraction. Sutures are placed in the mitral leaflets and gentle traction brings the valve into view. It is then easy to determine the feasibility of salvaging the valve. If resection is necessary, the septal leaflet is excised as close as possible to the aortic root to prevent a stump of thickened leaflet impinging upon the limited space available for the two prostheses. A definitive-traction suture is placed in the annulus near the posterior commissure. The remainder of the valve is resected including division of the papillary muscles and chordae tendineae. Double armed 2-0 teflon impregnated dacron sutures are placed in the liberated mitral annulus. Traction upon each succeeding suture is an important key to good exposure.

The selection of a proper size mitral prosthesis is especially important in patients with combined aortic and mitral disease. The size of the left ventricular cavity is the most important factor in making this selection. The smaller mitral prostheses are more frequently used in these cases than in isolated mitral valve replacement. The mitral prothesis is held incompetent with a Foley catheter through its orifice until bypass is to be discontinued. When the septal portion of a properly sized mitral prosthesis is in the usual sub-aortic position there is no impingement upon the aortic outflow tract.

Aortic valve replacement is performed secondly. If the aortic valve is replaced before the mitral, the subsequent exposure of the mitral valve is difficult. The selection of an aortic prosthesis which will pass easily into the aortic root is of prime importance;

a too large prosthesis causes difficult placement, malposition, or obstruction around the ball. The prosthesis is anchored in place with 3-0 teflon impregnated dacron vertical mattress sutures. The aortotomy is closed, air is evacuated from the proximal aortic root, and the aortic clamp is removed.

In patients with functional tricuspid regurgitation, a decision for replacement is withheld until bypass has been discontinued and the valve is again palpated in the filled beating heart. If organic tricuspid disease is discovered prior to bypass, defibrillation is delayed until the valve has been explored. With the caval tapes tightened the right atrium is widely opened and the decision is made to resect or repair the valve. Resection is begun by incising the attached margin of the anterior and posterior leaflets, and dividing the papillary muscles deep in the right ventricle. A broad attached margin of the septal leaflet and its chordal supports are left in-situ and 3-0 teflon impregnated dacron sutures are anchored in this residual tissue to avoid causing heart block. The size of the ventricular cavity is again the most important consideration in selecting the proper size prosthesis. Care is taken to avoid injury to the right ventricular endocardium by pressing the prosthesis into the decompressed ventricle.

Ventricular pacing wires are routinely implanted before the chest is closed. Atrial pacing wires are implanted in patients who have intact atrio-ventricular conduction either before operation or after defibrillation. A prophylactic tracheostomy is frequently performed. A high transverse incision helps to avoid communication with the median sternotomy. The bypass time ranged from 2 to 5 h with a mean time of 3 h and 17 min. Neither the total bypass time nor the period of aortic cross-clamping with intermittent coronary perfusion appeared to be a significant cause of mortality or morbidity.

Results

Multiple valve replacement has been performed upon 152 patients at this clinic with a 12% operative mortality and a 14% incidence of late death. Table 1 lists the combinations of multiple valve replacement which have been performed, and the early and late incidence of mortality for each combination. These statistics are compared with isolated mitral and aortic replacement. Table 2 compares early and recent results. The 1967 operative mortality of 4% indicates that these patients can be managed with a reasonable operative risk. Fig. 2 gives the age distribution of the

Table 1. *Operative and late mortality rates for isolated and multiple valve replacement during the past seven and one half years are listed and compared*

Sept. 1960 to Jan. 1968

	No of patients	Mortality operative	Mortality late
Isolated mitral	197	15%	10%
Isolated aortic	302	12%	15%
Mitral + Tricuspid	16	6%	6%
Mitral + Aortic	103	13%	16%
Triple	33	12%	12%
Total	651	13%	13%

patients and includes the operative deaths. 49 patients below 40 years of age have undergone multiple valve replacement without a mortality. This data is based upon a 100% follow-up of the 152 cases.

Table 3 lists the causes of the operative mortalities. Cardiac pacing, ventilatory assistance, and adequate blood volume have considerably diminished the incidence of low output deaths (STARR et al., 1964; FRIESEN et al.,; KLOSTER et al.). Five late deaths were clearly unrelated to the prostheses (Table 4). Table 5 lists the late deaths which may have been related to the prostheses. The timing of the late deaths is shown in Fig. 3.

Table 2. *The operative mortality following multiple valve replacement during the past year is compared with the preceding 5 years*

June 1962 to Jan. 1968

	No. of patients	Deaths			
		operative		late	
1962—1966	125	17	(14%)	21	(17%)
1967	27	1	(4%)	1	(4%)
Total	152	18	(12%)	22	(14%)

Table 3. *The causes of operative death following multiple valve replacement are tabulated*

Jan. 1962 to Jan. 1968

Low output	8
Failure to resuscitate	4
Hepatic failure	2
Thrombo-emboli	2
Primary Arrhythmia	1
Gastrointestinal infarction	1
Total	18

Table 4. *The causes of late death when the death is definitely unrelated to the prothesis are listed*

Jan. 1962 to Jan. 1968
134 Operative survivors

Myocardial fibrosis	2
Arrhythmia	1
Electrical pacemaker failure	1
Pneumonia	1
Total	5

Table 5. *The causes of late death when the death is probably or possibly related to the prosthesis are listed*

Jan. 1962 to Jan. 1968
134 Operative survivors

Coronary embolus	5
Cerebral Embolus	1
Thrombotic occlusion	3
Bacterial endocarditis	1
Ball variance	3
Sudden death — no autopsy	2
Reoperation — cardiac	2
Total	17

Table 6. *The incidence and significance of late leaks after multiple valve replacement are listed*

12 Cases (16 leaks) in 112 survivors

Susseccful reoperation	3
Reoperation — death	1
Leak not hemodynamically significant	8
Total	12

Complications were common in the early cases surviving multiple valve replacement. The majority were bleeding problems or arrhythmias. Electrical pacing has helped to solve the problem of arrhythmias. The major complications associated with prosthetic valve replacement are sepsis, leak, anemia, thromboembolism, and ball variance (HERR et al., 1965). Neither an endocarditis nor a wound infection has occurred in this multiple valve series. Table 6 shows the incidence of late leak and the significance of the leak.

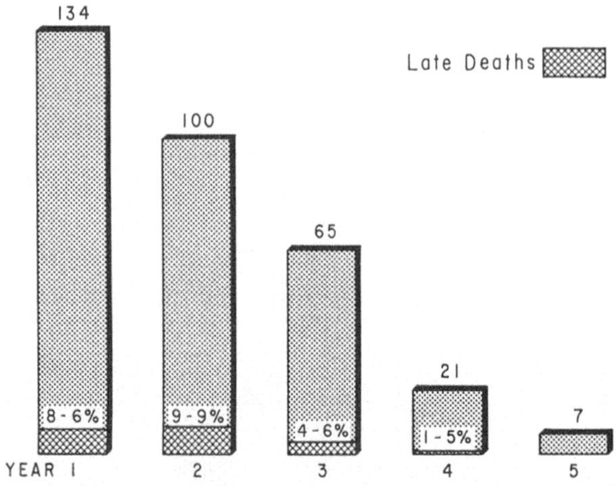

Fig. 3. The timing of 22 late deaths among 134 survivors of multiple valve replacement is demonstrated

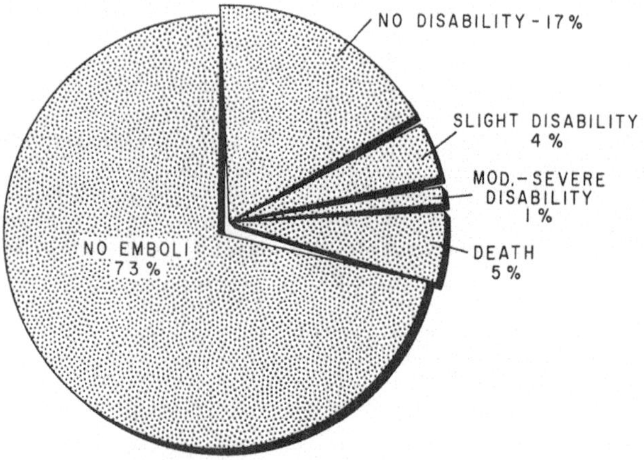

Fig. 4. The incidence and significance of thromboembolic complications after multiple valve replacement is shown in this pie graph. June 1962 to Jan 1968, 134 operative survivors

Thromboembolism is the most important late complication of prosthetic valve replacement. The incidence and severity of the thromboembolic complications following multiple valve replacement are shown in Fig. 4. There is no apparent increase in the risk of thromboembolism with multiple replacement compared to isolated mitral valve replacement. Fig. 5 illustrates the timing of the late thromboembolic complications which have been observed. The introduction of the extended cloth prostheses (Mitral no 6120, and Aortic no 1200) in 1965 has decreased the incidence of thromboembolic complications from 61% to 7% in isolated mitral replacement, and from 29% to 9% in isolated aortic replacement. It is too early to accurately predict the embolic potential of the completely cloth-covered prostheses (Model no 6300 mitral, and Model no 2300 aortic), which are now being used clinically (Tables 7 and 8). The necessity for long-term anticoagulant therapy is currently

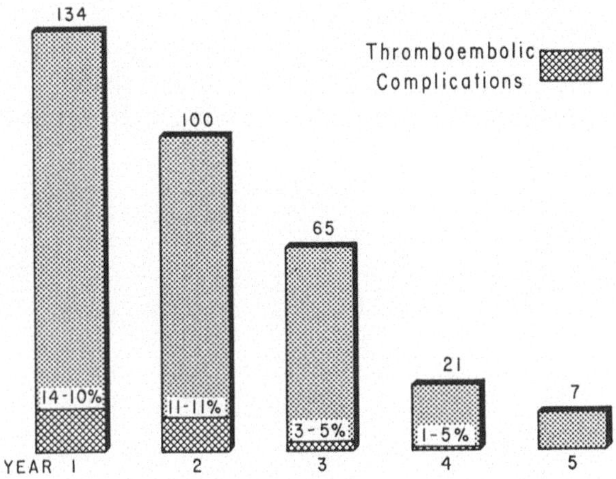

Fig. 5. The timing of the first thromboembolus after a multiple valve replacement is demonstrated

Table 7. *The incidence of emboli is related to the type of mitral valve* design and compared
Sept. 1960 to Jan. 1968

Valve series	Number of patients	Emboli early	late	total
Old	90	11 (12%)	44 (49%)	51 (61%)
6120	61	0	4 (7%)	4 (7%)
6300 Isolated	17	0	0	0
6300 Multiple	13	0	0	0
6500	2	0	0	0

Table 8. *The incidence of emboli is related to the type of aortic valve design and compared*
Sept. 1960 to Jan. 1968

Valve series	Number of patients	Emboli early	late	total
1000	157	9 (6%)	36 (23%)	45 (29%)
1200	95	3 (3%)	6 (6%)	9 (9%)
2300	20	0	0	0
2300 (Multiple)	14	0	0	0

being evaluated in a double blind study using these new prostheses. The majority of the patients who are unable to participate in this study are receiving routine anticoagulant therapy.

The destructive change in the silicone rubber ball, previously reported as ball variance, results from a unique and peculiar infiltration of the silicone rubber with fatty material from the blood (HERR et al., 1967, 1968). This deforms the ball and may lead to valve failure. Ball variance caused three deaths and five reoperations in multiple valve cases. Two patients had unsuspected mitral ball variance at reoperation 2 years after double valve replacement. After isolated aortic valve replacement the diagnosis of ball variance frequently can be made by auscultation. The opening click of the prosthesis is diminished or absent. Phonocardiography has helped to document

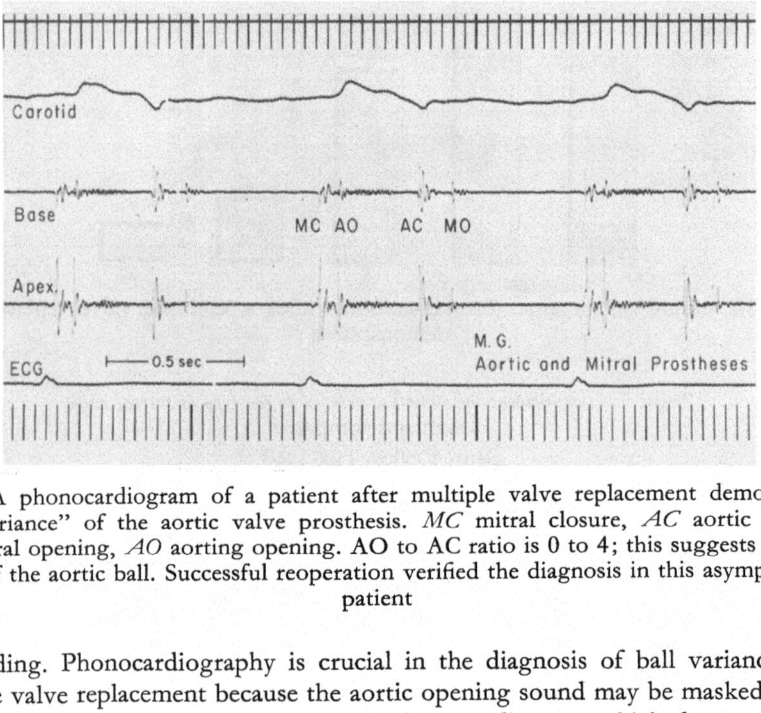

Fig. 6. A phonocardiogram of a patient after multiple valve replacement demonstrates "ball variance" of the aortic valve prosthesis. *MC* mitral closure, *AC* aortic closure, *MO* mitral opening, *AO* aorting opening. AO to AC ratio is 0 to 4; this suggests deterioration of the aortic ball. Successful reoperation verified the diagnosis in this asymptomatic patient

this finding. Phonocardiography is crucial in the diagnosis of ball variance after multiple valve replacement because the aortic opening sound may be masked by the closing sound of the mitral prosthesis. A phonocardiogram which demonstrates a marked diminution of the opening sound of the aortic prosthesis in a multiple valve replacement patient is shown in Fig. 6. Reoperation is necessary if the patient has symptoms suggesting obstruction of the aortic prosthesis or a complete absence of the prosthetic opening sound. The hollow Stellite ball of the current prostheses is designed to avoid this complication.

Functional Results

Representative cardiac catheterization findings following multiple valve replacement have been previously reported (BRISTOW et al., 1965, 1966; LEWIS et al.). Patients with preoperative pulmonary hypertension demonstrate a fall in pulmonary artery pressure. A profound fall is usually observed in the mean left atrial pressure, and despite the frequent use of small size mitral prostheses the left atrial end diastolic pressures are usually normal at rest. Left ventricular and systemic arterial pressures generally fail to demonstrate a gradient across the aortic prosthesis. Nine patients studied 6 months after multiple replacement including the tricuspid valve revealed a higher resting cardiac index than their preoperative values and a satisfactory exercise response in all but one patient.

Of the 112 current survivors of multiple valve replacement 100 are at least 6 months after operation. 64 patients are judged to be Class I by the New York Heart Association Classification. They are normally active, free of all cardiac symptoms, and eating a regular diet. Postoperative roentgenograms show a dramatic reduction in cardiac size. 34 patients are judged to be Class II. They require exercise restriction, but are greatly improved and are managed without severe salt restriction. Postoperative roentgenograms show a reduction in heart size, but mild cardiomegaly usually persists. Two patients remain Class III of IV, and require careful medical management including marked salt restriction and diuretics. Although these patients are improved, they represent unsatisfactory results because of continued cardiomegaly and limited exercise tolerance. Preoperatively they had massive cardiomegaly, severe right ventricular failure, and functional tricuspid regurgitation. This suggests that right ventricular dysfunction is an important factor in the poor results observed in these far-advanced cases. Severe myocardial fibrosis and coronary artery insufficiency are also frequently noted to contribute to a poor result (PETERSON et al.).

Discussion

The overall mortality for multiple replacement and for isolated replacement is comparable; however, a slightly greater late mortality is observed following multiple replacement. This result is only possible when all pathological valves are identified and corrected.

The criteria for surgical exposure of the aortic and mitral valves are clearly present in many patients but a significant number suspected of having either isolated aortic or mitral disease have coexisting valve disease completely missed unless careful hemodynamic studies and a complete surgical exploration are performed. A stenotic aortic valve with an insignificant preoperative pressure gradient may demonstrate marked obstruction and a high gradient after corrective mitral surgery has increased the cardiac output. Direct exploration may reveal a badly damaged valve which belies the mild hemodynamic findings. Uncorrected aortic regurgitation following mitral valve replacement often compromises the late functional result.

Severe aortic valve disease can overshadow coexisting mitral disease, especially in the presence of left ventricular failure with high end diastolic pressures. In patients with multivalvular disease it may be necessary to expose both the aortic and mitral valves before an accurate diagnosis can be made. The median sternotomy approach offers an excellent exposure for this purpose.

Tricuspid valve replacement was performed in 10% of the mitral replacement group, and in 27% of the mitral and aortic replacement group to make a total of 49 patients. Valve replacement is usually necessary for mixed tricuspid disease, although pure or predominant tricuspid stenosis can often be managed by direct vision commissurotomy. Such a valve must be repalpated to check for regurgitation after terminating the bypass.

Patients with pure tricuspid regurgitation secondary to right ventricular failure and mitral valve disease pose a difficult problem. Massive preoperative tricuspid regurgitation is usually greatly improved following mitral valve replacement. When it persists unchanged most patients require immediate operative correction if they are to survive and have a satisfactory late result. Annuloplasty is not always effective, and a tricuspid valve replacement is usually necessary. We have not observed significant tricuspid regurgitation present by palpation after bypass which disappeared either months or years after corrective mitral surgery. Tricuspid valve replacement is reserved for patients who require a mitral prosthesis for concomitant far-advanced destruction of the mitral valve. If the mitral valve can be repaired satisfactorily a marginal repair of the tricuspid valve may be acceptable because a later operation is a near certainty. Isolated tricuspid valve replacement for rheumatic valvular heart disease has not been performed in this clinic.

All patients routinely have ventricular pacing wires placed before closure of the chest. Patients with intact atrio-ventricular conduction either preoperatively or immediately after defibrillation routinely have a transatrial intracavitary pacing lead inserted just above the superior caval-atrial junction and a ground lead in the subcutaneous tissue. Arrhythmias or low cardiac output secondary to bradycardia are managed by atrial pacing at 100 to 120/min with marked improvement (FRIESEN et al.). Patients who are unable to follow the atrial pacer usually respond well to ventricular pacing, but the rise in cardiac output is approximately 30%. Fast arrhythmias have recently been managed by atrio-ventricular or simple ventricular paired pacing, but the experience is too brief to recommend its routine use. This liberal use of electrical pacing has nearly eliminated the use of myocardial depressant drugs in postoperative patients.

References

1. BRISTOW, J. D., C. FARREHI, C. W. MCCORD, A. STARR, and H. E. GRISWOLD: Circulation Suppl. **31**, 1—67 (1965).
2. —, F. E. KLOSTER, R. HERR, A. STARR, C. W. MCCORD, and H. E. GRISWOLD: Circulation **34**, 437—447 (1966).
3. FRIESEN, W. G., R. D. WOODSON, A. W. AMES, R. H. HERR, and D. G. KASSEBAUM: J. thoracic cardiovas. Surg. **55**, 271—278 (1968).
4. HERR, R., A. STARR, C. W. MCCORD, and J. A. WOOD: Ann. thorac. Surg. **1**, 403—415 (1965).
5. HERR, R. H., F. E. KLOSTER, Y. SEZAI, and A. STARR: Diagnosis and management of „ball variance" following aortic valve replacement. Abstract No. 860, American Heart Association, 1967.
6. —, A. STARR, W. R. PIERIE, J. A. WOOD, and J. C. BIGELOW: Ann. thorac. Surg. (In press).
7. KLOSTER, F. E., J. D. BRISTOW, A. STARR, C. W. MCCORD, and H. E. GRISWOLD: Circulation **32**, 415—424 (1966).
8. LEWIS, R. P., R. H. HERR, A. STARR, and H. E. GRISWOLD: Amer. Hearth J. **71**, 549—563 (1966).
9. PETERSON, C. R., R. H. HERR, R. V. CRISERA, A. STARR, J. D. BRISTOW, and H. E. GRISWOLD: Ann. intern. Med. **66**, 1—24 (1967).
10. PORTER, G. A., A. STARR, J. KIMSEY, and H. LENERTZ: J. surg. Res. **7**, 447—456 (1967).
11. STARR, A.: Surg. Forum **11**, 258—260 (1960).
12. —, M. L. EDWARDS, C. W. MCCORD, and H. E. GRISWOLD: Circulation **27**, 779—785 (1963).
13. —, C. W. MCCORD, J. WOOD, R. HERR, and M. L. EDWARDS: Ann. Surg. **160**, 596—613 (1964).
14. —, R. HERR, and J. WOOD: Surg. Gynec. Obstet. **122**, 1295—13010 (1966).
15. —, R. H. HERR, and J. A. WOOD: J. thorac. cardiovasc. Surg. **54**, 333—355 (1967).

Assisted Circulation and the Artificial Heart*

William H. Muller Jr.

Cardiopulmonary assistance has followed three general approaches. These are cardiopulmonary bypass with a pump oxygenator for open heart surgery or for temporary circulatory assistance, augmentation of the diastolic volume or partial ventricular bypass, and the totally implantable mechanical heart substitute.

The most frequently used type of cardiac assist device is the pump oxygenator, which is employed in hundreds of centers throughout the world to support the circulation during open heart procedures. However, with the constant improvement in design of oxygenators and the accumulation of data concerning the physiologic principles related to their use, the applications of extracorporeal circulation are becoming more diversified. Recently, an increasing amount of attention has been paid to perfusion systems not involving total bypass but designed to afford partial cardiorespiratory support. There are two principal types: veno-arterial perfusion and veno-venous perfusion.

Veno-arterial perfusion is directed toward support of the failing myocardium and might be applied to such clinical disorders as acute myocardial infarction, refractory congestive heart failure, and overwhelming shock. Whereas veno-arterial perfusion is best applied to myocardial insufficiency, veno-venous perfusion is most successfully used in the treatment of respiratory insufficiency. There are certain diseases of the respiratory system in which, although the disease process may be reversible, the clinical course is characterized by progressive hypoxemia, hypercapnia, and acidosis. Despite the usual means of ventilatory support, death may rapidly ensue. Examples are hyaline membrane disease of the newborn, overwhelming pneumonia, either primary or in association with pulmonary resection, and severe pulmonary contusion. An effective method of producing adequate gas exchange during the acute phase of the illness until the patient's pulmonary function has returned to a more normal range might allow a significant number of patients to be salvaged. Therefore, utilization of the pump oxygenator seems to be a logical answer to this problem. In veno-venous perfusion, the pump oxygenator is placed in parallel with the normal circulation, and provides pre-pulmonary oxygenation of the blood and is expected only to compliment respiratory function. Support of the failing heart is not a consideration, and thus elaborate triggering or monitoring devices need not be incorporated into the perfusion system.

In 1953, Melrose suggested the possibility of this type of treatment of respiratory insufficiency and performed a number of experiments which indicated that arterial oxygen saturation in the hypoxic animal could be elevated. Others, including Chadduck, Schramel et al., Krasna, Callaghan, and Zotti added information and data through experiments with this type of perfusing system. Various types of oxygenators were used, but the duration of the perfusion was limited because of the development of changes in the lungs, characterized by perivascular hemorrhage, constriction of vascular structures, and extravasation of blood into the alveoli in significant numbers of animals. In addition, nearly all of the blood elements were lowered to extremely low levels.

* From the Department of Surgery, University of Virginia Medical Center, Charlottesville, Virginia 22901. — Supported in part by USPH Grant HE 02038. Presented at the Amerikanisch-deutscher Chirurgenkongreß — ACS Meeting, Munich, June 1968.

In an effort to prolong the perfusion time and study changes in blood and viscera in a series of animals when perfused by the membrane oxygenator, HAKANSON and MULLER employed a Crystal-Day gravity flow membrane oxygenator. Using this system at perfusion rates of 40 to 60 cc per kg of body weight, animals could be perfused for much longer periods of time with minimal visceral and blood changes. One perfused for 48 h was alive and well several months later.

More recently, there has been much emphasis on the use of temporary assist devices to support the circulation. The first experiments by HARKEN and his associates were with counterpulsation. This system is based on the principle of diastolic augmentation of the volume and pressure during diastole, theoretically affording increased perfusion of the coronary arteries and viscera and at the same time reducing cardiac work. Although its basic principles underlie most of the heart assist devices, there is some question as to whether or not it has fulfilled all of its theoretical promises, and whether its application to the patient in cardiogenic shock or temporary low left ventricular function reduces the ultimate mortality rate in such patients.

DE BAKEY and his associates have designed a gas-activated, left ventricular bypass device, which is placed between the left atrium and the axillary artery. It is triggered from the electrocardiogram and synchronized with cardiac contractions in order to increase blood volume in the aorta during systole rather than during diastole, as in the case of counterpulsation. He has employed it in patients undergoing open heart operations whose ventricular function is temporarily reduced, and whose circulation cannot be maintained with the heart alone after cardiopulmonary bypass is discontinued. In one instance, he has dramatically demonstrated the value of such an apparatus in supporting the circulation until the patient's own heart had recovered sufficiently to maintain it. This patient was a 37 year old female with long standing rheumatic heart disease. She had marked enlargement of all of the heart chambers because of a severe mitral and aortic insufficiency. She had a fixed cardiac output of 1.9, a left ventricular end diastolic pressure of 20, and a left atrial pressure of 38. Both valves were replaced, and when it became apparent that the heart would not resume adequate cardiac output when bypass was discontinued, the left ventricular bypass pump was applied with a pump flow rate of 1200 cc per min. Using left atrial pressure as the chief criterion for determining the necessary pump flow rate, attempts were made from time to time during the first week to reduce the pump flow, and finally on the 9. postoperative day it could be reduced to 350 cc per min with maintenance of left atrial pressure at 10 mmHg. The pump was then stopped for 6 h with no increase of left atrial pressure and was therefore removed under local anesthesia. Cardiac catheterization studies 6 months after operation revealed markedly improved hemodynamic function, and the patient has resumed normal activities during the $1^1/_2$ years since operation.

DENNIS has passed a large caliber cannula attached to the end of a catheter through the ventricular septum, so that blood can be withdrawn and pumped back into a peripheral artery, thus bypassing the left side of the heart.

KANTROWITZ (1968) devised a curved, cylindrical pumping device with a collapsible, gas-activated pumping bladder inside of it, which is connected between the ascending and descending aorta with the intervening portion of this artery interrupted. Therefore, the entire blood flow passes through this pump in contrast to partial flow of blood which passes through other types of assist devices. Also, whereas other pumping devices employ valves, his pump depends upon the integrity of the patient's own aortic valve. Thus, in diastole, when the patient's aortic valve is closed and the pump is actuated, blood flow is in a forward direction. In addition, it should increase coronary blood flow, thus improving the work capacity of the heart and improved cardiac output in one patient for approximately 2 weeks. It has the obvious disadvantage that the tubes which activate the pump must pass through the patient's skin. Therefore, long-term circulatory assistance might be accompanied by the development of infection along the course of these tubes.

A similar device devised by BIRTWELL et al. is designed so that the pumping chamber is placed in a skin and subcutaneous tissue pedicle. It is activated by externally applied pressure, thus eliminating the necessity for the passage of power transmission tubes through the skin. Experimental studies of this device are encouraging; however, it seems likely that the skin and subcutaneous tissue overlying the pump might break down as a result of pressure applied over a long period of time.

One of the simplest and most effective assist devices is the intra-aortic pumping balloon initially described by MOULAPOULOS, TOPAZ, and KOLFF in 1962. It has been used infrequently until recently, when KANTROWITZ (1968) reported results with this device in the treatment of patients with cardiogenic shock. It consists of a polyurethene balloon mounted on the end of a hollow catheter which, when inflated, will displace approximately 31 to 32 cc of blood and is inserted through the femoral artery to a position in the superior portion of the descending thoracic aorta. The balloon is alternately inflated and deflated with helium, because of its low density allowing rapid inflation and deflation. It can be synchronized either through a pressure transducer or electrocardiogram, and pumping can therefore be augmented during any phase of the cardiac cycle, although diastole appears to be preferable. KANTROWITZ (1968) recently reported its use in 15 patients in refractory cardiogenic shock. There were six long-term survivors, six short-term survivors, and three immediate deaths. All of the short-term survivors died of causes unrelated to the cardiogenic shock, and two of the immediate deaths occurred due to interruption of the pumping. This device has certain obvious advantages in that it is relatively simple, and the balloon catheter may be introduced into the aorta through the femoral artery under local anesthesia, therefore eliminating the necessity for a major operation for its placement.

In an effort to evaluate several parameters related to left ventricular bypass, BESSINGER, LEFER, and MULLER designed experiments to evaluate 1) alterations with asynchronous partial left ventricular bypass and 2) the effects of pre-treatment with steroids in this system. Groups of animals included 1) a control series, 2) a low flow series of 15 to 45% of cardiac output, 3) a high flow series with 55 to 98% cardiac output, 4) a high flow series pre-treated with hydrocortisone, and 5) a high flow series pre-treated with hydrocortisone vehicle. A number of determinations were made 2 h after the animals were placed on bypass, including central venous and mean aortic pressure, arterial pO_2, pCO_2, and pH values, cardiac output, left ventricular minute work, and total peripheral resistance. Myocardial contractility was unchanged, because the dp/dt increased proportionately to left ventricular end diastolic pressure. Hydrocortisone treated dogs showed a significant decrease in dp/dt, with no change in left ventricular end diastolic pressure. This seemed to indicate decreased myocardial contractility. Dogs treated with hydrocortisone developed smaller excess lactate on bypass, and the left ventricular mean work recovered to a greater degree 30 min after bypass than in dogs not so treated. Left ventricular bypass apparently decreases left ventricular mean work in proportion to the degree of bypass while maintaining adequate tissue perfusion. It should be pointed out that bypass in these animals was asynchronous, thus making it appear that partial bypass does not favorably augment cardiac output.

A greater problem than the successful development and utilization of cardiac assist devices is the development of a completely implantable, mechanical, intracorporeal heart. Although recent success with homografted human hearts has currently overshadowed development in this field, a considerable amount of work which has been underway during the past decade continues. Much of the initial work was done by AKUTSU, KOLFF, and their associates. They made numerous models of injection molded silastic which simulate the atria and ventricles of the human heart. The ventricles were driven by an extracorporeal reciprocating pump, and the power transmitted through tubes attached to the intracorporeal heart. With such a heart, calves were kept alive for several hours.

Others have also contributed towards solving this problem. Intensive and progressive efforts are those of SHUMACKER, BURNS, and their associates, who have developed four models which have been reduced in size so that the final one fits into the lower lobe recess of the chest of a pig weighing approximately 200 pounds. This device weighs about 1200 grams and displaces 900 cc. It is powered by a DC brushless motor, employs a hydraulic mixed flow pumping system, is to some degree autoregulatory, and has a wide margin of control capability. Even so, the solution of control problems has been the most difficult. Out-of-phase pumping was used for the right and left ventricles in order to conserve power, and this asynchronous pumping system produced a relative mitral stenosis as the heart rate increased due to the greater demand on the left ventricle as compared to the right. Therefore, a new sequential hydraulic pumping system has been designed and is under construction. Pumping is achieved rotationally by distributing the hydraulic energy wave front about doughnut-shaped collapsible ventricles. The pump housing is sequentially rotated about the centrally located pump, thus distributing the energy more appropriately. Although it has not been tried experimentally, the investigators believe that it has several advantages not present in previous models. These include an atrial component behind the hydraulic wave front for venous filling, a smaller package, better flow characteristics, the elimination of inflow valves, decreased pumping energy losses, and a very low resistance to venous filling.

The problems which must be overcome in developing a long-term implantable total cardiac substitute appear insurmountable. However, from a technological standpoint, the development of such a device is within the realm of possibility. Many of these problems have been discovered, and some appear to have been at least partially solved. One of the greatest difficulties relates to an implantable power source so that wire conductors are not required to pass through the skin. Batteries with sufficient energy output which are now available are entirely too bulky for implantation. It is conceivable that by utilizing the piezoelectric principle sufficient electrical energy might be generated at least partially to recharge an implanted battery, and investigations by the Artificial Heart-Myocardial Infarct Program Office indicate that a satisfactory implantable power supply may be eventually achieved. Another possibility is an atomic power source. At the present time, however, such problems as shielding and heat generation seem insurmountable.

Electromagnetic induction through the chest wall without a direct wire connection is a possibility and has been used by GLENN and others for transmitting power to a cardiac pacemaker. There is evidence to indicate that significant amounts of electrical energy can be transmitted through the intact chest wall without discomfort. As yet, however, whether or not prolonged use would have detrimental effects on the skin and underlying tissues has not been determined.

Another problem has to do with the fatigue life of the materials used for the pump. However, the past decade has seen the development of many elastomuric flexible materials, many of which have great flex durability, and it is reasonable to suppose that this problem can be overcome.

By far one of the greatest challenges in the blood surface interface. This has been found to be true, especially in cardiac assist devices which have been applied for much longer periods than total heart replacements. It appears chiefly in two general categories: 1. the development of thrombus and subsequent embolization on the material surface and 2. alteration of many of the blood elements, particularly those concerned with clotting. The use of materials with non-wetable surfaces, even though polished as smoothly as possible, failed to eliminate these consequences. After first using this method unsuccessfully, DE BAKEY lined his device with dacron velour material, which traps blood elements and binds them to the surface, thus rapidly producing a pseudo-endothelium. Even though this improved the situation, he does not believe it answers this question completely for long term pumping required by assist devices or the implanted heart.

Attachment of the inlet and outlet vessels to the patient's venous and arterial structures is not as great a problem as initially believed because the use of synthetic tubular prostheses, which have been employed for many years as arterial substitutes and which can be attached easily to both the device and the patient's tissue, are thus far satisfactory.

The fabrication of a device with adequate output, but which at the same time is small enough for implantation without displacing other structures, is indeed important, but engineering refinements appear to have reduced it to a size for practical implantation and at the same time maintained efficiency criteria.

The dissipation of heat, both from the device itself and from an implantable power source, is a great one. Virtually all of the conceivable implantable energy sources generate significant amounts of heat, which would require dissipation. This could conceivably be done through the bloodstream itself but might require supplementary means of ridding the body of excessive heat.

One of the great problems is the control mechanisms, which must be built into such a device. When one is dealing with a multi-chambered heart substitute, even almost immeasurable differences become manifest after a prolonged period of pumping, particularly when one considers the enormous multiplication by the required number of pulsations per 24 h. Again, it appears that this can be overcome by means of autoregulatory mechanisms, which are in return controlled by various sensing devices.

Therefore, while the production of a satisfactory completely implantable heart and its power source seems remote at the present time, the combined efforts of engineers, basic scientists, and clinicians bring the reality of such a device into realistic feasibility and possibility. With proper financial support and coordinated effort, it is entirely probable that a mechanical heart will be forthcoming within the next decade.

Summary

Circulatory assistance has been approached from several different standpoints. The most frequently employed method is the use of the pump oxygenator for relatively short periods for the performance of open-heart operations. This modality has also been studied in the laboratory and applied infrequently in the clinical situation where circulatory assistance is needed. Veno-venous perfusion seems applicable in those cases where there is a temporary pulmonary insufficiency preventing adequate oxygenation. Veno-arterial perfusion is more appropriate where left heart failure is present. Neither of these methods is refined or developed to the point of prolonged clinical application because of the lack of an adequate perfusing system.

There are other assist devices which augment the diastolic volume by withdrawing blood during systole and replacing it during diastole. One device is placed so that the entire aortic flow passes through it, and diastolic pumping increases flow and pressure. A second type increases volume and pressure, while yet another variety augments the circulation by partially bypassing the left ventricle, thus reducing the work load of the heart.

Cardiac transplantation for total heart replacement is being done more and more frequently with increasing success. Work is progressing on the use of a mechanical totally implantable heart substitute. There are many problems, both from a biologic and engineering standpoint, related to its development. While it does appear feasible and possible to make a device capable of maintaining the circulation for prolonged periods of time, its perfection to clinical applicability does not appear to be imminent.

References

AKUTSU, T., and W. J. KOLFF: Trans. Amer. Soc. artif. intern. Org. **4**, 230—232 (1958).

BESSINGER, V. F., A. M. LEFER, and W. H. MULLER JR.: Circulation (Suppl. II), **XXXV** and **XXXVI**, 67—68 (1967).

BIRTWELL, W. C., H. S. SOROFF, F. GIRON, W. B. THROWER, T. TANAKE, N. TAKAYAMA, and R. A. DETERLING JR.: J. cardiovasc. Surg. (Torino) **9**, 31—42 (1968).

CALLAGHAN, J. C., D. CARDOZO, B. BORACCHIA, and A. ALELSINK: J. thorac. cardiovasc. Surg. **43**, 135 (1962).

CHADDUCK, W.: Amer. J. Physiol. **202**, 510 (1962).

DE BAKEY, M.: Partial support with artificial devices. Conference on Human Heart Transplants, Washington, D. C., May, 1968.

DENNIS, C., D. P. HALL, J. R. MORENO, and A. SENNING: Acta chir. scand. **123**, 267 (1962).

GIBBON, J. H., JR.: Surgery **59**, 1—5 (1966).

GLENN, W. W. L., A. MAURO, E. LONGO, P. H. LAVIETIES, and F. J. MACKAY: New Engl. J. Med. **261**, 948 (1959).

HAKANSON, C. M., and W. H. MULLER JR.: J. cardiovasc. Surg. (Torino) (In Press) (1968).

HARKEN, D. E., J. A. JACOBEY, W. J. TAYLOR, G. T. SMITH, and R. GORLIN: Surg. Forum **12**, 225—227 (1961).

KANTROWITZ, A., L. J. SHERMAN JR., and J. KRAKAUER: Progr. cardiovasc. Dis. **10**, (1967).

—, S. TJONNELAND, J. KRAKAUER, A. N. BUTNER, S. J. PHILLIPS, W. Z. YAHR, M. SHAPIRO, P. S. FREED, D. JARON, and J. L. SHERMAN JR.: Trans. Amer. Soc. artif. intern. Org. (In press.).

KRASNA, J. H., L. STEINFELD, I. KREEL, and I. D. BARONOFSKY: J. thorac. cardiovasc. Surg. **43**, 135 (1962).

MELROSE, D. G., J. W. BASSETT, P. BEACONSFIELD, I. G. GRABER, and R. SHACKMAN: Brit. med. J. **2**, 62 (1953).

SCHRAMEL, R., W. CHARMAN, E. WEIFFENBACH, and O. CREECH: J. thorac. cardiovasc. Surg. **42**, 804 (1961).
SHUMACKER, H. B., JR., W. H. BURNS, and N. J. GRIFFITH: Total mechanical cardiac replacement devices. Conference on Human Heart Transplants. Washington, D. C., May, 1968.
TOPAZ, S. R., S. D. MOULOPOULOS, and W. J. KOLFF: Am. Heart J. **63**, 669 (1962).
ZOTTI, E. F., S. IKEDO, A. M. LESAGE, W. C. SEALY, and G. YOUNG JR.: J. thorac. cardiovasc. Surg. **51**, 383—390 (1966).

Results of Intracardiac Pacing

HANS G. BORST* and A. SCHAUDIG**

Transvenous intracardiac pacing has been used as a temporary measure in the treatment of heart block for many years. By contrast, there has been some reluctance to accept this method for permanent therapy of cardiac conduction defects. This was due to certain difficulties in the placement and maintenance of stimulating electrodes in the heart. Intracardiac pacing has been considered by us the method of choice for permanent stimulation of the heart since 1963. Our experience with this method in more than 200 implantations forms the basis of this report.

Materials and Methods

Our series comprises 255 patients with complete and incomplete heart block treated at the Department of Surgery, Munich University, from 1962 through 1968. 230 cases have been analyzed for study, 207 of which received transvenous intracardiac pacemaker systems. The age ranged from 2 to 90 years. About one third of the patients was older than 70 years and nine were older than 80. While, originally, only patients with Adams-Stokes attacks were treated, the indication subsequently was extended to other complications of heart block (Table 1). 68% of the patients

Table 1. *Indications (230 patients)*

Heart block	Complications cerebral	Complications cardiac
total	49%	21%
intermittent and partial	18%	10%
sino-auricular	1%	1%
	68%	32%

complained of predominant cerebral sequelae such as Adams-Stokes attacks, dizziness or vertigo. Cardiac complications in the form of effort-intolerance, myocardial insufficiency and pectangina were prominent in the other patients. Included are five cases of surgical- and four of congenital heart block.

In $^4/_5$ of the 207 patients treated with transvenous systems the thin, pliable and non-elastic unipolar Elema-Schoenander electrode described by LAGERGREN et al. [*4*] was implanted. The electrode-cable consists of three bands of stainless steel wound around a Dacron core and is insulated with polyethylene tubing. It carries a

From the Departments of Surgery, Medical Schools of Hannover* and Munich**.

cylindrical platinum electrode-tip, considerably larger than the cable. The rest of the patients received Cordis intracardiac electrodes which are stiffer and more elastic because of silicone insulation and spring-coil wire. The electrode-head is of the same size or somewhat larger than the cable.

Elema-Schoenander impulse generators [3], type EM 137 and 139 were used in the early cases (Table 2). We then changed to the Vitatron unit [1] and, since 1966 to Cordis impulse generators.

Stimulation usually was of the constant frequency type. Only in 11% of the cases generators triggered by the R- or P-wave were employed.

The entire implantation-procedure routinely is done in local anesthesia. The permanent intracardiac electrode is inserted via either the right external or internal jugular vein, depending on the size and patency of the former.

To facilitate guidance and placement of the soft Elema-Schoenander electrode-cable it is threaded through a stiff, X-ray opaque Oedman catheter (size 7). This catheter is slightly bent at its tip and is slit longitudinally throughout. After proper intracardiac placement of guide catheter and electrode-cable the latter is grasped with forceps at its point of entry into the vein. The guide-catheter can now be withdrawn, simultaneously peeling it off the cable. Thus the electrode wire remains in its intended position and cannot be dislocated while extracting the guiding catheter. Should dislocation of the electrode occur subsequently, the cable can be withdrawn from the heart, reinserted into the slot of the Oedman catheter and reintroduced without disconnecting the cable from the pacemaker unit. The Cordis electrode-catheter is introduced with an intraluminal stylet. Should respositioning become necessary, rather cumbersome disconnection of the electrode from the pacemaker socket is necessary.

Table 2. *Impulse generators (230 first implantations)*

Elema-Schönander	40%
Vitatron	20%
Ventricor	23%
Ectocor	10%
Atricor	1%
Medtronic	4%
Electrodyne	1%
Biotronic	1%

Allowing for liberal slack of the electrode-wire on its way to the apex of the right heart turned out to be of prime importance in preventing later dislocation. The cable should follow the lateral atrial wall and then traverse the tricuspid anulus making a definite hump. Electrode threshold is measured at this point, a current less than 1 mA and less than 1.5 V being considered satisfactory. The free end of the electrode cable is connected to the impulse generator, generally located either in the abdominal or axillary subcutaneous tissue.

Results

Stimulation was maintained from 1 week to 6 years. There were 54 deaths (Table 3). Two of the fatalities occurred on the operating table, 10 in the hospital, and the rest after discharge. 24 of the latter fatalities were due to a failing heart without loss of pacemaker function, 15 were not related to the cardio-vascular system and in 15 sudden death occurred without evidence for its cause.

Pacemaker breakdown will only be discussed in passing. Briefly, the two earlier types of impulse generators implanted, i.e. the Elema- and Vitatron units, had a relatively short average life span of 18 and 11 months, respectively, with rupture of

Table 3. *Mortality (230 cases)*

Time of death		Cause of death		
		rel. to heart	not rel. to heart	unknown
Day of operation	2	2	—	—
Hospital	10	5	1	4
to 12 mos	23	10	9	4
over 12 mos	14	7	5	2
unknown	5	—	—	5
	54	24	15	15

the casing and leaks of the wire-input being the main causes of damage. Rapid rise of stimulating frequency was a particularly dangerous complication in the Elema units. By contrast only 1 of 50 Ventricor generators, functioning for an average of 10 months and none of 22 Ectocor units in operation for an average of 8 months have failed.

The electrodes performed rather well electrically. An increase of threshold, due to either a leaking insulation or an endocardial fibrous reaction was noted in 15 cases, while a wire break occurred only once. Dislocation of the intracardiac cable presented an annoying problem, not yet completely eliminated. 19% of the Elema cables and 36% of the Cordis cables had to be repositioned. These incidences have dropped somewhat with increasing experience but dislocation could not be prevented altogether. In only four cases repositioning of the electrode was ultimately impossible, necessitating implantation of myocardial wires. Other non-fatal complications are listed in Table 4. These included local infections and skin erosion over the pacemaker or cable, phrenic nerve stimulation, recurrent hematoma, and pain in the pacemaker pocket.

Table 4. *Complications – nonfatal (230 cases)*

Local infection	7
Skin erosion	4
Phrenic stimulation	4
Recurrent hematoma	3
Ventricular perforation	1

Discussion

The data presented demonstrate the value and safety of permanent transvenous intracardiac pacing. Total mortality in a group of patients observed up to 6 years was 24%, while hospital mortality was 5%. 15 patients died suddenly of unknown causes with impulse-generator and intracardiac electrode presumably functioning. Some of these patients must be suspected to have died as a direct result of cardiac pacing. In order to prevent sudden death from pacemaker-induced ventricular fibrillation, R-wave stimulation is now preferred in all cases of intermittent or partial heart block.

Failure of stimulation due to electrode dislocation was a most annoying complication in terms of efficiency of handling these patients. Early loss of pace may be due to three factors:

1. The heart may be very large and may have a relatively smooth inner surface, preventing engagement of the electrode-head. We encountered four such cases in which it was impossible to achieve permanent placement of the electrode. 2. The second important factor seems to be proper positioning of the electrode-wire in the right atrium and ventricle. Enough slack must be allowed for to prevent dislocation

of the tip during deep inspiration and body movements. 3. Finally, we feel very strongly that the electrode-cable must be soft and non-elastic in order to prevent jumping motions of its tip. Intracardiac electrodes with stiff silicone-rubber insulation and spring-coil core do not fulfill this postulate, resulting in a high incidence of dislocations. In our hands the Elema-Schoenander electrode has been far superior to other models, whether these had a large or small electrode head, an engaging shoulder or not.

Late failure of electrode function was due to threshold increase on the basis of either a leaky insulation or presumed endocardial fibrous reaction. Since these cannot be differentiated by measurement, the entire pacemaker-system generally was exchanged. It should be noted that the Elema-Schoenander electrode-head was not associated with a higher threshold current or voltage than smaller electrodes. This is probably due to the relatively small area of electrode contact with the myocardium, regardless of its dimensions.

Among the non-fatal, non-electric complications the following deserve mentioning: Infection occurred in 7 patients and could be handled by antibiotics in 3 and removal with replacement of the entire unit in another 4. Skin erosion over the pacemaker-cable in the neck could be treated by excision of granulation tissue with subsequent primary wound closure. Phrenic nerve stimulation occurred in 4 instances. It was corrected by repositioning the electrode. In 1 patient mild phrenic stimulation persisted and was found to be due to perforation of the ventricle, presumably having occurred at the time of first introduction of the electrode wire. In 3 patients on anticoagulants recurrent painful hematoma in and around the pacemaker was noted. In such cases discontinuation of the drug is the only effective way of treatment.

Summary

Of 230 patients treated with pacemakers at the Department of Surgery, Munich University, 207 cases were stimulated with permanent transvenous intracardiac systems, using Elema-Schoenander and Cordis electrodes and various types of impulse generators. This mode of cardiac pacing is considered superior to other types of heart stimulation, as evidenced by a low hospital mortality. Among the non-fatal complications of intracardiac pacing, early dislocation of the electrode-tip has been a problem. Its incidence can be reduced by using proper equipment and technique. The importance of using a thin, non-springy electrode-cable is stressed. The technique of efficient and proper placement of the electrode is described. Other complications of intracardiac pacing are discussed.

References

1. Berg, van den, Jw., J. N. Homan van der Heide, J. Nieven, R. Boonstra, and D. Klamer: Proc. kon. ned. Akad. Wet. C 65, 5, 407 (1962).
2. Borst, H. G., A. Schaudig and D. Alexitsch: Langenbecks Arch. klin. Chir. **313**, 595 (1965).
3. Elmqvist, R., J. Landegren, S. O. Pettersson, A. Senning, and G. William-Olsson: Amer. Heart J. **65**, 731 (1963).
4. Lagergren, H., and L. Johansson: Acta chir. scand. **125**, 562 (1963).
5. — —, H. Schüller, J. Kugelberg, G. Bojs, K. Alestig, E. Linder, H. G. Borst, A. Schaudig, O. Giebel, H. Harms, G. Rodewald, and K. D. Schepokat: Surgery **59**, 494 (1966).

Shock and Trauma

Statistics of Civilian Trauma*

Eberhard Gögler

More than 4 million persons were injured in traffic accidents within 10 years in Germany, 1.4 million of these severely. 142576 persons died. This number approximates to the population of Heidelberg. Thus Germany is the sombre road accident death rate champion of all comparable countries. Every year 25.4 fatalities occur per 100000 population. Every day 3331 accidents happen; every hour 53 persons are injured; every 30 min 1 person dies.

Table 1. *Traffic accidents 1965. Federal Republic of Germany 449243 persons injured and killed*

injured and killed		%
248523	motorcar	55
30921	motorcycle	6.9
25262	moped	5.7
43025	bicycle	9.6
24380	other vehicles	5.5
77132	pedestrians	17,3

Table 2. *Traffic accidents. Federal Republic of Germany. 1956—1965*

killed	142576
injured, total	4186974
seriously	1406120
slightly	2780852

Table 3. *Motor vehicle fatality rates USA compared with other countries, 1963*

	Fatalities per 100000 population
West Germany[1]	**25,4**
Australia	24.5
Austria	24.4
Canada[2]	23.6
USA[2]	**23.1**
France[3]	21.4
Denmark	17.9
Sweden[1]	15.7
Great Britain	13.6
Norway[1]	9.5

[1] 1962.

[2] Includes death occurring up to 1 year after the accident. Other data, unless noted, includes deaths occurring within 30 days.

[3] Includes only deaths occurring within 3 days of the accident.

* From the Surgical Hospital of Heidelberg University.

The extent of civilian trauma in the Federal Republic of Germany is completed when to the 148478 persons severely injured in traffic accidents, 100000 persons severely injured in labor accidents and again the same number of domestic and other

Table 4. *Motor vehicle fatality rates per 100 000 000 vehicle miles, 1963*

West Germany[1]	**12.9**
Netherlands[2]	12.6
Norway	9.1
Great Britain	8.4
Denmark	7.8
USA[3]	**5.0**

Source: Statistics of Road Traffic Accidents in Europe, 1963 (United Nations, ADL 1215); calculated from separate reports of fatalities and mileage of all types of vehicles.

[1] May be understated, since mileage figure includes West Berlin, but fatality figure may not.

[2] 1962.

[3] Accident facts (1965, ADL 195).

Table 5. *Civilian trauma. Federal Republic of Germany 1965*

seriously injured and deaths	
traffic	148478
labor	100000
other accidents	250000
total	500000
violent deaths	47587
80.6 per 100000 population	

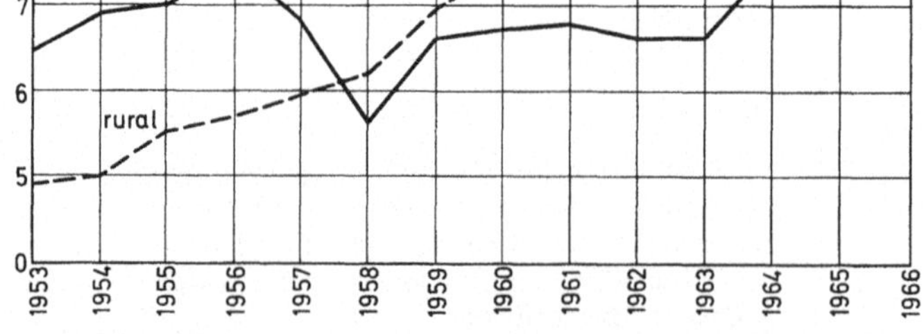

Fig. 1. Urban and rural deaths in traffic accidents in the Federal Republic of Germany 1953—1966 (Statistisches Bundesamt Wiesbaden)

accidents are added. This totals 500000 severely injured persons and 47587 fatalities due to trauma year after year, 80.6 per 100000 population.

As the increasing number of accidents and of injured persons is an almost mathematical function of the growing number of motor vehicles the decline of fatal accidents due to the renewal of the general speed limits law in urban areas since September 1, 1957, is as convincing as a laboratory experiment. In 1959 the number was rising again, but the level remains lower, i.e. 2000 fewer fatalities per year.

Table 6. *Traffic accidents. Federal Republic of Germany*

	accidents	injured	deaths
1960	610377	436100	14018
1967	1143503	461977	17079
1960 to 1967	+ 8.4%	+ 5.9%	+ 21.8%

This is still true in 1967; as compared with 1960, the accidents have increased 8.4%, the injured persons 5.9%, the fatalities 21.8%.

This experiment of law seems to indicate future trends. In Germany urban speed limits were suspended in 1953; it really was an experiment. While police tickets frustrate all endeavors for accident prevention, the law prescribing urban speed limits tends to incriminate the physical factor, speed, as the prime cause of accidents due to the physiological and psychomotive function of human beings, and as an injuryproducing factor due to the dynamic tolerance of man. It must be kept in mind that 66% of all road accidents occur in towns.

Considering this, K. H. Bauer has been agitating for 15 years for the general clearing of all roads and intersections. He also demands safety devices protecting from injury up to impact velocities of at least 50 km/h.

Excessive speed is the most important factor in 5 to 10% of all traffic accidents; persons are injured in 39% of these. However, 50% of accident causing behavior is observed to occur below 50 km/h.

Table 7. *Accident causation "speed". 5 to 10% of motor-vehicle accidents* (Meyer-Jacobi)

km/h	%
speed ranges	
25—50	44.7
50—80	46.7
80—100	4.8
> 100	0.7

39% with injured persons (average of all motor-vehicle accidents only 10%)

25% of those killed or injured in urban areas are pedestrians. As less protected road users, they suffer a high incidence of multiple injuries and the highest death rate. Although they are involved in only 6.6% of all accidents 81.4% of them are injured and 4.6% are killed.

Every second person injured or killed in urban traffic dies in a vehicle collision. Most of these collisions are front-to-side. The passengers are ejected on account of inadequate door latches. They are then crushed between the pivoting cars, as demonstrated by Severy's excellent crash tests. Safety belts do protect from ejection but they do not prevent the motion of head and thorax in the direction of deceleration.

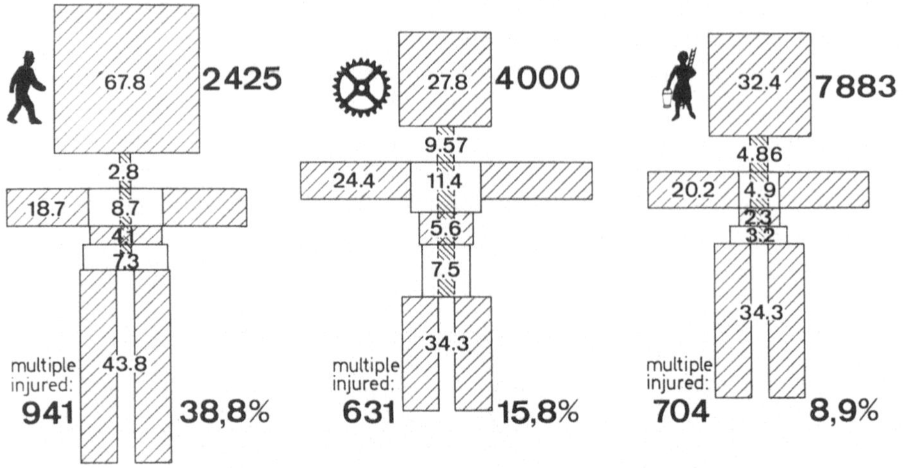

Fig. 2. Injured body areas of 2425 pedestrians, 4000 labor accidents, 7883 domestic accidents. Hospitalized patients. Surgical University Hospital Heidelberg 1953 to 1967

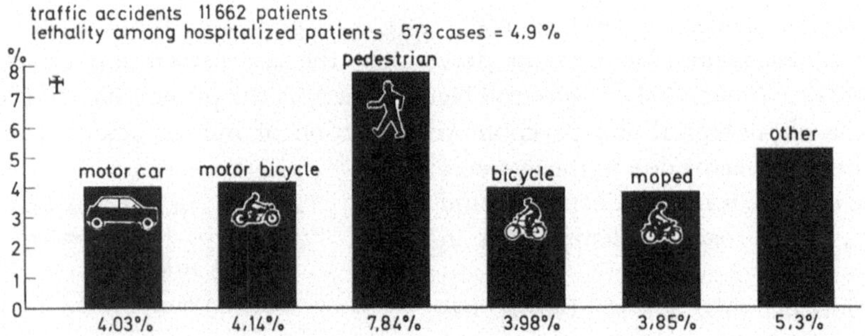

Fig. 3. Lethality of Hospitalized accident patients. Surgical University Hospital Heidelberg 1953 to 1967

Lethality — localization of the fatal injury — accident type. 1070 fatally injured patients

Localization of injuries	traffic accidents						domestic accidents	labor accident	fights, crime	suicide	total
	motor-car	motor-cycle	moped	bicycle	pedes-trian	total					
Head	40.32	67.0	72.5	68.7	56.8	57.6	27.7	37.3	81.8	64.1	512
Spine-Neck	2.4	0.9	2.5	1.5	1.1	1.4	0.7	3.9	—	—	16
Thorax	12.1	0.9	5.0	3.0	1.1	4.2	1.4	10.8	—	5.1	41
Abdomen	3.2	1.9	—	—	1.2	1.6	0.7	2.9	—	—	16
Pelvis	0.8	—	—	—	—	0.2	—	—	—	—	1
Limbs	—	0.9	—	—	—	0.2	—	—	—	—	1
external Hemorrhage	—	—	—	—	0.5	0.2	—	1.0	—	2.6	3
Complications	15.3	8.5	7.5	9.0	15.8	13.4	37.2	14.7	9.1	12.8	220
competitive and cumulative causes of Death	25.8	19.81	12.5	17.9	23.2	21.3	32.3	29.4	9.1	15.4	260
absolute number	124	106	40	67	190	573	282	102	11	39	1070

Example: Of 100 persons injured in cars 40.32 died from a head injury; 12.1 from a thorax injury. Of 100 persons fatally injured on mopeds 72.5 died from a head injury.

One third of the victims in collisions at intersections are motor and pedal-cyclists. It is a remarkable fact that 46.7% of intersection collisions occur in spite of priority signs and 8 to 10% at intersections with stop signs; 2.3% occur at light-controlled intersections.

In England there is no general priority from left or right. There are few priority signs. With the same density of traffic there are less than half as many fatalities as in Germany.

Table 8. *Traffic accidents 1966. Federal Republic of Germany. Urban: injured and deaths 295 537*

injured and killed	%
in collisions between moving vehicles	46.6
in collisions with stationary objects	13.5
in collisions with roadside objects	81.8
in collisions with pedestrians	25.0

Of each 100 fatalities, 12 die during transport, 43 at the scene of the accident and 45 in hospital. This means that in 1965 the ambulance set once with an injured person and arrived with a cadaver in 1890 cases. For each death at the scene of the accident there are 21 surgical emergency cases; of these, at least 41 will be surgical, anaesthesiological and intensive-care patients.

Table 9. *Traffic deaths 1967*

England	7985
Fed. Rep. Germany	17079

Table 10. *Traffic deaths 1965. Federal Republic of Germany*

total	15753	%
at scene of accident	6774	43
during transportation	1890	12
in hospital	7089	45

It becomes apparent how shocking the number of civilian trauma is in terms of surgical engagement, social product and suffering of the families. Road traffic is the number one factor in all violent deaths; in 30% of these alcohol is involved. We further recognize violent death as being the predominant cause of death in males 15 to 35 years of age. In the statistics of the labor and industrial associations the death rate from labor accidents is just half that of the road accident rate, i.e. 5.45% as against 10.5%. The social burden of this traumatology is even more striking when we take into consideration the completely disabled as well as the fatalities. Their number acumulates year after year. There are 15480 persons completely disabled solely as a result of labor and traffic accidents over a period of 10 years.

It should be emphasized that male persons 16 to 40 years of age, who are supposed to contribute to the social product, are those most frequently injured, killed or disabled in labor and traffic accidents.

On the other hand the pedestrians killed are mainly children, who have a whole life-span ahead of them, and elderly people. With this background of the official statistics and with Heidelberg's road accident rate exceeding that of all German towns with a population of over 100000 — i.e. 18.4 victims per 1000 — the Heidelberg clinical pattern of road accident injuries can be regarded as representative for the Federal Republic of Germany.

Corresponding to the multiphasic motion of car passengers such as knee-impact, impact of the thorax against the steering wheel and impact of the head with the upper frame and windshield, nearly every other car occupant has multiple injuries. One in three has injuries to the thorax, the abdomen or the urogenital organs and the pelvis; 72.6% have injuries to the facial soft tissues and facial bones, or brain concussions and skull fractures.

Table 11. *Civilian trauma. Federal Republic of Germany 1967*

violent death	47587
	%
road traffic	33.0
fall from height	25.8
suicide	24.6
labor, domestic, sport	11.0
poison	1.7
crime	1.4

With tempered glass in 95% of German cars we never had such problems of serious facial cuts as known in the United States due to the old laminated glass windshields. On the other hand, with tempered glass the edges of broken glass cause bad cosmetic lacerations and open facial bone fractures or even ocular injuries. Some injuries are due to the small glass particles of tempered glass.

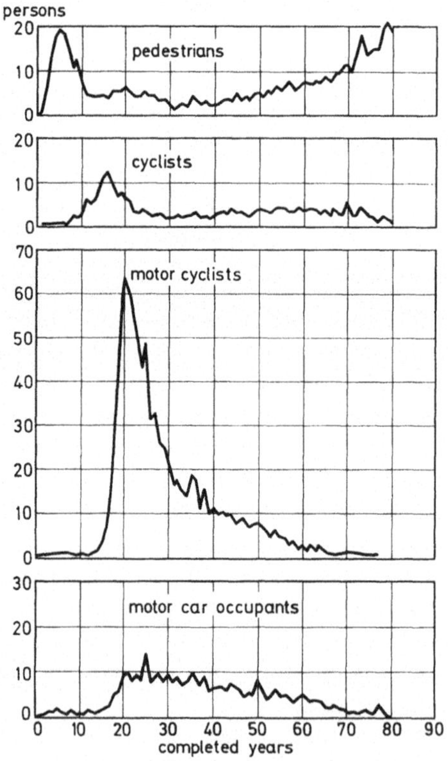

Fig. 4. Age distribution of those killed or seriously injured among various types of road users in Baden-Württemberg in 1955. (Per 10000 persons of the same age in the population) Statistisches Landesamt

Head injuries predominate in all types of traffic injuries. The incidence of head injuries among motor cyclists is twice as high as in domestic and labor accidents. The shift from bicycles to mopeds caused an increase in serious head injuries and abdominal lesions the latter caused by the handlebars. The shift from motor-cycles to small cars brought an even higher incidence of multiple injuries to limbs and

Table 12. *Causes of death 1965. Males, age 15 to 35. Federal Republic of Germany*

		%
total deaths, age 15 to 35	13196	100
of these due to diseases	4791	36.3
violent death	8405	63.6
of these traffic accidents	4666	35.4

Table 13. *Federal Republic of Germany. 1956—1965*

	seriously injured	fatalities		100% disabled	
traffic	1406120	142576	10.2%	9550	0.68%
labor	964553	52403	5.45%	5930	0.61%
				15480	

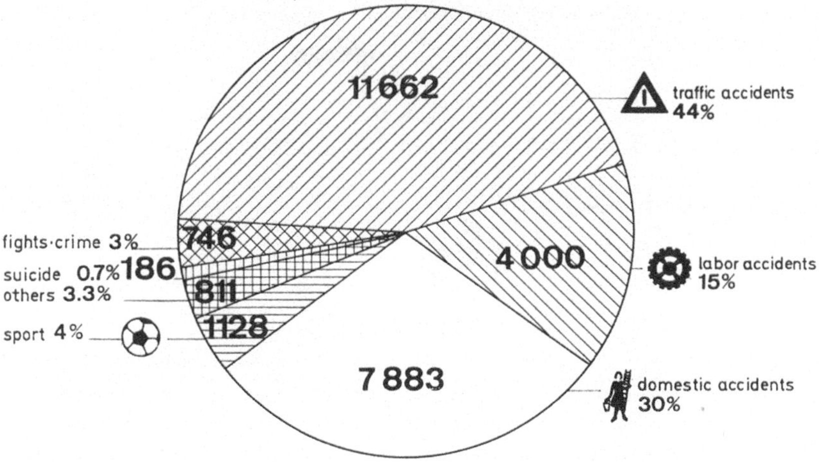

Fig. 5. Hospitalized patients. Surgical University Hospital Heidelberg 1953 to 1967

internal organs. In small cars, passengers are situated within the frontal impact and deformation zone of the car.

In accidents with moving machinery, the hands and arms of men in the 20 to 40 age group are exposed. In accidents with plant-operated transport, such as carts, trucks, lorries, caterpillars and tractors, men of the same age group are threatened by heavy masses which often strike limbs and trunk together. The lethality of 4.4% is undoubtedly an indicator of the seriousness of these injuries. It is nearly equivalent to 4.9% of traffic accidents.

The incidence of thoracic injuries in labor accidents (11% in 4000) is as high as in 11662 hospitalized traffic accidents. The incidence of 9.57% of injuries to the spinal

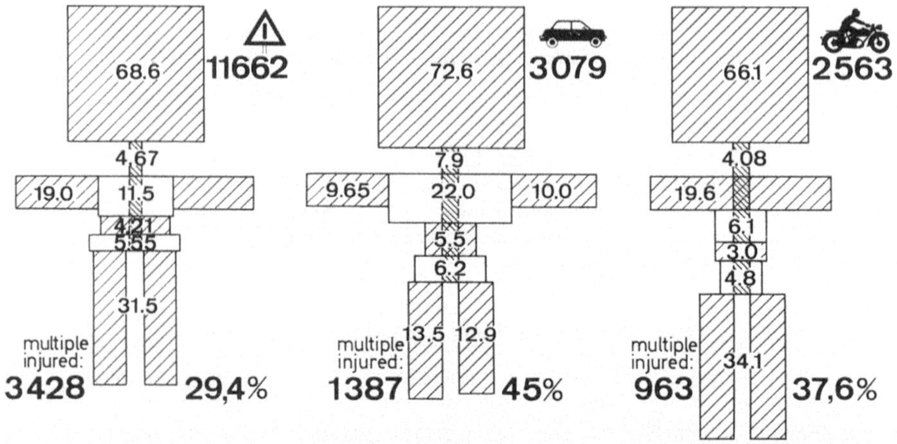

Fig. 6. Injuries to body areas of 11662 hospitalized traffic accident victims, 3079 hospitalized motorcar occupants, 2563 hospitalized motorcycle riders. Surgical University Hospital Heidelberg 1953 to 1967

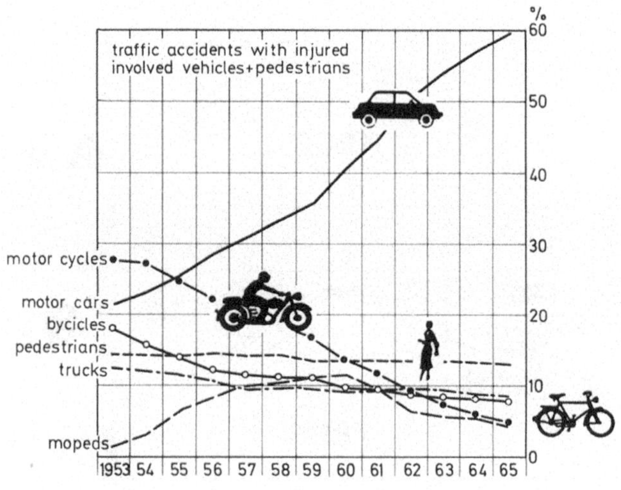

Fig. 7. Traffic accidents with injured. Involved vehicles and pedestrians. Statistisches Bundesamt Wiesbaden

column is due to falls from height in 30% of all labor accidents and in 29% of 14754 non-traffic accidents.

Types of accident and different mechanisms modify the clinical pattern of injuries in the total analysis.

Of 26416 hospitalized accident patients of the Surgical University Hospital of Heidelberg: 12671 have head injuries, of these 1690 dangerous brain concussions;

9544 have fractures, dislocations and fracture-dislocations of the limbs and the pelvis; 2354 have thoracic injuries; 1676 patients have an injury to the abdomen and urogenital organs, 354 of these have organ ruptures. 40% of the accident patients have injuries of the limbs, every 14th patient has a series of fractures in one limb or combinations of fractures in different limbs.

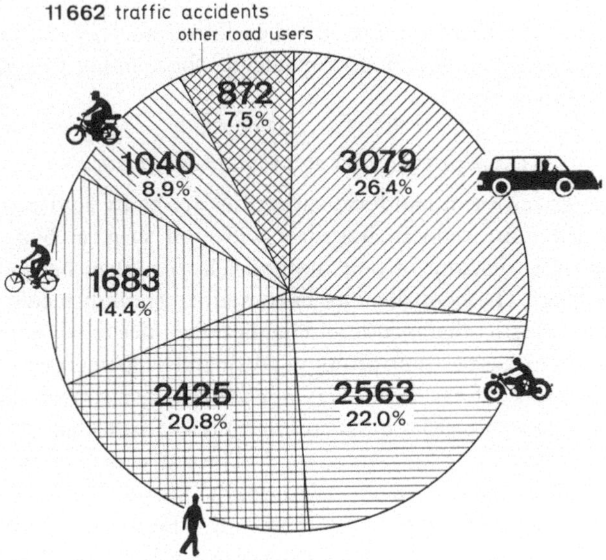

Fig. 8. 26416 hospitalized accident patients. Surgical University Hospital Heidelberg 1953 to 1967

But there is the remarkable fact that every 5th accident patient has multiple injuries. Every 4th patient with injuries of the limbs has additional injuries of the large cavities, in our sample 2803 out of the total number. Every 5th patient has injuries of the limbs *and* a severe head injury.

Table 14. *Surgeon's emergency car (1000 calls)*

1 000 calls	100%
with persons killed	16
with seriously injured	22
with moderately injured	42
with slightly injured	20

Table 15. *Surgeon's emergency car (1000 calls, 1291 injured)*

Peracute danger of life	106	
of these saved	34	= 32%
died	72	= 68%

Naturally this system is confined to local conditions. We are able to drive right across the city of Heidelberg in less than 6 minutes.

Of 1000 calls within 3 years, every 5th involved a seriously injured person. Out of 106 cases at death risk, 34 were saved. Otherwise these cases would have had no chance.

Report of a case: Perforation of the car and of the driver's thorax by a 2" railing piece of a bridge. Broad defect of the thoracic wall with destruction of five ribs, laceration of the lung, pneumothorax with shifting ventilation and fluttering mediastinum, severe shock, conscious.

As soon as he was freed by sawing trough the metal tube, an intravenous anesthesia with relaxation, intubation and infusion were commenced. During transportation lasting 30 min, the tube was held within the thorax — in a conventional ambulance this is impossible. Then immediate thoracotomy and tracheostomy were performed. After respirator-ventilation for 1 week the thoracic wall was stabilized. The patient was discharged within three and a half weeks.

2. The statistics of civilian trauma and the clinical analysis of injuries produce conclusions for the academic teaching of medicine, the training of surgeons and the structural planning of hospitals.

Specialization thrives only through coordination

Therefore, the government and local authorities are badly advised regarding new hospital plans when quite modern hospitals with 100 surgical bed units are constructed within a short distance of one another. This problem occurs in the United States as well as here. These small units have neither enough medical and nursing staff nor enough diagnostic, therapeutic and medical facilities to cover the complicated necessities of realistic acute traumatology adequately. Development must move towards clinical centers which have every specialized department under one roof. This is true not only for big cities but also for rural and suburban areas.

Table 16. *Federal Republic of Germany. Motorcar accidents 1965*

slightly injured	177953
severely injured	64303
killed	6062

3. The statistics of civilian trauma leave no doubt: prevention is better than cure. Through education, insight and through pragmatic follow-up action instead of by legal enforcement.

Some 3000 fewer fatally injured car drivers and passengers and 45000 fewer severely injured and roughly 100.000 fewer slightly injured would be the certain reward, year after year, if each and every one of us, as individuals and as a national and industrial community, would positively accept the idea of road safety, even if it were only in reference to the construction, use, and standardization of safety devices.

Some of these standard devices, imported from the United States, have been introduced into this country not because of better understanding of road safety but because of the financial interests of the export business.

Every 65th patient has a serious thoracic injury and 2.3% of the persons with multiple injuries have lesions of the abdominal and urogenital organs, excluding the so-called blunt abdominal trauma. Here, after some hours or days symptoms are completely relieved.

So traumatology does not essentialiy mean orthopedic surgery of the limbs, neither by number nor by seriousness

The clinical analysis requires many conclusions:

1. For the seriously injured the factor time is of utmost importance. This involves the system of information, the organization, the medical equipment of the ambulance, but first and foremost the willingness of surgeons to go to the scene of the accident.

This is the Heidelberg model: the doctor's emergency car, staying with the surgeon on duty day and night for 1 week, a specially equipped Red Cross ambulance and the police patrol car are called simultaneously through a well-functioning radio system so that they leave from any point in the same minute and arrive almost simultaneously (Fig. 9).

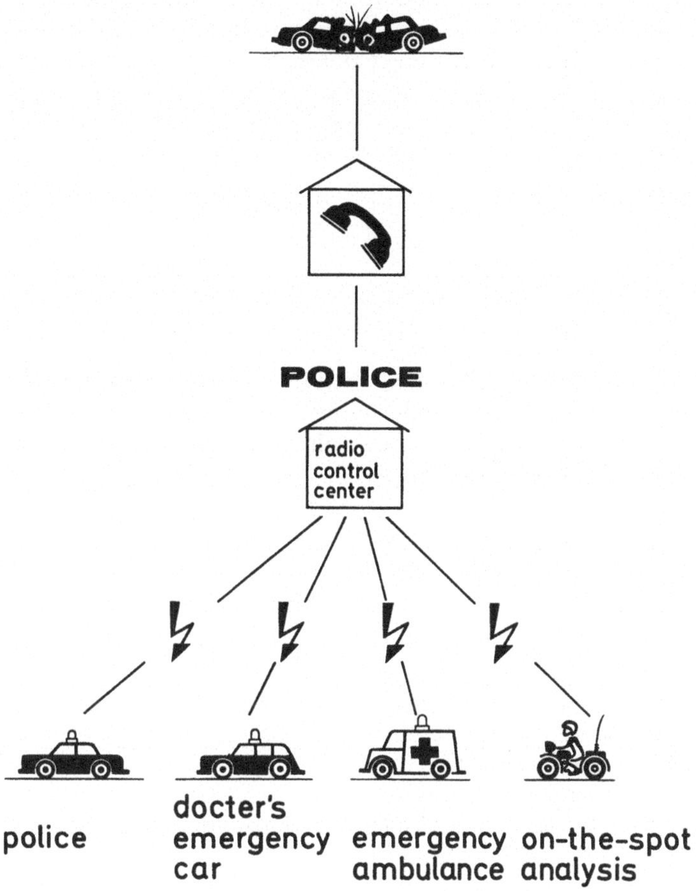

Fig. 9. Coordination of police call, medical emergency service and medical technological research groups by centralisation of the wireless System of information as it works for the area of surgical department of the University of Heidelberg i. e. (radius 10—15 miles)

The Current Management of Hypovolemic Shock*

G. Tom Shires

While shock has been recognized for over 50 years, a clear definition and dissection of this complex and devastating state has emerged slowly. An attempt will be made

* From the Department of Surgery, The University of Texas, Southwestern Medical School at Dallas, Dallas, Texas. — This investigation was supported by Research Grants GM-05428 and GM-14892 from the Division of General Medical Sciences, National Institutes of Health, U.S. Public Health Service.

here to summarize a clinical working classification of shock, to review several of our research studies, and finally, to outline the therapeutic concepts of management which have evolved in hemorrhagic shock.

Clinical Classification

A good physiological classification of shock was devised by the late Dr. ALFRED BLALOCK in the 1930's (BLALOCK). It is interesting that Dr. BLALOCK's contribution in the field of shock was a major turning point in the physiologic understanding of the shock syndrome. The working classification which he devised is still an excellent clinical classification of shock. The four forms of shock as described also conform to the later development in the pathophysiologic understanding of shock. BLALOCK suggested four categories:

1. Hematogenic.
2. Neurogenic.
3. Vasogenic.
4. Cardiogenic:
   a. Failure of the heart as a pump.
   b. Unclassified category (including diminished cardiac output from causes such as vena caval obstruction reducing venous return to the heart).

It is now clear that shock invariably results from failure of one or more of four separate but interrelated functions. These are:

1. The pump (heart).
2. The fluid which is pumped (blood).
3. Arterial resistance vessels (arteriolar tone).
4. The capacity of the venous bed (capacitance vessels or venous tone).

In the context of BLALOCK's etiologic classification, these functions may be correlated:

1. Cardiogenic shock. This implies failure of the heart as a pump and may be brought about by:
   a. (1) Myocardial infarction.
      (2) Serious cardiac arrhythmias.
   b. Miscellaneous causes would include mechanical venous obstruction such as occurs in the mediastinum with:
      (1) Tension pneumothorax.
      (2) Shift of the mediastinum.
      (3) Embolus in the vena cava ligation.
      (4) Cardiac tamponade.
2. Reduction in the blood volume. This loss of volume may be in the form of loss of whole blood, plasma or extracellular fluid in the extravascular space, or a combination of these three.
3. Changes in resistance vessels may be brought about by specific disorders which would include:
   a. Decrease in resistance.
      (1) Spinal anesthesia.
      (2) Neurogenic reflexes as in acute gastric dilatation.
      (3) Possibly the end stages of hypovolemic shock.
   b. Septic shock:
      (1) Change in peripheral resistance.

(2) Change in venous capacitance.

(3) Arteriovenous shunting.

Hypovolemic shock is the most common form seen clinically and is also the form which has been studied most intensively both clinically and in the laboratory. Most of our own studies have been carried out using hypovolemic shock as the model, produced by external blood loss.

The pathological physiology of shock, which is generally agreed upon, reflects a single hemodynamic common denominator: that is, the low flow state. Organ failure seems to be related ultimately to the low flow state. Similarly the biochemical aberrations which reflect evidence of anaerobic metabolism are all further evidence of reduced organ flow.

Experimental Studies

We become interested in studying body fluid volumes in an attempt to delinate changes in response to the low flow state. The method which was developed allowed us to simultaneously measure total body red cell mass with the use of ^{51}Cr — tagged red blood cells; and total body plasma volume with the use of ^{125}I, and later I^{131} — tagged human serum albumin. In addition, total body extracellular fluid can be measured simultaneously with the use of ^{35}S — tagged sodium sulphate (Shires et al., 1960).

These three isotopes are injected intravenously simultaneously, and by the use of appropriate energy differentiating counting instruments, all three isotopes can be determined following equilibration. Volumes are then determined by the dilution principle using multiple sampling.

A. In an early study, the three spaces were measured; splenectomized dogs were then bled a sublethal, subshock amount of 10% of the measured blood volume. 2 h posthemorrhage, the three spaces were again measured. The measured loss of red cells and plasma, removed during the hemorrhage, could be detected by the method used. It was shown that the decrease in extracellular fluid volume was only that which was lost as plasma removed during the hemorrhage (Shires, 1960).

Using the same model, spaces were measured before and after hemorrhage of 25% of the measured blood volume. This hemorrhage was again sublethal but did produce hypotension. It was shown in this group of animals that the loss of red cells and plasma can be measured by the method. In addition, however, the functional extracellular fluid volume as measured by the early ^{35}S — tagged sodium sulphate space decreased by 18 to 26% of the original volume. Since there was no measurable external loss of ^{35}S sulphate, this reduction was presumed to be an internal redistribution of extracellular fluid.

Subsequent studies of external bleeding of 35%, 45% and even above 50% hemorrhage, always produced the same reduction in functional extracellular fluid, as long as the animal was in shock.

B. In subsequent studies, splenectomized dogs were subjected to "irreversible" hemorrhagic shock according to a modified method of Wiggers, using a reservoir (Shires et al., 1964).

Return of shed blood in this severe preparation resulted in the return of blood pressure to near control levels followed by a fall in blood pressure within 1 to 16 h, with death in 80% of the dogs, a standard mortality.

In one group of animals, the three volumes were measured, the dogs were then subjected to shock by the Wiggers method. The three spaces were remeasured by reinjection during the period of shock, then shed blood was returned (Fig. 1).

The decrease in blood volume was that which had been removed. Concurrently, the functional extracellular fluid exhibited a marked reduction of 42%. Following the return of shed blood, the red cell mass returned to essentially normal levels, as did the plasma volume; however, there remained a deficit of functional extracellular fluid of 28%.

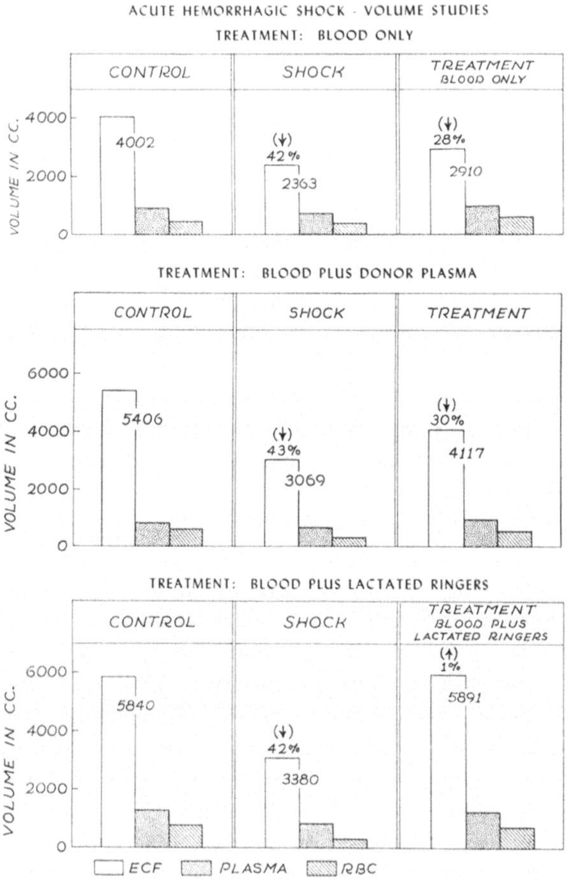

Fig. 1. Volume studies in acute hemorrhagic shock

In dogs treated with shed blood plus plasma, (10 cc per kg), the losses during shock were again similar. After therapy with plasma, plus return of shed blood, there was a return of blood volume to normal. However, there remained a 30% decrease in functional extracellular fluid volume.

Dogs treated with an extracellular "mimic" as a balanced salt solution plus shed blood have comparable losses during shock. As in the previous groups, the blood volume returned essentially to normal after treatment. Dogs treated with salt solution plus shed blood exhibited return of functional extracellular fluid volume to control levels.

In this study, only 20% of those treated with shed blood alone survived longer than 24 h. When plasma was used in addition to whole blood as therapy, 30% of dogs so treated survived. Of the animals treated with Lactated Ringer's plus shed blood, 70% survived.

So, the 80% mortality of a standard "irreversible" shock preparation was reduced to 30% by restoration of functional extracellular fluid volume in addition to return of shed blood.

C. All of our early studies on the measurement of the functional extracellular

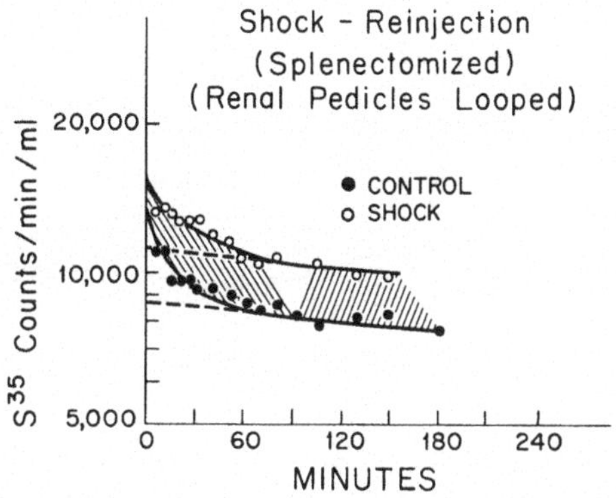

Fig. 2. Radiosulphate equilibration — acute renal pedicle looping, normalized, before and after hemorrhagic shock

fluid were based on volume distribution curves of sulphate being measured up to approximately 1 h. At any point in the course of the shock volume-distribution curve, there will be a reduction in extracellular fluid in the untreated state. The concentration at any time, compared to the control in the same animal, is used to divide into the amount injected to obtain an extracellular space.

Subsequent work has been done following these volume distribution curves out 5 h (Middleton et al.). In true hemorrhagic shock there is a reduction in the early equilibratable extracellular fluid. There is also a reduction in the total extracellular fluid, or final diluted volume of radiosulphate, when compared with pre-shock volumes (Fig. 2).

However, when a less severe shock preparation is used, there will still be a reduction in early equilibrating extracellular fluid, or early available extracellular fluid, whereas the total anatomical extracellular fluid may remain normal. Subsequent studies have shown that if shock is not of sufficient duration to produce reduction in both functional and total extracellular fluid, then the reduction may only be in functional extracellular fluid. Furthermore, if therapy is instituted quickly and blood pressure is returned to normal, a long sulphate equilibration curve may fail to reveal the acute reduction which was corrected very early.

Consequently, the current status of sulphate as a measure of the functional extracellular fluid must be interpreted in the light that early sulphate space measurement reveals "functional" or "available" extracellular fluid and that prolonged measurement of these curves will give "total" extracellular fluid values. It must further be remembered that if therapy has been instituted or has been completed, then the "total" or even the "available" extracellular fluid reduction may not be measurable (Fig. 3).

A working hypothesis was then necessary to explain the reduction in available interstitial fluid in response to hemorrhagic shock. There is no question that some plasma, or transcapillary, refilling does occur in response to hemorrhage and to hemorrhagic shock. This response, however, is initally rather limited and, in severe hemorrhagic shock, grossly inadequate to explain the reduction seen in interstitial fluid. Since there is no source for external loss, the question arose as to whether interstitial fluid might move into the cell mass in an isotonic fashion.

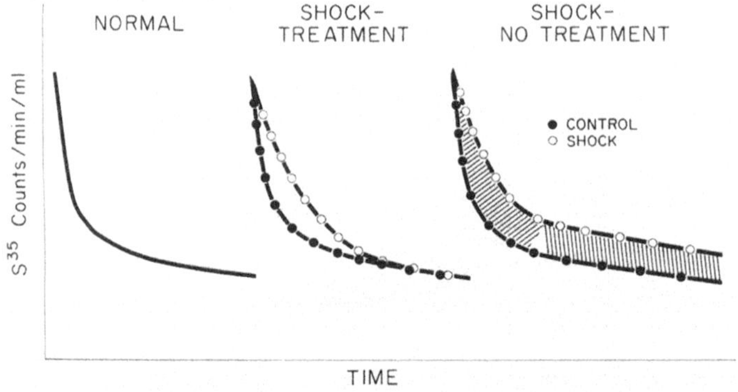

Fig. 3. Radiosulphate equilibration curve — semilogarithmic plot, summary model

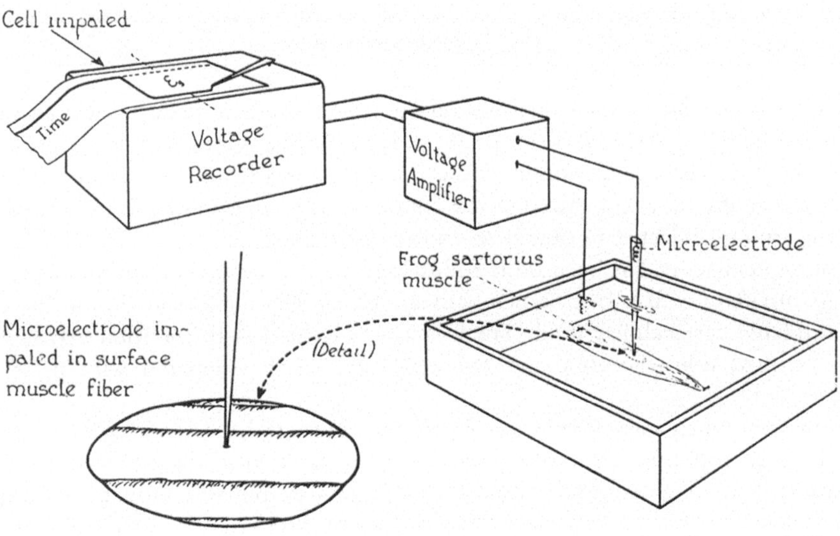

Fig. 4. Schematic of intracellular recording. [From Woodbury. In: Ruch and Fulton (Eds.): Medical Physiology and Biophysics 18th ed., Philadelphia: W. B. Saunders Company 1960]

D. More recently, we have been studying ion transport across cell membranes in order to determine the possibility of intracellular swelling in skeletal muscle in response to hemorrhagic shock (Shires and Carrico, 1966). Using a Ling-Gerard Ultramicroelectrode, intracellular transmembrane potential recording has been done with glass tip diameters of less than one micron. This electrode has been modified to record intracellular transmembrane potentials *in vivo* before, during and after shock (Carter et al.), (Fig. 4).

Skeletal muscle measurements in acute hemorrhagic shock demonstrate a constant and sustained fall in the normally negative intracellular transmembrane potential (Shires and Carrico, 1966), (Fig. 5).

This may represent a reduction in efficiency of the sodium pump induced by tissue hypoxia and is present only during shock producing hypotension. Additional studies in splenectomized dogs have shown that change in variables such as pH, pCO_2, and bicarbonate have been shown not to influence the transmembrane poten-

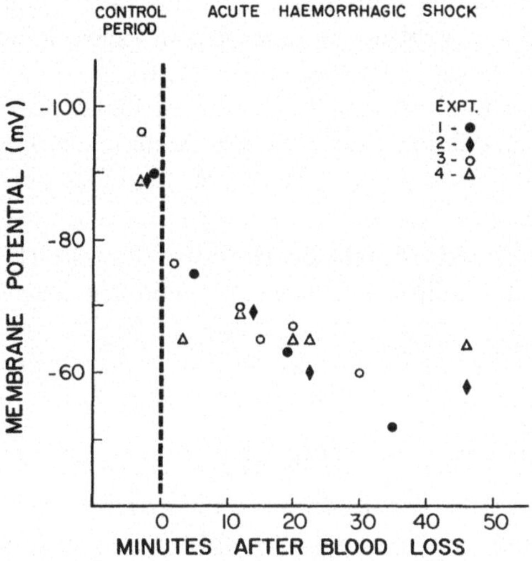

Fig. 5. Time course depolarization during hemorrhagic shock in rats

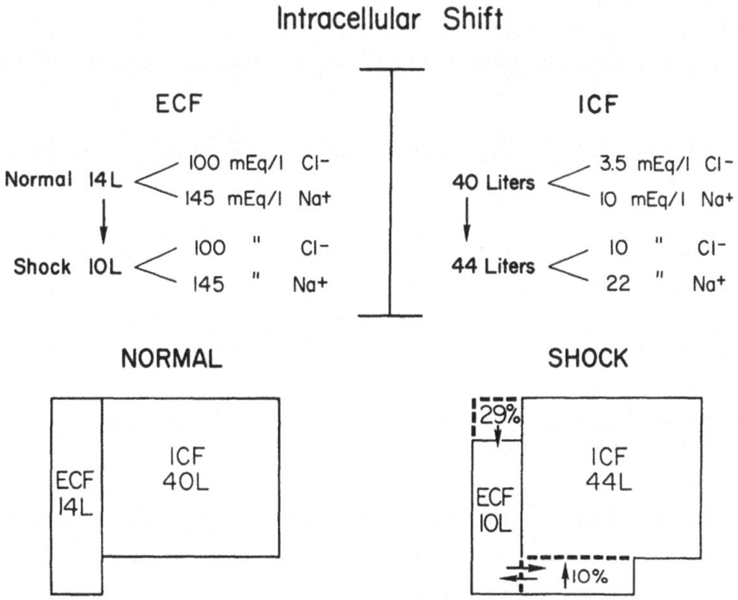

Fig. 6. Schematic of intracellular movement of extracellular electrolytes and water in response to hemorrhagic shock in man

tial in shock (Campion et al.). Even with progressive metabolic acidosis and its subsequent correction, the potential still follows the blood pressure and the shock state.

With a reset membrane potential, extracellular fluid electrolyte concentrations are unchanged. Consequently, from the Nernst equation, intracellular Cl^- must rise from 3.5 to 10 m.e.q., and intracellular Na^+ from 10 to 22 m.e.q.

For transposition of these data to the previously cited measurements in hemorrhagic shock in man, a model is shown (Fig. 6). This model shows a 10% isotonic swelling of muscle cells to explain the reduction in extracellular fluid measured in hemorrhagic shock. Studies are currently under way to determine the involvement of cell masses other than muscle during the course of hemorrhagic shock. However, muscle cell mass alone sustaining an intracellular swelling of 10% would be sufficient to explain the 25 to 30% reduction in extracellular fluid that has been measured.

Leaf and Whittam have shown *in vitro* evidence for cell swelling when energy metabolism is interfered with. Recent evidence by Rockert (Hagbert et al.) from Goteborg, Sweden, adds confirmatory data to this concept. This group has shown an accumulation of potassium in a direct extracellular fluid aspirate in muscle during shock. This would be expected if sodium and water have moved intracellularly as proposed.

Therapy

Since the concentrations of electrolytes in the extracellular fluid do not change, it is obvious that if volume reduction is to be replenished that an isotonic extracellular "mimic" should be used. For this replacement we have used a commercially available extracellular "mimic" in the form of Lactated Ringer's Solution. This fluid is essentially extracellular fluid without protein, with lactate serving as the source of bicarbonate. There is no question that the sodium ion is the most important component of the replacement fluid. However, a balanced salt solution will tend to prevent hypernatremia and dilution acidosis which may occur when isotonic saline alone is used.

Theoretical objections might include a worsening of the lactic acidosis which occurs in response to the low-flow state. Utilizing a standardized shock preparation removing 40% of the blood volume, measurements of lactate and pyruvate were made immediately and at 1 to 2 h after hemorrhage (McClelland et al.). When Lactated Ringer's Solution was given in addition to shed blood, the excess lactate returned to normal actually more quickly than when shed blood was used. In addition, there was no change in the rate of return of pH to normal when balanced salt solution was used in addition to whole blood. Several physiologic parameters, including: (1) stroke volume and cardiac output; (2) peripheral resistance also showed no detrimental, but conversely, a beneficial effect when balanced salt solution was used in addition to whole blood.

In view of the previously described studies, a therapeutic regimen has been used for the treatment of several thousand patients in hemorrhagic shock (Shires, 1965).

When patients are admitted to the Emergency Room in hemorrhagic shock, a large-gauge needle is inserted into an arm and a leg vein and an infusion of Lactated Ringer's Solution is begun immediately. Both veins are used so that all resuscitative fluid does not become lost in the peritoneal cavity if there is abdominal vessel injury.

At the same time, blood is drawn for type and crossmatching. The Lactated Ringer's Solution is run at a rapid rate so that in a period of 45 min between 1,000 and 2,000 cc have been given intravenously. This approach has several advantages:

(1) It has been found that this is a very effective therapeutic trial to determine the pre-existing degree of blood loss or the presence of continuing blood loss. It is often observed that blood pressure will return to normal, become stable and remain so in patients with marked hypotension, after infusion of 1 or 2 l of a balanced salt solution. When such a response is correlated with measurements of blood volume, it has been shown that the degree of pre-existing blood loss was relatively minimal. If blood loss has been minimal and hemorrhage is not continuing, then hemorrhagic hypotension can be alleviated simply by the infusion of a balanced salt solution.

(2) If blood loss has been severe, or hemorrhage is continuing, then the elevation of blood pressure and decrease in pulse rate that occurs with rapid intravenous infusion of Lactated Ringer's Solution will usually be a transient one. When this is manifest, whole blood that has been accurately typed and crossmatched is available and can be given immediately. Consequently, the initial use of the balanced salt solution allows time for accurate typing and crossmatching.

(3) In view of the reduction in the functional extracellular fluid, as demonstrated, it is felt that even though blood is needed, as it is in the majority of patients admitted in hemorrhagic hypovolemia, alleviation of the reduction in functional extracellular fluid is desirable. Current data also indicate a marked reduction in acute renal failure if balanced salt solution is given in addition to whole blood.

Using a combination of whole blood and balanced salt solution, it has been found that the use of plasma expanders has not been necessary (Shires, 1966). Similarly, we have found no experimental or clinical proof for the routine use of cortisone or vasodilators in the treatment of hypovolemic shock. Our own data, along with that of many others, would indicate that vasopressors are contraindicated in the treatment of hypovolemic shock in that they further depress plasma volume and extracellular fluid volume.

Work by Guntheroth (Guntheroth et al.) has shown that elevating the legs without depressing the torso is probably the preferable position for resuscitation in hypovolemic shock since abdominal organs do not impinge on the diaphragm. Oxygen is generally supplied, since there is frequently concomitant thoracic injury or pulmonary embarrassment with the trauma. Arterial transfusions seem to offer no advantage, provided the same volume of blood is given in the same period of time intravenously.

Other forms of shock are frequently seen in the traumatized patient. Often, combination types of shock may be seen requiring therapy for each. Not uncommonly, hypovolemic shock may co-exist with septic shock and even be complicated by cardiac tamponade. It is in these forms of multiple, or combination, or resistant shock that detailed patient monitoring is of most benefit. We have found urine volume to be the best clinical monitor of adequacy of resuscitation at the lower limits of acceptability. Central venous pressure, on the other hand, is of use only in terms of relative change to indicate an upper limit of volume repletion. We have learned that striving for a given level of venous pressure may lead to serious overload; whereas, a rapid rise in venous pressure is more important as a guide for slowing volume repletion or the use of inotropic adjuncts.

References

BLALOCK, A.: Principles of surgical care, shock and other problems. St. Louis: C. V. Mosby Company 1940.

CAMPION, D. S., L. J. LYNCH, F. C. RECTOR, JR., N. CARTER, and G. T. SHIRES: The effect of hemorrhagic shock on transmembrane potential. Surgery (In Press).

CARTER, N. W., F. C. RECTOR, JR., D. S. CAMPION, and D. W. SELDIN: J. clin. Invest. **46**, 920—933 (1967).

GUNTHEROTH, W. G., F. L. ABEL, and G. L. MULLINS: Surg. Gynec. Obstet. **119**, 345—348 (1964).

HAGBERTS, S., H. HALJAMAS, and H. ROCKERT: Ann. Surg. **168**, No. 2, August (1968).

LEAF, A.: Biochem. J. **62**, 241—248 (1956).

McCLELLAND, R. N., G. T. SHIRES, CH. R. BAXTER, C. D. COLN, and J. CARRICO: J. Amer. med. Ass. **199**, 830—834 (1967).

MIDDLETON, E. S., R. MATHEWS, and G. T. SHIRES: Radiosulphate as a measure of the extracellular fluid in acute hemorrhagic shock. Ann. Surg. (In Press).

SHIRES, T.: Surg. Clin. N. Amer. **45**, No. 2, April (1965).

SHIRES, G. T.: Care of the trauma patient. New York: McGraw-Hill 1966.

SHIRES, T., and C. J. CARRICO: Current status of the shock problem. Monograph, Chicago: Year Book Medical Publishers, March, 1966.

—, J. WILLIAMS, and F. BROWN: J. Lab. clin. Med. **55**, 776—783 (1960).

—, F. T. BROWN, P. C. CANIZARO, and N. SOMERVILLE: Surg. Forum **11**, 115—117 (1960).

—, D. COLN, and J. CARRICO: Arch. Surg. **88**, 688—693 (1964).

WHITTAM, R.: J. Physiol. (Lond.) **131**, 542—554 (1956).

Abdominal Injury*

P. FUCHSIG, E. KUTSCHA-LISSBERG and H. SPÄNGLER

Our report of abdominal injuries is based on an evaluation of aggregate statistical data collected in Austrian hospitals, as well as on the literature, and on our own experience.

Table 1: To begin I should like to show you the *incidence of non-penetrating abdominal injuries* and *of organ involvement* as seen from the aggregate statistics from six casualty hospitals under the General Casualty Insurance Scheme (Allgemeine Unfallversicherungsanstalt), two university clinics, and 22 general hospitals.

Table 2 shows the *causes of injuries*. "Horse kicks" and "tossing by bulls" are no longer significant statistically nowadays, where as "steering wheel injuries" and injuries due to compression sustained in road accidents or accidents at work are found to predominate. "Other causes" include such traumas as injuries due to falls (from trees, ladders, etc.) and to play in children as well as injuries of adults sustained at tavern brawls or falls from great heights (through windows).

Table 3 shows *the incidence of abdominal injuries* as compared with *injuries to other regions* of the body. These statistical data were compiled at two university clinics and 15 general hospitals in Austria.

Table 4 shows the *incidence of associated extra-abdominal injuries*. The figures clearly demonstrate the high proportion of multiple traumas. *Overall mortality was* 33.4%. This covers all deaths, including patients admitted in a moribund state. In view of the high frequency of fatal associated injuries, these figures are, of necessity, only relative.

Table 5 shows the *associated occurrence of injuries to abdominal organs*. The left column gives the figures of organs involved directly and most severely, compared with the figures of organs affected only indirectly. These data reveal that the potential involvement of other remote organs, which frequently occurs in such cases, should be considered in the diagnosis and particularly in intra-abdominal exploration.

---

* From the casualty ward (Head: Doz. Dr. H. SPÄNGLER), Surgical Service I, University Hospitals of Vienna (Head: Prof. Dr. P. FUCHSIG). Presented by H. SPÄNGLER.

The figures of exploratory laparotomies performed without yielding any positive findings range between 5 and 20%.

As a result of injuries to inner organs the life of the patient is gravely endangered either through severe hemorrhage or through peritonitis.

Table 1. *Pooled statistics from 6 casualty hospitals run by the Austrian general accident insurance establishment, 2 university clinics and 22 general hospitals in Austria*

175072 accident cases admitted of whom 2041 had abdominal injuries due to impact (1.16%)

Location of abdominal injuries
(total no. of cases: 2496)

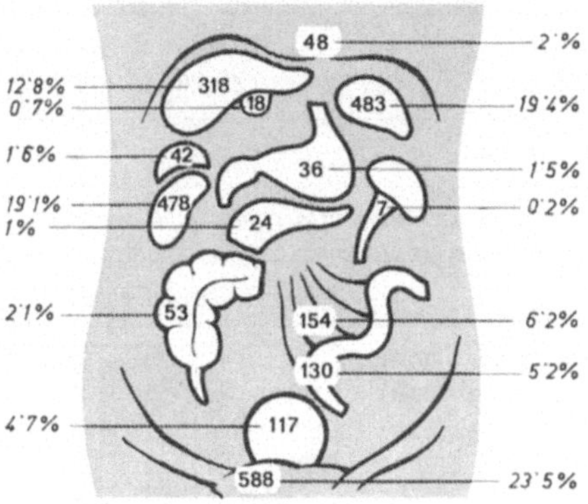

♂:♀ = 3:1

Table 2. *Pooled statistics from 6 casualty hospitals run by the Austrian general accident insurance establishment, 2 university clinics and 22 general hospitals in Austria*

175072 accident cases admitted of whom 2041 had abdominal injuries due to impact (1.16%)

Cause of injury		%
Road accidents	1030	50.5
Work	334	16.4
Sport	198	9.7
Other	479	23.4

Table 3. *Pooled statistics from 2 university clinics and 15 general hospitals in Austria*

92634 admissions with a total of 102531 injuries

Distribution of injuries	%
Head	30.2
Chest	7.4
Abdomen	2.3
penetration	0.6
impact	1.7
Spine, pelvis	7.2
Limbs	62.3

Penetrating abdominal injuries due to stabs, gunshot wounds, or dislacerations of the abdominal wall undoubtedly require prompt and systematic surgical intervention. We cannot subscribe to the view frequently expressed recently (BIJLSMA and SOROUR; RICHTER and ZAKI etc.) that minor penetrating wounds of the abdomen without any alarming signs do not require immediate surgical exploration provided the patients are kept under close observation. This is particularly true since the position of the organs at the time of the perforating impact may not have been the same as in the supine patient. For this reason wounds are routinely debrided at our department for purposes of verifying the diagnosis of a perforating injury. In positive cases laparotomies are extended so as to make possible a full exploration of abdominal organs

Table 4. *Pooled statistics from 6 casualty hospitals run by the Austrian general accident insurance establishment, 2 university clinics and 22 general hospitals in Austria*

175072 accident cases admitted of whom 2041 had abdominal injuries due impact (1.16%)

Additional non-abdominal injuries

2041 abdominal impact	1872 additional			
	head	chest	spine pelvis	limbs
	491 (24%)	515 (25.2%)	360 (17.6%)	506 (24.8%)

Fatal outcome: 33.4%

Table 5. *Pooled statistics from 6 casuality hospitals run by the Austrian general accident insurance establishment, 2 university clinics and 22 general hospitals in Austria*

Association of injuries

Worst or sole injured abdominal organ (without penetration of abdominal wall)	spleen	liver	kidney	small bowel	urinary bladder	mesent.	colon	diaphr.	stomach duod.	pancr.	renal gland	bile ducts	ureter	
424 spleen		30	47	6	3	13	5	11	5	4	7		1	132
267 liver	31		44	9	3	30	2	9	3	3	15	8	2	159
372 kidney	8	2		1		6	2				4			23
111 small bowel	1				2	30	8				1	1		43
104 urinary bladder		2	1	3		5	4		1			1		17
60 mesenterium	8	5	2		2						6			23
31 colon					2	4								6
25 diaphragma	5	2	4				1		2					14
24 stomach-duod.	1	3	1		1	1		2		2		1		12
15 pancreas	3	2	1			1			1					8
9 renal gland		1	4			3		1						9
7 bile ducts	2	3	1			1								7
4 ureter		1	1											2
total 1453													total	455

remote from the original wound. Whether or not the suggestion by Cornell and Ebert, as well as Steichen et al. to inject water soluble radiopaque substances into the site of the wound is helpful in detecting perforations on X-rays, remains to be seen. We do not have any personal experience of it.

Non-penetrating abdominal injuries are found to predominate.

The clinical signs and symptoms as well as a close observation of the patient will indicate whether surgery is necessary; if so, the surgical intervention should not be delayed even in cases of protracted shock, since this often can only be controlled by stopping the bleeding.

In intoxicated patients, as well as in patients with multiple injuries and organic injuries, which may initially be asymptomatic, it is often difficult to assess the extent of the injuries present.

There can be no doubt that early surgery is indicated in these cases. This is particularly true in injuries of the gastro-intestinal tract where a few hours' delay may lead to considerable worsening of the prognosis (BOSWORTH; SPATH; MINI and CAMPIONE et al., etc.).
Standard *blood counts* are no reliable diagnostic aid; only a rapid rise of *leukocytes* to *high levels* during the first few hours following the injury is suggestive of the presence of intra-abdominal injuries (SOMMER; BREIDENBACH; PATTERSON and BROMBERG; BERMANN et al.; MAURER and SCHÄFER etc.). Abdominal *paracentesis* described as early as in 1906 by SALOMON and *catheter paracentesis* in various modified versions to demonstrate the presence of pathological fluid in the abdomen by aspitarion (BAKER et al.; BRONFIN; THOMPSON and BROWN; STRICKLER et al.; WILLIAMS and ZOLLINGER; NEUHOF and COHEN; SCHLAG etc.) are further diagnostic aids; as is *laparoscopy* for direct inspection (FAHRLÄNDER; ROSSETTI etc.), and finally the method of *peritoneal lavage* described by ROOT et al. in 1965: through a catheter similar to that used for peritoneal dialysis Ringer's solution is injected and the irrigation fluid sucked off for purposes of microscopic, macroscopic; and chemical testing (VEITH et al.; GUMBERT et al.; ROOT et al.; 1967). *X-rays* and *enzyme* assays complement the battery of tests. As a negative paracentesis does not rule out any intra-abdominal injuries, we give preference to exploratory laparotomies whenever possible, all the more so as we do not have sufficient experience with peritoneal lavage.

Hemorrhagic shock, *peritoneal irritation*, and *upper abdominal pain* are characteristic symptoms of injuries to the spleen and liver. In cases where symptoms are scarce at the onset and where other pains due to chest involvement are superimposed, our observation that the pain slowly extends towards the middle and lower sections of the abdomen on *both sides* (cave appendicitis!) proved to be a reliable and diagnostic sign for inner hemorrhages (SPÄNGLER, 1963), which together with positive findings on palpation usually verifies the diagnosis.

In cases of *spleen involvement*, the *X-rays show* an elevation of the diaphragm as well as diminished diaphragmatic excursions (KNEISE; LAGHERO), and a displacement of the stomach towards the right associated with pronounced indentation of the greater curvatur (WYMAN). SCHORR and DANON reported on a new procedure: in positive cases the distance between the greater curvature and the abdominal wall is found to be considerable enlarged in the left lateral position after the administration of radiopaque substances. In doubtful cases *selective angiography* (Fig. 1) (FREY et al.; WENZ) and *scintigrams* (LITTLE et al.; SPINELLI RESSI; etc.) may give valuable diagnostic information. The problems presented by *delayed splenic ruptures*, whose incidence is relatively high (35%) are well known (WILLOX; SIZER et al.; KÜMMERLE 1959; etc.) The longest interval between trauma and rupture recorded so far was 54 days (KHANNA and HAYES): in our own material the longest interval was found to be 21 days. Rib fractures occur in about 10% of cases. The treatment of choice is splenectomy.
The operative mortality in our statistical material was 19.9% with a total mortality of 28.9%.

Similar problems are presented by *injuries of the liver* due to non-penetrating impacts. Selective celiacography (BOIJSEN et al.) as well as a rapid and significant rise in transaminase levels (SGOT, SGPT) immediately after the injury, which was demonstrated in animal experiments by SPÄNGLER (1963) and corroborated by clinical evidence, give reliable diagnostic information. The increase in transaminase activity is directly related with the extent of the injury.

Therapy is guided by the severity of the injury. In cases of isolated ruptures and minor foci suturing and tamponade with resorbable hemostyptic material as well as peritoneal drainage is the method of choice. If rupture of the parenchyme is extensive, a partial resection of the liver is indicated (BAKER et al.; JUDD and MOORE; ATIK etc.). Latent shock and severe hemobilia can be prevented if devitalized tissues are removed extensively (ATIK et al.). CLEMENS, SELIVALCOV and NIKITIN recommend tamponade with large omentum. MERENDINO et al.; PERRY JUN., and LAFAVE; JUDD and MOORE; STEICHEN and SHEINER etc. suggest to drain the hepatobiliary ducts for purposes of decompression.

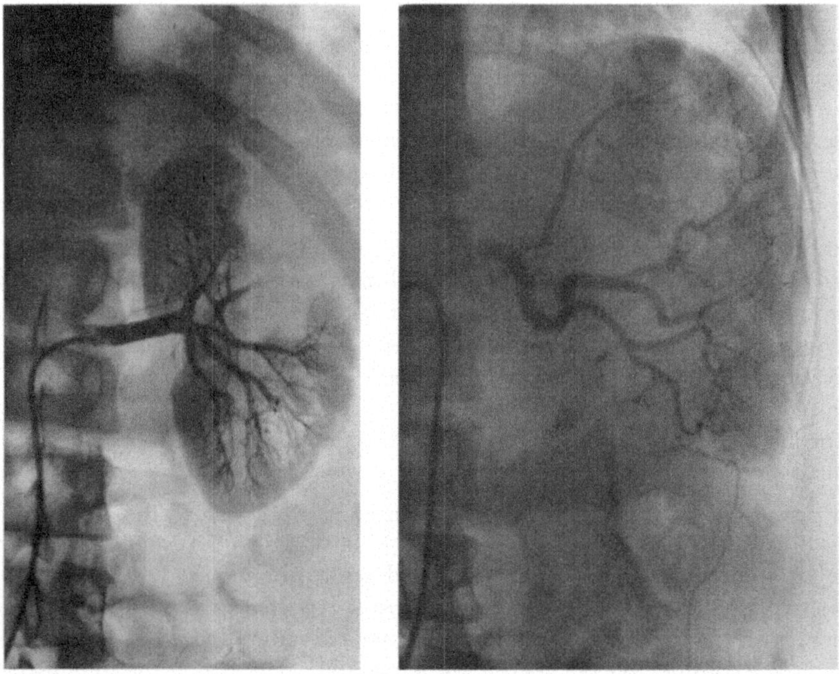

a b

Fig. 1. Selective angiography. a Rupture of the left kidney, b Rupture of the spleen. [From WENZ, W.: Die Arteriographie in der Diagnostik der Bauchorgane. Langenbecks Arch. klin. Chir. **322**, 134 (1968)]

The operative mortality in our statistical material is 35.8% with a total mortality of 60.3%.

Management of *lesions of the bile ducts*, which are rare and apparently favored by the presence of upper abdominal adhesions, will vary from case to case (BAUERS; DIETRICH et al.; FLETSCHER et al.; NOONE et al. etc.).

In *injuries of the pancreas*, which are typical consequences of "steering wheel injuries", early detection and diagnosis are paramount. The determination of serum and peritoneal amylase levels can be regarded as a standard method. The surgical procedure adopted will depend on the extent of the injury. Drainage and, if necessary, suturing of the capsula will be sufficient for simple contusions without extensive parenchyme damage. In extensive parenchyme lesions or ruptures distal pancreatectomy with exstirpation of the spleen is indicated, provided that the head of the pancreas is intact. In cases of extensive rupture involving the head of the pancreas it will be necessary to perform a partial resection with intestinal anastomosis or a total pancreatectomy. Postoperative treatment is similar to that of pancreatitis, and attention should be paid to the important role played by enzyme inhibitors.

Of the many publications in this field the work of STUCKE; KÄUFER; EHLERS and GRIMSEHL; WEITZMANN and SVENSON; NICK et al.; WILLSON et al.; HERVE and ARRIGH; JONES and SHIRES; BARNETT et al. etc.) might be particularly mentioned.

The operative mortality in our statistical material was 35.7% with a total mortality of 40%.

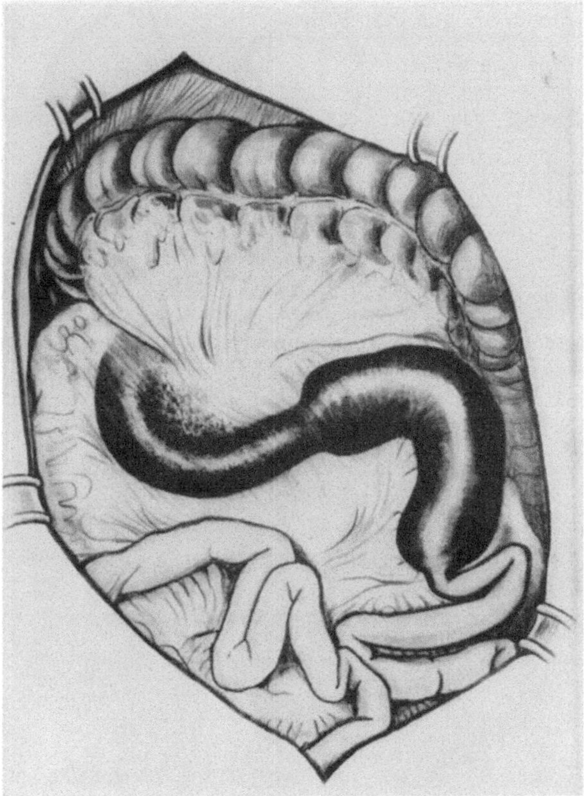

Fig. 2. Intramural hematoma of the duodenum. [From: FUNOVICS, J., u. H. SPÄNGLER: Zbl. Chir. **92**, 645 (1967)]

Surgical treatment of injuries of the *gastro-intestinal* tract and the *mesentery* usually does not present any difficulties. If there is the least suspicion of a *duodenal injury* with hemorrhagic suffusion, a careful inspection must always be made, particularly of the retroperitoneal portions in order to rule out perforations. A rather rare injury which, however, has frequently been described recently is the *intramural duodenal hematoma*, which is particularly difficult to detect, because it is often accompanied by a symptom-free interval of 24 h. (Fig. 2) (our own observation, FUNOVICS and SPÄNGLER).

Peritoneal irritation and signs of obstruction in the upper part of the small intestine are suggestive of this rare type of injury. Treatment usually consists of evacuation of the hematoma (DE NETTO and PIMSNER; HILL; WIDDERSHOVEN; MATHEWSON and MORGAN; TRIPPESTAD; LOUHIMO; FREEARK et al.; SCHNEIDER etc.).

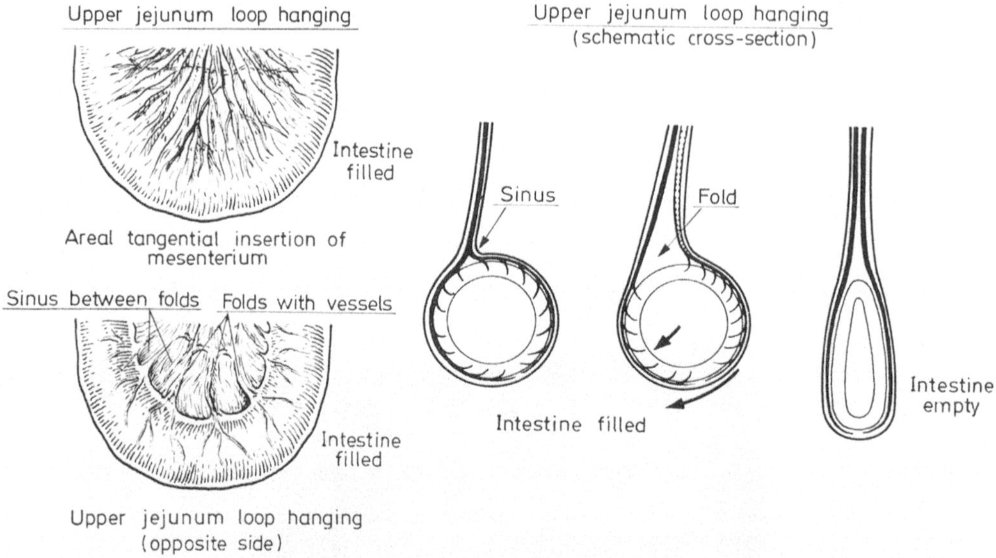

Fig. 3. View of mesenteric insertion of the upper small intestine. [From: SPÄNGLER, H. J. int. Coll. Surg. **39**, 499 (1963)]

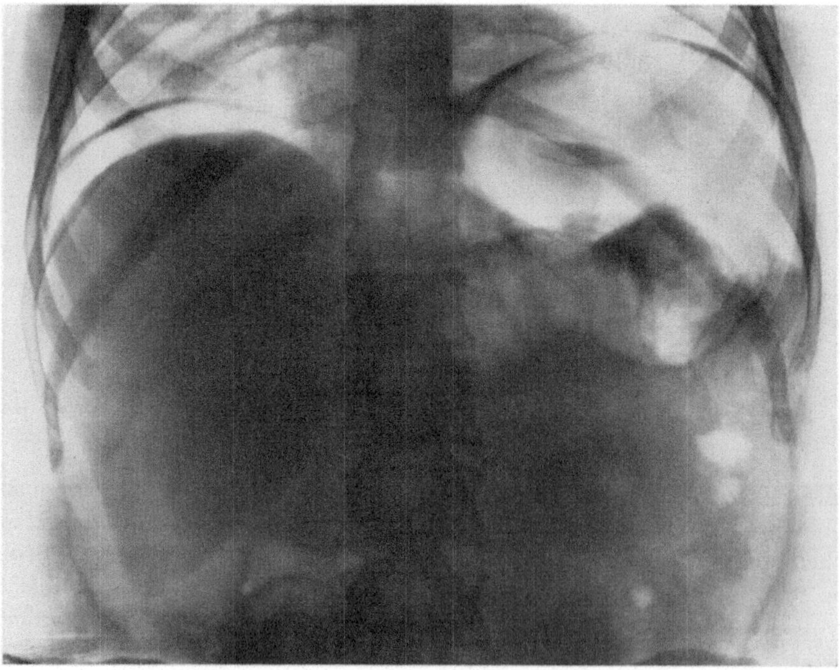

Fig. 4. Rupture of sigma with pneumoperitoneum after insufflation of compressed air (working accident)

Our observations that more than 50% of the *ruptures* of the *small intestine* due to non-penetrating injuries affected the upper jejunal portion approximately 40 to 60 cm below the duodenojejunal flexure have been explained by anatomical studies. These revealed that the upper intestinal loops normally lie in the region of the posterior abdominal wall and in the vicinity of the spine; in addition, the mesentery is oriented tangentially in this area (BENTENRIEDER; SPÄNGLER, 1958) (Fig. 3).

An unusual working accident due to insufflation of compressed air into the anus with sigma perforation is shown in Fig. 4.

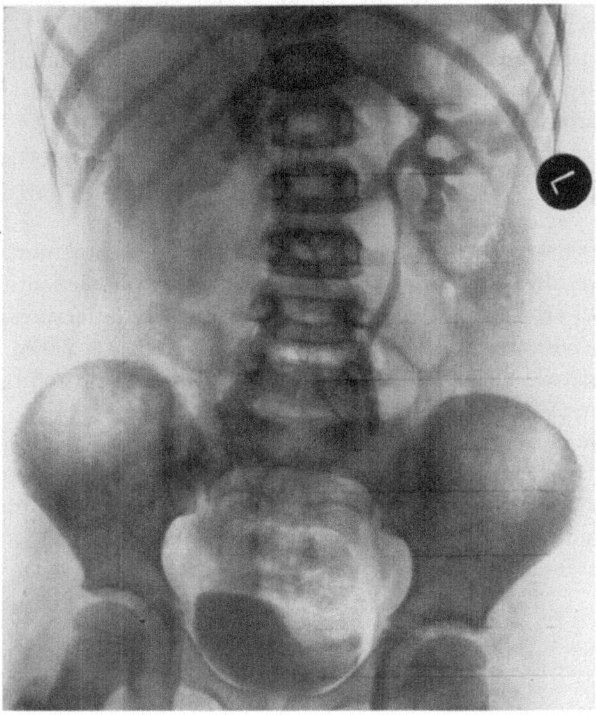

Fig. 5. Intravenous pyelogram, rupture of the right kidney (7 a, ♂)

(Fig. 4) Classical picture of a pneumoperitoneum, air scythe, prompt laparotomy, suturing of the defect and temporary transversotomy, uncomplicated postoperative course.

Another rarely observed injury is the rupture of the vermiform appendix as a result of non-penetrating abdominal injuries (SCHIMA).

The operative mortality in our statistical material was 18.6% for injuries of the small intestine (total mortality 25.2%), for injuries of the colon 36.0% (48.4%).

Ruptures of the diaphragm are usually due to thoraco-abdominal contusions. Correct interpretation of plain X-rays, possibly with the use of radiopaque substances, assists the diagnosis. The possibility of a delayed occurrence should be borne in mind (KÜMMERLE, 1967; NEVEUX et al.; HEBERER et al.; SUTTON et al.; EBERT et al.; FONTAINE et al. etc.).

Our observation of the rare case of a diaphragmatic rupture on the right side associated with a rupture of the liver was made only a few days ago, on the 14th of June, 1968 (demonstration of the case with three slides): road accident, severe throracoabdominal trauma of the right side with multiple rib fractures. Laparotomy: no pathological findings exept rupture of the diapharagm and liver prolapse. Right thoracotomy, suture of the damaged liver and diaphargma. Similar cases observed by DOBROWOLSKI, HARDY, etc.

The operative mortality in our statistics was 33.3% with a total mortality of 60.0%.

Renal injuries which are often associated with non-penetrating abdominal traumas and characterized by hematurie require only conservative treatment and close observation.

However, i.v. pyelograms should be taken in every case. Thus we can determine both the extent of the injury and the condition and excretory pattern of the contralateral kidney for later surgery, if required.

(Fig. 5) i.v. pyelogram of rupture of the right kidney. Undoubtedly selective renal angiography offers the affected parenchyme and the possibility of a successful surgical intervention.

In case of profuse and uncontrollable hemorrhage an early operation is necessary (RUMMELHARDT and SPÄNGLER; NICK et al.; BERGMANN; WRIGHT; SCHÄLLI and BETTEX).

The operative mortality in our statistics was 10.2%, the total mortality 8.6%.

Adrenal injuries always go almost undetected; they are only indentified by autopsy.

Bladder injuries are almost always associated with pelvic fractures. In the case of pelvic fractures with hematurie cystography with at least 300 cc of radiopaque material is indicated. Surgical management by sutures and careful drainage is the method of choice (WOLF etc.).

The operative mortality in our statistics was 6.3% and the total mortality 39.4%.

In the short time available we have attempted to give our own experience and to review briefly the existing knowledge of abdominal injuries. Inspite of the many diagnostic techniques available, careful clinical examination and continual observation remain essential.

References

ATIK, M.: J. Ky med. Ass. **64**, 143—144 (1966). Ref. Excerpta med. (Amst.) Sect. IX, 20/10, No. 4669, 873 (1966).

—, F. ISLA, R. GROSSMANN, and DE KERNIAN: Arch. Surg. **92**, 636—642 (1966).

BAILEY, W. C., and D. R. AKERS: Amer. J. Surg. **110**, 695—703 (1965).

BAKER, R. J., P. TAXMAN, and R. J. FREEARK: Arch. Surg. **93**, 84—91 (1966).

BAKER, W. N. W., D. B. MACKIE, and J. F. NEWCOMBE: Brit. med. J. **3**, 146—149 (1967).

BARNETT, W. O., J. D. HARDY, and R. L. YELVERTON: Ann. Surg. **163**, 892—899 (1966).

BAUERS, H. G.: Zbl. Chir. **85**, 654 —656 (1960).

BENTENRIEDER, A.: Z. Anat. Entwickl.-Gesch. **109**, 513—543 (1939).

BERGMANN, M.: Langenbecks Arch. klin.Chir. **307**, 21—26 (1964).

BERMANN, J. K., E. D. HABEGGER, D. C. FIELDS, and W. L. KLIMA: J. Amer. med. Ass. **165**, 1537—1541 (1957).

BIJLSMA, P. J., and U. E. SOROUR: Arch. chir. neerl. **18**, 185—193 (1966); — Ref. Excerpta med. (Amst.) Sect. IX, 21/12, No. 5722, 6795.

BÖHLER, J., M. GERGEN, B. LEITNER, E. LENER, L. MONSZPART, J. POIGENFÜRST und H. R. SCHÖNBAUER: Hefte Unfallheilk. **65**, (1960).

BOIJSEN, E., M. P. JUDKINS, and A. SIMAY: Radiology **86**, 66—72 (1966).

BOSWORTH, B. M.: Amer. J. Surg. **76**, 472—482 (1948).

BREIDENBACH, C.: Ref. BOSWORTH.

BRONFIN, G. S., J. P. LIEBLFR, and H. M. KATZ: Gastroenterology **21**, 426—428 (1952).

CLEMENS, M.: Zbl. Chir. **92**, 2376—2377 (1967).

COLOMBO, O.: Wien. med. Wschr. **116**, 343—348 (1966).

Cornell, W. P., and P. A. Ebert: Amer. J. Roentgenol. **96**, 414—417 (1966).
de Netto, F. O., and A. O. Pimsner: J. abdom. Surg. **4**, 83—90 (1962). Ref. Z. org. Chir. **172**, 69 (1963).
Dietrich, E. B., A. C. Beall Jr., G. L. Jordan Jr., and M. E. de Bakey: Amer. J. Surg. **112**, 756—759 (1966).
Dobrowolski, J.: Pol. Przegl. chir. **37**, 700—703 (1905).
Ebert, P. A., R. A. Gaertner, and G. D. Zuidema: Surg. Gynec. Obstet. **125**, 50—65 (1967).
Ehlers, P. N., u. H. Grimsehl: Langenbecks Arch. klin. Chir. **298**, 80—83 (1961).
Fahrländer, H.: Helv. Chir. Acta **32**, 54—59 (1965).
Fletcher, W. S., D. E. Mahnke, and J. E. Dunphy: J. Trauma **1**, 87—95 (1961). Ref. Z. org. Chir. **165**, 311 (1961).
Fontaine, R., C. Bollack, F. Jurascheck, J. C. Thibault et E. Papaevangelou: Poumon **22**, 1—47 (1966). Ref. Excerpta med. (Amst.) Sect. IX, 20/10, No. **4529**, 846 (1966).
Freeark, R. J., R. D. Corley, W. J. Norcross, and E. L. Strohl: Arch. Surg. **92**, 463—475 (1966).
Frey, C. F., C. Ernst, S. M. Lindenaufr, J. Barlett, and J. Bookstein: Amer. J. Surg. **113**, 137—148 (1967).
Funovics, J., u. H. Spängler: Zbl. Chir. **92**, 645—648 (1967).
Geisthövel, W., u. R. Zimmermann: Hefte Unfallheilk. **64**, (1960).
Gumbert, J. L., S. E. Frodermann, and J. P. Mercho: Ann. Surg. **165**, 70—72 (1967).
Hardy, K. J.: Aust. N. Z. J. Surg. **35**, 222—225 (1966). Ref. Excerpta med. (Amst.) Sect. IX, 20/11, No. **5003**, 941 (1966).
Heberer, G., A. Senno und A. Laur: Chirurg **38**, 410—416 (1967).
Hervé, P. A., et J. P. Arrigh: J. Chir. (Paris) **89**, 69—82 (1965). Ref. Z. org. Chir. **186**, 208 (1965).
Hill, M. C.: Amer. J. Roentgenol. **94**, 356—361 (1965).
Hoferichter, J.: Bruns' Beitr. klin. Chir. **214**, 58—70 (1967).
Holle, F.: Med. Klin. **58**, 293—312 (1963).
Jones, R. C., and G. T. Shires: Arch. Surg. **890**, 502—508 (1965).
Judd, D. R., and Moore: Ann. Surg. **163**, 149—152 (1966).
Käufer, C.: Zbl. Chir. **92**, 3074—3080 (1967).
Khanna, A. L., B. R. Hayes, and K. C. McKeown: Ann. Surg. **165**, 477—480 (1967).
Kneise, G.: Chirurg **20**, 427—430 (1949).
Kümmerle, F.: Pract. Chir. H. **55**, (1959).
— Chirurg **38**, 399—405 (1967).
Larghero, Y. P.: Surg. Gynec. Obstet. **92**, 385—404 (1951).
Little, J. M., J. McRae, N. Smitananda, and J. G. Morris: Surg. Gynec. Obstet. **125**, 725—729 (1967).
Louhimo, J.: Z. Kinderchir. **3**, 181—186 (1966).
Mathewson, C., Jr., and R. Morgan: Amer. J. Surg. **112**, 299—307 (1966).
Maurer, G., u. H. Schäfer: Chirurg **36**, 263—267 (1965).
Merendino, K. A., D. H. Dillard, and E. E. Cammoch: Surg. Gynec. Obstet. **117**, 285 to 293 (1963).
Mini, M., and G. Campione: Ref. Spängler, 1958.
Neuhof, H., and J. Cohen: Ann. Surg. **83**, 454—462 (1926).
Neveux, J. Y., E. Hazane, J. C. Lewaseur, J. J. Galey, and J. Mathey: Thorax **22**, 142 to 146 (1967).
Nick, W. V., R. W. Zollinger, and R. D. Williams: J. Trauma **5**, 495—502 (1965).
— —, and W. G. Pace: J. Trauma **7**, 652—659 (1967).
Noone, R. B., J. A. Mackie, and R. Stoner: Ann. Surg. **166**, 824—828 (1967).
Patterson, R. H., and B. Bromberg: Amer. J. Surg. **83**, 427—433 (1952).
Perry, J. F., Jr., and J. W. Lafave: Surgery **55**, 351—354 (1964).
Richtfr, R. H., and H. H. Zaki: Ann. Surg. **166**, 238—244 (1967).
Root, H. D., P. J. Keizer, and J. Perry Jr.: Arch. Surg. **95**, 531—537 (1967).
—, C. W. Hauser, C. R. McKinley, J. W. Lafave, and R. P. Mendiola: Surgery **57**, 633—637 (1965).
Rossetti, M.: Helv. chir. Acta **35**, 193—205 (1967).

RUMMELHARDT, S., u. H. SPÄNGLER: Öst. Ärzteztg. (in press).
SALOMON, H.: Berl. klin. Wschr. **43**, 45—46 (1906).
SCHÄRLI, A., u. M. BETTEX: Chir. Praxis **12**, 253—262 (1968).
SCHIMA, E.: Bruns' Beitr. klin. Chir. **208**, 343—345 (1964).
SCHLAG, G.: Akt. Chir. **2**, 17—20 (1967).
SCHNEIDER, O. H.: Aust. N. Z. J. Surg. **37**, 84—86 (1967). Ref. Excerpta med. (Amst.) Sect. IX, 22/4, No. **1807**, 286 (1968).
SCHORR, S., and J. DANON: Amer. J. Roentgenol. **99**, 616—624 (1967).
SCHRAMM, W.: Med. Welt (Stuttg.) **1964**, 706—709.
SIZER, J. S., E. R. WAYNE, and P. L. FRIEDERICK: Arch. Surg. **92**, 362—366 (1966).
SLANY, A.: Wien. Beitr. Unfallheilk. Wien: W. MAUDRICH 1948.
SPÄNGLER, H.: Wien. med. Wschr. **108**, 1014—1019 (1958).
— J. int. Coll. Surg. **39**, 499—503 (1963).
— Wien. klin. Wschr. **75**, 185—189 (1963).
SPATH, F.: Dtsch. med. J. 714—720 (1955).
SOMMER, R.: Zbl. Chir. **62**, 306—309 (1935).
SPINELLI-RESSI, F.: Minerva nucl. **9**, 184—187 (1965). Ref. Excerpta Med. (Amst.) Sect. IX, 20/6, No. **2833**, 510 (1966).
SUTTON, J. P., R. B. CARLISLE, and S. E. STEPHENSON JR.: Ann. Thorac. Surg. **3**, 136—150 (1967).
STUCKE, K.: Internist (Berl.) **8**, 135—140 (1967).
STEICHEN, F. M., and N. M. SHEINER: Arch. Surg. **92**, 838—847 (1966).
—, D. M. PEARLMAN, E. L. DARGAN, D. C. PROMMAS, and P. H. WEIL: Ann. Surg. **165**, 77—82 (1967).
STRICKER, D. H., P. D. ERWIN, and C. O. RICE: Arch. Surg. **77**, 859—863 (1958).
THOMPSON, C. T., and D. R. BROWN: Surgery **35**, 916—919 (1954).
TRIPPESTAD, A.: Acta chir. scand. **131**, 183—186 (1966).
VEITH, F. J., W. B. WEBBER, R. C. KARL, and M. DEYSINE: Ann. Surg. **166**, 290—295 (1967).
WEITZMANN, I. J., and O. SWENSON: Surgery **57**, 309—312 (1965).
WENZ, W.: Langenbecks Arch. klin. Chir. Kongreßbd. 1968. (in press).
WIDDERSHOVEN, G. M. J.: Ned. T. Geneesk **110**, 628—630 (1966). Ref. Excerpta Med. (Amst.) Sect. IX, 20/10, No. **4604**, 861 (1966).
WILLIAMS, R. D., and R. M. ZOLLINGER: Amer. J. Surg. **97**, 575—581 (1959).
WILLOX, G. L.: Arch. Surg. **90**, 498—502 (1965).
WILSON, R. F., I. P. TAGETT, J. P. PUCELIK, and A. J. WALT: J. Trauma **7**, 643—651 (1967).
WOLF, F.: Hefte Unfallheilk. **91**, 53—58 (1967).
WRIGHT, J. E.: Surgery **34**, 320—325 (1965).
WYMAN, A. C.: Amer. J. Roentgenol. **72**, 51—63 (1954).

Chest Injury

K. VOSSSCHULTE

Reports on the traumatological experience of large hospitals of this and foreign countries show that the number of severe thoracic injuries has steadily increased over the last years and that it has reached 6 to 8% of the admissions — 9% at our hospital. As far as causes are concerned, traffic accidents take the first place.

From 1951 to 1967 a total of 760 patients with thoracic injuries were admitted to the Giessen hospital. 51 of these patients had penetrating injuries. In addition to the increased number of cases with thoracic trauma, an etiological classification documents the importance of traffic accidents.

A detailed survey of the consequences of blunt trauma demonstrates the predominance of thoracic concussion. Multiple rib fractures are less frequent. 31 times we observed cases with depressed fractures and paradoxial breathing (Table 1).

A diagnosis of thoracic contusion includes the warning to look for more serious injuries.

Contusion of the thorax, painful restriction of ventilation, hemorrhagic alveolar effusions, inadequate expectoration, atelectasis, bronchopneumonia and respiratory insufficiency are the pathogenetic factors. Their consequences, particularly if they are bilateral, cannot always be prevented even by tracheotomy and additional measures. In this report it is not necessary to stress the value of bloodgas-analysis for therapeutic decisions.

The measures in patients with *rib fractures* are treatment of pain and its restricting effect on ventilation. If pharmacological blocking of the intercostal nerves is inadequate one should remember the cingulum which achieves far more than its reputation states.

Depressed fractures of the sternum — usually produced by the steering wheel of the car during frontal collisions — thus restrict the ability of the thoracic skeleton but they become more dangerous on account of the paradoxical respiratory movements

Table 1. *Type of injury in non penetrating chest injuries*

Type of injury	Number of cases
Concussion of thorax	213
Contusion of thorax	78
Compression of thorax	20
Rib fractures (< 3)	168
Multiple rib fractures (> 3)	199
Flail chest	31
Total	709

of the fractured area of the chest wall. The bandages and measures which were previously used for the fixation of the mobile chest wall have been replaced by tracheotomy and respirator treatment according to the suggestion of Avery, Mörch and Benson. In order to achieve the desired so-called "inner stabilization" single-phase positive pressure ventilation with muscle relaxants, which also maintains a positive pressure of approximately 5 mm Hg during expiration, is necessary. Krauss evaluates the indication according to the results of the bloodgas analysis and uses this method if the oxygen tension in the arterial blood falls below 60 mm Hg and the CO_2-value rises above 50. This is a practical rule of thumb.

In one of our injured patients this method did not produce the desired result and we were unable to find a convincing reason for its failure.

Fig. 1 outlines our surgical approach.

Clinical experience shows that a traumatic *hemothorax* can be controlled in many injured patients by aspiration or drainage. There can also be little argument that *surgery* is *indicated* if irreversible shock and massive blood accumulations in the pleural cavity necessitate an emergency thoracotomy.

The prognosis of intrathoracic hemorrhage determined by involvement of the lung or mediastinum and must be classified between these two extremes. It is frequently difficult to assess the extent of these internal traumatic lesions. Doubt regarding the intrathoracic situation cannot be eliminated by hesitating and waiting. We rely mainly on the effect of suction and we open the thorax if the lung does not completely re-expand under vacuum. Dense, basal, homogenous shadows after 1 or 2 weeks are an indication for surgical evacuation of the fluid or coagulated blood accumulations. The effect of instillations for the dissolution of the accumulated blood clots, according to all available experience, is not comparable to the results of surgical evacuation.

Pulmonary rupture may occur as a result of parietal or transtracheal trauma. An acutely life-threatening situation develops if explosive forces, via the airway, result in parenchymal tears and hemorrhage into the bronchial tree and thus endanger alveolar ventilation. In such cases immediate intubation is more important than

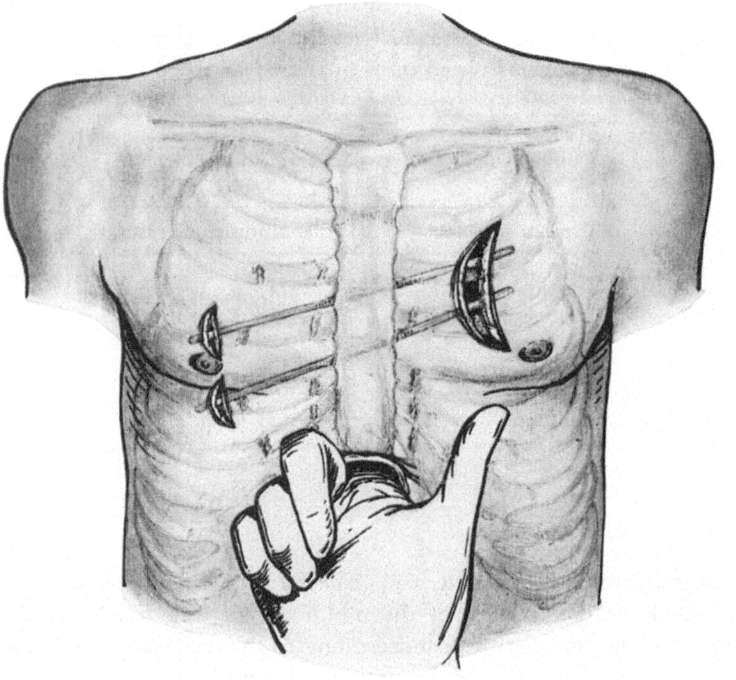

Fig. 1. Diagram showing procedure for chest wall stabilization

anything else. Years ago, during a small surgical procedure under mask-anesthesia with a closed system, we experienced an ether explosion and we were only able to control the severe intrapulmonary hemorrhage because everything required for intubation was immediately available. If surgical measures are required, their indication, according to the discussed rules, is based on the associated hemothorax or hemopneumothorax. Pulmonary wounds can usually be closed by suture. Lobectomy is rarely necessary, however, in cases with doubtful parenchymal healing it is to be preferred.

Rupture of a bronchus and *avulsion of a bronchus* are typical injuries of the main bronchi. Even though dyspnea and hemoptysis should make one suspicious and mediastinal emphysema with or without pneumothorax offers additional indications, according to BISHUP's statistical evaluation it was only possible to make a diagnosis in every 7th observed case with fresh injuries because bronchoscopy and bronchography were not used. Spontaneous healing has been known to occur, but it can only be regarded as the fortunate outcome of diagnostic omissions, not to mention total atelectasis of a lung with the functional late results due to obstruction of a main bronchus by scar tissue. The danger of waiting is adequately substantiated since BURKE, on the basis of statistical evaluations, states that the mortality of fresh bronchial injuries is 30% and OPDERBECKE observed 5 of 9 fatalities before the start of the planned procedure. For this reason every bronchus injury is an indication for surgical closure with interrupted sutures of chromic cat-gut. Thoracic surgery has taught us that a circular bronchus suture may occasionally later-on be subject to narrowing by scar tissue. Nevertheless, the functional result is always fully satisfactory. Figs. 2 and

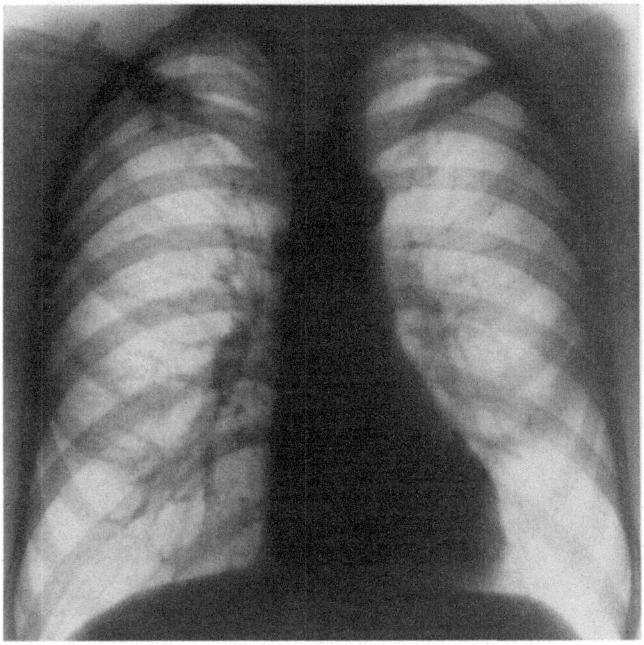

Fig. 2. Pat. K. H. Chest X-ray 1 year following operative repair of complete avulsion of the left main bronchus. Note good aeration of left lung

3 show an example of a circular avulsion of the left main bronchus 1 year after surgical treatment. This man is asymptomatic and he is fully and gainfully employed as a locksmith. Reconstruction of a bronchus which is occluded by scar tissue secondary to an undiagnosed circular avulsion is just as rewarding. In one injured patient SAMSON, 15 years after the accident, was able to re-expand the collapsed lung by resection of the scar tissue and end-to-end anastomosis of the bronchial stumps. We have used a similar surgical procedure in an injured patient after an interval of 14 years and the functional result of this patient now — at the 10th postoperative year — corresponds approximately to the age norm of this patient. However, return of respiratory function requires years and, according to the observations of KRAUSS, this is even the case if the atelectasis existed for a few months.

Of course, organ-preserving measures are contraindicated if infection and bronchiectasis have resulted in parenchymal destruction. With this indication NISSEN, in 1931, was the first to carry out a successful pneumonectomy.

In patients with circular avulsion of the *intrathoracic trachea* retraction of the distal stump may pose considerable difficulties to intubation. One female patient was sent to us as an acute emergency. An endotracheal tube had been inserted which had become impacted on the peritracheal wound. Thus, in an emergency, the broncho-scope temporarily must keep the airway patent until, by thoracotomy in the 3rd or 4th intercostal space, the injured stumps are exposed and the oxygen supply is assured by intubation from the surgical field. Then it is possible without haste to place the posterior layer of sutures and, after oral intubation, to continue it around

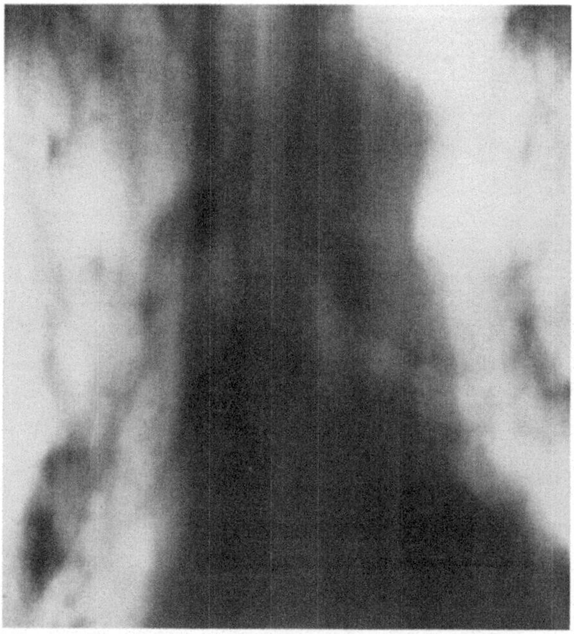

Fig. 3. Pat. H. Tomogram 1 year following operative repair of complete avulsion of the left main bronchus. Note concentric stenosis at the site of the anastomosis

the anterior circumference. A tracheostomy is advisable in order to protect the fresh suture line. If later stenosis due to scar tissue necessitates resection of the narrowed segment, defects up to 4 cm in length can be bridged, according to the experience of GRILLO, by mobilizing the right hilum and transection of the pulmonary ligament by direct end-to-end anastomosis.

According to studies by HEBERER *traumatic rupture of the aorta* is the cause of death of 3% of fatal traffic accidents. FISCHER even calculated 7%. Fig. 4 provides a survey on the regional location and frequency of this injury.

If the accident victim is still alive when he reaches the hospital, one finds, in addition to shock, typical but by no means regular symptoms, such as signs of ruptured hematoma, dyspnea, pain in the interscapular region, vascular bruit, pulse and blood pressure differences of the extremities and dysphagia due to compression of the esophagus. In the radiogram widening of the mediastinal shadow, double or triple aortic margins and displacement of the trachea are of diagnostic importance. Angiocardiography may support the suspicion, retrograde aortography is more reliable but is not without dangers.

To the extent to which it is hitherto possible to talk about experience, reality shows that diagnostic certainty in view of the quantitative and qualitative variability of symptoms cannot always be achieved, particularly in those accident victims who are most in need of immediate treatment. The rapidly enlarging mediastinal hematoma must then serve as an adequate indication for left thoracotomy which at least saves a part of the accident victims. However, it appears that hitherto a successful surgical intervention during the first 5 h has not been achieved. 2 of our accident victims died on admission and the other 2 died during emergency thoracotomy. The hospital in

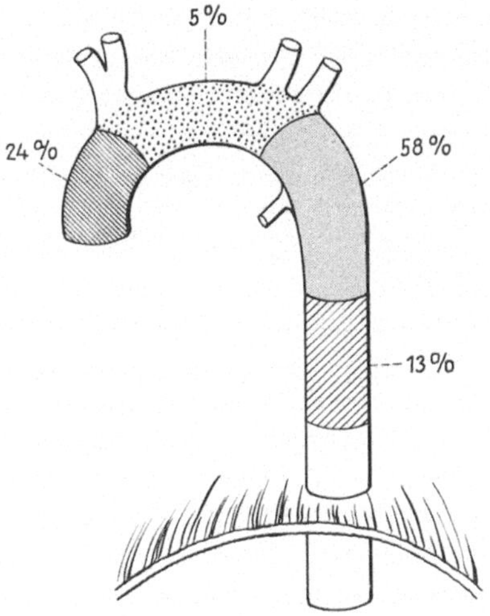

Fig. 4. Localization and frequency of traumatic aortic rupture

Düsseldorf has had similar experiences. In a group of 75 patients with aortic rupture who came to autopsy, HOLCZABEK only found 2 accident victims who had lived for more than 5 h. However, this is no reason to give up without trying.

In patients in whom treatment was possible after the 5 h-period, the surgical procedure was carried out a few times while the aorta was totally clamped. In one case of DE MUTH this was tolerated for 45 min without sequelae. However, the atrio-femoral bypass was primarily used with encouraging result. Table 2 summarizes a few individual observation.

For blunt thoracic trauma without severe associated injuries HEBERER has recently determined a mortality of 5 to 20% on the basis of statistical reports: We had a mortality rate of 14% one half of which is due to associated injuries and thus the mortality of isolated, closed thoracic trauma in our hospital was 6.9%.

For *perforating injuries* which account only for 1 to 5% of the cases with thoracic trauma, the same therapeutic principles which are used for closed injuries are valid. In general, surgical treatment is indicated more frequently than in cases with blunt trauma. In a group of 51 patients with perforating injuries 16 had to be treated surgically.

Among special problems I would like to mention perforating cardiac injuries. Statistical studies show that — depending on the transport and treatment facilities — approximately 40 to 50% achieve clinical significance and that of these more than 75% can be saved by immediate exposure and suture. This fact is so serious that a traumatic hemopericardium, if there is the least doubt about the type and extent of the source of the hemorrhage, should be approached surgically. Only in patients with slowly developing seeping hemorrhages can aspiration be regarded as a justifiable attempt, otherwise, by deciding on conservative treatment, one accepts a risk which can be considerably decreased by immediate surgical correction and suture of the injured wall. The admonishing remark that this rule results in overtreatment can be more readily accepted at the present level of surgical technique than the depressing recognition that a promising timely surgical procedure which can be performed by median sternotomy without special instruments has been missed.

Injuries which perforate the wall of the esophagus are far more frequently produced via the lumen than by external trauma. Iatrogenic instrumental measures show up in the

Table 2. *Results of early operation for aortic rupture*

Time of repair after trauma	Number of cases	Result	Protection
First 8 h	4	3 alive	2 none
		1 died	2 atriofemoral bypass
9 to 24 h	4	4 alive	1 none
			3 atriofemoral bypass
2 to 8 days	9	8 alive	7 atriofemoral bypass
		1 died	1 atrioiliac bypass
			1 aorta 45' crossclamped

Authors: De Muth, Dobell, Donovan, Fleischaker, Forsee et al., Heberer, Jahnke et al., Kraft-Kinz et al., Passaro et al., Rey-Baltar et al., Spencer, Stoney.

list of causes with particular frequency. Since initial manifestations are frequently absent, suspicion usually only starts when, after 12 or 24 h, mediastinitis which presents as mediastinal emphysema, develops. One exception is the infrequent spontaneous perforation which imitates the acute symptoms of a perforated gastric or duodenal ulcer.

Contrast examination with water-soluble substances is most valuable for diagnostic confirmation and location of the perforation. We do not trust esophagoscopy since this itself is not infrequently the unnoticed cause of the wall injury for the diagnosis of which it serves. We do not question its value for the endoscopic removal of foreign bodies.

Surgical treatment of a recent perforation of the esophagus by suture and solid coverage with adjacent pleura or lung is rewarding. In the terminal segment fundoplication according to *Nissen* assures particularly reliable closure. In patients with advanced mediastinitis one hardly has any resource other than the desperate attempt of suction drainage which has the depressing mortality of more than 50%.

Traumatic chylothorax is mainly seen after surgical procedures in the mediastinum. The danger of inanition and of susceptibility to infection due to fat, protein, fluid and lymphocyte loss in our opinion appears overrated in view of the fact that by continuous suction and re-expansion of the lung the secretion can usually be rapidly decreased and that healing can be achieved in at least 80% of the patients even though this may sometimes only be possible after 3 to 4 weeks. Only a chylothorax in a pneumonectomy cavity requires prompt surgical treatment by supradiaphragmatic plication of the thoracic duct. In other persistent cases the same measure which is to

Table 3. *Site of injury and mortality in 51 penetrating chest injuries*

Site of injury	stab	gunshot	other	total	deaths
Chest wall trauma without organ damage	22	5	6	33	1 13th postoperative day (due to pneumonia with lung abcess)
Lung	2	2	1	5	1 intraoperativ (shock due to rupture of upper and lower lobe)
Intrathoracic vessels	1	—	1	2	—
Heart	3	2	1	6	1 intraoperativ (heart contusion)
Esophagus	1	—	—	1	—
Concomitant injury of abdominal organs	3	1	—	4	1 intraoperativ (due to concomitant injury of diaphragm, transverse colon and left kidney)
Total	32	10	9	51	4 (7,8%)

be carried out on the ipsilateral side also achieves the desired result. A preoperative fatty meal to which Sudan III was added facilitates surgical exposure. Patients with a bilateral chylothorax are operated on through a right-sided surgical approach.

The primary results in patients with perforating thoracic injuries which were achieved in our hospital are demonstrated in Table 3.

The treatment of thoracic injuries is classical thoracic surgery, i.e., a field in which the exploration, care and promotion rests in surgical hands. As far as advocating, that traumatology be performed by orthopedic surgeons is concerned, I would like to state that I was unable to find a single contribution which, in this field, succeeded in achieving even minimal acceptance. This is enough reason not to withhold the helping hand which has learned the surgical rules and methods of thoracic procedures during surgical training from the patient with a thoracic injury.

Rigid Internal Fixation

M. Allgöwer

Some 10 years ago several general and orthopedic surgeons of Switzerland agreed that they were dissatisfied with their results of fracture treatment.

They formed the Association for the study of osteosynthesis (AO). In particular they were confronted with the following facts:

1. Fractures have an increasing importance in our modern Society of intensive traffic and increasing popularity of dangerous sports.

2. In many cases of fractures, restitution of the injured limb is not achieved.

3. Dystrophy of the injured limb, also freely called "fracture disease", is not primarily due to the initial injury but rather to the treatment necessitating long lasting inactivity of the injured limb.

4. Permanent damage very often does not result from the broken bone as such, but rather from this fracture disease leading to permanent impairment of adjacent joints and muscles.

5. Modern surgery has not fully unterstood the challenge which the fracture treatment constitutes. Integration of the work of some pioneers of fracture treatment has yet to be made: pioneer work which dates back to more than 50 years. By this we mean improvement of endresults by early active functional treatment. Such an improvement is possible in the conservative as well as in the operative approach to treatment of fractures. On the conservative side Böhler has shown early painless functional treatment to be a great advance in conservative fracture treatment.

Nothing however permits earlier postoperative functional treatment than adequate internal fixation of fractures and non-unions. This pioneer thought was brought forward at the end of the last century by the brothers Lambotte and later perfectioned by Danis.

It seemed a worthwhile challenge to take up the ideas of these pioneers and create an instrumentation using modern engineering and metallurgy. This allowed us to create an instrumentation integrating the various types of internal fixation [*1* to *4*]. It has to be clearly pointed out that internal fixation is no aim in itself but it has only one object, namely to allow immediate functional treatment of fractures and operated non-unions as early as possible in view of reducing discomfort, morbidity and permanent damage. If internal fixation would achieve this aim, we might well accept some delay in bone healing as the price of better endresults.

Extensive experimentation on dogs and sheeps as well as follow-up in more than 10000 patients have demonstrated that application of metal to bone, if biomechanically correct, does not necessarily interfere with bone healing. And this is especially true for the ideal case, i.e. hairline adjustment of two well vascularized fragments held rigidly together. Rigid apposition of cortical fragments brings the healing capacities of the cortex into play, specifically the direct bridging-over of the fracture line. Danis [*8*] some 25 years ago called this "soudure autogene" ("autogenic soldering"). In analogy to wound healing, we might call it "primary bone healing", where as the classical scheme of large callus formation might be called "secondary bone healing". What does this cortical regeneration look like and what is it based on? Bassett and others [*5* to *6*] under appropiate conditions saw direct formation of osteons out of the Haversian system.

In our group Schenk and Willenegger [*11*, *12*] studied cortical bone healing in fine osteotomies of the dog radius treated by compression plates. After osteotomy, they put on the plate and applied compression. Pressures of between 20 and 80 kg applied to the radius could be measured by the compression device. Immediately after operation, the fine gap was clearly visible roentgenographically, at 5 weeks the osteotomy appeared to be bridged over, and at 8 weeks "primary bone healing" seemed complete. Histologically the cortex adjacent to the plate is bridged over directly; the opposite cortex showed originally a small gap, and needed some filling in. The cortex was in full Haversian remodeling, 6 weeks after operation. The unit of this remodeling has three elements: (1) vascular sprout, (2) perivascular osteoblasts, and (3) "borehead" of osteoclasts.

If we study the normal radius by the *tetracycline technique*, 2,5% of the osteons are in regeneration, but 6 weeks after osteotomy 60% of the osteons are in regeneration. If accurate adjustment is not achieved, the orientation of the ingrowing bone is not optimal. The interposed granulation tissue and especially the interposed fibrocartilage cannot be penetrated by the Haversian units. This is the consequence of slight instability.

Wagner [*16*, *17*] has made careful studies on the biochemical response to various screws. In one experimental set-up, he inserted a cancellous screw into a growing tibia of a dog. Insertion of this screw consistently induced the laying down of new bone lamellae oriented along the lines of stress, with maximum bone formation localized at maximum pressure sites.

Perren with the use of strain gage monitored plates has followed the pressure decay of compression fixation over the course of several months in sheep. It is most interesting to know that there is no rapid decay but rather a very gradual disappearence of the pressure. This fact can only be explained by the slow remodeling of the bone cortex which slowly replaces the stressed bone. If a resorption at the bony end of only 10 μ would occur pressure would fall to 0 immediately after this resorption had taken place. The fact that such is not the case shows that internal fixation creates a biomechanical constellation which is well tolerated by the cortical bone and taken an advantage of by nature.

In general, the experimental studies on the regenerating capacity of bone support the rationale of very accurate reduction of fragments in order to induce an economical bone healing of the cortex itself, a capacity, that is not taken advantage of in the conservative approach to fracture treatment. It must be clear, however, that this capacity of the cortex is an extra benefit of and not the primary reason for advocating internal fixation. Unfortunately, the capacity for regeneration does not automatically enter into the healing process after every operation on cortical bone, and bad biomechanical planning or unfavorable fracture conditions may abolish it. Healing very often is of mixed types, with part of the fracture needing the help of endosteum and periosteum to fill in the gaps.

There are several ways of realizing the desired stability of internal fixation that allow immediate postoperative mobilization of the impaired limb without external fixation and that do not interfere with bone healing [*10*].

The *medullary nail* is probably the best known on the Continent. Reaming the medullary cavity increases later stability and it is possible to obtain primary bone healing with little radiological evidence of callus formation, although a slight instability usually remains that has to be overcome by a fixation callus.

Lambotte 50 years ago considered the *screw* to be the basic element of internal fixation [*9*]. Danis has taught us that biomechanics call for the *lag screw*, i.e., a screw that bites into the distal cortex only [*8*] and thus gives interfragmentary pressure.

To insert a screw, a large hole is first made in the exposed cortex; then a guide is inserted into the hole and a smaller hole is drilled in it; the thread is cut in the opposite cortex, and finally the screw can be put in. Screw fixation is adequate in long spiral fractures or in butterfly fractures where at least one screw can be placed between the two main fragments. The fracture lines usually disappear between the 8th and 14th week.

Plate fixation is appropriate when an extensive fracture area must be neutralized. It allows axial stability and even compression, and permits the insertion of compression screws for additional stabilization of longitudinal fracture lines.

In plating a fractured long bone, the plate is fixed with one screw to one fragment, the compression device is fixed to the other fragment, and then the compression device is removed. The histology of one patient who died from cerebral hemorrhage 12 weeks after internal fixation of a comminuted fracture of the tibia by lag screws and plating showed the same cortical healing with Haversian remodeling and direct union of fragments in hairline adjustment as seen in the osteotomised dog radius. PERREN found the same to be true in osteotomised tibias of the sheep, provided that internal fixation is adequate.

In fractures where traction is to be counteracted, a *traction-absorbing wire* is sufficient to give stability and even compression to the underlying bone. This allows immediate mobilization and is especially successful in fractures of the patella, the olecranon and the fibula.

In dislocated fractures of joints, hardly any treatment is acceptable other than open reduction, lest there be permanent damage or even total loss of function. This risk is especially common in transcondylar fractures of the femur and fractures of the distal end of the tibia. Traffic accidents and sport injuries have increased the incidence of these severe injuries considerably.

Four principles have been found useful in the treatment of injuries to the distal tibia involving the joint: (1) Reconstruction must begin with internal fixation of the fibula whenever the fibula is not comminuted. Axis and length of the tibia are thus restored. (2) The next step is the restoration of the distal joint surface of the tibia under good exposure from the medial side. Quite often we have to use preliminary fixation with Kirschner wires before plates or screws can be applied. (3) The third step consists of filling the cancellous defect with autogenous cancellous bone chips from the greater trochanter or from the iliac crest. (4) Finally, medial support must be provided by means of a plate to stabilize the whole fracture area, to prevent secondary varus deformity.

Open fractures with loss of integument constitute a major challenge in fracture treatment, and I can outline here only the most important principles. A stabilized bone defends itself well against infection and care of the patient after stabilization is greatly facilitated. In applying internal fixation in open fractures four rules must be followed strictly:

1. Prevent infection in the hospital. The wound should be inspected only under strict aseptic conditions. Cleansing of the wound as a completely aseptic procedure with sterile instruments also helps to prevent hospital germs from being introduced into the wound.

2. Metal implants should be minimal and must be covered by vital tissue, preferably muscle.

3. Damaged skin should never be jeopardized only for the purpose of covering exposed bone, covering exposed bone is not imperative.

4. Immediate skin closure should never be attempted when viability of the skin is

questionable. In open fractures with extensive contusions, operation may be delayed for 8 to 10 days.

As to the results of internal fixation in fresh fractures, we can report on four series of consecutive cases that totaled 617 tibial fractures [*7*, *13* to *15*]. Primary bone healing was observed in 70% of the cases. Of 535 closed fractures, six had some minor permanent damage.

This indicates that internal fixation did not expose these patients to an unduly high risk and compares favorably with the results of other fracture treatment in our country. Of 37 fractures of the lower tibia involving the joint, permanent damage resulted from three; this seems satisfactory. The results with the open fractures also compared favorably with other treatment of similar fractures, although in many cases medullary nails have been inserted after reaming of the medullary cavity. We now tend to avoid this procedure in open fractures; the large dead space of the nail and the reduced vitality of the reamed medullary cavity make the bone very prone to infection.

Treatment of non-union by operation is well accepted throughout the world. It is however generally appreciated that the hypertrophic non-union with its enlarged bony ends ("elephant foot") needs no major removal of "interposed" tissue and does not require bone transplants. It goes on to uneventful healing following rigid internal fixation without requiring external fixation. The hypotrophic avascular non-union is best treated by combining internal fixation with autologous cancellous transplants.

In the light of these results we conclude that open reduction and internal fixation have something to offer in the treatment of fresh fractures and non-unions. However, that holds true only if those responsible are willing to plan and execute such operations properly and to use adequate instruments. The open treatment of fractures has a certain fascination, and we must remember that this is not in itself a justification for its use. There is only one proper justification: to achieve full functional recovery of the injured limb.

References

1. Allgöwer, M.: Langenbecks Arch. klin. Chir. **319**, 383 (1967).
2. — Langenbecks Arch. klin. Chir. **308**, 423 (1964).
3. —, A. Huggler und G. Segmüller: Z. Unfallmed. Berufskr. **4**, 276 (1966).
4. —, M. E. Müller, R. Schenk und H. Willenegger: Langenbecks Arch. klin. Chir. **305**, 1—14 (1963).
5. Bassett, C. A.: J. Bone Jt. Surg. **44-A**, 1217 (1962).
6. —, D. K. Creighton, and F. E. Stinchfield: Surg. Gynec. Obstet. **112**, 145 (1961).
7. Corrodi, E.: Die Ergebnisse der Behandlung frischer Unterschenkelfrakturen Erwachsener mittels Zugschraubenosteosynthese. Dissertation Basel, 1962.
8. Danis, R.: Théorie et pratique de l'ostéosynthèse. Paris: Masson & Cie. 1949.
9. Lambotte, A.: Chirurgie operatoire des fractures, Paris: Masson & Cie. 1913.
10. Müller, M. E., M. Allgöwer, and H. Willenegger: Technique of internal fixation of fractures. Rev. English Edition. Berlin-Heidelberg-New York: Springer 1965.
11. Schenk, R., and H. Willenegger: Experientia (Basel) **19**, 593 (1963).
12. — — Langenbecks Arch. klin. Chir. **308**, 440 (1964).
13. Segmüller, G., u. M. Allgöwer: Chirurg **36**, 504 (1965).
14. —, E. Corrodi und G. Kessler: Z. Unfallmed. Berufskr. **57**, 252 (1964).
15. —, C. Wieser und M. Allgöwer: Radiol. clin. (Basel) **36**, 254 (1967).
16. Wagner, H.: Langenbecks Arch. klin. Chir. **305**, 28 (1963).
17. — Neue Osteosyntheseschrauben und ihre Gewebsverträglichkeit. Verh. dtsch. orthop. Ges., p. 419, 1962.

Management of Acute Arterial Injuries

Frank Cole Spencer

Introduction

This presentation summarizes clinical experiences with arterial injuries in both military and civilian populations in the past 17 years. For brevity, experiences are summarized as didactic statements, without specific reference to experimental or clinical data.

Historical Considerations

The feasibility of routinely repairing injured arteries in military casualties was first demonstrated in the Korean War in 1952. Earlier ettempts in World War II were generally unsuccessful, and rather pessimistic conclusions were reached concerning the possibilities. Following the Korean War experiences, injured arteries have been repaired almost routinely, for ligation of major arteries has an overall incidence of subsequent gangrene of about 50%. The advances in therapy in the Korean War were due to several factors. The most significant was the almost routine prevention of infection in traumatic wounds by extensive debridement, followed by antibiotics and secondary wound closure 4 to 10 days later. Familiarity with techniques of vascular surgery, in combination with the availability of vascular instruments, was also important. The prompt evacuation of wounded men by helicopter, often bringing a wounded patient to the hospital within 2 to 4 h after injury, was also a significant factor.

Pathogenesis

Etiology. Most arterial injuries result from penetrating wounds which disrupt partly or completely the wall of the artery. Non-penetrating injuries, usually associated with a fracture in an adjacent bone, are less frequent but often have a more serious prognosis, partly from extensive crushing injury to the wall of the artery and partly from delay in diagnosis.

Pathology. Most injuries are either lacerations or transections of the arterial wall. Uncommon injuries include arterial spasm, arterial contusion with thrombosis, and arteriovenous fistula. With lacerations or transections, the extent of injury varies with the type of trauma, which is an important consideration in subsequent debridement and surgical therapy. With clean, incised wounds, such as those made by a knife or an ice-pick, injury to the arterial wall is minimal. By contrast, trauma from a high velocity missile disrupts the intima and media for a short distance away from the actual laceration in the arterial wall and requires a wider debridement at the time of surgical repair.

Contusion or spasm often occurs in association with fractures and extensive soft tissue injuries from blunt trauma. The presence of multiple injuries obscures recognition of the arterial injury, especially with extensive comminuted fractures. With the frequency of automobile accidents, arterial injuries in association with fractures in an extremity are increasing in frequency. Arteriography has been found of particular value in such problems.

Arterial spasm is an infrequent injury in which sustained contraction of the smooth muscle in the wall of the artery may obstruct blood flow and precipitate thrombosis. The etiology is obscure, for the spasm results from direct muscular contraction and not from a neurogenic stimulus. It is most frequently seen in the brachial artery with a fracture of the humerus. An arterial contusion from a blunt injury has multiple areas of fragmentation of the arterial wall with intramural hemorrhage. The intima may become detached and prolapse into the lumen, creating an intraluminal obstruction similar to an intussusception in the intestine. This can be detected only by performing an arteriotomy and inspecting the intima. A serious error occurs when a contusion is misdiagnosed as "spasm." The delay in treatment as a consequence of this diagnostic error can result in gangrene. The well known VOLKMANNS ischemic contracture of the muscles of the forearm is due to an untreated spasm or contusion of the brachial artery in association with a supracondylar fracture of the humerus.

Pathophysiology. The severity of the ischemic injury following an arterial injury varies with the tolerance of different tissues for anoxia. In the extremity the peripheral nerves are the most sensitive to anoxia; hence, paralysis and anesthesia quickly develop when arterial blood flow is seriously decreased. Striated muscle is almost equally sensitive to anoxia and will usually become necrotic if arterial blood flow is decreased to such a degree that anesthesia and paralysis are present. Skin, tendon, and bone all have a greater tolerance for anoxia and may survive an ischemic injury which has produced irreversible extensive muscle necrosis. This is seen in an extremity in which an arterial repair is performed several hours after injury. The skin may appear viable, but the extremity is anesthetic, paralyzed, and after a period of time will be found to have widespread necrosis of the muscles.

The tolerance of striated muscle for ischemia is in the range of 6 to 8 h. Experimental studies by MILLER and WELCH found arterial repair successful in about 90% of experiments when performed within 6 h after injury, but the success rate decreased to 50% when repair was delayed for 12 h. Therefore, every effort should be made to complete arterial repair within 6 h after injury if anesthesia or paralysis are present, indicating a severe degree of anoxia. A definite time limit does not exist, however, beyond which arterial repair is futile, for the importance of the time interval varies with the collateral circulation. The collateral circulation, in turn, varies with the artery injured, the degree of soft tissue injury which has interrupted collateral circulation, associated shock, and ambient temperature. In some patients with little disturbance of collateral circulation, arterial repair has been successfully performed 12 to 15 h after injury, but in general, successful repairs were obtained much more frequently when accomplished within 6 h after injury because of the tolerance of striated muscle for anoxia.

Clinical Manifestations

Shock, from loss of blood, was present in over 50% of patients with an arterial injury, either from hemorrhage from the injured artery or from associated injuries. The degree of shock varied, of course, with the severity of the blood loss or the severity of other injuries. When profound shock was present, the severe peripheral vasoconstriction often concealed the presence of an arterial injury until blood pressure was restored to near normal levels.

With blunt trauma, multiple organ injuries were commonly present, such as skull fractures, rib fractures, or blunt abdominal injuries. Careful assessment of each injury present, with subsequent assignment of priorities in therapy, is a critical part of initial evaluation of the patient.

In the injured extremity, fractures and nerve injuries were commonly present with either penetrating wounds or following blunt trauma. The presence of a fracture or extensive soft tissue injury greatly influences the prognosis of an arterial injury. For example, in one series of arterial injuries the presence of a fracture of a femur in association with an injury of the femoral artery raised the incidence of gangrene from 11 to 55%.

In the extremity, the arterial injury frequently produced four abnormal findings, conveniently remembered as four P's: loss of Pulses, Paralysis, Paresthesias or anesthesia, and Pallor. Of these four, the neurological findings are the most important, for as previously stated loss of neurological function indicates a degree of tissue ischemia which will progress to gangrene unless arterial blood flow is improved. Absence of a pulse in the presence of a normal pulse in the contralateral extremity immediately suggests an arterial injury. If serious vasoconstriction is present from hypotension, evaluation of peripheral pulses may be difficult until blood volume is restored. It is important to emphasize, however, that the presence of a peripheral pulse does not exclude an arterial injury. This was frequently seen with a tangential laceration of the wall of an artery which was sealed by a blood clot with preservation of some flow through the arterial lumen.

With penetrating wounds, bright red bleeding, even in small amounts, immediately suggests an arterial injury. In the absence of hemorrhage, a tense hematoma may be palpated around the wound, evolving from extravasation of blood under significant pressure beneath the fascia. Occasionally a systolic bruit may be audible over the wound, or rarely a continuous bruit if an acute arteriovenous fistula has been produced.

It should be emphasized, however, that an arterial injury can be present with virtually no abnormalities in the extremity. Hence, the presence of a penetrating injury near a major artery should alert the physician to the possibility that an arterial injury may be present. In a recent series of 85 arterial injuries reported by DILLARD and associates, the correct diagnosis was delayed in 15 of the patients. Usually the diagnosis is missed if serious hemorrhage is not present, or if a peripheral pulse can be felt. Unrecognized cases may subsequently develop a secondary hemorrhage from the wound, or may form a false aneurysm or an arteriovenous fistula in the area where the hematoma has formed around the lacerated artery.

With uncertain cases, an arteriogram should be performed. This has been of particular value with blunt trauma producing a fracture of the extremity. A critical question in such patients is whether a decreased or absent pulse is due to an arterial injury or to angulation of the artery from fractured bone.

Treatment

Preoperative Considerations. Control of bleeding is the most urgent immediate problem. This was usually done by tightly packing the wound with gauze and applying a pressure dressing. A large amount of packing was often required, for the efficacy of packing depends upon compression of the artery between the overlying skin and the underlying bone. Tourniquets were avoided for most injuries. When used they were carefully padded to avoid the risk of permanent injury to a peripheral nerve.

Shock, present in 50 to 60% of patients, was treated by the rapid infusion of fluids (500 ml every 5 to 10 min) until the systolic blood pressure rose to 80 mm Hg, after which additional fluids were infused more gradually as needed. Usually 1000 to 2000 ml of fluid was required. Blood is preferable, but until the necessary crossmatching has been done, Ringer's lactate solution, plasma, or Dextran may be used.

Antibiotic therapy was started promptly and appropriate prophylactic therapy for tetanus begun. Sympathetic blocks and anticoagulant therapy had no significant role in preoperative care.

Operative Considerations. An important basic attitude regarding arterial trauma is that almost all injuries can be repaired successfully with available surgical techniques. The prognosis then becomes a question of whether or not the repair was performed before irreversible muscle necrosis developed. The only special instruments required are atraumatic vascular clamps and arterial silk, sizes 4-0 or 5-0, with swaged needles. The surgical incision was placed to expose the artery proximal and distal to the site of injury in order to avoid hemorrhage when clots were evacuated from the wound. Once proximal and distal control of the artery had been obtained, the hematoma surrounding the injury was widely opened and the site of injury mobilized. Most injuries were treated by excision of the injured area followed by end-to-end anastomosis. With injuries from high velocity missiles, 2 to 4 mm of adjacent arterial wall were excised. Tangential repairs of lacerations are deceptive in that suture of the laceration often results in constriction and subsequent thrombosis. Usually excision followed by direct anastomosis was found preferable.

With transection of an artery, elastic recoil will separate the two ends of the vessel for one or more centimeters, giving the erroneous impression that a segment of artery has been destroyed. In most instances application of gentle traction on the ends of the artery with vascular clamps demonstrated that direct anastomosis could be performed. Normally, 1 to 2 cm of a peripheral artery can be excised and the vessel ends still approximated after limited mobilization of the two ends. For example, in 180 arterial reconstructions for civilian injuries reported by PATMAN, grafts were necessary in only 20 patients. Similarly, in a series of 190 arterial reconstructions reported by MORRIS, primary repair was done in 167 patients and vascular grafts in 23. In the author's personal experience with 25 civilian injuries, repair was almost always done by direct anastomosis, although in the Korean War grafts were needed much more frequently. Before the anastomosis was performed, the degree of back-bleeding from the distal artery was noted and any blood clots present removed with a catheter. The anastomosis was performed with 4-0 or 5-0 arterial silk, using a continuous suture interrupted in two or three areas to avoid a purse-string effect. Individual sutures were 1.0 to 1.5 mm in depth and a similar distance apart. With small arteries, interrupted or horizontal mattress sutures were employed. Either a continuous over-and-over suture or an everting suture was satisfactory (Fig. 1).

A vascular graft is needed only when direct anastomosis cannot be performed because of loss of two or more centimeters of artery; this occurs in about 10 to 15% of injuries. An autogenous vein is the preferred graft, reversing the ends of the vein which is employed, usually the saphenous. If for some reason a vein cannot be utilized, a graft of knitted Dacron is preferable. If a prosthetic graft is used, the diameter should rarely be less than 8 mm, for thrombosis occurs much more frequently with smaller grafts.

With contaminated wounds, the best protection from infection following adequate debridement and arterial reconstruction was found to be approximation of the adjacent soft tissues over the arterial repair and leaving the remaining wound open, to be closed by secondary suture 4 to 7 days later. This technique almost routinely prevented the development of infection.

Ligation of an injured artery should only be performed for minor arteries, such as a radial or an ulnar artery which is clearly not essential to survival of the limb. Back-bleeding is an inadequate guide to ligation of major arteries, indicating that some collateral circulation is present but not guaranteeing that collateral flow will be large enough to prevent gangrene. In the Korean War "good" or "fair" back-bleeding was recorded in nine of 20 arterial ligations performed in one group of patients, all of which resulted in gangrene.

Arterial spasm, an unusual injury, may be treated by the topical application of 2 to 5% papaverine. Another technique reported by MUSTARD has been the forceful

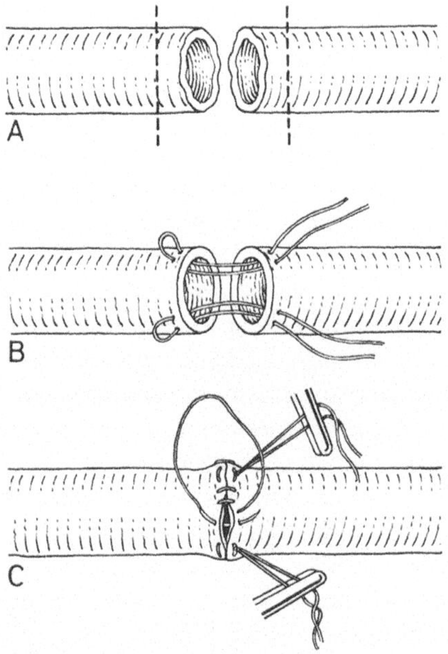

Fig. 1. Steps followed in the repair of a traumatic transection of a peripheral artery. A. Initially the edges of the injured artery are debrided, removing 1 to 2 mm. of normal arterial wall, especially if the injury was from a high velocity missile which would traumatize adjacent segments of arterial wall. B. The two ends of the artery are aligned with mattress sutures of 4-0 or 5-0 silk placed about 180 degrees apart. C. Anastomosis is then performed with a continuous suture of 4-0 or 5-0 silk, usually as a simple over-and-over suture. Alternately, an everting suture can be employed. With small vessels, simple interrupted or horizontal mattress sutures can be used to lessen the risk of constriction of the lumen

dilatation of the area of spasm by the injection of saline into the lumen of the artery. The importance of differentiating spasm from contusion with disruption of the wall of the artery has been mentioned previously. Unless the area of constriction can be satisfactorily corrected, it should be excised and continuity re-established by direct anastomosis or a vascular graft.

Postoperative Care. Anticoagulant therapy is not recommended after arterial repair, for it provides little protection from thrombosis but does increase the risk of bleeding into the wound. Sympathetic blocks are similarly of little value. The most important consideration following operation is the presence of peripheral pulses, indicating satisfactory restoration of arterial flow. If pulses cannot be detected, or if previously palpable pulses disappear, an arteriogram should be performed, or alternately the site of anastomosis should be re-explored. The important principle to re-emphasize is that with modern vascular techniques a traumatic injury of a normal artery can almost always be successfully repaired.

When a femoral artery was repaired several hours after injury, ischemic swelling often occurred in the leg muscles in the anterior and posterior tibial compartments. Such swelling can progress to a degree that ischemic necrosis results. Prompt fasciotomies over the muscle compartments, decompressing the edematous, turgid muscles, were of great value.

When an arterial repair was performed several hours after an injury, a peripheral pulse might be restored, but the extremity remained paralyzed and anesthetic. In such patients the skin may be viable, but the status of the underlying muscles is uncertain. Such patients must be carefully observed, because extensive muscle necrosis will result in serious toxic manifestations, with high fever and occasionally renal insufficiency. A decision to amputate such extremities, as opposed to widespread debridement of the necrotic muscles, is a difficult one to make, and must be evaluated carefully for each individual patient. Some patients may be salvaged following extensive debridement of necrotic calf muscles, with preservation of a limited but useful foot.

The development of a postoperative infection around the site of arterial repair is a grave complication, because frequently the anastomosis will disrupt with life-threatening hemorrhage. The infection should be promptly treated by widespread drainage, for it is usually due to inadequate removal of necrotic tissue. If infection involves the arterial reconstruction, ligation of the artery is usually required to prevent fatal hemorrhage or sepsis. Occasionally bypass grafts may be inserted through channels circumventing the area of infection, performing an anastomosis between the artery proximal and distal to the point of injury. As mentioned earlier, the Korean War experiences well emphasized that despite massive contamination, the policy of widespread debridement, followed by secondary wound closure, almost always prevented postoperative wound infections.

Summary

With present vascular techniques, arterial reconstruction can almost always be successfully performed if undertaken within 6 h after injury. In a recent group of 209 patients with arterial injuries reported by PATMAN, the amputation rate was 3.8%. In another series of 67 arterial reconstructions reported by DILLARD, only two amputations were necessary. In the author's personal experience with 25 civilian injuries gangrene developed in one patient with a fracture of the femur in whom the correct diagnosis of laceration of the femoral artery was missed for 4 days. If a vein graft is needed for arterial reconstruction, the long-term patency is probably in the range of 80 to 85%, varying with the experience of the surgeon and the circumstances of the injury. If subsequent occlusion of a vein graft does occur, viability of the extremity is rarely jeopardized, although claudication may develop. In such patients a subsequent vascular reconstruction may be electively performed.

References

DILLARD, B. M., D. L. NELSON, and H. G. NORMAN: Surgery **63**, 391 (1968).
HUGHES, C. W., and A. COHEN: Surg. Clin. N. Amer. **38**, 1529 (1958).
MORRIS, G. C., JR., A. C. BEALL, JR., W. R. ROOF, and M. E. DE BAKEY: Amer J. Surg. **99**, 775 (1960).

Morton, J. H., W. A. Southgate, and J. A. de Weese: Surg. Gynec. Obstet. **123**, 611 (1966).
Mustard, W. T., and C. A. Bull: Ann. Surg. **155**, 339 (1962).
Patman, R. D., E. Poulos, and G. T. Shires: Surg. Gynec. Obstet. **118**, 725 (1964).
Spencer, F. C.: Vascular injury and arteriovenous fistula. In: Lewis-Walters, Practice of Surgery, Vol. XI, Chap. 8, Hagerstown, Md.: W. F. Prior Co. 1965.
—, and R. V. Grewe: Ann. Surg. **141**, 304 (1955).
—, and R. K. Tompkins: Postgrad. Med. **28**, 476 (1960).

Mechanism and Prevention of Design-Related Injuries in Automobile Collisions*

Alan M. Nahum

The time has arrived in which rather confident predictions of diagnostic value can be made regarding accidental collision trauma. The implications of this for the teaching and the practice of surgery should prove to be dramatic and far reaching. Clinical and experimental studies of trauma have now reached the point where it is possible to predict the location, nature, and severity of traumatic injuries sustained in vehicular collisions. While my remarks will apply here only to motorists, information is also available for cyclists and pedestrians and will be the subject of later publications. The implicat:on of predicting trauma may well affect not only diagnosis and treatment and the planning of emergency medical systems, but methods of controlling trauma causation by such means as altering highway environments and changing vehicle design.

The critical variables in the prediction of trauma may be devided into three groups:

A. *Human Variables*
 1. age,
 2. anthropometric characteristics, e.g., height, weight,
 3. pre-existing medical conditions,
 4. restraints,
 5. seating location

B. *Vehicle Variables*
 1. weight and size,
 2. design characteristics,
 3. model year.

C. *Collision Variables*
 1. configuration,
 2. pre-impact speed and force characteristics.

Only a few of the many variables have been listed. Of these the most crucial are *speed*, *weight of car*, *collision configuration*, *use of restraints*, and *vehicle design*.

* Supported in part by grants from the Automobile Manufacturer's Association; the National Highway Safety Bureau, U.S. Department of Transportation; and the Injury Control Branch, Bureau of Disease Prevention and Environmental Control, U.S. Public Health Service.

The data presented here are the result of 6 years of intensive investigation by a medical-engineering team at the University of California, Los Angeles. The team consists of physicians and engineers who collect data from many sources to complete the analysis of a particular accident (Fig. 1).

Data are collected from the accident scene, from the hospital, and from the vehicles, and are correlated to provide an accurate reconstruction of the mechanisms by which injuries were produced and the roles of the important variables. For accidents of particular interest a special team is on call at all times of the day and night to provide the type of microscopic analytic approach which was formerly used in our country only for aircraft accidents. For example, several months ago a passenger bus with 31 occupants collided at a high speed with a passenger car which was travelling the

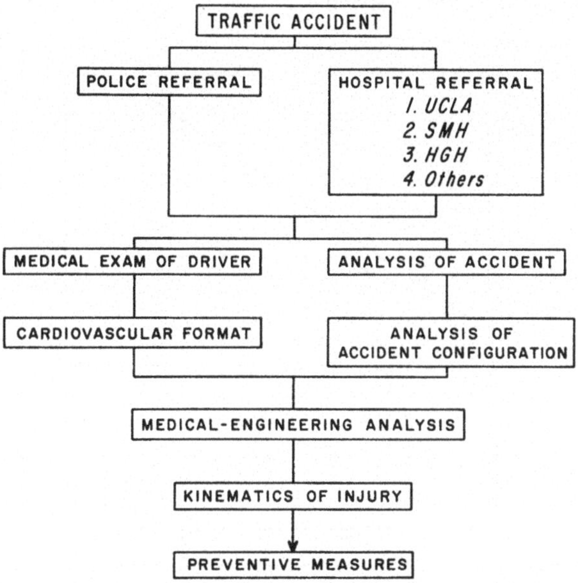

Fig. 1. Organization and methodology of UCLA research

wrong way on a highway. The collision resulted in a disastrous fire in which 20 persons were burned to death. Serious questions were raised not only about the cause of the collision and the fire, but how to prevent such fires and how to save persons if such a fire occurs. Within minutes after the fire a helicopter was carrying the medical-engineering team towards the site of the accident. Special surveys and analyses of the accident site were performed from the air. Then the investigation team landed and completed a precise detailed analysis of all aspects of the accident. This comprehensive approach has already indicated a potential for analysis and prevention of motorist deaths — a problem which far exceeds the deaths which occur in aircraft accidents.

Detailed information is also derived from studies of experimental decelerations using human volunteers, and from collisions which utilize anthropometric dummies.

From research of this type it is possible to understand how the important variables affect the production of traumatic injuries.

Speed and vehicle deformation are estimates of the forces involved in a collision, forces which put the motorist in motion and which are transmitted to him abruptly when the vehicle decelerates in a collision. It is known that such force parameters as duration, peak force, and rate of onset may be important. In addition, the area where the force is applied and the area over which it is distributed are also important.

An accident may be divided into three or more collisions: the *primary:* That between the vehicle and its environment; the *secondary*: that between the occupant and the inside of the vehicle.; the *tertiary*: that between the internal organs and the body shell.

This latter collision may be of crucial importance for areas such as the heart and aorta which contain blood under pressure.

As would be expected, the total number and the severity of injuries (Fig. 2) increase with the collision speeds. At the same time, significant injuries frequently occur at surprisingly low impact speeds.

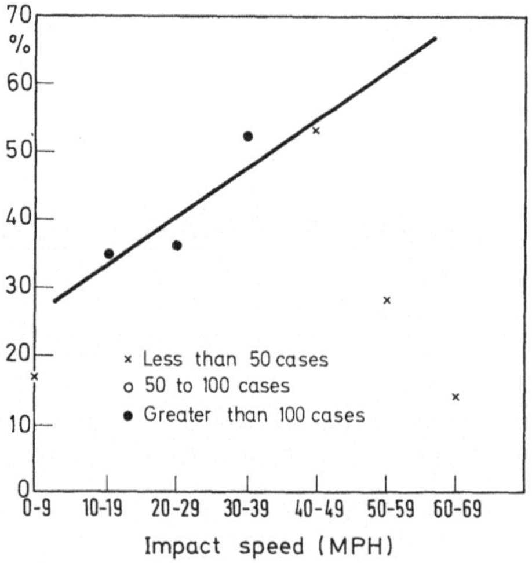

Fig. 2. Percent of occupants injured according to speed at impact (frontal collisions)

An example of the interplay of crucial variables is demonstrated in Case no. 637. A 1967 Plymouth weighing 3300 pounds was struck left front side by a 1966 Ford weighing 3400 pounds. The pre-impact speeds were about 50 mph. In the Ford were three young males in their early 20's who were all unrestrained. The driver sustained fractures of the left femur and pelvis which would have been survivable. But, in addition, he sustained multiple cerebral contusions when his head struck the A pillar. And when his chest struck the unyielding wheel-column system, it resulted in a laceration of the right lower lung and a $^1/_2$ cm linear laceration of the dorsal aspect of the midabdominal aorta. There were no other intraabdominal injuries, suggesting the susceptibility of the aorta to certain dynamic impact situations which fulfill critical force-time relationships.

The right front seat passenger sustained a severe skull fracture and concussion when his head struck the header, but he survived. The rear seated passenger struck his head against the roof and sustained a fatal head injury.

Restraints could have prevented the majority of these injuries. The addition of an energy-absorbing wheel-column system would have decreased the driver's chest and abdominal injuries and he would have survived even without a restraint.

In the struck car there was a 31 year old male driver and a 7 year old female in the right front seat. Both occupants were wearing seat belts. The driver sustained a mild concussion when his head hit the A pillar. As he moved forward and somewhat to the left of the steering wheel, his chest contacted the wheel column which was of an energy-absorbing type, and it collapsed, partially absorbing some of his energy of motion. However, at this same time the left door was being pushed inward on him. He sustained multiple bilateral rib fractures, a fractured pelvis, and a fracture of the left femur. An electrocardiogram showed flattening and inversion of the T waves in leads I and II with slight ST depression, ST depression and inverted T waves in lead AVF, and flat T waves in lead V 6. The findings were consistent with a diagnosis of myocardial contusion. His off-center impact did not allow him to take full advantage of the new wheel-column system. His major chest and abdominal injuries were due to the intrusion of the door into his left side. If he had not been wearing a seat belt, he would have suffered fatal head and chest injuries, that common fatal combination of injuries occurring to drivers.

It is interesting to note that he was 6 feet 4 inches in height and weighed 205 pounds, while the fatally injured driver of the opposing vehicle was 5 feet 3 inches in height and weighed 155 pounds. This means that the driver of the striking car who was fatally injured would have weighed *4650* pounds during a 30 G deceleration, while the surviving driver of the struck car would have weighed *6150* pounds for a comparable deceleration. However, he survived and made a full recovery.

The child seated in the right front seat sustained a mild concussion and facial contusions when her head struck the instrument panel.

Another type of problem is illustrated in Case no. 779. A 1967 Buick was struck on its left side by a 1968 Dodge which was travelling about 35 mph. The Buick, the struck car, is of particular interest here. The driver, who was alone in the vehicle, received multiple left-sided rib fractures, a cardiac contusion, a ruptured spleen, and a traumatic rupture of the left diaphragm. He received his injuries when the striking car intruded into the motorist compartment, forcing his door toward him at the same time that the collision forces were pushing him toward the opposing car. The man in the striking car was wearing a seat belt and received only minor injuries. The side impact collision is particularly critical. It is a soft frontal collision for the striking car, but for the struck car it is the most critical collision configuration since it occurs at the weakest point in the motorist compartment where the motorist has the least distance between him and an oncoming car. In a collision, motorists move in the direction of the collision, except in rollovers, and invariably strike that portion of the vehicular interior which is directly in their path.

For this reason, in an analysis of over 500 collisions (Fig. 3) it is possible to say with certainty that front seat passengers will strike the wheel column, panel, and windshield most frequently and the injuries will be distributed over the body according to the objects struck. The head, chest, and abdomen will receive most of the injuries. Rear seated occupants will sustain significantly less head, chest, and abdominal injuries and a great increase in trauma to the lower extremities. The objects struck will be primarily the back of the front seat and the doors and result in an entirely different spectrum of injuries.

For the front seat passengers the significant head injuries will be concussions with rare fatal contusions usually associated with fractures. Chest injuries will occur either due to contact with the wheel or the door resulting in rib fractures, cardiac

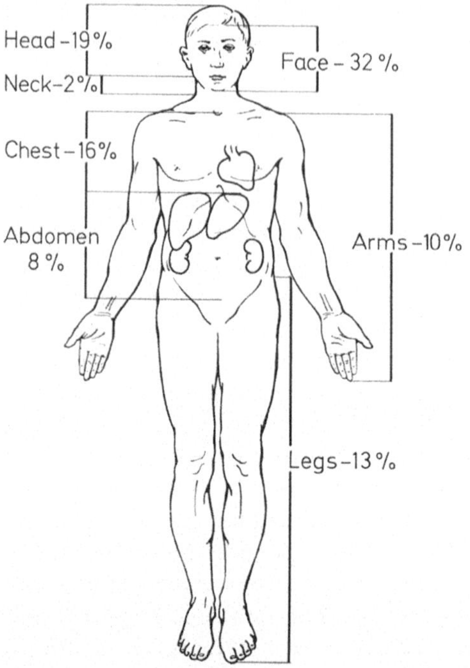

Fig. 3. Distribution of significant (no minor injuries included) injuries by body area

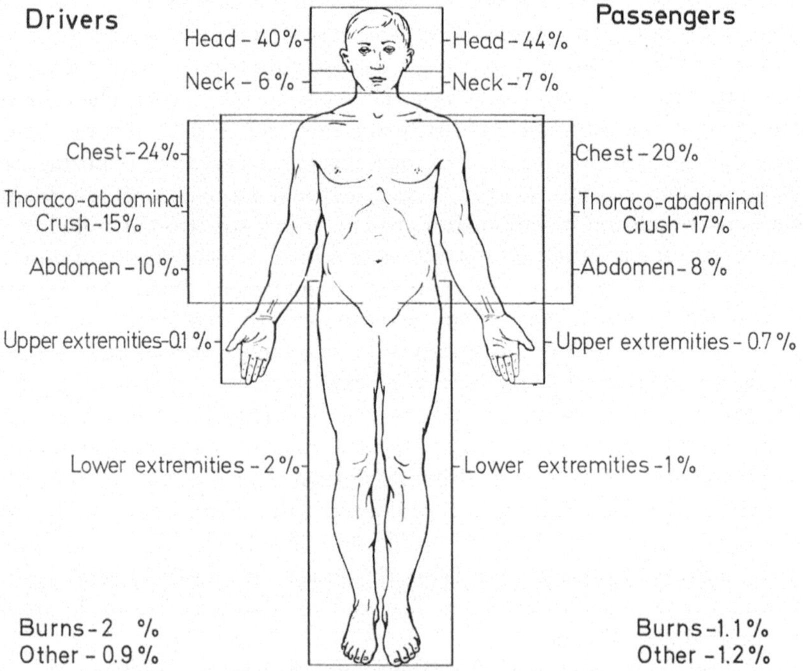

Fig. 4. Distribution of fatal injuries among drivers and passengers (for 2 years) (Courtesy Dr. Thomas T. Noguchi, Medical Examiner of Los Angeles County)

bruising, aortic rupture, and pulmonary lesions. Cardiac contusion may occur without rib fractures, but the other lesions ordinarily would not. Abdominal trauma follows a distinct pattern. Frontal impact to the driver produces abdominal trauma only if he contacts the steering wheel. This may vary from tear of the mesentery to liver laceration or blunt trauma to pancreas or a fixed area of the intestines. Left side impacts produce splenic lesions and rarely renal trauma. Right side impacts again may produce renal trauma or liver trauma. The right front seat passenger sustains blunt chest trauma against the panel, but rarely abdominal injury, except in the right side

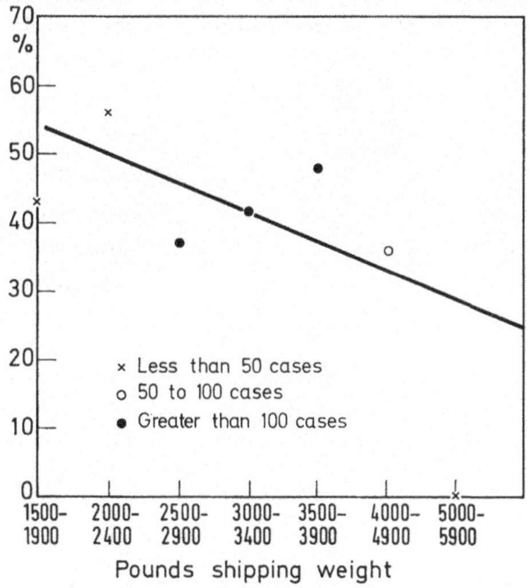

Fig. 5. Percent of occupants injured according to weight of car (frontal impacts)

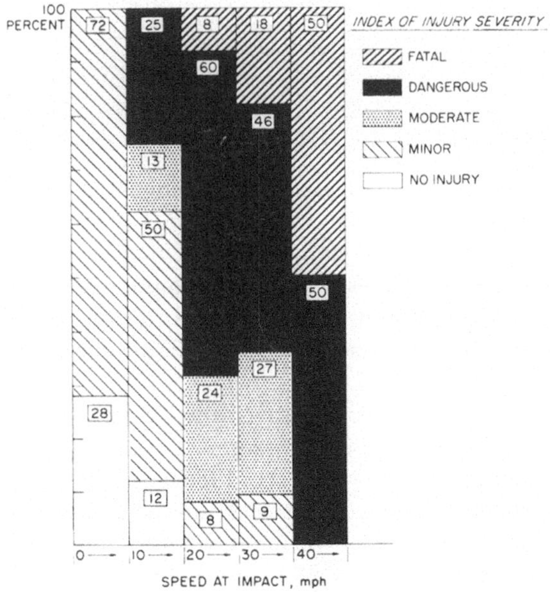

Fig. 6. Index of injury severity for chest contact against non-energy absorbing wheel-column (pre 1967)

impact in which the liver and kidney are particularly susceptible. The head injuries are the same as for the driver, but more common. Fractures of the pelvis occur only in side impacts, but lower extremity fractures may occur with any configuration.

Rear seat passengers rarely have abdominal trauma, except in side impact collisions which produce the same spectrum seen for front seat occupants. Blunt head trauma from contact with roof or header also occurs.

Mortality data collected on the computer of the coroner-medical examiner[1] tend to support these findings. Motorists were injured in a variety of collision situations. Injury patterns for drivers as opposed to (Fig. 4) passengers shows the slightly higher incidence of chest and abdominal injuries due to driver contacts with

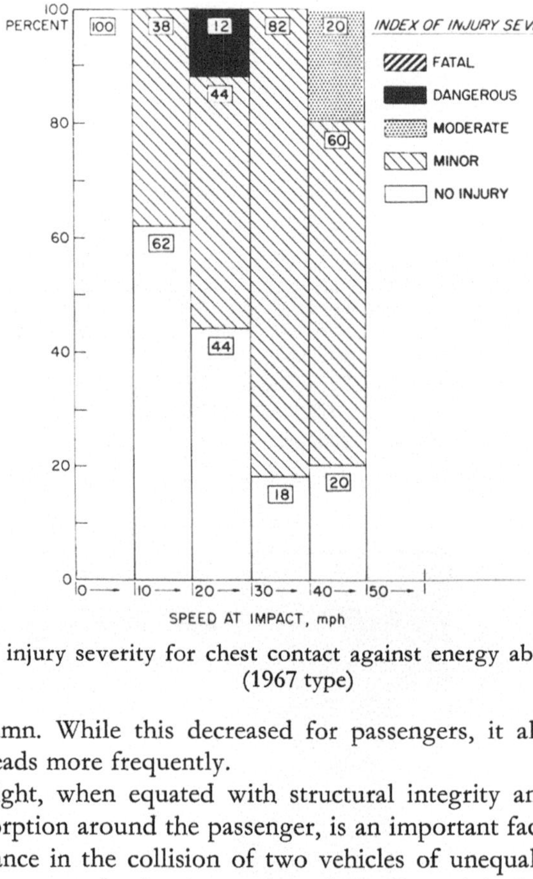

Fig. 7. Index of injury severity for chest contact against energy absorbing wheel-column (1967 type)

the wheel column. While this decreased for passengers, it also allowed them to contact their heads more frequently.

Vehicle weight, when equated with structural integrity and material available for energy absorption around the passenger, is an important factor. It assumes even greater importance in the collision of two vehicles of unequal weight and size. A tabulation supports a reduction in number of significant injuries with an increase in car weight (Fig. 5).

On the other hand, remarkable improvements in vehicle design through the years is serving to reduce the numbers of injuries. One example of this, the energy-absorbing steering column may cause a marked reduction in cardio-thoracic trauma. A tabulation of injuries (Fig. 6) in vehicles with and without this device show before a very significant (Fig. 7) proportion of injuries which appear to increase with an increase in speed. Measurements of collisions involving cars which have this new device show a remarkable decrease in the incidence of severe chest injuries.

[1] Courtesy of Thomas T. Noguchi, M. D., Los Angeles County Medical Examiner

Summary

The location, nature, and severity of much trauma can be predicted on the basis of a few facts about the accident, the vehicle, and the occupants. This information should be collected and made immediately available to the responsible physician. Important implications are noted in the diagnosis of blunt trauma and the education of surgeons.

References

NAHUM, A. M., Ed.: Early management of acute trauma. A Symposium. St. Louis: C. V. Mosby Co. 1966.

—, D. M. SEVERY, and A. W. SIEGEL: Automobile accidents correlated with collision experiments: Head-on collisions. Ninth Stapp Car Crash Conference Proc., Chap. 18, pp. 303—316, 1966.

—, and A. W. SIEGEL: Report to committee on commerce, U.S. Senate, April 1968.

— —, and P. V. HIGHT: Injuries to rear seat occupants in automobile collisions. Eleventh Stapp Car Crash Conference Proc., pp. 159—174, 1967.

— — —, and S. H. BROOKS: Lower extremity injuries of front seat occupants, SAE paper No. 680483, May 1968.

— —, and S. B. TRACHTENBERG: Causes of significant injuries in nonfatal traffic accidents, Tenth Stapp Car Crash Conference Proc., pp. 182—196, 1966.

LASKY, I. I., A. W. SIEGEL, and A. M. NAHUM: Automotive cardio-thoracic injuries: A medical-engineering analysis. SAE Auto Engineering Cong., paper No. 680052, (Jan.) 1968.

Physiology and Surgery of Peptic Ulcer

The Physiology of Duodenal Ulcer with Special Emphasis on Gastric Acid Secretion

Andrew W. Kay

Why should the duodenal mucosa in a minority of individuals be susceptible to the digestive action of gastric juice whereas in the majority it possesses a remarkable resistance? Many have sought the answer to this question believing that therein lay the solution to the peptic ulcer problem. Even to-day, our armamentarium strengthened by many new research tools and techniques, the explanation of the variable vulnerability of the duodenal mucosa evades us. By contrast knowledge of the physiology of gastric secretion has increased, modestly in relation to the pepsin moiety, considerably in relation to the acid moiety. And so, at the present time, the surgical management of duodenal ulcer has as its physiological basis the control of gastric acid secretion; an appreciation of the intricate mechanisms involved in acid production and of the effects of surgical operations on these mechanisms is desirable.

In a review of gastric acid secretion three elements merit consideration: the parietal cell mass, mechanisms which stimulate secretion, and inhibitory mechanisms.

The Parietal Cell Mass

Before the early 1950's the various tests of gastric acid secretion had taken no account of individual susceptibility to the stimulus used and, in all, the stimulus was short of maximal. In consequence, the tests lacked reproducibility and the stomach acquired the reputation of being a rather capricious organ. The augmented histamine test (Kay, 1953), the histalog test (Kirsner and Ford, 1955) and the maximal pentagastrin test (Abernethy et al., 1967) have now almost completely replaced all other gastric secretion tests based on sub-maximal stimulation.

The following important basic information, which is probably applicable to the histalog and pentagastrin tests, has been determined for the augmented histamine test. Firstly, it has an acceptable degree of reproducibility; secondly, the quantities of acid produced are within the range that can be released by physiological mechanisms (Gillespie and Masters, 1966); thirdly, the acid output achieved correlates closely with the actual number of parietal cells in the gastric mucosa and thus provides an index of the parietal cell mass (Card and Marks, 1960). These features have made tests of maximal acid secretion a valuable investigative tool, the use of which has added greatly to our knowledge of human gastric secretion.

It soon became evident that the parietal cell mass, as reflected in the results of augmented histamine tests, varied from individuals to individuals; the question of whether it was immutable for each individual had still to be answered. Crean (1968), using the rat as an experimental model, has studied the effects of duodenal obstruction and of chronic administration of pentagastrin. Moderate stenosis, produced by tying a ligature around the duodenum about 1 cm distal to the pyloro-duodenal junction, led to a marked hyperplasia of the gastric mucosa which was characterised by increased of the order of 60 to 70% in the surface area and volume of the mucosa, both in the fundus and antrum of the stomach; the population of both the parietal and peptic cells increased by about 60%. It would seem that the hyperplasia produced by duodenal obstruction represents the overgrowth of an otherwise normal mucosa with normal dimensional and cellular proportions so that the increases in parietal and peptic cell populations were proportional to the increase in the mass of the stomach mucosa as a whole. It seems possible that the effect may be analogous to the hyperplasia of the gastric mucosa which occurs in patients with long standing duodenal ulcer.

The effects of prolonged stimulation with pentagastrin were in sharp contrast. Hyperplasia of the parietal cells was produced without any increase in the peptic cell population and without any other major change in the gastric mucosa. This effect presumably represents a work hyperplasia associated with chronic hypersecretion and may be analogous to the situation in some patients with the Zollinger-Ellison syndrome. It is emphasised that the analogies drawn are only tentative and are offered as suggestions for future investigation rather than as firm conclusions. Meantime it can be concluded that the parietal cell mass is *not* immutable.

The Physiological Control of Gastric Acid Secretion

Stimulation of the parietal cell mass is under both nervous and hormonal influences. The nervous control is mediated through the vagus nerves; the hormonal influence is mediated mainly by gastrin secreted from the pyloric gland area and to a lesser extent by gastrin secreted from the mucosa of the upper reaches of the small intestine. Gastrin is also produced by pancreatic tumors in the Zollinger-Ellison syndrome but there is no direct evidence that it is released from the normal pancreas.

Inhibition of the parietal cell mass is mediated by influences acting on the mucosa of the antrum, the duodenum and, to a lesser extent, of the small intestine.

It will be seen that the vagus nerves and the pyloric antrum have a major part to play in the control of gastric acid secretion and it is these at sites that surgical attack is able to modify physiological mechanisms to reduce the acid hypersecretion characteristic of duodenal ulcer. It is therefore appropriate to consider firstly, the way in which vagal and antral influences control acid secretion and, secondly, the alterations effected by vagal nerve section and by antrectomy.

The Vagus and Gastric Acid Secretion

The vagus nerves facilitate the secretion of acid by the stomach in at least five ways and also participate in gastric acid inhibitor mechanisms.

Firstly, the vagus permits the direct transmission of stimuli to the acid secreting cells. It should be noted, however, that although psychic factors such as the sight, smell and anticipation of food are potent stimulants of gastric secretion in the dog, available evidence indicates that these factors alone stimulate only small amounts of acid secretion in man (NORING, 1951).

Secondly, there is now good evidence that intact vagal innervation to the parietal cell mass is essential for the full secretory response to circulating humoral stimuli, such as histamine and gastrin. The injection of either substance produces a good response in the presence of intact vagi, but lesser responses to the same dose after nerve section. Of particular interest is the finding in man that even the response to an augmented dose of histamine or a maximal stimulating dose of pentagastrin is reduced by approximately 70% after vagotomy. The demonstration by PAYNE and KAY (1962) that a stable choline-ester restores the post-vagotomy maximal histamine response to preoperative levels, emphasises the permissive role of vagally released acetylcholine at the gastric mucosal level with regard to histamine stimulation. Preliminary observations in man suggest that vagally released acetylcholine has a similar function with regard to gastrin stimulation.

Thirdly, vagal impulses reaching the pyloric antrum can directly release gastrin into the circulation. It is difficult to estimate the contribution made by this mechanism to the production of acid because, as is mentioned below, the acid released will acidify the antral mucosa and so tend to inhibit the further release of gastrin.

Fourthly, the vagus facilitates the local release of antral gastrin in response to chemical and mechanical stimuli and FORREST (1956) has shown that the fully innervated antrum in dogs responds better to such stimulation than does the denervated antrum.

Fifthly, the vagus may exert a controlling influence over the potentiating effect of distension of the fundic gland area. This mechanism was elucidated by GROSSMAN (1961) who showed that the response of a separated pouch in the dog to a small dose of stimulant, such as gastrin, can be greatly potentiated by the synchronous gentle distension of the pouch during the administration of the stimulant. The fact that this potentiation can be abolished by atropine indicates its cholinergic nature; as the pouches studied have been denervated, it seems likely that the cholinergic activity resides within the sub-mucosal plexuses. Although further evidence is required, it seems likely that the intact vagus would exert a controlling influence on this potentiating mechanism.

Finally, it is likely that the vagus nerves also modify inhibitor mechanisms of acid secretion. When acid from the stomach passes through the pylorus into the first part of the duodenum, the response to further stimulation of the parietal cells is inhibited. Clarification must await further studies but meantime it is of interest that JOHNSTON and DUTHIE (1964) have shown that the effectiveness of duodenal acid inhibition is reduced after vagotomy in man.

The Antrum and Gastric Acid Secretion

We have already seen that gastrin can be released from the pyloric antrum as a result of direct vagal stimulation. However more potent mechanisms exist and it is clearly established that gastrin can also be released by mechanical and by chemical stimulation of the antrum. Distension is the effective mechanical stimulus and is facilitated by an alkaline pH (WOODWARD et al., 1954). Effective chemical stimulation is exemplified by the local application of acetylcholine or ethanol, and by the introduction into the stomach of meat or liver extracts whose secretagogue action is due to their content of amino acids and choline.

The possibility that the presence of the pyloric antrum is essential for the full response of the parietal cells to direct vagal stimulation was first raised by UVNAS in 1942. He had shown that excision of the pyloric antrum reduced the response of the fundic glands in animals to electrical stimulation of the vagus nerve in the neck. The concept that the antrum may provide a background tone of circulating gastrin which plays a permissive role in the responsiveness of the acid secreting cells is supported by our own findings in man that antrectomy reduces the response of the stomach to an augmented dose of histamine (GILLESPIE et al., 1960). It is likely that the responses to acetylcholine, vagal impulses and other stimuli would similarly be reduced after antrectomy but there is not yet direct evidence for this in man.

The inhibitory effect on further secretion of acid by the stomach of acidifying the gastric content was observed over 60 years ago by SOKOLOV (1904). However almost a half century was to elapse before DRAGSTEDT made his inspired suggestion that the effect was due to inhibition of gastrin release, and subsequent work with his colleagues clearly estabilshed the antrum as the gastric site of the mechanism. It is indeed a striking paradox that antral inhibition is exerted from the site of a powerful excitatory mechanism for gastric acid secretion.

The Surgical Control of Gastric Acid Secretion

It is evident from this brief review of the intricate physiological mechanisms involved in the control of gastric acid secretion that vagal and antral influences can no longer be considered to be entirely separate in their actions. From the surgical standpoint this is fortunate in that a greater reduction in acid output is achieved from vagotomy alone and from antrectomy alone than would be expected if the two mechanisms were unrelated.

The effects on acid secretion of the operations commonly employed in the management of duodenal ulcer can be deduced from the information presented in this review. It should be borne in mind, however, that direct evidence in man for some of these effects is still awaited.

Effects of truncal vagotomy. Complete division of the vagus nerves can be expected to abolish the direct stimulation of the acid secreting cells by nervous stimuli and the direct vagal release of gastrin from the pyloric antrum. The local release of gastrin by distension and chemical stimulation is likely to be impaired by the absence of vagal influence. Again, the reduction in the cholinergic permissive background resulting from vagotomy will diminish the responsiveness of the parietal cells to most stimuli. Finally, the potentiation of chemical stimulation which occurs from distension of the fundic part of the stomach may be diminished in the absence of central vagal control. On the debit side, the inhibition of gastric acid secretion which occurs on acidification of the duodenum can be expected to be reduced after denervation.

Gastric secretion studies before and after vagotomy have shown that the overall effect of vagal nerve section is to reduce the maximal acid output of the stomach by about 70%.

Effects of antrectomy. The production, storage and release of gastrin by the mucosa of the pyloric antrum is inevitably lost after resection of that part of the stomach. Although more evidence is required in man, it seems likely that small amounts of gastrin may continue to be produced and released by the mucosa of the upper small intestine. Again, the action of gastrin in providing a permissive background without which vagal and perhaps all forms of stimulation cannot exert a full effect on the parietal cells will be absent or greatly reduced. Finally, on the debit side, the powerful inhibitory influence which functions when acid comes into contact with the antral mucosa will be lost.

The overall effect of antrectomy is to reduce the maximal acid output of the stomach by about 65%.

Partial gastrectomy can be expected to have the same effects as antrectomy but a further reduction in maximal acid output will occur and this will vary with the extent of resection of the acid secreting mucosa.

Antrectomy with vagotomy has a profound effect on the production of acid by the parietal cell mass. All major stimulatory mechanisms are thereby removed and this operation has the overall effect of reducing the maximal acid output by between 85 and 90%.

Conclusion

The past few decades have seen a considerable extension of our knowledge of the physiological mechanisms controlling the secretion of acid by the stomach. The surgical attack on these mechanisms is scarcely worthy of their delicacy but nevertheless it is usually effective in reducing acid secretion to levels at which duodenal ulcers can heal and remain healed. While research on physiological mechanisms should and will continue, the precise causation of duodenal ulceration is unlikely to be discovered by this approach alone. The time has come to increase our understanding of this disease by reaching right back into the cells of the duodenal mucosa in normal subjects and in those with peptic ulcer. In this context the application of biology at the cellular level is both desirable and mandatory.

References

ABERNETHY, R. J., I. E. GILLESPIE, J. H. LAWRIE, A. P. M. FORREST, R. A. PAYNE, A. BARABAS, I. D. A. JOHNSTON, G. P. BURNS, K. E. F. HOBBS, R. T. CLEGG, H. L. DUTHIE, and J. D. FITZGERALD: Lancet **1967 I**, 291—295.

CARD, W. I., and I. N. MARKS: Clin. Sci. **19**, 147—163 (1960).

CREAN, G. D., D. F. HOGG, and R. D. E. RUMSEY: Hyperplasia of the gastric mucosa produced by duodenal obstruction. In press.

FORREST, A. P. M.: The importance of the innervation of the pyloric antrum in the control of gastric secretion in dogs. XXth International Congress of Physiology. Abstract of communications **20**, 299 (1956).

GROSSMAN, M. I.: Gastroenterology **41**, 385 (1961).

JOHNSTON, D., and H. L. DUTHIE: Brit. J. Surg. **51**, 71 (1964).

KAY, A. W.: Brit. med. J. **1953 II**, 77—80.

KIRSNER, J. B., and H. FORD: J. Lab. clin. Med. **46**, 307—311 (1955).

MASTER, S. P., J-P. GOVAERTS, and I. E. GILLESPIE: Brit. J. Surg. **52**, 626 (1966).

NORING, O.: Gastroenterology **18**, 413 (1951).

PAYNE, R. A., and A. W. KAY: Clin. Sci. **22**, 373 (1962).

SOKOLOV, A. P. (1904): Quoted by B. P. BABKIN, New York, HOEBER: Secretory mechanism of the digestive clands. 1950.

UVNAS, B.: Acta physiol. scand. **4**. Suppl. 13, 1., (1942).

WOODWARD, E. R., E. S. LYON, J. LANDOR, and L. R. DRAGSTEDT: Gastroenterology **27**, 766 (1954).

Selective Vagotomy

CHARLES A. GRIFFITH

For the past 10 years the late HENRY N. HARKINS and I have claimed that selective vagotomy is a worthwhile refinement of Dragstedt's total vagotomy. This claim has not met general acceptance, and the vast majority of surgeons in the United States perform total vagotomy. I assume that the same holds true in Germany, although HOLLE and HART (1967) of Munich have reported their preference for selective vagotomy.

In comparing the two types of vagotomy by the standard criteria of mortality, recurrent ulcer, and gastrointestinal dysfunction, the only disadvantage of the selective technic is that it is more tedious and difficult to perform. This greater technical difficulty is of particular significance in obese and poor-risk patients undergoing urgent operation for bleeding or perforation. In these adverse circumstances we often perform the easier and quicker technic of total vagotomy. In patients of good risk undergoing elective operation we perform selective vagotomy because the technic is not overly difficult. This discriminate application of selective vagotomy has not increased our rates of postoperative morbidity and mortality. However, we caution that the indiscriminate performance of selective vagotomy upon all patients by inexperienced surgeons may well increase mortality.

The cardinal advantage of the selective technic over Dragstedt's technic is a lower rate of incomplete vagotomy and consequently a lower rate of recurrent ulcer. This advantage is based on the following anatomic considerations. Fig. 1: This diagram

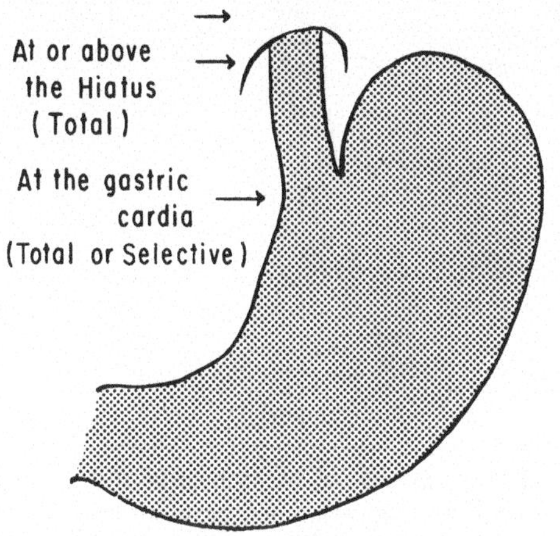

Fig. 1. The anatomic levels of the various technics of vagotomy. (From GRIFFITH and HARKINS, 1968)

shows the essential differences in the various technics of vagotomy. Dragstedt's technic of total vagotomy is performed at or just above the hiatus. In contrast, the selective technic is performed at the lower anatomic level of the gastric cardia. It is noted that at the gastric cardia either selective or total vagotomy may be performed. Fig. 2: This diagram shows that the vagal system consists of three constant components — the esophageal plexus, the two trunks, and the four truncal divisions (the hepatic, the celiac, and the anterior and posterior gastric divisions). However, by virtue of the fact that there is no anatomic relationship between the vagal system and the diaphragm, the vagi may descend through the hiatus as the esophageal plexus or the two trunks or the four truncal divisions. Failure to recognize this fundamental anatomic fact has led to the anatomically meaningless concept of "multiple vagus nerves". With this concept the surgeon performing vagotomy at the hiatus may not know how many nerves there are or where they are, and therefore may fail to find one or more nerves. Fig. 3: In this figure the anterior vagal system is shown as a single trunk at the hiatus in the diagram on your left and as the esophageal plexus in the diagram on your right. Both diagrams show that the anterior trunk or a branch of the esophageal plexus contributing to the anterior trunk may lie far away from the esophagus and adjacent to the patient's left hiatal margin. The arrows indicate the finger encircling the esophagus and the vagal fibers. In the diagram on your left the encircling finger at the hiatus does not include the anterior trunk, but failure to find this trunk should lead to continued search for it. However, in the diagram on your right, the encirclement of one branch of the esopgaheal plexus at the hiatus may

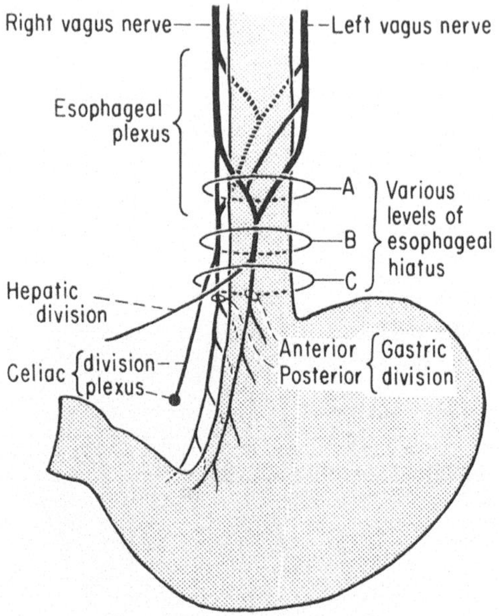

A. "Multiple nerves" of esophageal plexus
B. Two trunks (anterior and posterior)
C. "Multiple nerves" of truncal divisions

Fig. 2. The vagal system and the diaphragm. [From GRIFFITH, 1968 (1)]

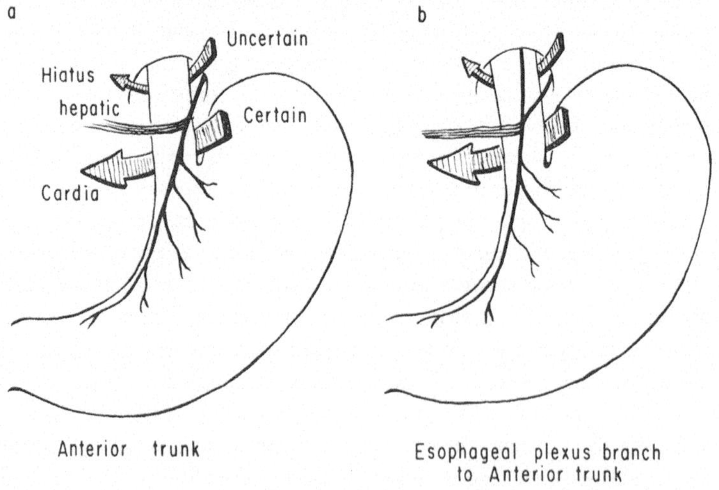

Fig. 3. The encirclement of the anterior vagi. (From GRIFFITH and HARKINS, 1968)

dissuade further search and the remaining branch is overlooked. In contrast to this uncertain encirclement at the hiatus, the encirclement at the gastric cardia is certain because all anterior gastric vagi always gather together at the cardia to innervate the stomach, and the anterior gastric truncal division always assumes a constant position adjacent to the lesser curve. Fig. 4: In this figure the posterior vagal system is

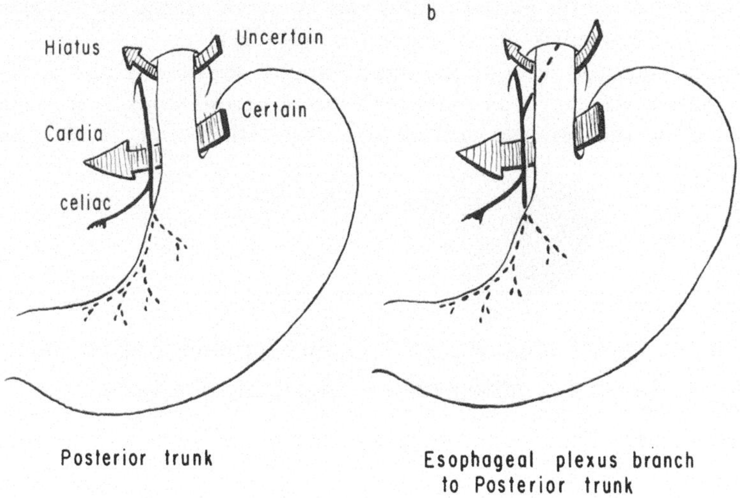

Fig. 4. The encirclement of the posterior vagi. (From GRIFFITH and HARKINS, 1968)

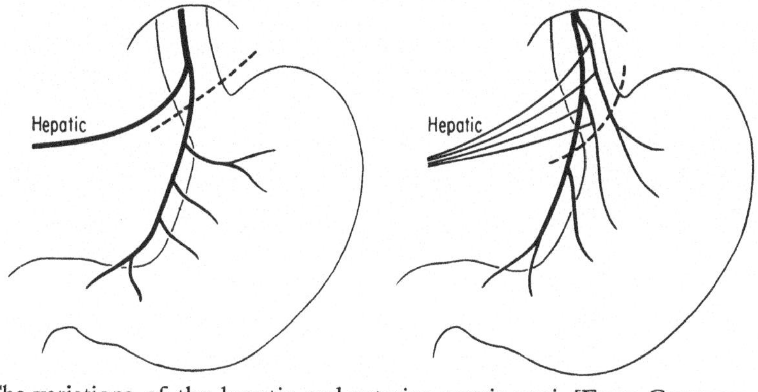

Fig. 5. The variations of the hepatic and anterior gastric vagi. [From GRIFFITH, 1968 (2)]

shown as a single trunk at the hiatus in the diagram on your left and as the esophageal plexus in the diagram on your right. Both diagrams show that the posterior trunk or a branch of the esophageal plexus contributing to the posterior trunk may lie far away from the esophagus in an extremely dorsal position adjacent to the right diaphragmatic crus and aorta. In this circumstance the encircling finger at the hiatus may fail to include the posterior trunk or a branch of the esophageal plexus for the same reasons as discussed in the previous figure. This error is probably the most frequent cause of incomplete vagotomy in the United States today, but does not occur at the gastric cardia because at the lower level of the cardia the continuation of the posterior trunk as the celiac division may be identified with certainty by palpating its constant course to the celiac autonomic plexus. By including the celiac division with the encircling finger, all posterior gastric vagi are encircled because all posterior gastric vagi always lie ventral to the celiac division. Fig. 5: This figure shows the variations that account for another anatomic type of incomplete vagotomy. In the diagram on your left the hepatic and celiac vagi exist as single fibers but in the diagram on your right as multiple fibers. Even though all of these multiple gastric vagi are encircled at the cardia, a small fiber to the gastric fundus may be overlooked if the distal esophagus is not carefully dissected as a final step in the operation.

The significance of recognizing these various anatomic types of incomplete vagotomy lies in the fact that vagal innervation of the stomach is segmental, as demonstrated by our studies with electric vagal stimulation in the presence of

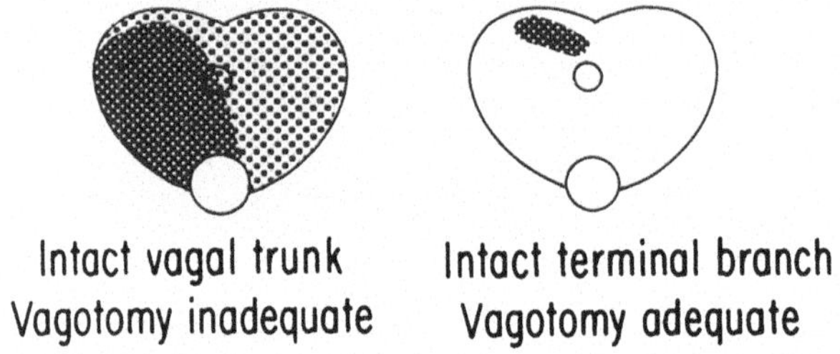

Fig. 6. The residual secretion after incomplete vagotomy of an intakt trunk and an intact terminal branch to the fundus. (From Pritchard et al., 1968)

Table 1. *Effects of various anatomic types of incomplete vagotomy in pyloric ligated shay rats*
[From Legros and Griffith, 1968 (*1*)]

	Both trunks intact (control)	One trunk intact	Fundic branch intact	Both trunks transected (control)
Gastric secretion	100%	65%	25%	20%
Gastric ulcer	100%	75%	0%	0%
Classification	—	Inadequate incomplete	Adequate incomplete	Adequate complete

circulating neutral red (Pritchard et al., 1968). Fig. 6: This figure shows the differences between an incomplete vagotomy of an intact trunk and an incomplete vagotomy of an intact terminal branch to the gastric fundus. In the diagram on your left, stimulation of one trunk elicits an initial secretion localized to the ipsilateral wall of the stomach (as indicated by the darker shading). With continued stimulation a delayed secretion appears from the contralateral wall (as indicated by the lighter shading). This contralateral secretion has been proven to be due to the vagal release of gastrin from the innervated antrum. The results of stimulating one branch of the esophageal plexus are similar, because the fibers of an esophageal plexus branch are distributed to a large area (approximately two-thirds) of the ipsilateral stomach including the antrum. In contrast, as shown in the diagram on your right, stimulation of a terminal branch to the fundus elicits a secretion localized to a small area in the fundus. No delayed generalized secretion appears because this fundic branch does not innervate the antrum.

In subsequent studies we have confirmed that an intact trunk is an *inadequate* vagotomy and an intact fundic branch is an *adequate vagotomy* [LEGROS and GRIFFITH, 1968 (*1*)]. Table 1: This table shows the comparative results in pyloric ligated Shay rats. After incomplete vagotomy of an intact trunk, gastric secretion is lowered to 65% of the control level and 75% of the rats develop gastric ulcer. In contrast, after incomplete vagotomy of an intact fundic branch, secretion is lowered to 25% and no rats develop ulcer. Table 2: This shows the results of insulin tests in dogs. After incomplete vagotomy of an intact trunk, the secretory response does not decrease but remains as large in amount and occurs as early in onset as the control response before vagotomy. In contrast, a significant decrease and delay in the response occurs after incomplete vagotomy of an intact fundic branch. Subsequent studies in each dog with

Table 2. *Secretory responses to insulin with incomplete vagotomy of an intact trunk and intact fundic branch*

[From LEGROS and GRIFFITH, 1968 (1)]

	Percentage of decrease in acid response from control response before vagotomy	Time of occurrence of maximal acid response after insulin	Percentage of residually innervated mucosa (by neutra red)
Dogs with one trunk intakt			
1	0%	30—60 min	50%
2	12%	30—60 min	50%
3	0%	30—60 min	50%
Dog with a fundic branch intact			
4	40%	90—150 min	8%
5	84%	90—150 min	4%
6	89%	90—150 min	4%

the method of neutral red permit a correlation between the type of response and the area of residually innervated mucosa.

ROSS and KAY (1964) have provided some evidence that patients with large and early insulin responses develop recurrent ulcer, whereas patients with small and delayed responses do not. In applying these criteria to the results of insulin tests after selective vagotomy reported by several surgeons to date (HEDENSTEDT and LUNDQUIST, 1966; BANK et al., 1967; AMDRUP et al., 1967; GRIFFITH, 1967; SAWYERS et al., 1968; SCHEINEN and INBERG, 1968), the over-all rates of positive responses are quite low and furthermore, the vast majority of the positive responses are of the small and delayed type indicative of adequate vagotomy.

The permanence of the adequacy of an adequate incomplete vagotomy may be questioned on the basis of vagal innervation by the phenomenon of sprouting (MURRAY, 1959; CLARK, 1964). By this phenomenon the small area of residual innervation due to an intact fundic branch may increase in size and result in an inadequate vagotomy. This possibility is currently under study in our laboratory by the method of neutral red in both rats and dogs. Preliminary results indicate no significant enlargement of the size of the residual area of innervation after 7 months, and therefore sprouting with this specific anatomic type of adequate incomplete vagotomy may be insignificant. Furthermore, we have observed the small and delayed insulin response up to 5 years after vagotomy, which indicates that an adequate vagotomy may remain adequate and not become inadequate due to sprouting.

Another reason for a lower rate of recurrent ulcer with selective vagotomy concerns the function of the hepatic and celiac fibers to the antrum. We have shown that the hepatic and celiac vagi have neither efferent motor fibers for antral motility (STAVNEY et al., 1963) nor efferent secretory fibers for the release of gastrin [LEGROS and GRIFFITH, 1968(*2*)]. Their function remained unknown until HART (1967) demonstrated that the antral branches from the hepatic and celiac vagi inhibit gastric secretion. This inhibitory function suggests that selective vagotomy lowers gastric secretion more effectively than total vagotomy. Table 3: This table shows the results of a recent study (SHIINA and GRIFFITH, 1968) comparing the effects of selective and total vagotomy upon the secretion from Heidenhein pouches in dogs. After selective vagotomy there is a small increase in secretion over the control level. After total vagotomy there is a large increase in secretion, and statistical analysis with the Student t Test confirms that this large increase is quite significant. In this study tests with insulin and with neutral red demonstrated that the degree of completeness of gastric vagotomy was the same after selective and total vagotomy, and X-rays with barium meals showed a definite gastric stasis after selective vagotomy and only a slight increase in gastrointestinal stasis after total vagotomy. Therefore, the results of the pouch secretions can only be explained by inhibition of gastric secretion by the hepatic and celiac vagi preserved with selective vagotomy and elimination of this inhibition by transection of the hepatic and celiac vagi with total vagotomy.

Table 3. *Means and standard deviations of titratable acid (mEq) from Heidenhain Pouch Secretions for 30 days before and after selective and total vagotomy*

(From SHIINA and GRIFFITH, 1968)

	Control	Selective vagotomy	Total vagotomy
Grouped data (five dogs)	43.88 ± 16.72	53.59 ± 22.20	93.33 ± 32.96

Statistical comparison of operative procedures with student t test

Control with selective	Control with total	Seclective with total
$t = 4.28$ $p < 0.001$	$t = 16.38$ $p < 0.001$	$t = 12.25$ $p < 0,001$

This inhibition of gastric secretion by the hepatic and celiac vagi to the antrum is of no clinical significance when the antrum is removed with antrectomy, but may well be quite significant when the antrum is preserved with pyloroplasty. With this concept in mind, LOEWENECK and his colleagues in the Anatomic Institute at the University of Munich studied the variations of the hepatic and celiac vagal branches to the antrum. In most cadavers these branches run a course quite separate from the gastric vagi and therefore are preserved by the technic of selective vagotomy. In a few cadavers however, these branches run to the antrum in close association with the gastric vagi and would be transected with the gastric vagi by selective vagotomy. These anatomic variations of the hepatic and celiac branches to the antrum may be a factor in the variable results of selective and total vagotomy in decreasing gastric secretion. Table 4: This table shows the results of 62 patients with duodenal ulcer operated upon consecutively by selective vagotomy plus Finney pyloroplasty during the years 1963 through 1965. Of these 62 patients, 40 had no free acid in their fasting basal gastric secretion. The remaining 22 patients had variable amounts of free acid. In regard to the presence of free acid after vagotomy, I must state parenthetically that many American surgeons have the erroneous concept that complete vagotomy of the stomach is always followed by no free acid. How this erroneous concept came about I am unable to state, for DRAGSTEDT has repeatedly emphasized that complete vagotomy only lowers the acid in the fasting secretion but does not always lower it to the state of no free acid. At any rate, all of the 22 patients with free acid in this table underwent one or more insulin tests and all tests were negative. The majority of these patients with free acid showed a significant reduction of preoperative hypersecretion to a level of normal secretion. However, three patients, particularly the patient with an hourly secretion of 8.9 milliequivalents of free acid, did not show any reduction in gastric secretion despite a complete vagotomy as determined by negative insulin tests. This phenomenon of persistent hypersecretion with complete vagotomy was first reported by DRAGSTEDT's group (WOODWARD et al., 1949) and has since been confirmed by other investigators (GELB et al., 1961; GILLESPIE and KAY, 1961). GILLESPIE and KAY proposed that this persistent hypersecretion is due to antral hyperfunction. The question may be raised that this antral hyperfunction is related to a loss of antral inhibition, and that in patients with persistent hypersecretion the hepatic and celiac vagi to the antrum were transected with the gastric vagi by virtue of the anatomic variations described by LOEWENECK and his colleagues. It may be significant that none of our patients with selective vagotomy has developed recurrent ulcer, and the three patients with persistent hypersecretion have been followed for 4 to 5 years. In contrast, one of nine patients operated upon during this period of study with total vagotomy plus pyloroplasty has developed recurrent ulcer with a negative insulin test. However, the drawing of definite conclusions concerning the over-all rate of recurrent ulcer must await further studies of more patients with longer follow-ups.

Table 4. *Postoperative basal secretions in 62 patients with selective vagotomy plus pyloroplasty* (From GRIFFITH, 1967)

Number of patients	mEq free acid/h
40	0
17	0—1.5
1	1.76
1	1.99
1	2.78
1	3.70
1	8,93

Although the foregoing considerations suggest the advantage of preserving the hepatic and celiac vagi in order to preserve the inhibition of the antral phase of gastric secretion (and also the inhibition of the intestinal phase of gastric secretion as demonstrated by KELLY et al., 1964 and MIDDLETON et al., 1965), the advantage of preserving the hepatic and celiac vagal phases of secretions from the viscera of the mid gut has not been confirmed. In most comparative studies of selective and total vagotomy, no significant differences in digestion and absorption and over-all nutrition have been established. However, we remain concerned about the differences in motility of the viscera of the mid gut. For example, the gall bladder dilates after total anterior vagotomy but does not dilate after selective anterior vagotomy (Rudick and Hutchison, 1965). In one patient with a normal preoperative cholecystogram, selective hepatic vagotomy was done to facilitate exposure of the diaphragmatic hiatus in order to repair a hiatal hernia. 4 years later this patient returned with symptoms of biliary colic. Cholecystography demonstrated poor visualization of a markedly dilated gall bladder, which was removed in the subsequent year because of repeated attacks of biliary colic. The gall bladder contained thick biliary sludge and mud but no stones. Another example is the occasional result of severe and prolonged postoperative ileus. In one patient with a severe ileus 8 days after selective anterior-total posterior vagotomy, barium enema showed a dilated and flaccid mid gut denervated by celiac vagotomy but a normal tonus of the hind gut (descending colon) innervated by the sacral parasympathetics. The long-term significance of this hypomotile change in the mid gut after total vagotomy remains unknown (Isaac et al., 1950; Ballinger, 1966).

Table 5. *Selective vs. total vagotomy*

	Selective at cardia	Total at cardia	Total at hiatus
Rate of incomplete	same		higher
Technical difficulty	more	same	
Side effects	less	same	

In summary (Table 5) we recognize three technics of vagotomy — selective at the gastric cardia, total at the cardia, and total at the hiatus. By virtue of the certain encirclement of all gastric vagi at the cardia and the uncertain encirclement at the hiatus, the rates of incomplete vagotomy by the selective and total technics at the cardia are the same but lower than with total vagotomy at the hiatus. The selective technic is more difficult and therefore we do not perform it upon all patients. The technical difficulties with total vagotomy at the cardia and at the hiatus are equal. Therefore, when we do perform total vagotomy, we perform it at the cardia in order to insure the result of complete or adequate vagotomy. The undesirable side effects are less with selective vagotomy because sparing the hepatic and celiac vagi preserves the motility of the biliary tract and intestine, and also preserves the inhibition of the antral and intestinal phases of gastric secretion.

From these considerations, and in conclusion, we continue to claim that the selective technic is a worthwhile refinement of the total technic, and continue to perform selective vagotomy whenever the specific operative circumstances indicate its safe performance.

References

Amdrup, E., T. Clemmesen, and J. Andreassen: Amer. J. dig. Dis. **12**, 351—355 (1967).
Ballinger, W. F., II: Surg. Clin. N. Amer. **46**, 455—462 (1966).
Bank, S., I. N. Marks, and J. H. Louw: Gut **8**, 36—41 (1967).
Clark, C. G.: Brit. J. Surg. **51**, 539—542 (1964).
Gelb, M., I. D. Baronofsky, and H. D. Janowitz: Gut **2**, 240—245 (1961).
Gillespie, I. E., and A. W. Kay: Brit. med. J. **1961 I**, 1557—1560.

Griffith, C. A.: Amer. J. dig. Dis. **12**, 333—350 (1967).
— (1) Anatomy, in surgery of the stomach and duodenum. Ed. by Harkins, H. N., and L. M. Nyhus, 2nd ed. Boston: Little Brown & Co. 1968.
— (2) Selective gastric vagotomy, in surgery of the stomach and duodenum. Ed. by Harkins, H. N., and L. M. Nyhus, 2nd ed. Boston: Little Brown & Co., 1968.
—, and H. N. Harkins: Selective gastric vagotomy, in abdominal operations. Ed. by R. Maingot, 5th ed. New York: Appleton-Century-Crofts 1968.
Hart, W.: New aspects on the antral inhibition and their significance for ulcer surgery. Presented to the International Society of Surgeons, Vienna, 1967.
Hedenstedt, S., and G. Lundquist: Acta chir. scand. **131**, 448—459 (1966).
Holle, V. F., and W. Hart: Med. Klin. **62**, 441—450. (1967).
Isaac, F., R. E. Ottoman, and J. A. Weinberg: Amer. J. Roentgenol. **63**, 66—75 (1950).
Kelly, K. A., L. M. Nyhus, and H. N. Harkins: Gastrioenterology **46**, 163—166 (1964).
Legros, G., and C. A. Griffith: (1) The anatomic basis for the variable adequacy of incomplete vagotomy. (Submitted for Publication) (1968).
— — (2) The anatomic pathways for vagal innervation of the antrum. (Submitted for Publication) (1968).
Loeweneck, H. v., M. v. Ludinghausen, and W. Mempel: Münch. med. Wschr. **109**, 1754—1762 (1967).
Middleton, M. D., K. A. Kelly, L. M. Nyhus, and H. N. Harkins: Gut **6**, 296—300 (1965).
Murray, J. G.: J. roy. Coll. Surg. Edinb. **4**, 199—217 (1959).
Pritchard, G. R., C. A. Griffith, and H. N. Harkins: Surg. Gynec. Obstet. **126**, 791—798 (1968).
Ross, B., and A. W. Kay: Gastroenterology **46**, 379—385 (1964).
Rudick, J., and J. S. F. Hutchinson: Ann. Surg. **162**, 234—240 (1965).
Sawyers, J. L., H. W. Scott Jr., W. H. Edwards, H. J. Shull, and D. H. Law: Amer. J. Surg. **115**, 165—171 (1968).
Scheinin, T. M., and M. V. Inberg: Acta chir. scand. **133**, 533—537 (1968).
Shiina, E., and C. A. Griffith: Selective and total vagotomy without drainage. (Submitted for Publication). (1968).
Stavney, L. S., T. Kato, C. A. Griffith, L. M. Nyhus, and H. N. Harkins: J. surg. Res. **3**, 390—394 (1963).
Woodward, R. R., P. V. Harper Jr., E. B. Tovee, and L. R. Dragstedt: Arch. Surg. **59**, 1191—1212 (1949).
Yamagishi, M., T. Okubo, T. Yonemoto, T. Kasagawa, and S. Morita: Stomach and Intestine **2**, 195—202 (1967).

Treatment of Bleeding Gastric and Duodenal Ulcers*

Ludwig Zukschwerdt and Eduard Farthmann

The frequency of massive hemorrhage from peptic ulcers generally has increased (Edelmann), due partly to extragastric ulcerogenic factors (Table 1) often combined with coagulation defects, partly to long-term administration of anticoagulants. The following *principles of treatment* for massive bleeding from peptic ulcerations have emerged:

1. The results of strictly conservative or operative management are poor. Individual evaluation is necessary.

2. Operations to remove the peptic ulceration carry a considerably lower risk when performed during the interval. The mortality of gastric resection during hemorrhage amounts to 20 to 30% (Blanc et al.; Brooks and Eraklis; Dalichau

* From the Department of Surgery, University Hospitals, University of Hamburg, Germany.

et al.; FOSTER et al., 1963). Control of bleeding by conservative means should be attempted whenever possible.

3. The older the patient, the more dangerous are the consequences of protacted hemorrhagic shock.

4. Prognosis is impaired by every recurrence.

5. Unrelieved pyloric obstruction increases the danger of recurrent hemorrhage.

6. Definite preoperative diagnosis reduces the operative risk.

7. Operation should be performed only after clotting defects have been corrected.

8. Intractable hemorrhagic shock despite adequate volume replacement (2000 ml) demands immediate operation. Simultaneous treatment of shock sequelae is imperative.

9. Massive hemorrhage not infrequently leads to overtransfusion. Continuous monitoring of venous pressure is necessary.

10. The use of vasopressors in shock not responding to volume replacement may further impair the blood supply of liver and kidneys.

Table 1. *Peptic ulcers of extragastric origin*

1. *Curling's ulcer* following burns
2. *Cushing's ulcer* following tumor, operation or trauma at the midbrain-pituitary area
3. *Stress ulcer*
4. *Ulcer of hepatic origin*
5. *Drug-induced ulcer* (salicylates, phenylbutazone, reserpine, adrenal steroids)
6. *Ulcer combined with endocrine adenoma*
   a) pancreatic adenoma (Zollinger-Ellison syndrome)
   b) adrenal cortical adenoma
   c) parathyroid adenoma
   d) pluriglandular adenomata (Wermer's disease)

The initial therapeutic measure is *treatment of shock* by volume replacement. At the same time *baseline data* should be established for impaired parameters: arterial and venous pressure, blood volume, urine output, hemoglobin, hematocrit, serum minerals, blood pH, clotting mechanism, bilirubin, blood urea nitrogen. Later evaluations may be difficult due to the lack of initial data.

This principle holds true especially for *primary and secondary clotting defects* (Table 2). The latter occur frequently following massive transfusions. If overlooked they lead to unnecessary operations, increase operative risk, and often cause immediate postoperative rebleedings. *Acidosis* not infrequently causes unsatisfactory reaction to sufficient volume replacement and should therefore be corrected.

The administration of hypotensive drugs inducing *peripheral vasodilatation* is debatable and not recommended prior to transfusion of a least two pints of blood in 30 min. Blood pressure should not fall below 100 mmHg. Indication for this type of treatment may be considered in case of unstable arterial pressure, high venous pressure, and lack of acidosis. BLANC et al. report surprising results.

At the beginning of treatment a *nasogastric tube* is passed. A stomach full of clots should be emptied to reduce distension of the walls with impairment of spontaneous hemostasis. Severely ill patients require an *indwelling catheter* to check urine output. We were able to resuscitate three pulseless patients by intraarterial and, in one case, intraaortal transfusion.

Vital signs having stabilized, the *source of bleeding* should be localized as exactly as possible.

1. *Clinical evaluation.* History (earlier hemorrhages and X-ray examinations), physical findings, and laboratory data will establish the diagnosis in about two thirds of the patients. Differential diagnosis of peptic ulcer vs. esophageal varices has leading importance. Possible ulcers of hepatic origin (LIPP and LIPSITZ) demand examination of the stomach even in the presence of proven esophageal varices.

2. *Radiology.* "Steroid ulcers" should be examined by a plain film of the abdomen to rule out simultaneous perforation causing few symptoms if any. Prior to X-ray examination — using water soluble contrast media instead of barium — the stomach should be emptied. Failure to do this frequently results in missed diagnosis. Radiological and clinical evaluation will lead to the right diagnosis in about 70% of patients.

3. *Esophago-gastroscopy* is indicated after negative X-ray examination and in case of suspected bleeding at the esophago-cardiac junction (Mallory-Weiss syndrome etc.).

Table 2. *Coagulation defects in gastric or duodenal hemorrhage*[a]

Bleeding lesion	No of patients	Primary[b] defect	Secondary[c] defect	Total	%
Peptic ulcer	24	2	15	17	71
1. gastric ulcer					
2. duodenal ulcer	16	—	8	8	50
Ulcer of hepatic origin					
and/or erosive gastritis	6	—	6	6	100
Stress or drug-induced ulcer	5	—	5	5	100
Total	51	2	34	36	71

[a] Patients with complete analysis of coagulation mechanism only.
[b] Hemophilia A and thrombocytopenia.
[c] Impaired factor synthesis, fibrinolysis, and/or defect secondary to diffuse intravascular coagulation.

Immediate (peracute) operation is indicated by intractability of life-threatening shock despite massive volume replacement. The indication should be narrow, however. Mortality is high because the source of bleeding is unknown and impaired functions cannot previously be corrected. Intraoperative evaluation often is difficult. We observed intrathoracic cysts and diverticula lined by gastric mucosa penetrating into the heart and aorta, aneurysms penetrating into the duodenum etc.

Urgent operation is the most frequent acute procedure and indicated by instability of vital signs despite continuous volume replacement, i.e. by bleeding not responding to conservative treatment. Prognosis deteriorates with the duration of this situation. The dominant problem therefore is recognition of continuous bleeding. Clues can be derived from (1) gastric secretion, (2) behavior of vital signs, (3) blood volume, (4) hemoglobin and hematocrit. Additional determination of venous pressure is necessary.

Internists frequently attach greater value to vital signs than to hemoglobin and hematocrit which are thought to lag behind. Surgeons tend to rely more on hemoglobin and hematocrit because centralized circulation and volume replacement can keep blood pressure and pulse within normal limits even after hemoglobin and hematocrit are already altered (ZUKSCHWERDT et al.). The importance of blood volume determinations is questioned by physiologists (blood depots). Therefore hemoglobin, hematocrit, pulse, arterial and venous pressure, and — if possible — blood volume should be measured. A single determination only points to the dependency of mortality from the impairment of initial values. Indication for operation is derived from *continuous registration in short intervals* (Fig. 1) demonstrating the tendency and turning-point to operative therapy (ZUKSCHWERDT and GIEBEL).

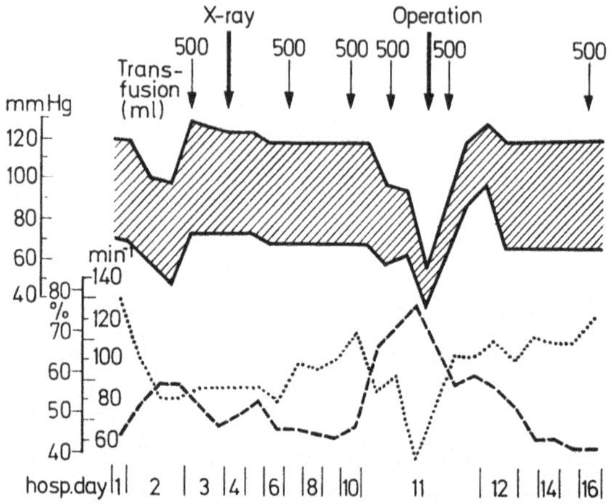

Fig. 1. Blood pressure (=), pulse (— —), and hemoglobin (. . . .) in case of bleeding duodenal ulcer (male, 47 years)

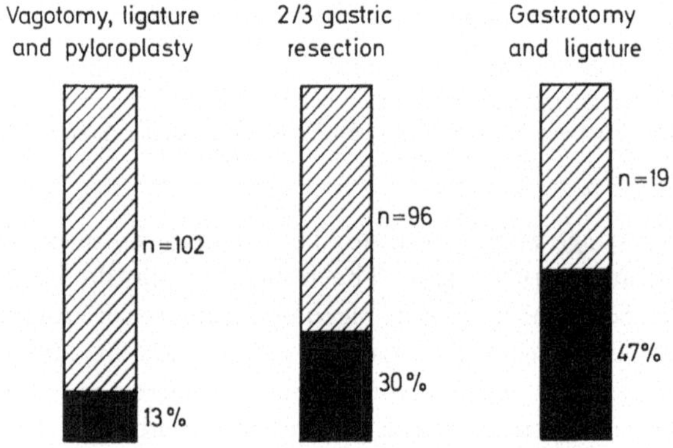

Fig. 2. Operative mortality of different procedures for bleeding peptic ulcer. (n = number of patients) (After FOSTER, J. H. et al., 1966)

Patients with massive hemorrhage in medical as well as in surgical departments should be kept in intensive care units for at least 48 h after definite hemostasis. Close observation by a doctor throughout the night is indispensible because recurrences otherwise are noted not before the morning, explaining the lesser mortality of gastrointestinal hemorrhage in private patients (MAYO and OWENS).

Among *operative procedures* two thirds resection and vagotomy with pyloroplasty or antrectomy should be considered. Primary mortality is lower following vagotomy (Fig. 2). We observed postoperative hemorrhage in only 2% after 112 resections, however. They subsided after correction of clotting defects. FOSTER et al. (1966) report 8% recurring hemorrhages following vagotomy, ligation, and pyloroplasty with two deaths. In addition the long-term higher incidence of recurrent ulcerations after vagotomy as compared to resection should be considered because not infrequently they require second operations with corresponding mortality. Both procedures may therefore be regarded as equally acceptable for the time being. Simple ligation of the bleeding vessel is unsatisfactory even in combination with gastroenterostomy. In desolate cases splanchnic infiltration seems to yield surprising results (MIALARET et al.). Gastric cooling has not fulfilled original expectations. We were able to control bleeding from a huge subcardiac ulcer by local application of carbon dioxide snow via an esophagoscope.

Special Problems

No diagnosis of bleeding source by non-operative diagnostic procedures:

1. The complete *clotting system* should be investigated at first. Correction of defects will control two thirds of these bleedings.

2. *Exploratory laparotomy* with gastrotomy. Even after opening the stomach 10 to 15% bleeding sites remain obscure (BIRKE and ENGSTEDT, FOSTER et al., 1966; RETZLAFF et al.). In 49 of 191 cases BIRKE and ENGSTEDT later found an ulcer, in 6 a benign, and in 24 a malign tumor. Still, 86 patients did not rebleed following laparotomy. As for operative procedure: revision of stomach and duodenum first (posterior wall, cardia); if negative: revision of the entire gut; if negative: gastrotomy.

Following questions may arise:

a) How to proceed in case of "*bleeding gastritis*"? Hypochlorhydria is not infrequently found explaining rebleeding after resection or vagotomy (WADDELL). Coagulation defects (ZUKSCHWERDT and THIES) may cause massive bleeding from tiny erosions. Therefore treatment should be conservative. High acid levels are indicative of gastritis accompaning an ulcer and justify acid-reducing operations.

b) How to proceed if repeated interventions, even "blind" resections, failed to reveal the source of bleeding? Gastric manifestation of *Osler's disease* (SMITH et al.) should be suspected. We were able to confirm the diagnosis in three patients using the following method: a white woolen thread is passed into the duodenum and left in place over night. After removal the hight of bleeding can be identified by aspect, chemical blood identification, isotopes or fluorescence. Resection can than be carried out. Retroperitoneal arterio-venous hemangioma involving the stomach may cause severe hemorrhage. Identification by angiography and operative removal of the cardiac half of the stomach proved successful to us.

c) How to proceed in case of "*innocent*" *diverticula* of the stomach, duodenum or jejunum? They should be removed because hemorrhages as a rule do not recur (RETZLAFF et al.).

Bleeding from special ulcer types:

1. The *steroid ulcer* has a tendency to bleed and perforate (MIALARET et al.). Operative mortality is high because of underlying disease. The atrophied adrenal cortices are exhausted by hemorrhagic shock and require high dosage substitution.

2. *Stress ulcer*, frequently found in patients hospitalized and operated upon, carry a high operative risk, too, because of concomitant disease (septic infections, operations of long duration) (FOSTER et al., 1966). Frequent impairment of liver function explains simultaneous clotting defects. Conservative treatment should be tried.

3. *Ulcers of hepatic origin* are more frequent than suspected. Normally gastrin reaching the liver via the portal vein is partly inactivated. In liver disease the regulation may be deficient (DUBUQUE et al.; LEBEDINSKAJA; STELZNER), explaining the frequency of gastritis with or without ulcer, impairment of clotting mechanism, and bleeding tendency. Following portocaval shunt gastrin regulation by the liver is completely absent, as shown experimentally (SKILLMANN et al., STELZNER) and clinically. Resulting hyperchlorhydria justifies acid-redusing operations.

Management following conservative hemostasis: Intensive care should be continued for at least 48 h. Premature transferal is dangerous. In case of recurrent bleeding immediate operation should be performed.

In summary, following points deserve attention: the bleeding tendency in ulcers of extragastric origin; the frequency of primary or acquired clotting defects; the importance of acidosis in hemorrhagic shock, and the necessity of intensive care with graphic registration of all parameters. Detection of the right moment for operative intervention determines the prognosis. Therefore the results of operative treatment of bleeding ulcers are a further test of cooperation between internist and surgeon.

References

BLANC, J. F., B. CONSTANTIN, V. BAQUE et A. HERVÉ: Mém. Acad. Chir. **92**, 695 (1966).
BIRKE, G., u. L. ENGSTEDT: Gastroenterologia (Basel) **85**, 97 (1956).
BROOKS, J. R., and A. J. ERAKLITS: New Engl. J. Med. **271**, 803 (1964).
DALICHAU, H., E. UNGEHEUER und G. SCHADE: Med. Klin. **63**, 587 (1968).
DUBUQUE, T. J., L. V. MULLIGAN, and E. C. NEVILLE: Surg. Forum **8**, 208 (1958).
EDELMANN, G., P. BOUTELIER et J. BRENOT: Mém. Acad. Chir. **92**, 304 (1966).
FOSTER, J. H., D. F. HICKOK, and J. E. DUNPHY: Surg. Gynec. Obstet. **117**, 257 (1963).
—, A. D. HALL, and J. E. DUNPHY: Surg. Clin. N. Amer. **46**, 387 (1966).
LEBEDINSKAJA, S. J.: Z. ges. exp. Med. **88**, 264 (1933).
LIPP, W. F., and M. H. LIPSITZ: Gastroenterology **22**, 181 (1952).
MAYO, H. W., and J. K. OWENS: Surgery **36**, 412 (1954).
MIALARET, J., H. CHARLEUX, M. JULIEN et M. THOMAS: Mém. Acad. Chir. **92**, 744 (1966).
RETZLAFF, J. A., B. A. HAGEDORN, and L. G. BARTHOLOMEW: J. Amer. med. Ass. **177**, 104 (1961).
SKILLMAN, J. J., W. SILEN, H. A. HARPER, J. C. NEELEY, and E. L. SIMMONS: Surg. Forum **12**, 276 (1961).
SMITH, C. R., L. G. BARTHOLOMEW, and J. D. CAIN: Gastroenterology **44**, 1 (1963).
STELZNER, F.: Langenbecks Arch. klin. Chir. **308**, 439 (1964).
ZUKSCHWERDT, L., u. M. G. GIEBEL: Die Indikation zur Behandlung der massiven Magenblutung. In: Chirurgische Indikationen. Stuttgart: Thieme 1956.
—, u. H. A. THIES: Internist (Berl.) **8**, 62 (1967).
—, W. HAHN und I. PETERSEN: Dtsch. med. Wschr. **78**, 1725 (1953).
WADDELL, W. R.: Surg. Clin. N. Amer. **46**, 397 (1966).

High Gastric Ulcers

CLAUDE E. WELCH and JOHN F. BURKE

High Gastric Ulcers

Ulcers located in the upper part of the stomach have demanded increasing attention in recent years. Not only have they become more common, but they also frequently are accompanied by serious complications that require difficult surgery to correct. For these reasons, it has seemed wise to consider this group of ulcers as an entity.

In order that factual data might be presented, approximately 1 000 gastric ulcers observed in the records of the Massachusetts General Hospital during the past 10 years have been studied. 50 cases have been identified and will form the basis for this study.

Definition. The word "high" will have different connotations to various observers. In this paper, it will denote either those ulcers arising in the proximal third of the stomach or which are present in a hiatus hernia. It is apparent that the definition must be somewhat flexible; for example, an ulcer in a para-esophageal hernia that contains the entire stomach may be found, after reduction of the hernia, to be near the angularis. The diagnostic and technical problems, however, are no different than occur with the

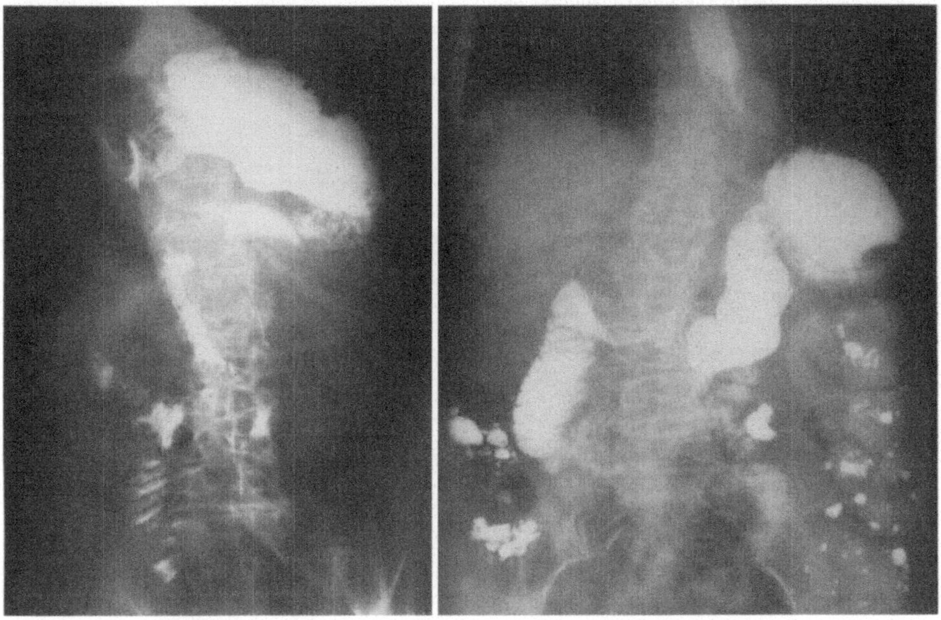

Fig. 1. left: Large gastric ulcer on lesser curvature in a para-hiatal hernia. right: The hernia has been repaired. Three weeks later volvulus at the site of the ulcer scar required gastric resection

other ulcers which, in the absence of a hiatus hernia, are situated just below the esophagus.

Such ulcers occur at or above the level where the left gastric artery reaches the lesser curvature or on the greater curvature above the lower two or three of the vasa brevia. The upper margin of the ulceration provides the important technical consideration. Obviously, large ulcers may extend well down into the body of the stomach.

Types of ulcers. These ulcerating lesions may be of several types that fall into distinct clinical groups. The majority can be classified as typical chronic gastric ulcers. Small groups include erosive fundal gastritis, ulceration secondary to a cirsoid aneurysm, stress ulcers, lacerations or perforations secondary to the Mallory-Weiss syndrome, and gastric cancers masquerading as benign ulcers. Of much more importance is the fact that any of these lesions may appear in hiatus hernias. The distribution in this series is shown in Table 1.

Incidence. This group of 50 represents approximately 5% of all gastric ulcers seen in this hospital in the last 10 years. On the other hand, because of the frequency of severe hemorrhage, they included 12% of all operations for gastric ulcers during this period. It is thus apparent that this group is comparatively small—a rather fortunate feature. It is of interest that nearly twice as many gastric ulcers appeared in the M. G. H. in the years 1958 to 1967 as in the previous decade. This disease is one of old age,

Table 1. *High gastric ulcers, clinical groups*

	Number of patients
Chronic gastric ulcers	30
Hiatus hernia with ulcer erosions	9
Erosive fundal gastritis	4
Cirsoid aneurysm	1
Mallory-Weiss laceration	0
Stress ulcer	0
Possible cancer	6

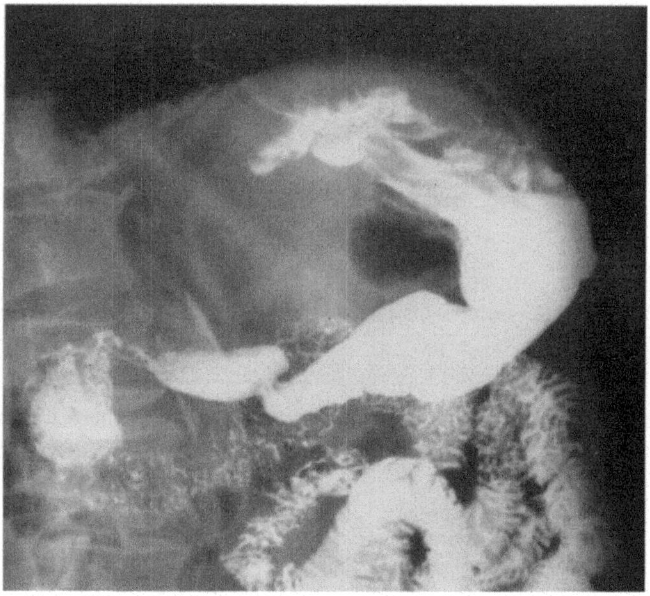

Fig. 2. Juxta-esophageal ulcer treated by the Madlener procedure

equally applicable to both sexes. Thus, the median age was 62; only two patients are included who were under 40, while the oldest was 89. There were 24 males and 26 females in the series.

While it seems that the absolute number of these lesions in increasing, it also seems there is a comparative increase in the percentage of high ulcers. Thus, in the previous decade (1948 to 1958), we found that only 2% of the resections for gastric ulcers required other than distal gastrectomy [*1*]. In the present series, the comparable figure is 6%.

Symptoms. In general terms, the symptoms could be divided into those which required early surgery (severe, acute bleeding in twelve) and those which persisted over a long period (continued or recurrent pain, or persistent lowgrade bleeding in three). In a number of instances, the possibility of cancer posed an additional threat.

Diagnosis. While it is not the intent of this paper to include a discussion of symptoms or diagnostic methods, a few statements will be made. Radiographs have been the standard method of diagnosis. However, the gastroscope has proved to be of inestimable value in diagnosis in recent years. The introduction of the fiberoptic gastroscope has made this procedure much safer. It is now used frequently particularly in cases with massive hemorrhage when bleeding can be stilled long enough by ice-water irrigations. In elective cases, the gastroscope may display lesions not seen by X-ray; the reverse is occasionally true, particularly with lesions near the esophageal hiatus.

Esophagoscopy is also valuable if bleeding is suspected from a hiatus hernia. Gastric cytology, though it is still used, is not in great favor because negative smears have been obtained in many patients with proved cancer.

The problem of cancer. It is clear that the possibility of cancer exists in these lesions just as it does with any other gastric ulcers. Theoretically, it would seem that the diagnosis of benignancy versus malignancy should be more difficult because the rib cage prevents the radiologist from making as adequate an examination as can be obtained at a lower level.

On the other hand, this is a fortunate period in the history of gastric ulcer because, for some unknown reason, there has been a great decline in the number of gastric cancers. Coupled with the corresponding increase in the number of benign ulcers, misdiagnosis of cancer has become less common than it was years ago.

On the other hand, this danger cannot be overlooked. In a recent case in our hospital, an apparently benign ulcer of the antrum was treated by vagotomy and pyloroplasty; the lesion failed to heal by X-ray and at a second operation a year later, the resected specimen was an ulcerated cancer. This difficulty in differentiation should be even more difficult in the upper portion of the stomach.

Frozen section diagnosis of four-quadrant biopsy specimens from the ulcer has been urged by some surgeons, provided that the ulcer is not removed. Untorfunately, we have found these examinations are difficult and reports may be erroneous. Diagnosis on the basis of the entire ulcerating lesion may be difficult also, and in some instances, only serial sections have shown cancer it what was apparently a benign ulcer.

For these reasons, when a patient with a gastric ulcer is submitted to operation, we believe the best course is to excise the ulcer.

In this series of 50 cases, confusion with cancer occurred six times. In two instances, the lesion was believed to be benign at the time of operation, but final sections proved them to be cancer; both of these patients had inadequate cancer operations. In four instances, preoperatively and at the time of operation, the surgeon believed he was dealing with cancer; but the resected specimens were found to be benign; in two of these cases, a less radical resection could have been used.

At present, it seems impossible to avoid some errors in the differentiation of ulcer and cancer. On the other hand, the error is less common than in the past. We believe that with these high lesions the surgeon should avoid extensive cancer operations in questionable cases; after a conservative resection he will obtain a good deal of help from the pathologist who can examine the entire lesion. If malignancy should be found, a more extensive procedure can be carried out immediately.

Type of therapy. In the absence of symptoms indicating urgent operation, these patients usually have been given a trial of medical therapy. A second barium study has been made at the end of a 10 day period; if there is definite improvement, further medical therapy has been carried out. Relapses under therapy have been frequent.

Ultimately, 12 patients during the study period (24% of the whole group) improved with medical therapy. 38 patients (76%) have required surgery. It is possible that protracted medical management might have produced a few more satisfactory results at the price of inadequate treatment of a few cancers.

While there were 2 deaths in the group treated medically, both had other underlying fatal diseases; death occurred from gastric hemorrhage. 5 deaths occurred in the 38 patients who had operations.

Of the 38 patients with surgical therapy, 13 required urgent operations for hemorrhage. There were 2 deaths after emergency operations and 3 after elective resections.

These figures indicate that operations are required more frequently for high ulcers than they are for those lower in the stomach, and that the response to medical treatment is poor in the great majority of cases. On the other hand, the mortality from surgical therapy is higher than it is for the low ulcers, and surely high enough to warrant a short period of medical therapy if urgent symptoms do not contraindicate it.

Medical therapy will not be discussed further in this paper, except to note that protracted treatment in the hospital has become impractical in recent years. The follow-up on many of these patients has been quite cursory indicating, perhaps, that the physician does not share the surgeon's worry about this disease. However, in the last decade in our hospital, approximately 50% of all patients with gastric ulcers have been treated medically.

Surgical therapy. It is with surgical therapy that we will be concerned in detail. It is apparent that at this time surgeons are employing a variety of techniques and approaches to deal with gastric ulcers; these concepts apply to the high ulcer as well as to those in more accessible parts of the stomach. Since surgeons do not agree on the proper therapy, the authors will list their beliefs and attempt to justify them. They are as follows:

1. Operations for gastric ulcer preferably should include removal of the lesion. The reasons for this statement are: a) that only in this way can the occasional ulcerating cancer be diagnosed and b) that, in the case of acute hemorrhage, this is the most certain way to control bleeding.

2. These operations also preferably should include removal of the antrum. Though the cause of gastric ulceration is not clear, it seems certain that nearly all surgeons would agree with Woodward [*2*] that the antrum is, for some reason, the most likely key to formation of gastric ulcer. Removal of the antrum even with retention of the ulcer, as in the Madlener operation, will lead to cure of the ulcer. On the other hand, excision of the ulcer itself will invite recurrence, as Moynihan [*3*] emphasized 40 years ago.

3. Vagotomy and pyloroplasty alone is not a satisfactory operation for gastric ulcer. There is a good deal of question about its efficacy for duodenal ulcer; for gastric ulcer where gastric acid levels are much lower, it has even less theoretical justification. This statement is made despite the favorable results reported by Dorton

[4], FARRIS [5], and KRAFT [6]. We believe we are dealing in many instances with a more severe type of ulcer than that encountered by these authors. Only in this way can the highly unsatisfactory results reported by WOODWARD [7], by SCOTT [8], and by HARRINGTON [9] be explained. The last author has found an 18% recurrence rate after vagotomy and pyloroplasty for peptic ulcer.

Fundal gastritis with acute erosions is not an uncommon cause of severe gastric hemorrhage. WADDELL [10] believes that the operation of vagotomy and pyloroplasty is specific for this lesion. While we have seen dramatic cessation of bleeding with this operation, in some instances in this series, it has offered no relief.

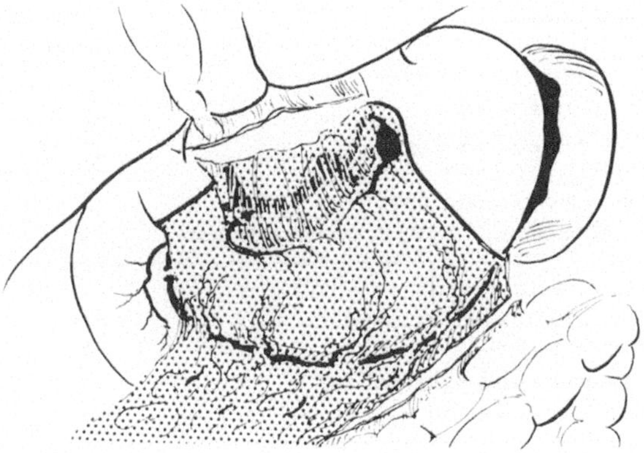

Fig. 3. High gastric ulcer removed by distal partial gastrectomy

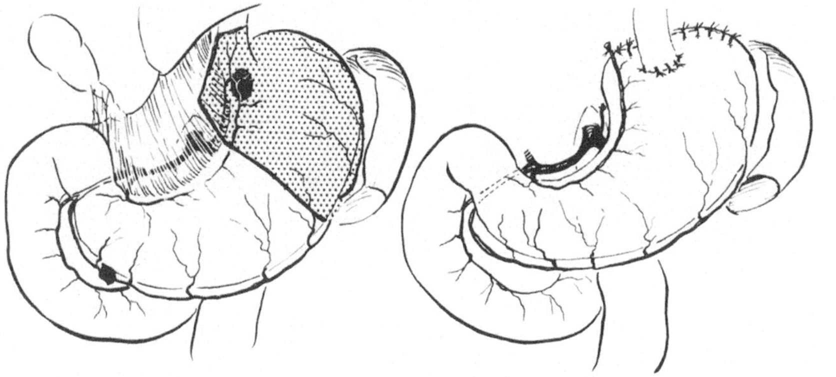

Fig. 4. Proximal gastrectomy, for high ulcer, followed by esophago-gastrostomy

When these general tenets are transferred to the high ulcer, these additional conclusions seem to be justified.

4. If there is a choice between a proximal resection (with esophago-gastrostomy) and distal resection (followed by either a BILLROTH I or II anastomosis) we believe the choice should be in favor of the latter. In the hands of most surgeons, any anastomosis involving the esophagus is more hazardous than in any other part of the gastrointestinal tract. Furthermore, the end results are not likely to be so good, since reflux esophagitis may occur and be very troublesome. Though this may be avoided in part by a pyloroplasty, it is an ever-present threat.

5. In many instances an ulcer that appears very high on the radiograph is readily exised by a distal gastrectomy at the time of operation. MARSHALL [11] and many others have emphasized this method in the past.

6. When a hiatus hernia and massive hemorrhage occur simultaneously, the hernia must be repaired and the bleeding controlled in some fashion. Several measures are available. Vagotomy and pyloroplasty may provide enough protection for cure; local excision of the ulcer or gastric resection may be necessary.

Table 2. *Types of operations*

Ulcer removed	27	Number of patients
Distal gastrectomy		11
Proximal gastrectomy		5
Total gastrectomy		2
Extended gastrectomy		2
Local excision (± V, P, or H.H. repair)		7
Ulcer not removed	11	
Repair hiatus hernia alone		2
Plication ulcer		1
Vagotomy and pyloroplasty		3
Madlener resection		5

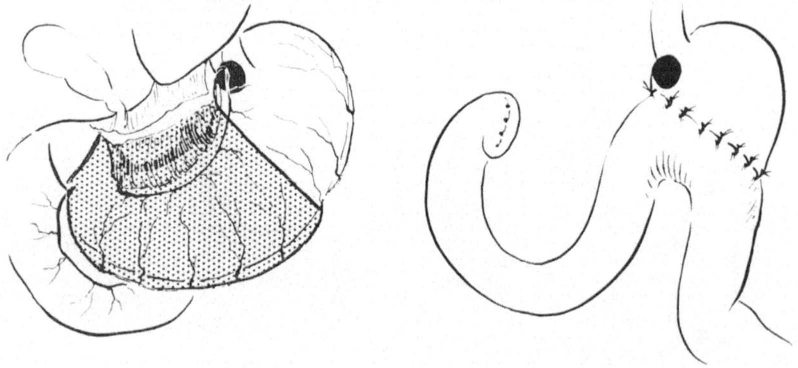

Fig. 5. Distal gastric resection with retention of ulcer. (Madlener procedure)

In this series, 38 patients had operations (Table 2). In 20 of the patients, the ulcer was removed by some type of gastrectomy. It was of interest that 4 (or 15%) of these had severe complications, 1 of which was recurrent bleeding (Table 3). In 7 patients the ulcer was excised, usually with vagotomy and pyloroplasty; 1 rebled and required gastrectomy. In the other 11 patients, the ulcer was not removed; 4 of them (36%) had severe complications, 2 of which were recurrent bleeding. While there does appear to be some advantage when the ulcer is removed, the number of patients in each group is small, and there is no clear advantage of one operation over another. It seems that technical problems with high ulcers are serious enough because of the anatomic location of the ulcer with any type of operation to counterbalance the advantages of one procedure over another.

The relative merits of competing operations cannot be assessed on the basis of these figures. The authors personally prefer excision of the ulcer preferably by distal gastrectomy or otherwise by proximal gastrectomy. The Madlener operation is reserved for poor risk patients who do not have acute hemorrhage and in whom the chances of cancer appear low. Pyloroplasty and vagotomy is reserved for patients with acute mucosal ulcerations or fundal gastritis. Stress ulcers are treated by distal resection. Whenever a hiatus hernia is present and contains an ulcer or is the site

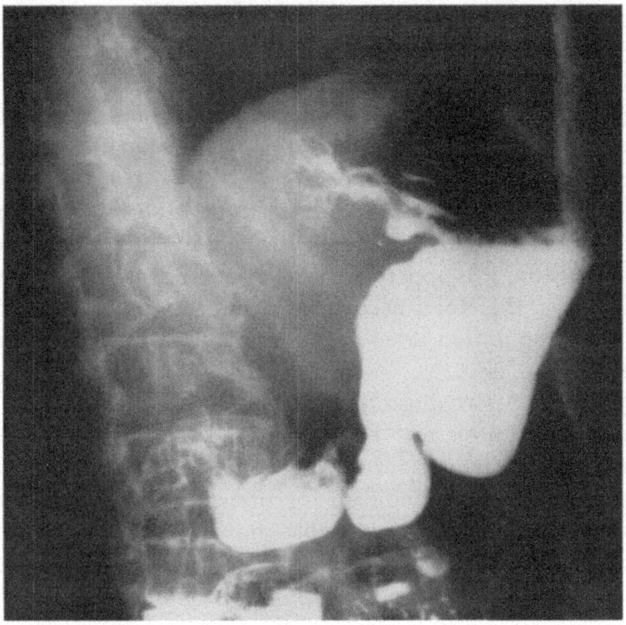

Fig. 6. Carcinoma of stomach, mimicking benign ulcer

Table 3. *Severe complications*

Operation	Complication	Second operation	Result
Ulcer removed			
Distal gastrectomy	Cardiac arrest	Thoracotomy	Died
Distal gastrectomy	Subdiaphragmatic abscess	I + D	Died
Extended gastrectomy	Subdiaphragmatic abscess	I + D	Died
Local excision	Recurrent bleeding	Distal gastrectomy	Recovered
Ulcer not removed			
Repair para-esophageal hernia	Pyloric obstruction	Distal gastrectomy	Recovered
Plication bleeding ulcer	Recurrent bleeding	None	Died
Vagotomy and pyloroplasty	Subdiaphragmatic abscess	I + D	Died

of bleeding, the hernia is repaired as well. All operations have their disadvantages. Thus, the only operation that offers complete freedom from recurrent bleeding is total gastrectomy; however, it nearly always is followed by severe loss of weight. Distal resections of high ulcers have not been followed by anastomotic ulcers in this series, though such ulcers have followed distal resection for gastric ulcers near the pylorus. Proximal resections, even with the addition of pyloroplasty, may invite regurgitation and oesphagitis. Pyloroplasty and vagotomy neglect the possibility of cancer, do not always relieve bleeding (three patients bled after this operation in this series), and do not regularly lead to healing of the ulcer. Balanced judgment, therefore, is of extreme importance in the selection of an operation for the high ulcers.

Complications and mortality. The important complications of operations are given in Table 3. They consist chiefly of recurrent hemorrhage and of sepsis. Since minor complications are not included in the table, it is apparent that the complication and mortality rate is much higher than for the usual gastric ulcer. Thus, serious complications occurred in nearly a third of all the cases; a second operative procedure was necessary in nearly all of these.

The overall surgical mortality rate was 13% (5 of 39 patients). The mortality for emergency operations was 17% (2 of 12 patients), and for elective operations, 12% (3 of 26 patients). All of these samples are too small to be of significance except to point out the hazards of all types of operations.

Discussion. The high gastric ulcer is difficult to treat both from the point of view of the internist and of the surgeon. Since the failures of medical therapy will be delivered to the surgeon, it is apparent that the surgeon must bear the brunt of the mortality figures. It is, therefore, necessary for him to consider methods by which he may lessen the complication rate. The most important details by which this can be accomplished will be listed.

Emergency operations. Approximately a third of all operations will be performed as emergencies, so that diagnosis may be difficult and the operation often performed under less than optimum circumstances. In general terms, if the patient has had five transfusions or more, he is a candidate for immediate operation. Preoperatively, esophagoscopy and gastroscopy are valuable; however, unless the stomach can be freed of clots and bleeding essentially stopped by ice-water irrigation, gastroscopy will be useless and will merely embarrass the surgeon by excessive inflation of stomach and gut with air.

A preoperative central venous pressure system must be established; and, except in dire circumstances, the pressure raised to 6 cm of H_2O before the operation is started. This is particularly important with these high lesions where a transthoracic or thoracoabdominal approach will be time-consuming. ZUIDEMA [*12*] has reported a drastic improvement of results from operations for bleeding ulcers due to this method alone. Fresh blood should be available at the rate of one for every five citrate transfusions.

A cuffed intratracheal tube should be inserted under local anesthesia before inducing general anesthesia. The stomach is often full of clots; and, if vomiting occurs during induction, aspiration is certain if the cuffed tube has not been placed previously.

While an abdominal approach is usually the best, the build of the patient may dictate an initial transthoracic or the conversion of the abdominal into a thoracoabdominal incision. The stomach usually will be found full of clots and must be emptied manually through a gastrostomy incision.

The surgeon's choice of operation often will be difficult. It will be necessary for him to balance absolute control of bleeding with the extent and difficulty of the operative procedure. The purpose of the operation is to stop the hemorrhage; prevention of any future ulcer recurrence is of secondary importance.

It should be noted that there were many combined operations. Thus, there were ten hiatus hernia repairs, eight which were combined with other operations. It should also be observed that poor results occurred indiscriminately with various operations. However, the results were worse when the ulcer was not removed (4 of 11 or 36% poor results) than when it was removed (4 of 27 or 15% poor results).

Elective operations allow the surgeon more leisure to carry out a proper procedure that preferably will prevent ulcer recurrence, eliminate cancer when present and, if possible, to retain enough stomach to maintain adequate nutrition and weight. With these high ulcers very radical distal resections were the rule formerly. The tendency has not shifted to less extensive resections. Frequently, at least a half of the greater curvature can be saved even when the lesser curvature is excised nearly up to the esophagus. A BILLROTH I anastomosis also is desirable in many of the patients, since it will aid in maintenance of nutrition.

The *late results* of medical therapy approximate the figures produced by CAIN et al. [*13*] for the treatment of all gastric ulcers, in that 24% of the patients have been able to continue without surgery though a number have recurring symptoms. The late results following operation have not yet been investigated in detail. The most serious late complications have included persistent loss of blood from erosive gastritis (though none has developed a true anastomotic ulcer), and severe loss of weight. It is apparent that many of these patients will never return to a productive existence because of age alone, since the mean age at the time of operation is 62.

Conclusions. A series of 50 cases of high gastric ulcers from the M.G.H., observed in the past 10 years, has been presented. It is contended that they are serious lesions that respond poorly to medical therapy. They are prone to bleed severely. Surgical therapy is difficult not only because of the frequent occurrence of massive bleeding but because of the location of the ulcer and the confusion with cancer.

References

1. WELCH, C. E., and J. F. BURKE: Surgery **44**, 943—958 (1958).
2. WOODWARD, E. R.: Personal communication.
3. MOYNIHAN, B.: Abdominal Operations. 4th ed. Philadelphia: W. B. SAUNDERS Co., 1926.
4. DORTON, H. E.: Surg. Gynec. Obstet. **122**, 1015—1020 (1966).
5. FARRIS, J. M., and G. K. SMITH: Ann. Sulr. **158**, 461—480 (1963).
6. KRAFT, R. O., W. J. FRY, and H. K. RANSOM: Arch. Surg. **92**, 456—462 (1965).
7. WOODWARD, E. R., M. M. EISENBERG, and L. R. DRAGSTEDT: Amer. J. Surg. **113**, 5—12 (1967).
8. SCOTT, H. W.: Personal communication.
9. HARRINGTON, J. L., JR.: Personal communication.
10. SULLIVAN, R. C., R. B. RUTHERFORD, and W. R. WADDELL: Ann. Surg. **159**, 554—562 (1964).
11. MARSHALL, S. F.: Personal communication.
12. FISHER, R. D., P. A. EBERT, and G. D. ZUIDEMA: Arch. Surg. **92**, 909—916 (1966).
13. CAIN, J. C., G. L. JORDAN, M. W. COMFORT, and H. K. GRAY: J. Amer. med. Ass. **150**, 781—874 (1952).
14. KELLING, G.: Langenbecks Arch. klin. Chir. **109**, 775 (1918).
15. MADLENER, M.: Zbl. Chir. **50**, 1313 (1923).

The Pancreas

Management of Acute Hemorrhagic Pancreatitis*

Karl H. Grözinger

Patients suffering from acute hemorrhagic pancreatitis are usually treated medically by surgeons. This sounds paradox, but there are plausible reasons. The patients are admitted to the hospital in many instances for a yet undefined acute upper abdominal illness which could possibly require an urgent surgical intervention. When the diagnosis is certain treatment should be strictly conservative unless surgery is necessitated. This can be caused by complications such as formation of abscess, tissue sequestration or intractible hemorrhage. In such cases only, delayed selective surgery is applicable for acute pancreatitis (Hess, 1961; Howard and Jordan, 1960).

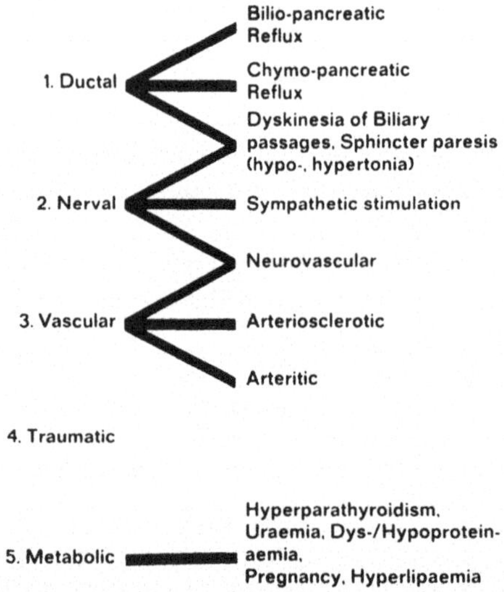

Fig. 1. Etiopathogenesis of acute pancreatitis

Throughout the world a higher standard of living and a steady increase of life expectation have led to a higher frequency of pancreatic diseases. This is also observed in other diseases of gastrointestinal organs. The clinical diagnosis of acute pancreatitis has not been improved to such a degree. Clinical, X-ray or laboratory possibilities to diagnose pancreatic disorders remained limited despite the many technical advances medicine has achieved. This discrepancy is, in part, caused by the well-known various etiology and pathogenesis, and even more by the unknown pathologic factors (Fig. 1).

---

* From the Chirurgische Universitäts-Klinik 6900 Heidelberg (Director: Prof. Dr. F. Linder).

These factors can be considered to be established: metabolic disorders in alcoholics, hyperlipidemia, uremia, hyperparathyroidism and pregnancy; canalicular causes such as biliopancreatic (OPIE, 1901) or chymopancreatic reflux.

The importance of neurovascular lesions is doubtful, for such lesions are present in many autopsy findings; without an acute pancreatitis ever to have occurred before. Hormonal, infectious, allergic, anaphylactic actions and trauma effects are objects of discussion.

The clinical forms of acute pancreatitis do not in all instances seem to be influenced by these different causes. Once the pathologic process is initiated it often proceeds in somewhat like a pre-determined pathway. The original causation cannot always be differentiated in the morphological substrate. At any time in the course of the disease the pathologic process can be disturbed, retarded or interrupted entirely by the body's own defense mechanisms. If this counteraction fails, and if a possibly instituted therapeutic intervention remains without effect the result may finally be the complete destruction of the pancreas.

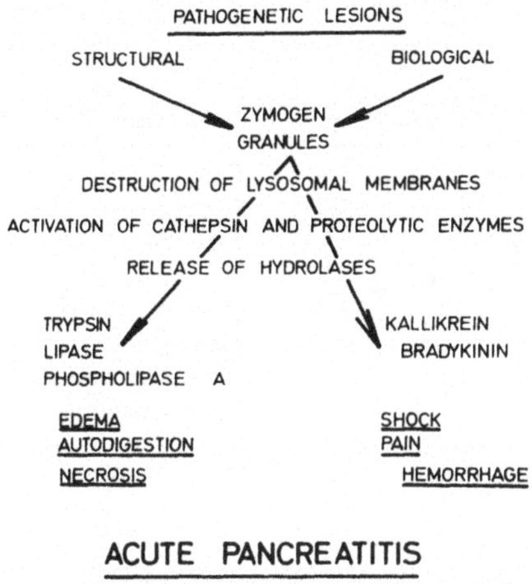

Fig. 2. Release of enzymes and of vasoactive substances are causes for local and general lesions in the course of acute pancreatitis

Severe lesions of distant parenchymatous organs originating from locally effective pathologic reactions in the pancreas may ultimately cause the patient's death. These lesions are believed to be called forth by the intrusion of highly active substances into the general circulation (Fig. 2).

Prematurely activated enzymes like trypsin, chymotrypsin and phospholipase A as well as lipase are supposed to be the agents of hemorrhagic necroses in the pancreas. They are released from the zymogen granules in the acinar cells after a decrease of tissue pH. The zymogen granules, well defined as suicide bags, are probably influenced by various structural, biological and circulatory disorders. These are caused by canalicular, neurovascular, metabolic, hormonal, infectious, allergic or sometimes traumatic processes. Enzymes liberated from the zymogen granules start, almost at once, the following pathobiological consequences:

1. an activation of the cathepsin system,
2. an activation of proteolytic enzymes,
3. a release of lipolytic enzymes.

Trypsin, lipase and phospholipase A become effective in the pancreas. The respective substrates are attacked consecutively, according to the prevalence of lipolytic or proteolytic enzymes. The lipolytic lesion of the pancreas is regularly followed by a secondary proteolytic tissue digestion.

Normally, a circulatory increase in the pancreas is observed after each meal. In the beginning of an acute pancreatitis, this elsewhere reversible alteration may progress to a consecutive condition with formation of edema and with subsequent tissue destruction. Progressive expansion of these digestive centers will lead to a breakdown of the exocrine pancreatic function. In case of a very extensive dissemination the endocrine function of the gland may also be involved.

Processes decisive for the further course of the disease are observed during the early phase of acute pancreatitis. The congested gland is flooded by blood from extremely dilated and permeable vessels. The produced enzymes will not be transported into the duodenum due to an outlet obstruction of the secretory ducts. There is also an isthmic blockade in the acinar intermediate tubules. Therefore, these enzymes penetrate through the basal membranes of the acinar cells into the postinsular capillaries and lymph vessels.

Table 1. *Symptoms in acute hemorrhagic pancreatitis*

Abdominal pain:		Palpable tumor
upper circular	35%	Amylasemia, -uria
right	35%	Lipasemia
upper central	15%	Hypocalcemia
left	15%	Hyperglycemia
Nausea		Jaundice
Vomitus		Hypovolemic shock
Fever		Liver damage
Abdominal distension		Renal insufficiency
Dehydration		ECG changes

Some of the enzymes which have been secreted into the general circulation exert no as yet known pathologic action. An example of this is α-amylase. Its increase in the serum, however, is considered to be a valuable diagnostic means; even though there are doubts to its actual importance [Trapnell and co-workers, 1967 (1)].

The pathologic action of some enzymes being secreted into the blood stream is as yet unknown; for instance of elastase and of pancreatic ribonuclease.

Enzymes having a noteworthy systemic action are for instance

trypsin, which may cause characteristic lesions in distant parenchymatous organs,

the fat splitting lipase, the action of which can be observed in fat tissue necroses, or

kallikrein which liberates vasodilating, pain releasing, and permeability increasing kinins from the α_1 and α_2 globulin fractions. Their action causes circulatory insufficiency. In some cases they can cause protracted irreversible shock.

The combined action of this enzyme derailment finally produces the clinical symptoms of acute hemorrhagic pancreatitis. According to the intensity of the enzyme action the different symptoms are more or less pronounced (Table. 1).

In the beginning, the diagnosis of acute pancreatitis is based, to a high degree, on suspicion (Black and co-workers, 1967). This is supported by a careful questioning of the patients's history.

Upper abdominal pains, vomitus, jaundice as well as heat and reddishness of the face are prevalent complaints. The physical examination shows the following main symptoms: hypotension, upper abdominal tenderness, sometimes defense, eventually adynamic ileus and occasionally jaundice. Along with the not always typical increase of the α-amylase, the ESR is accelerated, with or without leucocytosis.

In some instances, a pleural effusion which can be caused by a fat tissue necrosis is the only objective finding.

Treatment of acute pancreatitis must take into account the etiopathogenesis of the disease (CREUTZFELDT, 1963; DEMLING, 1961). Operative treatment, as recommended by KÖRTE (1911), SCHMIEDEN and SEBENING (1927), did not give favourable results. Total pancreatectomy as decribed in our modern times had no success even in the few cases in which it was deemed necessary. After the abandonment of the surgical management of acute pancreatitis (NORDMANN, 1938) the mortality of the disease was decreased to less than 20%.

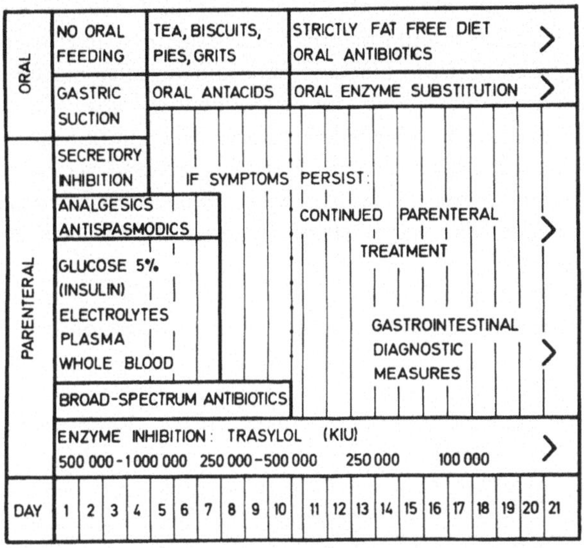

Fig. 3. Synopsis of treatment in acute pancreatitis

The most important principles of conservative internal management of acute hemorrhagic pancreatitis are decribed as follows (Fig. 3):

With the aim of a blockade of the pancreatic secretory functions there are different ways to put the pancreas at complete physiologic rest. One of the practicable measures considered to be important and also effective is the continuous gastric suction through a nasoesophageal tube. This condition does not permit any oral nourishment. Pharmaceutical suppression of enzyme production and secretion can be achieved by anticholinergic drugs. Atropine, Banthine and Pro-Banthine seem to exert such a beneficial effect.

Antihistamines may be applied to influence the histamine response of gastric cell secretion. Parenteral acetazolamide suppresses bicarbonate and water excretion by means of an inhibition of the carboanhydrase synthesis. It should, however, not be administered since an increase of the pancreatic juice viscosity has a bad influence on the course of acute pancreatitis. This might disagree with the opinions of many authors.

ACTH and cortisone are able to initiate acute pancreatitis by their own action. They should be restricted to cases of intractible shock and be used only as an ultimate reserve.

Relief of severe pains can constitute a major problem. Analgetics which also suppress respiration or peristalsis should be avoided. Morphine and its derivatives must not be given since these alkaloids may cause spasms of the sphincter of Oddi. Mepiridine and papaverine exert a reasonable analgetic effect, like the antispasmodics nitroglycerine and chloropromazine. Analgetics should be given in sufficient doses as often as they are needed. Some surgeons have emphasized that paravertebral blockades of sympathetic or splanchnic nerves are as effective as the epidural anaesthesia. In addition, the intravenous administration of procaine is believed to relieve pains.

Shock affords the most urgent care in some instances. It frequently requires a combination of different therapeutic measures (BARTHOLOMEW and CAIN, 1961). Intravenous cardiac glycosides are recommended to support the severely attacked cardio-circulatory system, particularly in foudroyant forms of acute pancreatitis. Peripheral analeptic agents should be omitted. Circulatory insufficiency is frequently caused by a discrepancy between blood volume and vascular capacity. A better treatment, therefore, consists of an adequate replacement therapy. The appropriate fluid and electrolyte balance can be achieved by classical salt solutions in conjunction with electrolyte solutions which have been especially prepared according to individual laboratory tests (WARREN and co-workers, 1967). Sometimes, plasma substitutes such as low molecular weight dextran are helpful due to their at the same time diuretic action.

Relatively large amounts of blood and plasma are lost in the retroperitoneal space. They must be replaced by regularly repeated blood transfusions, for example 250 ml every 1 or 2 days.

We recommend for prophylaxis a broad-spectrum antibiotic even though there is usually no infection in most cases of acute pancreatitis. Moreover, tetracyclin and its compounds have the advantage of inhibiting pancreatic lipase.

Numerous experimental studies have given evidence that prematurely activated and liberated pancreatic enzymes are responsible for the local destruction of pancreatic tissue and for the manifold systematic lesions. It is true that all of the pathophysiologic mechanisms could not be elucidated. It seems to be established that minute amounts of trypsin, kallikrein, and further pancreatic enzymes may sustain these dangerous signs. Only recently (DE HAAS, 1968) it became evident that trypsin also activates phospholipase A. Phospholipase A acts via the lysolecithin mechanism.

In the case of the edematous pancreatitis the body's own enzyme inhibitor is completely sufficient for the blockade of this undesirable enzyme action. A larger enzyme inflow into the general blood stream can be less completely compensated. In these cases, where the body's own inhibitors are not sufficient the polyvalent inhibitor Trasylol may have a therapeutic value. This substance which was developed during the past decades has a proved counteraction against trypsin, kallikrein, fibrinolysin and several other enzymes. Experimental and clinical studies have demonstrated the physical, chemical and biological identity of this substance and of the natural enzyme inhibitor. For this reason, this inhibitor can be substituted by a simple intravenous injection. To exert its entire working spectrum the enzyme inhibitor must be administered early and in sufficient doses (GRÖZINGER and BODEM, 1964; WARREN and co-workers, 1967).

With Trasylol a better clinical success can be expected in acute pancreatitis the earlier its medication is started. Of course, Trasylol must be given in addition to the classical management. The initial dosage is 500000 to 1000000 KIU intravenous. Equal amounts of the substance must be given in the following days, preferably in the running infusion. Trasylol medication should not be ceased abruptly. Its dose should be gradually decreased as the clinical condition improves (MAURER and ASANG, 1961).

There were some controversies related to the actual effectiveness of Trasylol since it has been introduced to clinical therapy (SKYRING and co-workers, 1965; TRAPNELL and co-workers, 1967). These controversies are, to some extent, justified due to the complexity of diagnosing acute pancreatitis. The problem becomes clearer if the single case-reports and double-blind studies of inhomologous patient groups are eliminated. Then, as demonstrated by BACHRACH and SCHILD (1966) in Los Angeles, NODINE and GREBERMAN (1966) in Philadelphia, and PETROW and BELJAJEW (1966) in Moscou, the additional treatment with Trasylol shows better clinical results.

By impending death we have tried with marked success pancreatic perfusion with Trasylol (GRÖZINGER and WENZ, 1965). This was later attempted in many cases throughout the world.

Table 2. *Therapeutic results in acute pancreatitis*
(10 years selected world literature 1958 to 1967)

Treatment	Total No.	Deaths	Mortality
Operative	305	87	28.5%
Medical	1010	161	15,9%
Medical + enzyme inhibition	1542	102	6.6%

Reviewing the world literature of the past decade (1958 to 1967) a selection of therapeutic results in a rather homogenous group of patients has demonstrated that the additional treatment of acute pancreatitis with Trasylol has led to a marked decrease of mortality (Table. 2).

It should be clarified whether the disease has been caused by an involvement of the extrahepatic bile ducts when the acute signs have disappeared. Cholecystectomy, eventually combined with an inspection of the bile ducts and the pancreas may be curative and, in many instances, prevent recurrent attacks.

In reference to the timing of an operation for pancreatic or biliary lesions it should be emphasized that many are done too early and too extensively (WARREN and co-workers, 1967). If done later they are generally too late and not extensive enough.

A listing of therapeutic measures in a condition as complex as acute pancreatitis can never be complete. The purpose of this presentation is primarily to emphasize widely established clinical applications. Therefore, procedures or medications in the state of progress or discussion, for example propylthiouracil, local, or general hypothermia, have not been touched.

References

BACHRACH, W. H., and P. D. SCHILD: A double-blind study of Trasylol in the treatment of pancreatitis. Conf. Chemistry, Pharmacology, and Clinical Application of Proteinase Inhibitors. N.Y. Acad. Sci. New York, 12.—13. Sept. 1966.

Bartelheimer, H.: Dtsch. med. J. **11**, 1 (1960.
Bartholomew, L. G., and J. C. Cain: J. Amer. med. Ass. **175**, 299 (1961).
Black, W. S., T. C. Sutterfield, and J. D. Martin: Amer. Surg. **33**, 94 (1967).
Child, C. G., and D. R. Kahn: J. Amer. med. Ass. **179**, 1 (1961).
Creutzfeldt, W.: Fortschr. Med. **81**, 563 (1963).
Demling, L.: Ther. d. Gegenw. **100**, 194 (1961).
Elmslie, R. G.: Med. J. Aust. **1967**, 211.
Grözinger, K.-H.: Die Inhibitorentherapie der akuten Pankreatitis. In: Marx, R., H. Imdahl und G. L. Haberland, Neue Aspekte der Trasylol-Therapie, Bd. 2. Stuttgart, New York: F. K. Schattauer 1968.
—, u. G. Bodem: Med. Klin. **59**, 1969 (1964).
—, u. W. Wenz: Z. Gastroent. **3**, 77 (1965).
Haas, G. de.: In press.
Hansen, H. T., H. C. Drube, W. Brüning und D. Borm: Med. Klin. **61**, 1254 (1966).
Hess, W.: Die Erkrankungen der Gallenwege und des Pankreas. Stuttgart: Thieme 1961.
Howard, J. M., and G. L. Jordan: Surgical diseases of the pancreas. Philadelphia und Montreal: Lippincott 1960.
Körte, W.: Langenbecks Arch. klin. Chir. **96**, 557 (1911).
Lataste, J.: Presse méd. **74**, 1875 (1966).
Maurer, G., u. E. Asang: Chir. Praxis **1961**, 169.
Nodine, J. H., and M. Greberman: Proteinase inhibitors in human pancreatitis: digital computer analysis of clinical research data. Conf. Chemistry, Pharmacology, and Clinical Application of Proteinase Inhibitors. N.Y. Acad. Sci. New York, 12.—13. Sept. 1966.
Nordmann, O.: Langenbecks Arch. klin. Chir. **193**, 370 (1938).
Nugent, F. W., W. A. Atendido, and S. P. Gibb: Amer. J. Gastroent. **47**, 511 (1967).
Opie, E. L.: Bull. Johns Hopk. Hosp. **12**, 182 (1901).
Petrow, B. A., u. A. A. Beljajew: Zbl. Chir. **91**, 257 (1966).
Schmieden, V., u. W. Sebening: Langenbecks Arch. klin. Chir. **148**, 319 (1927).
Skyring, A., A. Singer, and P. Tornya: Brit. med. J. **1965**, II, 627.
Trapnell, J. E., and M. C. Anderson: (1) Ann. Surg. **165**, 49 (1967).
—, C. H. Talbot, and W. M. Capper: (2) Amer. J. dig. Dis. N.S. **12**, 409 (1967).
Warren, K. W., M. C. Veidenheimer, and G. A. Kune: N.Y. St. J. Med. **67**, 1174 (1967).
Ziegler, A., u. M. Schamaun: Schweiz. med. Wschr. **96**, 967 (1966).

Surgical Treatment of Chronic Relapsing Pancreatitis

James T. Priestley and William H. ReMine

There are few patients with abdominal disease who present more problems to the surgeon than those who have chronic relapsing or progressive pancreatitis. Etiology of this disease may be obscure or basically of a nonsurgical nature as exemplified by the patient who uses alcohol to excess. The surgeon is always handicapped in his therapeutic efforts under these circumstances. Not infrequently we find ourselves in the position of relieving complications of this disease rather than correcting its cause. True, complications such as obstruction of the pancreatic duct may perpetuate the process if not relieved, but may actually be the result rather than the primary cause of the disease.

Many reports concerning surgical treatment of patients with chronic pancreatitis review the author's experience with one particular type of operation. Frequently the extent and nature of findings in the pancreas are not clearly described in relationship with the operation performed or result obtained. We firmly believe that the surgical procedure to be performed should be selected for each individual patient depending on clinical and surgical findings. A prolonged period of follow-up is essential to determine the surgical result.

Unfortunately, experimental studies on the pancreas have not been as rewarding as they have in some other areas such as the stomach and duodenum. Frequently the experimental setup may involve situations that are not encountered in patients. Chronic relapsing pancreatitis has not been produced in the experimental animal by use of alcohol or production of abnormality only in the biliary tract.

Etiology

Obstruction to free drainage of pancreatic juice into the duodenum has long been recognized as a possible cause of pancreatitis although pancreatic obstruction alone does not produce pancreatitis in the experimental animal. Under certain conditions, however, evidence indicates that ductal obstruction may be an important factor in the production of pancreatitis. This obstruction may occur any place in the ductal system from the tail of the gland to the sphincter of Oddi. It may occur at single or multiple sites. It may be caused by stone. It requires surgical relief.

Reflux of bile into the pancreatic duct is frequently mentioned as a cause of pancreatitis. On the other hand, cholangiographic studies made through a T-tube often reveal reflux of radiographic media into the pancreatic duct and therefore presumably bile in patients with no evidence of pancreatitis. It is true that under certain experimental conditions bile or a mixture of bile and pancreatic juice can cause pancreatitis when injected into the pancreatic duct. One wonders just how often these experimental conditions are encountered in the patient. It is known that pancreatic secretory pressure is usually higher than that in the biliary tree. If reflux of bile were a frequent cause of pancreatitis, should we not see bile in the pancreatic duct more often when the duct is aspirated or opened? In our experience this has been a rare occurrence. Does it not seem rather unlikely that nature would have placed the outlets of the common bile and pancreatic ducts in such proximity if reflux, per se, from one to the other would cause such serious disease as chronic relapsing pancreatitis?

The development of pancreatitis in association with disease in the biliary tract has been recognized since the turn of the century. This occurrence may not be too difficult to understand when one encounters a stone or stones in the ampulla of Vater that obstruct the pancreatic duct and also to a greater or lesser degree the common bile duct. How often is this found in patients with chronic pancreatitis? In our experience, it is rather uncommon. Organic obstruction of the sphincter of Oddi can likewise result in biliary and pancreatic obstruction. Again, this is not a common finding in our experience.

Spasm of the sphincter of Oddi has frequently been mentioned as a cause of recurring pancreatitis. It is difficult to understand how spasm of such weak musculature as exists in this area could cause such a serious disease as chronic relapsing pancreatitis. We have never been able to determine with satisfaction at the time of operation that spasm of this musculature actually has occurred preoperatively. Supposition and conjecture always seem to play a part in such a diagnosis.

It is generally agreed that any disease in the biliary tract may be a factor in the production of pancreatitis. The mechanism of this relationship is not entirely clear, however, when disease in the biliary tract appears to be confined to the gallbladder.

All agree that excessive use of alcohol may lead to chronic relapsing pancreatitis. Although there are various explanations for this sequence of events, the exact manner in which use of alcohol leads to pancreatitis has not been well documented.

The fact remains that even a small amount of alcohol may initiate an episode of pancreatitis. It is also true that any surgical procedure, short perhaps of total or subtotal pancreatectomy, may not protect the patient against recurring attacks of pancreatitis if the patient continues to use alcohol.

Other causes of pancreatitis have been suggested. These include metabolic disorders such as hyperlipemia, prolonged administration of cortisone, hyperparathyroidism, and malnutrition. Hereditary pancreatitis, associated with abnormalities of amino acid metabolism, is a recognized clinical entity. Other conditions such as vascular insufficiency, abnormal circulation of certain enzymes, allergic phenomena and infection are said to be infrequent causes of pancreatitis.

Surgical Treatment

There are many different views regarding surgical treatment of chronic relapsing pancreatitis (Bartlett, 1965; Bartlett, 1967; Cox and Gillesby, Doubilet and Mulholland, Duval and Enquist, Egdahl and Hume, Fry and Child, Gillesby and Puestow, Keddie and Nardi, Lempke et al., Madding et al., Marks, Priestley et al., Puestow and Gillesby, and Warren et al.). The following comments will present our own opinions.

Operation on the biliary tract. The status of the biliary tract is determined first and any abnormality that is found there is corrected. The gallbladder is not removed unless it contains stones or is significantly diseased. The common duct should be explored if it is enlarged or if there is any question whether stone or obstruction is present. We do not believe that any abnormality at the sphincter of Oddi can cause such a serious condition as chronic pancreatitis without causing simultaneous and recognizable changes in the biliary tract.

If preoperative cholecystography has revealed a normally functioning gallbladder, without stones, if there is nothing in the patient's history to suggest biliary obstruction, and if the common duct appears to be normal at the time of operation, exploratory choledochotomy is not performed. Nor do we usually perform operative cholangiography under these circumstances.

If, however, there is reason or evidence to suggest any pathologic change in the biliary tree, the common duct is explored. If organic obstruction of the sphincter of Oddi is demonstrated, this may be relieved by sphincterotomy. It is our practice to use a long-limbed T-tube, the lower end of which enters the duodenum, if sphincterotomy is performed. We have not observed complications from its use if the tube is not too large. Sphincteroplasty, as suggested by Jones et al., may be a superior operation to sphincterotomy but we have had no experience with this operation. If sphincteric obstruction has caused significant enlargement of the common duct, we frequently perform choledochoduodenostomy rather than sphincterotomy. This procedure is also used if compression by a diseased pancreas is causing obvious obstruction of the common bile duct. We have rarely seen cholangitis follow this operation if the anastomotic stoma remains adequate. It is not our usual practice to expose the papilla of Vater transduodenally unless there is reason to think that there is some organic abnormality in this area. Routine transduodenal pancreatography is not employed.

Operation on the pancreas. After one is satisfied about the biliary tree, attention is turned to the pancreas. The entire gland is examined and the type, extent, and degree of involvement are determined. In some patients the major area of involvement is confined to the tail or to the tail and body. This is one of the most favorable situations to find. The involved area is resected and the cut end of the pancreas is sutured if there is no evidence of pancreatic ductal obstruction. If the head of the gland is extensively involved and the remainder of the gland is virtually normal and if the patient has had severe symptoms, we may proceed with a Whipple operation, although we do not often do this as a primary procedure. If this is not done, the condition of the pancreatic duct is determined by pancreatography or direct exploration and one then proceeds according to the findings.

During recent years, interest has developed in subtotal pancreatectomy — so-called 90 or 95% pancreatectomy (Fry and Child). Our experience with this procedure has been too limited to permit significant comment on this operation. It would seem, however, that this operation should be reserved, at least as an initial procedure, for the patient who has an advanced form of pancreatitis with significant loss of pancreatic function. The same might be said for total pancreatectomy, which we have seldom used.

Various types of pancreatic drainage operations are performed. These are primarily designed to relieve pancreatic ductal obstruction. For this purpose, varying amounts of the tail or the tail and body of the pancreas may be resected until a dilated duct is encountered. A Roux-Y type of pancreaticojejunostomy is then established. Preferably this operation is performed only when exploration of the duct or pancreatography reveals just one site of obstruction in the head of the gland. Our preference for a drainage procedure, if it does not seem advisable to resect any pancreatic tissue, is for the so-called mid-ductal drainage (Priestley et al.). The pancreatic duct is identified by aspiration or incision in the midportion of the pancreas. The duct is opened as widely as need be to relieve sites of obstruction or to remove calculi. Depending on the length of the opening in the duct, a Roux-Y type of anastomosis is then made with the end or side of the jejunum. We have not performed the so-called filleting operation of Puestow and Gillesby. Likewise, we have seldom employed ductal ligation (Madding et al.). Two of three patients in whom this operation was performed had poor results.

Other operations. Internal drainage of a pseudocyst is one of the most satisfactory procedures for chronic pancreatitis. The cyst may be drained into the stomach, duodenum, or jejunum. Our preference is for a dependently placed stoma and a Roux-en-Y type of jejunal anastomosis. In the occasional patient if the cyst wall is thin and friable or because of location of the cyst, external drainage may be safer. In a few patients, resection of the cyst with some adjacent involved pancreas may be the procedure of choice. One of the most satisfactory causes of recurrent episodes of pancreatitis for the surgeon to find is the single ductal calculus. Removal of this stone usually provides complete relief. In our experience, operations planned solely for relief of pain seldom give a lasting favorable result and in recent years we have rarely used these procedures.

Review of Cases

We have recently reviewed the records of 137 patients that our colleagues and we have operated on for chronic relapsing pancreatitis. With a few exceptions these patients were operated on in the period 1962 to 1965. There were approximately twice as many males as females in this group. Five postoperative deaths occurred, a mortality of 3.6%. 95 patients (69%) had had some previous operation for pancreatitis. Most of these procedures were performed on the biliary tract, including those on 17 patients on whom sphincterotomy had been performed.

Clinical findings. 95 (69%) of the 137 patients used alcohol in varying amounts. Diabetes was present in 37 (27%), definite steatorrhea in 21 (15%), and calcification in 54 (39%). Some patients had two or all three of these findings. The relationship between the use of alcohol and these findings is shown in Fig. 1. It is noted that pancreatic calcification is more common (44%) in the patients who use alcohol but that it did occur in patients who did not use alcohol (29%). In our opinion the occurrence of calcification is related more to the severity and duration of the disease than to any specific etiologic factor. A higher incidence of calcification in patients who use alcohol might be explained by the usually more severe disease seen in these patients than in those who do not use alcohol. Definite steatorrhea occurred twice as often in patients who used alcohol as in those who did not (18% and 9%). In contrast it was found that diabetes occurred with about equal frequency in both groups of patients (26% and 29%). If obstruction of the pancreatic duct, per se, were always responsible for development of chronic pancreatitis, one might reasonably expect that steatorrhea rather than diabetes would occur more frequently in these patients. As noted, this

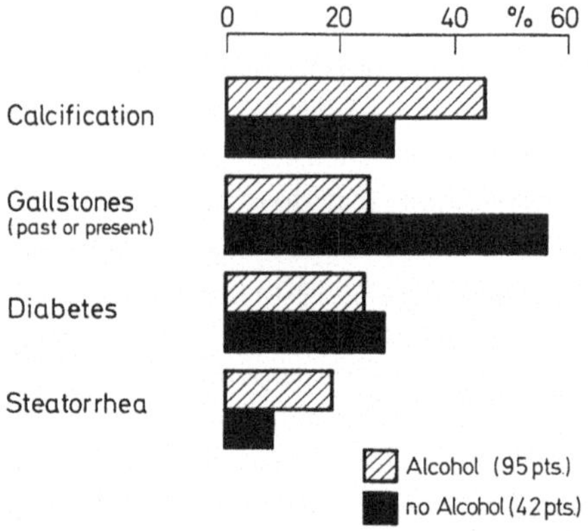

Fig. 1. Incidence of pancreatic calcification, gallstones, diabetes, and steatorrhea in patients who did and patients who did not use alcohol

was not the case with our patients. Perhaps the incidence of steatorrhea was not documented as well as that of diabetes but this appears to be a rather unlikely explanation. Microscopic study that evidences a significant degree of chronic pancreatitis may sometimes reveal extensive destruction of the islets but in other patients these may even appear to be hypertrophied. It is not understood why these variations occur.

Those patients who had tests of pancreatic function such as the glucose-tolerance test or stimulation of external pancreatic secretion with secretin or pancreozymin usually showed decreased function even though gross clinical insufficiency was not evident.

Pancreatic calcification is considered to indicate extensive disease. Thus, it is not surprising to find (Fig. 2) that steatorrhea occurred in 31% of patients with calcification and in only 5% of those without calcification. Similarly diabetes was present in 48% of those with calcification and in only 13% of those without this finding. Although the use of alcohol was noted both in patients with and in patients withou calcification, its incidence was somewhat greater (78%) in the former than in the latter group (64%). Gallstones, past or present, were found in 20% of those with calcification and in 43% of those without calcification. This suggests that pancreatitis is commonly less severe in patients who have disease in the biliary tract than in those who do not.

Surgical findings in the pancreas. A wide variation in degree, extent, and type of reaction in the pancreas was found. While it is difficult to categorize these findings in a simple and arbitrary manner, our effort to do so is shown in Fig. 3. We believe that such an evaluation at the time of surgery is important in selecting the most appropriate procedure. The entire pancreas was virtually uniformly involved in the largest number of patients in the present series (41%). Involvement that was most pronounced but not necessarily solely present in a localized area of the pancreas was noted

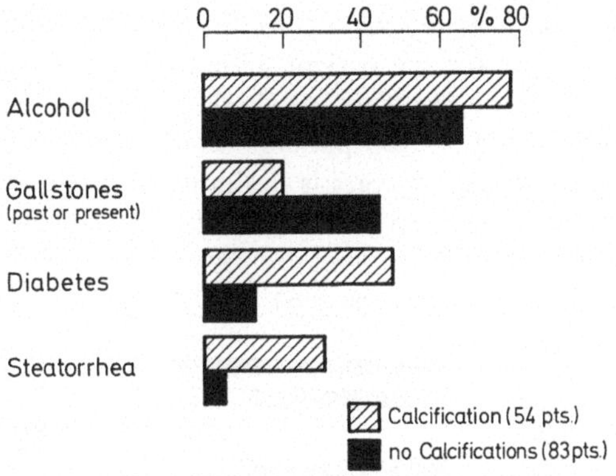

Fig. 2. Incidence of use of alcohol and presence of gallstones, diabetes, and steatorrhea in patients who did and patients who did not have pancreatic calcification

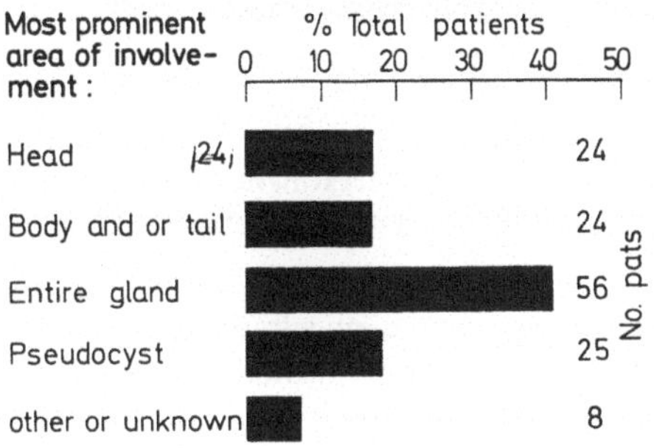

Fig. 3. Incidence of most prominent area of involvement in pancreas (not significantly influenced by alcohol or gallstones) in patients treated surgically for chronic pancreatitis

in a total of 34% of patients. Pseudocysts were found in 18% with varying degrees and types of involvement of the pancreas. In a small number (7%), findings in the entire pancreas were not noted because of conditions that made examination of the entire pancreas inadvisable.

Selection of surgical procedure. As would be expected, a wide variety of surgical procedures were used in treatment of the 137 patients of the series. Some portion of the pancreas was resected in 54 patients. In 44 of these the tail or the tail and body of the pancreas were removed. In some patients this included removal of a pseudocyst. In 24 of these 44 patients an anastomosis was made between the cut end of the pancreas and the intestinal tract. This was almost always done with a Roux-en-Y type of pancreaticojejunostomy. In the remaining 20 of these 44 patients there was no evidence of pancreatic ductal obstruction and the cut end of the pancreas was sutured. In 7 of the 54 patients a Whipple operation was performed and in the remaining 3 total pancreatectomy was carried out.

In 15 of the 137 patients a Roux-en-Y pancreaticojejunostomy was performed by opening the pancreatic duct for varying lengths in the neck and body of the gland without resection of any pancreatic tissue. Internal drainage of a pseudocyst was established in 23 patients, and 30 patients had operation only on the biliary tract. Some type of operation on the biliary tract was also performed on a number of other patients but this was not considered the major procedure in these patients. In the remaining 6, various other procedures were performed.

Surgical procedures related to late results. Frequently more than one procedure is performed at the same time for the patient with chronic relapsing pancreatitis. It is difficult therefore to relate the result to one single procedure. However, an effort has been made to do this in Fig. 4. 128 patients were followed for an average of 44 months. A follow-up of at least 5 years is desirable in discussing results of surgical treatment of chronic pancreatitis. In fact we have had patients who did well for more

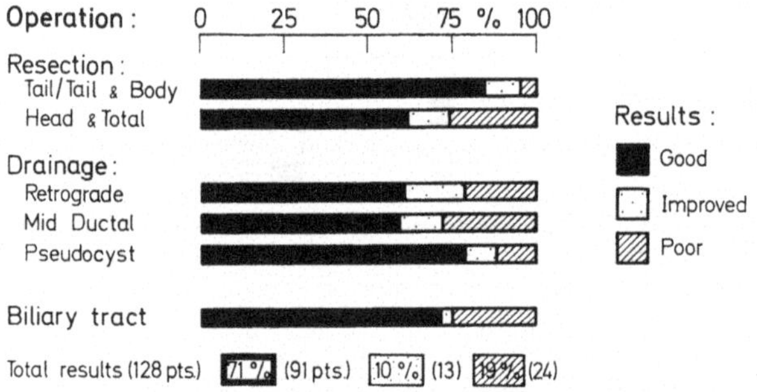

Results for Figs. 4—6

Fig. 4. Relation of late results in surgical treatment of patients with chronic pancreatitis to type of operation performed

than 5 years and then had recurrence of symptoms, but this is uncommon. Most patients who have poor results can be identified within the first 6 to 12 months after operation although some do well for 2 or 3 years and then have recurrent symptoms.

In the evaluation of results, patients listed as having a poor result had no significant benefit from surgery. Those listed as improved had definitely fewer and less severe attacks. Those listed as having a good result were virtually or completely symptom-free. In many instances failure to discontinue the use of alcohol was associated with persistent or recurring symptoms. Patients addicted to narcotics and the confirmed alcoholic were most likely to have unfavorable results.

One must remember that the result obtained cannot necessarily be related directly to the type of operation performed, as the type and degree of the pathologic findings usually determine the type of operation performed. For what it is worth, then, it is noted (Fig. 4) that the highest proportion of good results (85%) was obtained in those patients who had resection of the tail or the tail and body, which was usually performed for predominant disease in these areas. A similar incidence (80%) of good results was obtained following internal drainage of a pseudocyst. When disease was found in the biliary tract and only this was corrected, 73% had good results. Drainage operations performed under other circumstances produced a lower incidence (60 to 62%) of good results. The Whipple operation was performed on only 7 patients. 5 of these had a good result. Total pancreatectomy was performed only 3 times and only 1 of these patients did well. This operation was performed only under most unfavorable conditions when multiple previous procedures had failed and the patient was in a most undesirable state from the standpoint of morale and physical condition. Possibly the result would be different under more favorable circumstances. Some patients who had a poor result after the initial operation underwent reoperation and obtained a more favorable result.

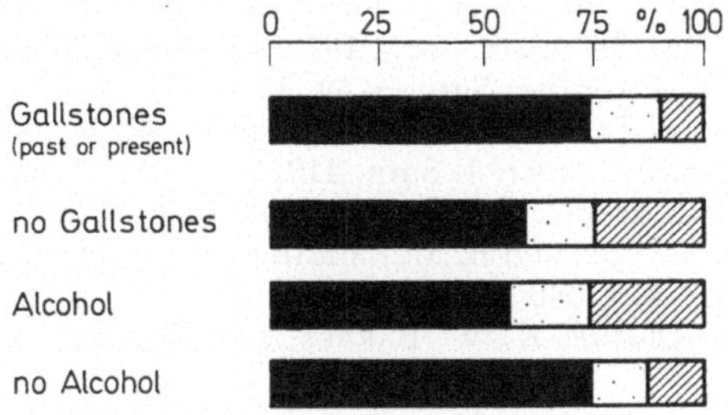

Fig. 5. Relation of late results in surgical treatment of chronic pancreatitis to presence of gallstones and use of alcohol

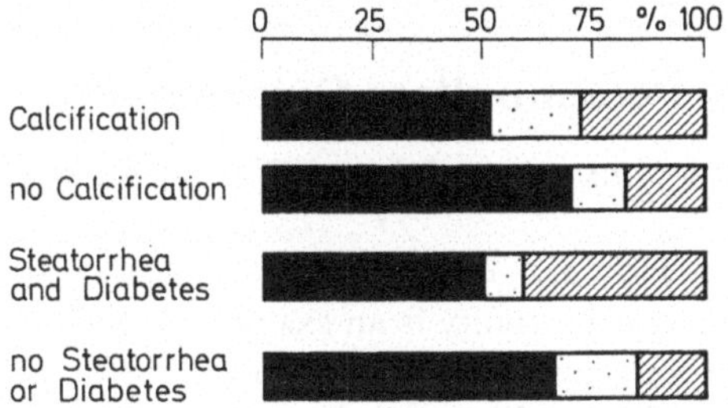

Fig. 6. Relation of late results in surgical treatment of patients with chronic pancreatitis to presence of calcification, diabetes, and steatorrhea

Other factors related to late results. Patients who had or had had gallstones experienced a greater incidence of good results (74%) than did those who had no gallstones (58%) (Fig. 5). Quite similar figures were found for those who did not use alcohol (74%) compared with those who did (55%). This same was true for those who did not have pancreatic calcification (70%) compared to those who did (52%) (Fig. 6). Comparable findings were also noted for those who did not have steatorrhea or diabetes (67%) compared with those who had both of these conditions (50%). From these data it is seen that use of alcohol, absence of gallstones, existence of pancreatic calcification, and presence of steatorrhea and diabetes militate against a favorable result.

Late deaths. Unfortunately patients with chronic pancreatitis appear susceptible to serious disease other than that related directly to the condition of the pancreas. It was found that 25 (20%) of the 128 patients who were followed for an average of 44 months died during this period. In slightly less than half of these patients (11 patients) death was attributed to complications that resulted in one way or another from chronic pancreatitis. The next most frequent (5 patients) cause of death was cardiovascular in nature. As a group, patients who died during the period of follow-up had a lower incidence of good results after operation than did the entire group that was followed. It is true, however, that 10 of these 25 patients had been relieved of symptoms related to the pancreas prior to the time of death.

References

BARTLETT, M. K.: Amer. Surg. **31**, 773—780 (1965).
— Arch. Surg. **95**, 887—891 (1967).
COX, W. D., and W. J. GILLESBY: Arch. Surg. **94**, 469—472 (1967).
DOUBILET, H., and J. H. MULHOLLAND: J. Amer. med. Ass. **175**, 177—182 (1961).
DUVAL, M. K., JR., and I. F. ENQUIST: Surgery **50**, 965—969 (1961).
EGDAHL, R. H., and D. M. HUME: Amer. J. Surg. **106**, 471—475 (1963).
FRY, W. J., and C. G. CHILD, 3rd: Ann. Surg. **162**, 543—548 (1965).
GILLESBY, W. J., and C. B. PUESTOW: Surgery **50**, 859—862 (1961).
JONES, S. A., L. L. SMITH, and G. GREGORY: Ann. Surg. **147**, 180—190 (1958).
KEDDIE, N., and G. L. NARDI: Amer. J. Surg. **110**, 863—865 (1965).
LEMPKE, R. E., R. D. KING, and G. C. KAISER: Arch. Surg. **87**, 90—98 (1963).
MADDING, G. F., P. A. KENNEDY, and B. MCLAUGHLIN: Ann. Surg. **165**, 56—60 (1967).
MARKS, C.: Amer. J. Surg. **113**, 340—345 (1967).
PRIESTLEY, J. T., W. H. REMINE, K. W. BARBER, and E. E. GAMBILL: Ann. Surg. **161**, 838—844 (1965).
PUESTOW, C. B., and W. J. GILLESBY: Arch. Surg. **76**, 898—905 (1958).
WARREN, K. W., M. C. VEIDENHEIMER, and G. A. KUNE: N.Y. St. J. Med. **67**, 1174—1180 (1967).

Periampullary Carcinoma*

WILLIAM P. LONGMIRE, JR., and WALTER L. BRUCKNER

The recent report of HOWARD of 41 consecutive pancreatoduodenectomy procedures without an operative mortality is an example of the continued improvement in the immediate operative results of this resection.

Although it is still a formidable procedure, the operation cannot be excluded from the surgical armamentarium solely on the basis of a prohibitive mortality rate. Significant progress is being made in reducing the number of deaths from operation, and the current long-term results must be considered.

MORRIS and NARDI compared the results of 152 patients with periampullary carcinoma treated at the Massachusetts General Hospital from January 1951 through December 1960 with the results of treatment during the previous decade at that institution.

They concluded that in the decade from 1951 to 1960 there was an encouraging increase in the number of long-term survivors after resective surgery for pancreatic or duodenal cancer, and that resection increased the survival time.

Despite these encouraging findings, the 5-year survival rate of patients following resection for carcinoma of the head of the pancreas leaves much to be desired in that it has ranged from 10 to 15% in most current series. The 5-year survival rate following pancreato-duodenectomy for the other three malignant lesions in this area (carcinoma of the lower end of the bile duct, the ampulla of Vater and the duodenum), however, is about 35%.

* From the Department of Surgery, UCLA School of Medicine, Los Angeles, California 90024. — This work was supported in part by the Janis G. Greims Trust Fund.

Differentiation of the various types of periampullary tumors on clinical and gross evidence alone is frequently impossible.

Many surgeons feel it is unnecessary and at times even unwise to attempt to obtain, by biopsy, histological evidence of the malignant character of the lesion, contending that a diagnosis of malignancy can usually be established on the basis of the clinical history and the findings at the time of operation.

Therefore, the decision to proceed with resection rests primarily on the presence or absence of distant metastases or local tumor extension (which would preclude total removal of all gross tumor by pancreatoduodenectomy) rather than upon the nature of the tumor and its primary site, despite the considerable difference in ultimate survival rate with primary pancreatic cancer as compared to other periampullary malignancies.

Case Material

The present review is based upon an analysis of the 106 patients with a periampullary type carcinoma at the UCLA Hospital from 1955 to the present.

Primary site. Carcinoma of the head of the pancreas was by far the most frequently encountered neoplasm; there were 81 cases. The primary site of the tumor was in the distal end of the bile duct in 10 patients, and the ampulla of Vater in 15 (Table 1).

Table 1. *Primary site of tumor and treatment*

	Head of pancreas		Bile ducts		Ampulla	
	No. cases	Deaths	No. cases	Deaths	No. cases	Deaths
Resection	28	3	7	0	11	2
Palliation	35	2	1	0	4	2
Exploration	7	1	2	0	—	—
No operation	11	0	—	—	—	—
Total	81	6	10	0	15	4

46 Pancreato-duodenal resections 5 deaths (10.8%)
40 Palliative procedures 4 deaths (10%)

There were approximately twice as many males (69) as females (37) in the series. Although the average age of these patients was 62.5 years (excluding one 3-year-old male), there were 25 patients 70 years of age or above and 4 over the age of 80. Even when the localization of the neoplasm would seem to meet the requirements for resection, the surgeon may well hesitate to embark upon this extensive procedure in patients of such advanced age.

Diagnosis

As indicated in an earlier publication (Longmire and Shafey) jaundice and upper abdominal pain are the most common symptoms of the disease initially identified. Such symptoms, particularly with tumors arising in the head of the pancreas, may indicate that the tumor has advanced beyond its original site and that it has spread in either gross or microscopic form to areas beyond the limits of resection.

Vague symptoms of bloating, eructation, epigastric fullness, loss of weight, weakness, anemia, and onset of mild diabetes are present in 50% of patients prior to the onset of pain or jaundice (Longmire and Shafey). Relating such symptoms to a well localized pancreatic tumor, however, remains a most difficult task with the diagnostic technique currently available. Photoscanning of the pancreas with the γ emitting radioisotope ^{75}S Selenomethionine (BLAU and MANSKE) or selective arteriography (ÖDMAN) with catheterization of the celiac axis and the superior mesenteric artery, have not been sufficiently discriminating in our experience to be of value in the diagnosis of small localized lesions in the periampullary area. Atonic, double contrast duodenography seems to be a promising technique for evaluating the status of the duodenal mucosa and ampullary area, but our experience with the procedure is limited.

Surgical Management

Throughout this period an attempt has been made to assess the extent of the tumor carefully before embarking on a definitive resection. Particular attention is directed toward examination of the area along the hepatic artery and the cephalad border of the pancreas and the region of the superior mesenteric vessels along the caudal margin of the pancreas both for metastasis to lymph nodes as well as direct tumor extension. Direct invasion into the wall of the portal vein or the superior mesenteric vein unfortunately cannot be determined with certainty until dissection of the area between these veins and the undersurface of the pancreas is begun. Some indication of invasion may be suggested by the size of the tumor, its extension into the uncinate process and the adherence of the gland or tumor to the vein at either border of the pancreas.

Some attempts were made to extend operability by removing a segment or a part of the wall of the portal vein when invaded by tumor, but we have abandoned the procedure. Three of five patients so treated promptly developed extensive hepatic metastases indicating tumor embolism in the portal system either before or during operation.

Extensive fibrosis associated with chronic pancreatitis may make it difficult to distinguish the extent of tumor invasion into the body of the pancreas and for this reason as well as the possibility of a multicentric origin of pancreatic cancer, removal of the entire pancreas when performing a pancreatoduodenal resection has been suggested (ROSS). Total pancreatectomy has been performed only once in the present series, for the benefits to be derived from this extension of the procedure have not been established. When there is question of the adequacy of the level of pancreatic resection, tissue sections from the cut surface are examined and if necessary additional gland substance removed.

In two patients in the present series the cut end of the distal pancreatic segment was oversewn without a pancreato-enteric anastomosis. The immediate postoperative course of 1 patient was uncomplicated; the other developed an alimentary fistula from the gastroenterostomy which closed spontaneously. One lived for 7 months; the other for 9 months. The moderate postoperative steatorrhea was controlled in part with pancreatic supplement. Routine closure of the pancreatic stump has been recommended by RABWIN and KARLAN who pointed out the substantial reduction in serious postoperative complications when the pancreatojejunal anastomosis was eliminated. They reported that the exocrine deficiencies so created have not been difficult to control. A leak at the pancreatojejunal anastomosis, always a serious, potentially fatal complication, was encountered 11 times in the 46 resections but was a factor in only 1 of the 5 deaths following resection. Even when all anastomoses are healed it may be difficult to be certain that the pancreatojejunal anastomosis remains patent.

Closure of the pancreatic stump may be considered in patients who have local lesions highly favorable for resection, but in whom a lesser procedure would be desirable due to advanced age or accompanying illness regardless of the anticipated exocrine deficiency. On the other hand, when total restoration of alimentary continuity is achieved with well functioning anastomoses of the pancreas, bile duct and stomach to the jejunum, a normally functioning alimentary tract may be regularly anticipated within 3 to 6 months after operation and such is the usual goal if resection is to be done.

Contrary to the recommendation of certain previous authors (MAKI et al.), the experiences gained in the present series suggest that a two-stage operation has certain definite disadvantages and is rarely indicated. Patients so ill as to require immediate biliary decompression frequently have tumors that have advanced beyond the limits of resectability, or their general condition due to concomitant diseases is so poor that resection would usually be contra-indicated.

With careful management of the usual preoperative measures it has been possible to establish a reasonable metabolic state before operation in patients who are candidates for resection.

Resections

Forty-six pancreatoduodenal resections were performed. The primary site of the cancer was in the head of the pancreas in 28, the bile duct in 7 and the ampulla of Vater in 11 cases. There were 5 postoperative deaths, an operative mortality rate of 10.8%. No deaths have occurred in the last 29 consecutive resections (Table 2).

A positive biopsy of malignant tumor tissue was obtained prior to resection in 30 patients. Tissue was removed through the opened duodenum in 6 of these patients. Regional nodes were found to be positive in 4. The biopsy specimens in the other patients were taken from the region of the head of the pancreas. Clinical and gross evidence of malignancy was so convincing in 4 patients that resection was performed in spite of a negative biopsy report, and in 11 patients no attempt was made to obtain tumor tissue for biopsy (Table 3).

The extensive fluid shifts which follow this operation with loss of protein rich fluid into the peritoneal cavity and the retroperitoneal tissues make fluid and electrolyte management a critical issue in postoperative care, particularly in the elderly patient with reduced cardiac reserve. Three of the 5 deaths that occurred in this series were specifically related to hypovolemia, or pulmonary edema and electrolyte imbalance. One death was directly related to a leak at the pancreatojejunal anastomosis and the other to thrombosis of the superior mesenteric artery and intestinal gangrene. The average period of survival following resection for carcinoma of the head of the pancreas was 11 months, the same as that achieved by a simple bypass procedure. The average was 40 months, however, following resection for ampullary cancer and 20 months for cancer of the bile duct.

Ten patients are currently alive; 6 have survived for over 5 years. Eight are alive 2 years or more following resection. The longest survivor is alive 16 years following resection for carcinoma of the ampulla of Vater.

The 10% operative mortality rate which accompanied the 40 palliative procedures is indicative of the poor general condition of many of these elderly patients.

Table 2. *Results in 46 pancreatoduodenal resections*

Primary site	No complications	Fistula	Bleeding	Delay in gastric emptying	Abscess, pneumonia, other complications	Time of operative death and cause	Survival	No. of patients alive
Head of pancreas (28 cases)	16	5	3	3	2	5 days-shock 21 days-pul. edema; electrolyte imbalance 8 days-gangrene of intestine	3—6 mo. = 4 6—12 mo. = 11 1—2 yrs. = 6 2—5 yrs. = 2 Avg. = 11 mo.	7 yrs. = 1 7 yrs. = 1
Ampulla (11 cases)	4	4	1		3	5 days-shock 9 days-leak of panjej. anastomosis	6—12 mo. = 1 1—2 yrs. = 2 2—5 yrs. = 0 5—10 yrs. = 1 Avg. = 40 mo.	$1^1/_2$ mo. = 1 4 mo. = 1 8 yrs. = 1 11 yrs. = 1 16 yrs. = 1
Bile duct (7 cases)	4	2		1			6—12 mo. = 1 1—2 yrs. = 2 2—5 yrs. = 1 Avg. = 20 mo.	2 yrs. = 1 3 yrs. = 1 $9^1/_2$ yrs. = 1
Total	24	11	4	4	5	5		10

Survival following palliative operations ranged from 5.5 months to 11 months. Combining gastroenterostomy with biliary decompression did not seem to significantly alter the period of palliation (Table 4).

The operative technique employed has previously been described and is similar to that generally utilized today. Continuity of the alimentary tract is reestablished by

Table 3. *Preresection diagnosis*

From positive biopsy	
Transduodenal	6
Regional nodes	5
Region of head of pancreas	20
	31
From clinical evidence and gross examination	
No biopsy	11
Negative biopsy	4
	15

Table 4. *Survival following palliative operation*

Bypass	No. cases	Average survival (months)	Operative deaths
Choledochojejunostomy	16	11.0	
Choledochoduodenostomy	3	10.7	
Cholecystojejunostomy	6	5.5	2
Cholecystoduodenostomy	6	6.5	
Biliary-enteric with gastroenterostomy	9	7.4	2
Total	40		4

an end-to-end pancreatojejunal anastomosis, an end-to-side choledochojejunal anastomosis, followed by a Hofmeister gastrojejunostomy. Vagotomy is performed and approximately 50 to 60% of the stomach excised in order to reduce the acid gastric secretion if an anastomotic fistula occurs.

References

Blau, M., and R. F. Manske: J. nucl. Med. **2**, 102—105 (1961).

Howard, J. M.: Pancreatico-duodenectomy: forty-one consecutive Whipple resections without an operative mortality. Presented 1968 Meeting American Surgical Association, Boston, Mass. (April 17—19, 1968).

Longmire, W. P., Jr., and O. A. Shafey: Amer. J. Surg. **111**, 8 (1965).

Maki, T., T. Sato, and G. Kakizaki: Arch. Surg. **92**, 825 (1966).

Morris, P. J., and G. L. Nardi: Arch. Surg. **92**, 834 (1966).

Ödman, P.: Acta radiol. (Stockh.) Suppl. **159**, 1—168 (1958).

Rabwin, M. H., and M. S. Karlan: Calif. Med. **104**, 437 (1966).

Ross, D. E.: Amer. J. Surg. **87**, 13 (1954).

Diagnosis and Therapy of Islet-Cell-Tumors

R. Zenker, H. Hamelmann, A. Grabiger, and R. Bedacht*

There are three problems concerning diagnosis and therapy of hyperinsulinism:

1) the differentiation of the symptoms of the disease and the proof of diagnosis,
2) the preoperative localisation of islet-cell-tumors,
3) the choice of operation.

Hyperinsulinism is seldom recognised because this diagnosis is rarely thought of. The majority of patients with hyperinsulinism receives treatment for exhaustion, epilepsy, delerium, schizophrenia or brain tumor and is admitted at a hospital for psychiatric patients or a neurosurgery department. All diagnostic means like angiography, pneumoencephalography et al. do not reveal any diagnosis. A clear picture will be obtained only when blood sugar determination is done during an acute phase of the disease. Therefore the determination of blood sugar is a very important test in patients with neurologic and psychiatric symptoms as well as sedimentation rate and Wassermann reaction.

The consequences of non-treated hyperinsulinism are as follows: severe brain damage according to organic cerebral changes, — which might be indicated by dilated ventricles — further increasing psychic and mental disorders. One reason for this is that the CNS takes the metabolic energy mainly out of glucose. Non-treated organic hyperinsulinism is letal. Referring to pernicious anaemia Katsch talks in terms of pernicious hyperinsulinism.

The disease starts very often with non-characteristic symptoms, which can be subdivided in three groups:

1) vegetative nervous disturbance,
2) central nervous symptoms,
3) psychic symptoms.

Since these symptoms may appear in varying combinations, the diagnosis of hyperinsulinism is rarely thought of. The classical symptoms of hyperinsulinism are weakness and somnolence in the morning, which recur after longer fasting periods and after physical strain. In more than 80% of our patients these symptoms were present. A short unconsciousness — appr. in half of the cases — was another symptom. Quite often patients were aware of the fact that by intake of carbohydrates the attacks were softened. Therefore some of the patients were gaining weight tremendously.

First step to diagnose hyperinsulinism is the consideration of the Whipple-trias, id est:

1) appearance of symptoms of hypoglycemia in fasting state or after physical activity,

2) the proof of hypoglycemia during such an event,

3) sudden amelioration of symptoms after oral or intravenous administration of glucose.

The diagnosis hyperinsulinism can be established by means of a so-called fasting-test, e.g. repeated determination of blood sugar during fasting for 36 h. Mostly a significant decrease of blood sugar will occur. Further diagnostic means are tests with betacytotropic substances like Tolbutamid, Glucagon or Leucin, which cause

* Department of Surgery, University of Munich. Director: Prof. Dr. med. R. Zenker.

even in small doses a significant decrease of blood sugar with all signs of hypoglycemia, whenever an islet-cell-tumor is present. It is necessary to perform the test during EEG registration in order to recognise a hypoglycemia the earliest possible and to meet its dangers (BOTTERMANN, KOLLMANNSBERGER et al.). Characteristic changes in the EEG occur already before the appearance of clinical symptoms. They disappear after glucose intake.

Organic hyperinsulinism can be confirmed only by decrease of blood sugar with simultaneous increase of the serum insulin level. Therefore it is advisable to perform at the same time the very sensitive biological or immunobiological methods for "insulinactivity" or "immunoreactive Insulin" (IMI = immunological measurable insulin = IRI = immunoreactive insulin) (Fig. 1).

Examining the reaction of islet cell apparatus one should not forget that in the course of hyperinsulinism there may be periods of inactivity of the adenoma without response to the test. For this reason the diagnostic procedures should be repeated for control in case of doubtfull results.

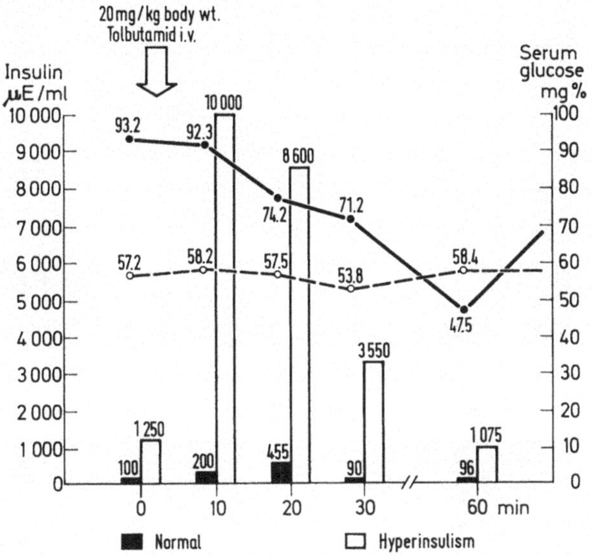

Fig. 1. Tolbutamidtest with insulin-determination

The preoperative localisation of islet cell adenoma is very important for the surgeon. We prefer the simultaneous angiography of the art. coeliaca and the art. mesenterica cranialis with Seldinger catheter according to BOYSEN, OLIN and ALLE OLSSON (Fig. 2). Using this method we were able to localize the tumor in eight cases in cooperation with Dr. ZIMMERMANN of the Rieder-Institut. Bigger tumors may be recognised by *pancreas-scintigraphy* with Seleno^{75}-Methionine, but pancreas scintigraphy does not state as well as angiography.

A few words concerning the pathologic anatomy of islet-cell-tumors. 70% of the cases are islet cell adenomas. As single adenoma they appear in all segments of the pancreas, but are seen with 40% in pancreas-tail and only 28% in pancreas-body or with 26% in the pancreas-head. In only 3% of the cases the adenoma is found in organs as stomach, duodenum, omentum etc.

During the last years we operated on 16 cases. The adenoma was 3 times in the pancreas-head, 5 times in pancreas-body and 7 times in pancreas-tail. In one case a diffuse islet cell hyperplasia was present. Referring to literature multiple adenomas appear in appr. 10 to 15% of the cases.

The histological differentiation between adenoma suspect of malignancy or intermediary adenoma and the benign ones is in many cases very difficult. Not too seldom, however, they show an increased number of mitosis, vascular invasion and metastases.

Recently we have seen such a case of islet cell adenoma with secondary growth in the liver (Fig. 3). Both the pancreas tumor and the metastases in the liver have been removed. One year after operation the patient is still well.

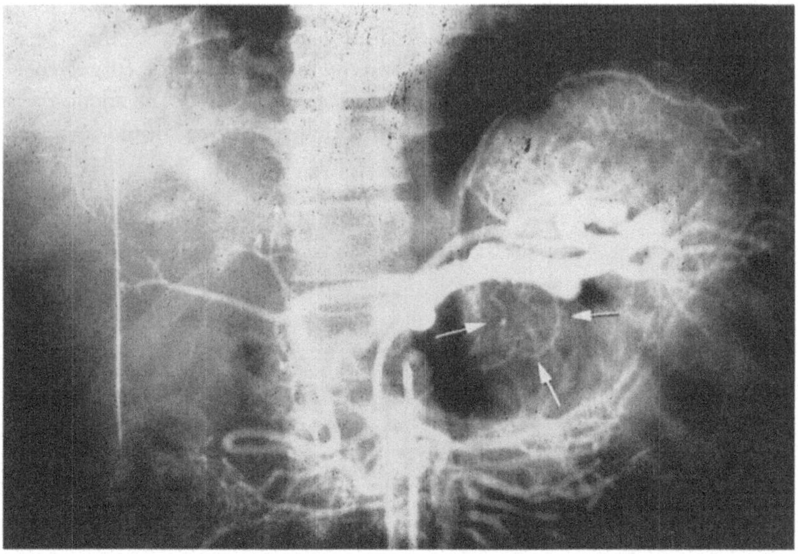

Fig. 2. Angiogram of art. coeliaca and art. mesenterica cranialis. The arrows indicate an adenoma

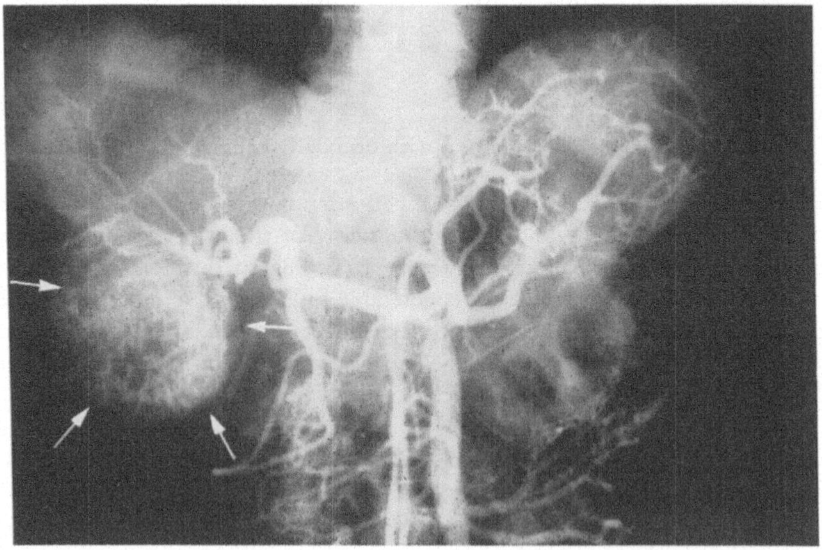

Fig. 3. Representation of liver metastasis in the angiogram (arrows) with intermediate islet cell adenoma

True islet cell carcinomas are more seldom than benign adenomas. In 16 patients with hyperinsulinism we observed three carcinomas with widespread metastases. The majority of the carcinomas of the islet cell apparatus were endocrinologically highly active. Most of them metastased into regional lymphatic nodes and into the liver, sometimes also in the gastro-intestinal tract, the lungs, adrenals, and brain.

The therapy of hyperinsulinism consists in removing the adenoma or the islet cell tumors. The curved transverse laparotomy in the upper abdomen and dissection of the gastrocolic ligament allows the best survey of the pancreas. By cutting the dorsal peritoneal leaflet the dorsal part of the pancreas is free. Using this technique body and tail of the pancreas can be palpated between the fingers and tumors may be felt. In order to find adenomas in the head of the pancreas it may sometimes be necessary to mobilize the duodenum according to the technique of KOCHER. In general the tumor is enucleated. A partial resection of the pancreas may be necessary if the adenoma can not be removed in toto or if some additional adenoma or suspicious nodules are present in the pancreas, or if the simultaneous histological examination reveals malignancy. In nine of our operated patients a partial resection has been done.

The situation may become critical if on one hand an islet cell tumor cannot be found by inspection or palpation, on the other hand all tests seem to prove the presence of such a tumor. Under these conditions histologic dissections should be made according to the technique of HOLTQUITH and BECKER, which determines the relationship between a- and b-cells. If a b-cell adenoma is present in the residual Langerhans islets the a-cells should be increased. If histological examination of such a slide shows an increased number of a-cells a hormon active b-cell tumor may be exspected without knowing anything about the localisation. This result should stimulate the continuation of intensive search for a tumor.

It should be emphasized again, that if no tumor can be found the head of the pancreas should be controlled again very carefully. In one case we could not find the tumor, though head and tail of the pancreas were dissected. However the symptoms of hyperinsulinism are still present.

The recurrence in the strict term of a newly developed adenoma is very rare. If the symptoms reveal the presence of an islet cell tumor most probably parts of the tumor remained.

In 1963 in one patient an islet cell tumor was removed from the head of the pancreas. This patient was without symptoms during the following 4 years. Then acute hypoglycemia developed again. In 1967 the patient was operated again and the rest of the pancreas was removed. The histologic examination showed an adenoma in the head of the pancreas which could not be peeled off.

Only if a malignant islet cell tumor is present a duodenopancreatectomy seems to be indicated. If the tumor cannot be found during operation and the clinical symptoms of hyperinsulinism are without any doubt the same operative intervention seems necessary.

After total resection of the pancreas due to islet cell tumor a survival rate of 4 to 8 years has been observed, so the diagnosis carcinoma might not be justified. Metastases should be removed too.

In the postoperative course it is very rarely necessary to administer insulin. However, it is absolutely necessary, as everybody knows, after pancreas resection to begin with a substitution of hormon.

A conservative treatment may be necessary if age and condition of the patient do not permit an operation or if carcinoma with metastases is established. The conservative treatment consists of a special diet with low carbohydrate and high fat and protein content. The latest medical treatment is the administration of "Diazoxid". This drug, which originally is used against hypertension, increases the glucose level in the blood by means of inhibition of insulin secretion.

Our medical colleagues have used this drug in the preoperative course of very obese patients without any side-effect. It is said that high doses and long time administration affect the hematopoesis.

Prognosis and results of the operated islet cell tumor are good. According to the literature 80 to 90% of all cases, treated by operative enucleation or partial resection are cured permanently.

In our hospital 13 patients with hyperinsulinism were operated upon. One patient suffered from an intermediate adenoma, another from diffuse islet cell hyperplasia. 11 patients are still alive. 1 died and 1 could not be followed up.

References

Becker, W. H.: Bruns' Beitr. klin. Chir. **179**, 291 (1950).

Beyer, J., H. Ditschuneit, F. Melani und E. F. Pfeiffer: Verh. dtsch. Ges. inn. Med. **73**, 1079 (1967).

Bottermann, P., K. Kollmannsberger, K. Schwarz und K. Kopetz: Verh. dtsch. Ges. inn. Med. **73**, 1082 (1967).

Boysen, E., u. T. Olin: Zöliakographie und Angiographie der A. mesenterica superior. In: Schinz, H. R., R. Glauner und A. Rüttigmann, Ergebn. med. Strahlenforsch. N. F. **1**, 112 (1965). Stuttgart: Thieme 1965.

Breidahl, H. D., J. T. Priestley and E. H. Rynearson: Ann. Surg. **142**, 698 (1955).

Büngeler, W.: Diskussionsbeitrag z. Vortrag W. Creutzfeld am 8. 6. 1967 beim Ärztl. Verein München.

Creutzfeldt, W.: Die Behandlung hypoglykämischer Zustände durch pharmakologische Hemmung der Insulinsekretion. Vortrag am 8. 6. 1967 am Ärztl. Verein München.

David, V. C.: Surgery **8**, 212 (1940).

Harris, S.: J. Amer. med. Ass. **83**, 729 (1924).

Howard, J. M., and G. L. Jordan: Surgical diseases of the pancreas. Philadelphia: Lippincott 1960.

Hultquist, G. T., M. Dahlen und C. G. Helander: Schweiz. Z. Path. **11**, 570 (1948).

Jalow, R. S., and S. A. Berson: J. clin. Invest. **39**, 1157 (1960).

Joseph, L., and H. S. Bhat: Indian J. Surg. **28**, 1 (1966).

Katsch, R.: Zit. nach Meythaler, F., u. A. Müller.

Kooreman, P. J.: Arch. chir. neerl. **17**, 1 (1965).

Labhart, A.: Klinik der inneren Sekretion. Berlin-Göttingen-Heidelberg: Springer 1957.

Maingot, R.: Abdominal operations. Fourth Edition 1961. New York: Appleton-Century-Crotts, INC.

Marshall, S. F.: Surg. Clin. N. Amer. **3**, 775 (1958).

Meythaler, F., u. A. Müller: Pancreopathia hypoglycaemica. Ärztl. Forsch. **7**, 337 **9**, 467 **10**, 518 (1966).

Olsson, O.: Acta chir. scand. **126**, 346 (1963).

Pfeiffer, E. F., M. Pfeiffer, H. Ditschuneit und Akn Chang-Su: Klin. Wschr. **37**, 1239 (1959).

Renold, A. E., D. B. Marten, J. M. Dagenais, J. Steinke, R. J. Mickerson, and M. C. Sheps: J. clin. Invest. **39**, 1487 (1960).

Schultis, K., u. F. X. Sailer: Med. Welt (Stuttg.) **22**, 1213 (1966).

Sendrall, M., u. M. Cahnzag: Physiologie der inneren Sekretion. Leipzig: Thieme 1936.

Terbrüggen, A.: Virchows Arch. path. Anat. **315**, 407 (1948).

Vossschulte, K.: Verh. dtsch. Ges. Verdau.- u. Stoffwechselkr. **16**, 193 (1953).

—, u. W. H. Becker: Dtsch. med. Wschr. **78**, 105 (1953).

WHIPPLE, A. O.: J. int. Chir. **111**, 1 (1938).
WILDER, R. H., F. N. ALLAN, M. H. POWER, and H. E. ROBERTSON: J. Amer. med. Ass. **89**, 348 (1927).
ZENKER, R.: In: KIRSCHNER-GULEKE-ZENKER, Allgem. u. Spez. Chir. Op.-Lehre, 2. Aufl., Bd. VII/1 S. 778. Berlin-Göttingen-Heidelberg: Springer 1951.
—, u. A. GRABIGER: Bruns' Beitr. klin. Chir. **214**, 41 (1967).
—, u. H. J. PEIPER: Münch. med. Wschr. **100**, 1094 (1958).
—, u. R. PICHLMAYR: Wien. med. Wschr. **47**, 795 (1961).
—, R. BEDACHT und H. ZIMMERMANN: Münch. med. Wschr. **108**, 1691 (1966).

Non-Insulin-Secreting Islet Cell Tumors

ROBERT M. ZOLLINGER*

Islet cell tumors of the pancreas have been confirmed to have the potential for producing a variety of clinical syndromes. Certain non-insulin-secreting islet cell tumors exert a strong functional influence on the gastrointestinal tract, either in the form of a fulminating ulcer diathesis, a fulminating diarrhea or a combination of both. These clinical variants have given rise to considerable speculation that more than one hormone is involved. Those islet cell tumors producing a potent gastric secretagogue responsible for a fulminating ulcer diathesis, as well as those producing a secretin-like hormone responsible for achlorhydria, watery diarrhea and hypokalemia will be discussed.

Approximately 600 clinical cases have been reported to substantiate the clinical triad proposed in 1955 which consisted of: (1) fulminating ulcer diathesis, (2) marked gastric hypersecretion, and (3) a non-β islet cell tumor of the pancreas (ZOLLINGER and ELLISON). Additional emphasis has subsequently been placed on associated endocrine adenomata involving particularly the parathyroid glands, and the familial polyglandular syndrome described by WERMER. Originally it was postulated that an ulcerogenic humeral factor of pancreatic islet origin was responsible for the gigantic gastric hypersecretion resulting in recurrent ulcerations until all the acid-secreting surface had been removed by total gastrectomy. Within 5 years, Professor GREGORY and his associate, Dr. TRACY, found that these tumors as well as their metastases were producing a potent gastric secretagogue similar to gastrin in amounts 35 times greater than a similar weight of hog antrum (GREGORY et al.). This demonstration renewed interest in the mechanisms of gastric hypersecretion and methods for its control. However, the problems of establishing the presence of such a tumor preoperatively and how best to treat it remain a challenge.

Gastric hypersecretion continues to be the dominating feature in approximately 95% of those patients having a gastrin-producing islet cell tumor (Fig. 1). A fulminating ulcer diathesis occurred in 59% of the cases, and in another 30%, the ulceration was accompanied by a diarrhea described as either watery or steatorrhea. It has been difficult to understand the absence of ulcer in approximately 6% of the patients who have only severe diarrhea. 5% of the patients with non-insulin-secreting islet cell tumors have had a fulminating diarrhea so severe as to be called pancreatic

* Professor and Chairman, Department of Surgery, The Ohio State University College of Medicine.

Supported by a grant from The John A. Hartford Foundation, Inc., New York, N.Y.

"cholera" (MATSUMOTO et al.) and accompanied by achlorhydria rather than gastric hypersecretion.

Studies of gastric secretion are invaluable in establishing the diagnosis of an ulcerogenic tumor. The diagnosis is suspected if 1,000 cm^3 or more of gastric juice containing 100 mEq free hydrochloric acid is produced by an unobstructed stomach during a 12 h overnight aspiration. Further support is given to the diagnosis if the ratio of the basal acid output to the maximal acid output after histamine stimulation is greater than 0.6. Of even greater significance, according to RUPPERT and associates is the concentration of acid output regardless of the volume (RUPPERT et al.). Once again, after histamine stimulation the ratio of basal acid concentration to maximal acid concentration is greater than 0.6 in the presence of a tumor. They have found this high ratio to have great diagnostic significance.

The roentgenologists are recognizing the tell-tale signs of this syndrome which result from the marked gastric hypersecretion. The important diagnostic signs include: markedly hypertrophic gastric rugae and the presence of large amounts of

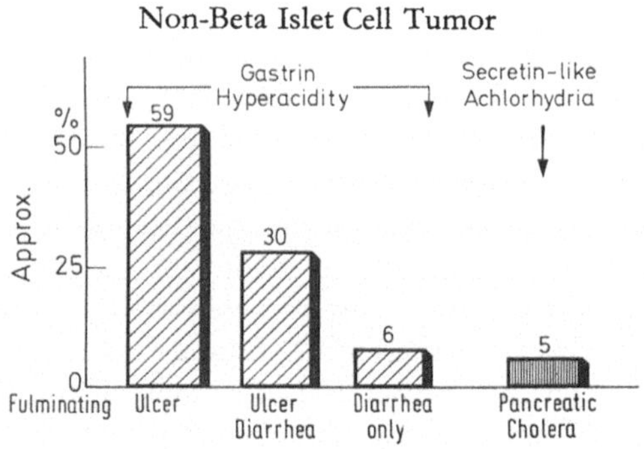

Fig. 1. Distribution of presenting symptoms in reported cases with non-insulin-secreting islet cell tumor

gastric fluid despite fasting, continuous overnight aspiration and the lack of any obstruction. A primary ulcer beyond the ligament of Treitz is almost pathognomonic of ulcerogenic syndrome; however, peptic ulcerations usually occur in the duodenum. The duodenal bulb is often dilated while the remainder of the duodenum has a shaggy appearance. Less specific signs are small bowel hypermotility, edema and inflammation. Ulcers recurring after previous gastric resection tend to be located along the mesenteric border in the efferent loop rather than in the usual marginal location (CHRISTOFORIDIS and NELSON).

In addition to the previously mentioned studies, visualization and localization of the tumor by arteriography or isotope scan using ^{75}Selenium may prove valuable. Because of the high incidence of malignancy, a scan of the liver with ^{99m}Technetium may also be indicated. Further confirmation of the diagnosis may be obtained by a search for excessive amounts of gastric secretagogue in specimens of early morning, fasting serum, gastric juice or urine. The bioassay method of LAI as utilized by SIRCUS and BONFILS (BONFILS et al.) can provide diagnostic verification of the presence of an ulcerogenic tumor. Recent studies by SCHNEIDER (SCHNEIDER et al.), STREMPLE (STREMPLE et al.), MCGUIGAN and others have sought a more sensitive indicator for the presence of excessive amounts of gastrin by radio-immunoassay.

This interesting advance should eventually enhance the accuracy and earlier diagnosis of those tumors producing a gastric secretagogue.

As in the original recommendation, total gastrectomy remains the most satisfactory treatment for the majority of patients regardless of age. FRIESEN has recently given additional support to this concept with the suggestion that metastases and residual ulcerogenic tumor have tended to disappear after removal of the target organ by total gastrectomy. 1 of the original 2 patients with metastatic islet cell tumor in the adjacent lymph nodes has remained symptom-free 14 years after total gastrectomy and has had 2 children, 7 and 8 years after the operation. While there have been reports of sporadic successes after local excision of a tumor of the pancreas or the duodenal wall, a high incidence of recurrence must be anticipated because of the ulcerogenic tumor's high rate of malignancy and its tendency to be multiple and microscopic.

When the surgeon is unable to find gross tumor after a very careful search of the entire pancreas as well as the lumen and wall of the duodenum through a duodenotomy and frozen section examination of adjacent lymph nodes, a blind resection of the left half of the pancreas should be considered. In addition, the output of gastric juice should be continuously monitored during the procedure to observe the effects of vagotomy and resection of the antrum along with an inch of duodenum with the patient in the supine position and the tip of the tube in the fundus of the stomach. Unless the output of gastric juice is markedly reduced, total gastrectomy should be performed. The nutrition of these patients following total gastrectomy has been unexplainedly good, in contrast to the patient who has had total gastrectomy for another disease.

Although watery diarrhea was noted in one of the first patients, it remained for PRIEST and ALEXANDER in 1957 to call attention to its potential seriousness. In 1958, VERNER and MORRISON defined the renal lesion which could cause death in those few patients with severe watery diarrhea and hypokalemia. They suggested this entity was a variant of the ulcerogenic syndrome and theorized that two different tumors existed, each associated with a different clinical syndrome. That same year, MAYNARD and POINT described steatorrhea on the basis of gastric hyperacidity.

The diarrhea was commonly believed to result from the neutralizing effects of the extreme gastric hypersecretion, which also caused irritation of the bowel. It has also been suggested that the diarrhea could be explained by the direct stimulatory effect that gastrin has on bowel motility. Although a separate mechanism was suspected, it was not until 1961 that MURRAY called attention to achlorhydria in the group of patients with watery diarrhea and hypokalemia (MURRAY et al.). This small group of patients numbers approximately 25 or less in the literature, with only 13 having documented achlorhydria. This syndrome has been termed pancreatic "cholera" by MATSUMOTO in 1966 (MATSUMOTO et al.). More recently MARKS of Capetown in 1967 called this entity the WDHA Syndrome, which represents the first letter of the primary clinical and laboratory findings, i.e. *W*atery *D*iarrhea, *H*ypokalemia and *A*chlorhydria (MARKS et al.). There is no evidence of gastrin activity by bioassay in either the serum or in extracts of the tumor in these patients.

A recent study (ZOLLINGER et al.) of two patients, one from the Ohio State University Hospitals (Columbus, Ohio) and the second from The Emory University Hospital (Atlanta, Georgia), has suggested that these diarrheogenic tumors produce a secretin-like hormone. These patients were both married women, 24 and 47 years of age, and the mothers of several children. Both patients presented with the classical syndrome of fulminating diarrhea, which approximated 2 to 4 l a day. There was a tremendous loss of potassium in the stool which resulted in severe hypokalemia. Their serum potassium levels were invariably lower than 3 mEq/l despite the administration of 200 mEq potassium every 24 h. The diarrhea was watery in nature, with no evidence of steatorrhea. The potassium loss was dramatic and far in excess of that usually encountered. Both patients were demonstrated to have absence of free hydrochloric acid by gastric analysis. Lai rat serum bioassay for the presence of a gastric secretagogue was negative in both cases. The younger patient had a strong family history of ulcer disease, hyperparathyroidism and her father and one uncle had ulcerogenic tumors of the pancreas. She previously had evidence of hyperparathyroidism which was treated by removal of 3.5 parathyroid glands. Microscopically these glands demonstrated hyperplasia.

The diarrhea in the younger patient had recurred intermittently in cycles over a 4 year period. This was in contrast to the second patient who had a constant diarrhea for 9 months.

At surgery, the younger patient had a large, discrete islet cell tumor in the mid-portion of the pancreas, as well as a smaller tumor in the tail and diffuse micro-adenomatosis. The body and tail of the pancreas were removed, but nothing was done to the stomach. The older patient had evidence of extensive metastases to the liver, and within 30 days succumbed to her disease. There was a small non-β islet cell tumor found deep in the head of the pancreas at postmortem examination. The microscopic appearance of the tumors was similar in both cases.

During the operation on the younger patient, it was observed that the duodenum appeared to refill with secretions. The gallbladder was noted to be markedly distended. A sufficient amount of bile (30 cc) was aspirated to ensure complete chemical analysis. Several biopsy specimens were taken from the small intestine and stomach for microscopic study.

The first clue to the possibility that the non-β islet cell tumors of the younger patient were producing a secretin-like hormone became apparent within 5 days after operation. Careful, repeated gastric analyses performed before surgery had shown achlorhydria, which could be overridden by the administration of histamine. Within 5 days after removal of the tumors, with nothing having been done to the stomach, gastric analysis showed the appearance of 55 mEq/l of free hydrochloric acid without stimulation. This suggested that a gastric acid inhibitory factor had been removed by surgery. Follow-up studies performed as long as 8.5 months later have continued to show the presence of free hydrochloric acid. As pointed out by Dragstedt, secretin inhibits the production of hydrochloric acid, but this inhibition can be overridden by the administration of histamine as shown in this patient (Greenlee et al.). Because of the metastatic disease, such observations were not possible in the second patient.

The second clue supporting the concept that these non-β islet cell tumors were producing a secretin-like hormone came from the subsequent analysis of the bile aspirated from the dilated gallbladder of the younger patient at the time of surgery. The bile was indeed dilute. Despite this dilution, however, the bile was found to contain 2.5 times the normal amount of sodium chloride and 4.5 times the normal amount of bicarbonate. Previous experience with the analysis of gallbladder bile from ten patients, without gallstones, were used for comparison. The presence of a dilated gallbladder containing dilute bile, rich in chloride and bicarbonate concentrations, is consistent with the biliary effect of secretin as described by Agren and Wheeler.

Dr. J. RICHARD AMERSON of The Emory University Department of Surgery aspirated bile from the distended gallbladder of the second patient with parallel chemical findings.

Proof to support the presence of secretin, short of amino acid sequence determinations, would be to show that an extract made from these tumors had a classical secretin stimulating effect on pancreatic and hepatic secretions. Using the method provided by LIN (Eli Lilly Research Laboratories), hydrochloric acid extracts of the tumors were prepared for intravenous injection. Dogs were prepared according to the method of LIN with the pylorus ligated and extraduodenal cannulation of the pancreatic and common bile ducts (LIN and ALPHIN). Under phenobarbital anesthesia, pure natural *(Jorpes)* and synthetic secretin *(Bodanszky)* were injected in 25 unit amounts to establish the typical pancreatic response for comparison with the tumor

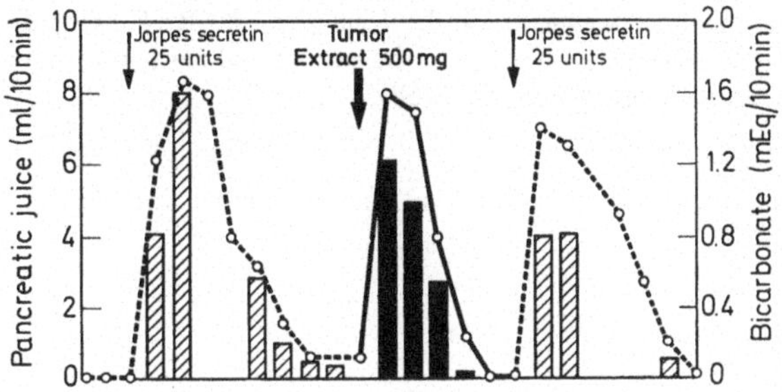

Fig. 2. The pancreatic juice volume *(line)* and bicarbonate output *(bar)* after intravenous injection of *Jorpes* secretion and extract made from "diarrheogenic" non-beta islet cell tumor are similar

extracts. The volume and bicarbonate response of the extract made from the metastasis of the older patient was parallel to that of the natural and synthetic secretin. A positive response was obtained in five different animals (Fig. 2). No response was obtained from the extracts of the firm, smaller tumor removed from the younger patient.

Further studies on adequate amounts of primary tumors or their metastases will be required to confirm or deny these observations. It is not unreasonable to assume that the non-β islet cells of the pancreas can produce secretin as well as gastrin since they have a common cell of origin with the antrum and the duodenum, which normally produce these hormones.

References

AGREN, G., and H. LAGERLOF: Acta med. scand. **92**, 359—366 (1937).

BONFILS, S., J. P., BADER, M. DUBRASQUET et A. LAMBLING: Arch. Mal. Appar. dig. **54**, 647—662 (1965).

CHRISTOFORIDIS, A. J., and S. W. NELSON: J. Amer. med. Ass. **198**, 511—516 (1964).

FRIESEN, S. R.: A gastric factor in the pathogenesis of the Zollinger-Ellison Syndrome. Ann. Surg. (In press).

GREENLEE, H. B., E. H. LONGHI, J. D. GUERRERO, T. S. NELSEN, A. L. EL-BEDRI, and L. R. DRAGSTEDT: Amer. J. Physiol. **190**, 396—402 (1957).

GREGORY, R. A., H. J. TRACY, J. M. FRENCH, and W. SIRCUS: Lancet **1960 I**, 1045—1048.

LAI, K. S.: Gut **5**, 327—341 (1964).

LIN, T. M., and R. S. ALPHIN: Amer. J. Physiol. **203**, 926—928 (1962).

MARKS, I. N., S. BANK, and J. H. LOUW: Gastroenterology **52**, 695—708 (1967).

Matsumoto, K. K., J. B. Peter, R. G. Shultze, A. A. Hakim, and P. T. Franck: Gastroenterology **50**, 231—242 (1966).
Maynard, E. P. III, and W. W. Point: Amer. J. Med. **25**, 456—459 (1958).
McGuigan, J. E.: Clin. Res. **16**, 288 (1968).
Murray, J. S., R. R. Paton, and C. E. Pope II: New Engl. J. Med. **264**, 436—439 (1961).
Priest, W. M., and M. K. Alexander: Lancet **1957 II**, 1145—1147.
Ruppert, R. D., N. J. Greenberger, F. M. Beman, and F. M. McCullough: Ann. intern. Med. **67**, 808—815 (1967).
Schneider, D. R., G. L. Endahl, M. C. Dodd, J. E. Jesseph, N. J. Bigley, and R. M. Zollinger: Science **156**, 391—392 (1967).
Stremple, J. F., P. Abramoff, J. C. van Oss, S. D. Wilson, and E. H. Ellison: Lancet **1967 II**, 1180—1182.
Verner, J. V., and A. B. Morrison: Amer. J. Med. **25**, 374—380 (1958).
Wermer, P.: Amer. J. Med. **35**, 205 (1963).
Wheeler, H. O.: Inorganic ions in bile. In: W. Taylor, Ed., The biliary system. Philadelphia: F. A. Davis Co. 1965.
Zollinger, R. M., and E. H. Ellison: Ann. Surg. **142**, 709—722 (1955).
—, R. K. Tompkins, J. R. Amerson, G. L. Endahl, A. R. Kraft, and F. T. Moore: Identification of the diarrheogenic hormone associated with non-beta islet cell tumors of the pancreas. Ann. Surg. (In press, 1968).

Portal Hypertension

Hepatic Blood Flow and Portal Hypertension

W. Dean Warren

Introduction

Cirrhosis of the liver is one of the ten great killers in the United States. In spite of an enormous effort in the investigation of therapeutic modalities, there is little evidence that the basic outlook for the cirrhotic has been improved. This has been admirably demonstrated in a report by Garceau and Chalmers, who found death from bleeding to be the greatest single threat to patients with cirrhosis and esophageal varices. Yet, in the randomized studies by Callow et al., and Conn and Lindenmuth, the effectiveness of prophylactic portacaval shunt in prolongation of life was not confirmed; no significant difference has been demonstrated between the control, or non-operative group, and those undergoing portacaval shunt. An analysis of this data by Warren et al., reveals that the shunt successfully prevents death from bleeding, but an increased death rate from hepatic failure is substituted in the surgical group. By comparison, in an analysis of a non-shunting procedure by Johnson et al., re-bleeding was quite common, but hepatic failure did not appear to be accelerated in the survivors of the operation. Because of our belief that change in hepatic hemodynamics is one of the major factors influencing the fate of persons undergoing portacaval shunt, extensive hemodynamic studies have been carried out in over 150 patients with various complications of cirrhosis of the liver. There is a growing conviction that a thorough understanding of the hemodynamic implications of any operative procedure must be achieved before optimal therapy can be chosen for the individual patient. This work is presented as a brief survey of our current knowledge in this important field of clinical investigation.

Hepatic Blood Flow in the Normal

Although our group has not been extensively involved in the study of normal liver blood flow, a great amount of work has been carried out in this field by many other investigators. Until recently it was generally believed that the two afferent pathways perfused essentially the same group of capillary vessels, except for the biliary ductules which receive only arterial blood. However, studies by Birtch et al., utilizing a wash-out technique of radioactive gases have seemed to indicate that the portal venous blood perfuses all of the hepatic sinusoids while a lesser number receives both arterial and venous inflow. While the significance of this is not fully understood at present, it would seem likely that sudden, complete diversion of portal blood by portacaval shunt would leave some sinusoids with markedly diminished perfusion. A—V shunts in the pre-sinusoidal region have been demonstrated by a number of anatomic techniques and perhaps these are involved in the redistribution of flow under such circumstances. These rather unique characteristics of hepatic blood flow are still incompletely elucidated and contribute to the generally inadequate understanding of the effect of operative procedures involving the portal system.

Another characteristic of the hepatic circulation of clinical significance is the sinusoidal nature of its capillary bed. It is now thoroughly documented that the size of particles crossing the membrane of the hepatic sinusoid is much larger than seen in an ordinary capillary system. One manifestation is an increased albumin content of the hepatic lymph; with sinusoidal hypertension there is a marked increase in the lymph of cellular components as well as protein. This is of significance in the development of two well-known aspects of cirrhosis, the occurrence of ascites and a markedly increased thoracic duct flow as measured by thoracic duct cannulation. The significance of these normal physiologic characteristics of liver circulation will be discussed later in relation to the implications of various therapeutic endeavors.

Effect of Operative Changes upon the Normal Liver

Portal Venous System

It has long been known that portacaval shunt in experimental animals is tolerated poorly and followed frequently by delayed hepatic failure and death. This has been extensively studied in dogs and has been well documented in laboratories throughout the world. This was thought by some to be an idiosyncrasy of the canine species with little application to other animals or to humans. However, in studies with the spider monkey, WARREN and FOMON obtained results very similar to those seen in the dog. Although the initial operative procedure was tolerated well, the animals began a downhill course which was characterized by a loss of appetite, weight loss and death from hepatic failure. The mechanism of this demise is poorly understood. Although instances of portacaval shunt in a non-cirrhotic man are few and frequently complicated by other considerations, it would appear that portacaval shunt in the presence of an unobstructed portal vein and a normal liver is fraught with hazard. The studies of HUBBARD emphasized this problem, and were supported by other reports. It is worth noting that the studies by MIKKELSEN et al. on so-called hepatoportal sclerosis add supportive data in this regard. In a group of 17 patients, characterized by a patent portal vein and essentially normal liver chemistry, portacaval shunt was followed by delayed hepatic death in five and encephalopathy in an additional five. This also adds strength to the impression that the normal liver tolerates a portacaval anastomosis poorly.

By contrast, thrombosis of the portal vein appears to be tolerated relatively well. One evidence of this is the lack of hepatic failure and hepatic disability seen in children who have been found to have spontaneous thrombosis of the portal vein. This conceivably could be due to the thrombosis of the vein in the neonatal period when the hepatic circulation has not fully changed from its fetal environment. However, ALDRETE et al., showed that in experimental animals complete obstruction of the portal vein was tolerated much better than was portacaval shunt. Although the portal flow to the liver is lost in both groups, it is apparent that there is a markedly divergent vascular pattern in the two situations. In one there is a normal or below normal portal pressure with normal intrahepatic pressure whereas in the other the intrahepatic pressure remains normal but there is a marked hypertension in the portal venous system. Recent data from the laboratory of PRICE et al., would indicate that following portacaval anastomosis there is a more rapid absorption of metabolic products, such as ammonia, which raises the question of a toxic factor.

Hepatic Artery

The outlook following hepatic artery ligation is markedly different. Although there is a definite mortality associated with the ligation of the hepatic artery in experimental animals, due to the precipitation of hepatic necrosis, animals which survived suffered little disability. RESTREPO and WARREN found the liver blood flow of the dog acutely depresssed to a moderate degree with a return to normal within a few days following hepatic artery ligation. In survivors there was no evidence of disability and there was no impairment of long-term survival. It appears that loss of the hepatic artery, if not fatal due to acute hepatic necrosis, carries little disability so long as the portal vein is open and continues to perfuse the liver.

Cirrhosis and Portal Hypertension

The proper utilization of surgical procedures in the management of complications of cirrhosis is greatly facilitated by an understanding of the overall vascular physiology of this condition. The table is a summary of the features of cirrhosis and portal hypertension that we have documented over a number of years in the study of many patients. Although some of the techniques are still somewhat inexact, the utilization of large numbers of patients and repetitive examinations in an individual patient has allowed us to develop results which are highly significant when analyzed statistically. A brief summary of these parameters is in order:

Hepatic Sinusoidal Pressure

The wedged hepatic vein pressure has now been well documented to reflect closely the sinusoidal pressure. This has been shown by WARREN et al., utilizing simultaneous catheterization through the portal venous and hepatic venous systems, and by CHALMERS et al., who determined the intrahepatic pressure by percutaneous transhepatic needle puncture. Consequently, we can be fully confident that the data obtained by these studies are highly significant and extremely reliable in terms of the analysis of the group of patients. There is no doubt that the hepatic sinusoidal pressure is increased in cirrhosis of the liver. This has been demonstrated to be true in virtually 100% of cases in our own studies as well as those of many other investigators. Although this may range from only a few millimeters of mercury above central venous pressure to levels of 40 to 50 millimeters of mercury, the occurrence of a true cirrhosis of the liver without sinusoidal hypertension is extremely rare. By contrast, extrahepatic obstruction of the portal vein in the non-cirrhotic is characterized by normal hepatic sinusoidal pressure. The techniques available do not allow us to make a judgment between normal and subnormal pressures, and it is quite conceivable that there actually is a minute depression of sinusoidal pressure in this latter circumstance.

Portal Vein Pressure

A number of studies have now compared the level of portal vein pressure with the hepatic sinusoidal pressure in cirrhosis and delineated a very close correlation. It is obvious that when portal blood continues to perfuse the hepatic sinusoids there has to be a slight pressure gradient from the portal vein through the hepatic sinusoids but this has been found to be quite small. In marked contrast is the non-cirrhotic extrahepatic obstruction in which there is a marked elevation in portal vein pressure but a normal sinusoidal pressure. Consequently hepatic vein catheterization allows for a clear delineation between cirrhosis and non-cirrhotic extrahepatic portal vein obstruction.

Portal Venous Flow to the hiver

It is universally accepted that a marked reduction in portal venous flow to the liver is seen in cirrhosis. This can be substantiated in a number of ways. Splenoportographic examination has graphically demonstrated the large amounts of dye flowing around the liver to various collateral channels connecting the portal and the systemic venous systems. This angiographic portrayal of the progressive diminution of portal venous flow to the liver was recently climaxed by reports of WARREN et al., which demonstrated spontaneous reversal of flow in the intrahepatic portion of the portal vein. In such patients the obstruction to outflow from the liver raises the intrahepatic

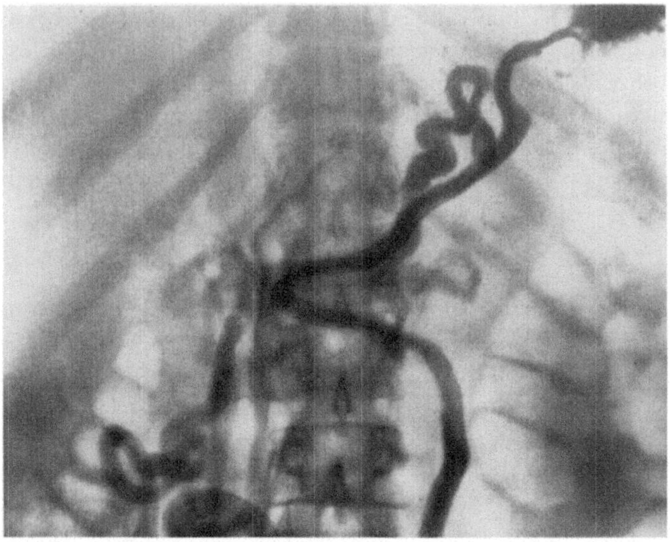

Fig. 1. Splenoportogram showing large collateral veins and absence of portal flow to the liver. Radiologic diagnosis was thrombosis of portal vein. (Reprinted by permission of Surgery, Gynecology and Obstetrics)

pressure to levels that exceed that in the portal vein, which is limited due to marked collateral vein development. In this circumstance the portal vein will appear to be thrombosed on splenoportography yet be patent and show *hepatofugal* flow through the portal vein on wedged hepatic venography (Figs. 1 and 2). This demonstration of the conversion of the portal vein to an outflow tract in the spontaneous evolution of cirrhosis is irrefutable evidence for the marked diminution in portal venous perfusion of the liver in cirrhosis. However, additional studies have been carried out to demonstrate this point; among them are studies which demonstrate little fall in the total hepatic blood flow following a total portacaval shunt in the far-advanced cirrhotic. Although the technique of measurement of venous flow by the electromagnetic flowmeter is especially subject to criticism around a side-to-side portacaval anastomosis, there are a number of studies which have demonstrated the markedly increased flow through the portal vein *following* an end-to-side portacaval anastomosis, indicating markedly restricted flow to the liver parenchyma pre-shunt.

The development of venovenous collateral between the portal vein and the central hepatic vein is a characteristic of the cirrhotic liver which is of real significance. Although it was widely held that hepatic artery-portal vein fistula was the major vascular shunt in the cirrhotic liver, it now appears from studies of SHALDON et al. and others that the major bypass of the hepatic parenchyma is accomplished by veno-venous shunts rather than by arteriovenous shunts. Using the technique of injection of macro-aggregates of human serum albumin, those authors have calculated that such shunts in cirrhotic patients may divert 25% of the total hepatic blood flow.

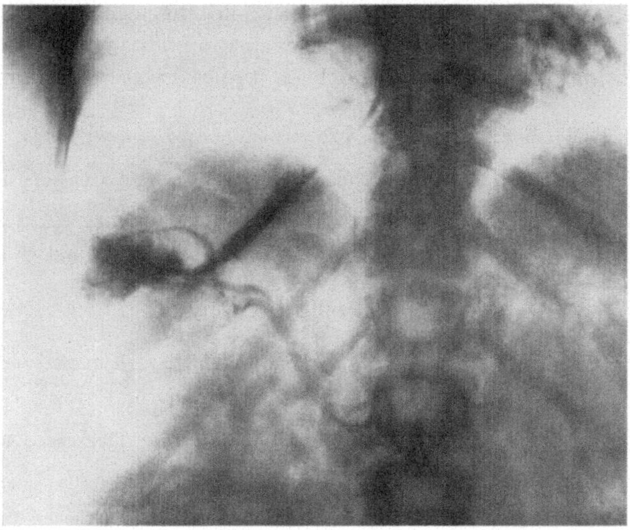

Fig. 2. Wedged hepatic venogram in same patient as Fig. 1 showing patent portal vein with hepatofugal portal flow

Hepatic Arterial Flow

The arterial system lends itself to measurement by the electromagnetic flowmeter to a far more satisfactory degree than does the venous system. Consequently, such studies of the hepatic arterial flow in cirrhosis are more reliable and reproducible than those of portal venous flow. Excellent data, both experimentally and clinically, reveal that hepatic arterial flow may actually increase in cirrhosis. There are also instances in which the hepatic arterial perfusion is markedly restricted either by the vascular lesion of cirrhosis or actual obstruction to the major hepatic radicals. It is evident, therefore, that in any given patient the hepatic arterial flow may be essentially normal, increased or decreased. This factor would appear to be of great importance in the pre-operative evaluation of patients for portacaval shunting but, thus far, satisfactory techniques for the *pre-operative* assessment of these various factors of flow to the liver are not available.

Total Hepatic Blood Flow — Estimated Hepatic Blood Flow (EHBF)

One of the great needs in the study of the human with cirrhosis is the development of better techniques for the assessment of total hepatic blood flow and its various components. All currently utilized methods have serious drawbacks in terms of inherent error. These stem largely from the 1) extrahepatic uptake of either colloidal or BSP-like materials, 2) the presence of intrahepatic arteriovenous and venovenous shunts which mitigate against the measurement of true sinusoidal blood flow by utilizing the Fick principle, 3) the unknown efficiency of the hepatic cell in cirrhosis for extraction of tracer substances. In spite of this and utilizing groups of patients so that statistical data of high significance have been attained, it is well documented that the total hepatic blood flow is decreased in the majority of patients with hepatic cirrhosis. Although the EHBF may be normal or even increased in an occasional patient with cirrhosis it is usually depressed, sometimes to levels which are one-third or less than that seen in the normal. Because the inherent direction of the error may be anticipated with the use of radioactive colloidal gold, this technique has proven to be especially useful to us as clinical tool in the evaluation of patients with cirrhosis and portal hypertension. In a large number of such studies it was found that patients with

Table. *Some general hemodynamic changes in portal hypertension*

	Cirrhosis Pre-shunt	Cirrhosis Post-shunt	Extra hepatic portal Vein obstruction
Hepatic sinusoidal pressure	Elevated	Decreased from pre-shunt level. Still higher than normal	Normal
Portal vein pressure	Elevated	Normal to sub-normal	Elevated
Portal venous flow to liver	Decreased to absent	Absent	Decreased to absent
Hepatic arterial flow	May be either decreased or increased	May be either decreased or increased	Increased
Total hepatic blood flow	Decreased	Decreased further	Usually decreased

cirrhosis and esophageal varices have an estimated total hepatic blood flow depressed to about two-thirds of the mean of the unoperated, normal human. In the normal experimental animal, RESTREPO and WARREN clearly showed that total hepatic blood flow is markedly altered by total deviation of portal venous blood. In such a circumstance the flow in the hepatic artery increases by about 100%. However, as the portal vein — hepatic artery ratio is about 3 to 1 in the normal, this would indicate that a 50% level of flow is to be expected following total deviation of portal venous blood. This indeed has been measured utilizing several different techniques in different laboratories with essentially similar findings being obtained. The recent utilization of radioactive gases and the washout technique has many theoretical advantages and may help clarify some of the uncertainties which persist in any study of patients with cirrhosis.

In summary, the portal hypertension of cirrhosis can be clearly shown to be an outflow block with the production of an elevated hepatic sinusoidal pressure. This, in turn, regulates the level of portal venous pressure, as long as the portal vein continues to perfuse the liver. As the pressure in the portal vein rises, the extrahepatic collateral venous circulation increases, which is a factor tending to decrease portal venous flow to the liver as well as limit the degree of pressure elevation in the portal vein. Of great importance metabolically is the large volume of portal venous blood which completely bypasses the liver. The estimated total hepatic blood flow is then moderately to markedly decreased in most instances due to severe reductions in hepatic portal venous flow. The hepatic arterial flow may increase in partial compensation for loss of portal flow but only rarely is the compensation complete.

Effect of Portacaval Shunt in the Presence of Cirrhosis and Portal Hypertension

Several investigations have found that a portacaval shunt in the cirrhotic results in a definite diminution of the *hepatic sinusoidal pressure* from the preoperative levels. This can be readily measured and has been found to be more profoundly depressed following a side-to-side portacaval shunt than after an end-to-side shunt. This is

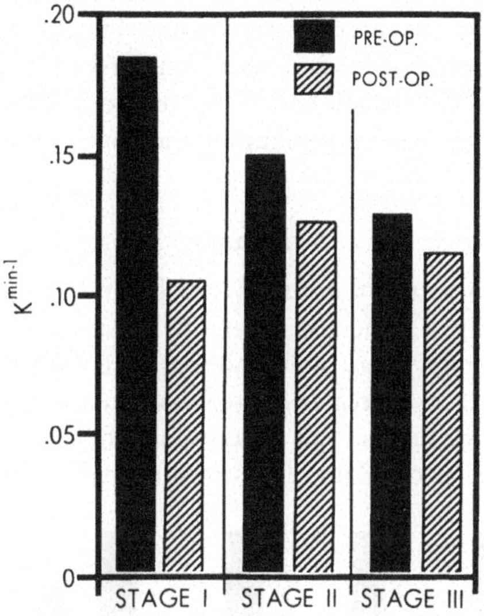

Fig. 3. Stage I is least severe portal hypertension. Note marked fall in the postoperative period, which is more severe than in Stage II or III. [Warren et al., Ann. Surg. **158**, 393 (1963)]

entirely predictable as the side-to-side portacaval anastomosis converts the portal vein to an outflow tract from the liver, whereas the end-to-side portacaval shunt does not alter the hepatic outflow venous system. A fall in pressure following an end-to-side shunt is proportional to the fall in EHBF which follows the portacaval anastomosis. The portacaval shunt procedures have had marked success in the control of bleeding from esophageal varices, and portal vein pressure post-shunt in our patients has been entirely normal with very rare exceptions. An occasional failure may be seen when a very large, caudate lobe results in compression of the vena cava and the so-called "reverse ECK fistula" with shunting of inferior vena caval blood in a reverse fashion through the shunt. Fortunately, however, these instances are quite uncommon. Although clinical studies are not very precise in this regard, there are at least some patients in whom hepatic-arterial flow seems to increase following a portacaval anastomosis. There are other instances, however, in which this does not occur and the work of Smith et al., would seem to indicate that there is reflex vasomotor control which may actually limit arterial compensation. The complete fall in pressure in the intestinal bed while hypertension continues in the hepatic sinusoids might account for the failure to compensate fully for loss of hepatic flow.

In a study of more than 75 side-to-side portacaval shunts, we have never obtained angiographic evidence that portal blood continues to perfuse the liver. It might then be said that following a portacaval anastomosis of any type no perfusion of portal blood through the hepatic sinusoids can be expected. However, there can be instances in which the size of the anastomosis is so small as to incompletely decompress the portal system and in this instance perfusion might be seen.

As the portal venous flow to the liver can be quite high preoperatively and then be totally absent postoperatively, it follows that there should be a decrease postoperatively in the total hepatic blood flow. This has been documented and the data are unequivocal in this regard. The level of postoperative blood flow as seen in Fig. 3 is markedly similar in all postoperative patients following a portacaval anastomosis while being dissimilar in the preoperative state. This, again, adds confirmatory of evident 1) the completeness of portal venous diversion post-shunt and 2) the inadequate compensation of the hepatic artery for total loss of portal venous flow. Both factors are of great importance in understanding the physiology of portal hypertension and portacaval shunt.

Summary

In cirrhosis the portacaval anastomosis usually induces the following changes graphically depicted in Fig. 4. There is a definite lowering of the hepatic sinusoidal pressure. However, this rarely returns to normal, even with the side-to-side shunt which lowers this pressure to a greater degree than an end-to-side shunt. The portal vein pressure is lowered to normal; all portal blood bypasses the liver parenchyma, which means that there is a total loss of gastrointestinal venous blood perfusing the

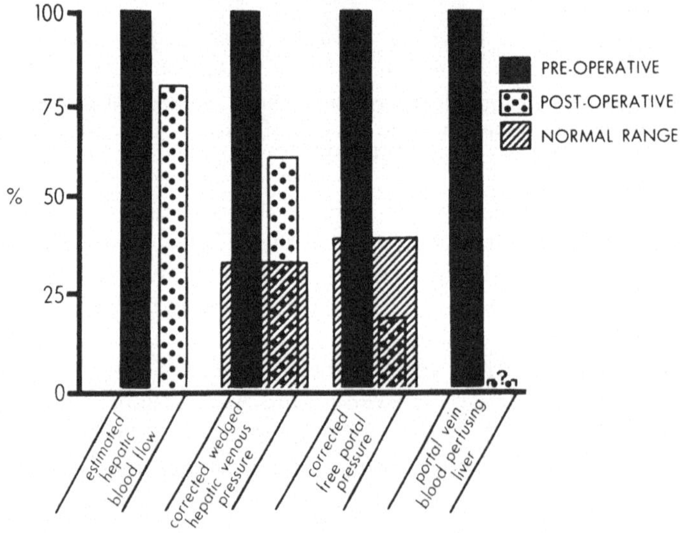

Fig. 4. Average of changes induced by portacaval shunting. Corrected pressures indicate differences from central venous pressure. Note the subnormal post-shunt free portal pressure. [Warren et al., Ann. Surg. **158**, 395, (1963)]

liver. The hepatic artery flow may increase following a portacaval anastomosis and becomes the sole source of perfusion of the hepatic sinusoids following a portacaval shunt. The total hepatic blood flow suffers a definite fall which is most pronounced in those patients having high preoperative portal flow to the liver but may be slight in those patients with spontaneous diversion of most of the portal flow prior to the shunt. The patient with extrahepatic thrombosis of the portal vein will suffer no change in hepatic sinusoidal pressure, will have a marked drop in the portal venous pressure, but will have little change in portal venous flow or portal perfusion of the liver except in the occasional case in which collateral veins have contributed significantly to the pre-shunt hepatic sinusoidal flow.

Comment

Any analysis of the results of therapy in cirrhosis of the liver is complex because of the multiple factors of importance in determining the ultimate outcome. Of paramount importance appears to be the cessation of alcohol intake in those cases in which the disease appears to be related to chronic alcoholism. As pointed out by Powell et al., the prognosis in patients who abstain totally from further alcohol consumption is markedly improved over those in whom continued alcohol intake is found. However, in patients with varices this difference is not as clearcut, which emphasizes the basic hazard of gastrointestinal bleeding. As pointed out in several recent studies, the danger of severe hemorrhage from esophageal varices continues to be one of the major threats facing patients with cirrhosis and varices. Although a successful portacaval anastomosis greatly lessens the risk of bleeding, the excellent review by Grace et al. has emphasized the failure to demonstrate any prolongation of life by successful portacaval shunting. It had seemed likely to most observers that the mortality from hepatic failure related to portacaval shunting procedures would be in the immediate postoperative period. However, these authors have not found this to be the case and this group of randomized prophylactic shunts has demonstrated an increased rate of hepatic failure following successful portacaval anastomosis. There appeared to be no difference between the groups in the other important variables, such as hepatocellular function, so that selection of patients with more far-advanced disease for operative intervention is unlikely as the explanation for this severe complication. Hemodynamic data from these studies is not sufficient to allow a comparison of the patients who did well following a shunt with those who had either severe morbidity or delayed mortality. Data from our laboratory have indicated that one group of patients in whom marked physiologic changes seemed to occur were those with so-called early portal hypertension. In this group the preoperative hepatic blood flow was more nearly normal than in the average cirrhotic patient, but the postoperative flow was depressed just as severely as in more far-advanced cases. This apparently resulted in a sudden, great change in hepatic vascular physiology including a marked change in hepatic blood flow. In general, these patients have not done well and have appeared to have higher incidence of encephalopathy, prolonged weakness, peripheral edema or delayed hepatic death than patients with stable but more far-advanced disease. The numbers are too small in this series, reported by Warren et al., to allow thorough evaluation and the patients were not randomized but, rather, were selected relative to the physiologic stage of the portal hypertensive process. Of equal significance has been the failure to find an increased incidence of encephalopathy or death from hepatic failure in the excellent study by

Johnson et al. In their patients, extensive devascularization of the stomach was carried out, but portal systemic shunting was not utilized. Although there was high immediate mortality and re-bleeding occurred in about 40% of the survivors, the problems of encephalopathy and delayed hepatic death were almost non-existent.

These when analyzed together would seem to give a strong circumstantial case for the potentially harmful effects of portacaval anastomosis. Recent laboratory studies by Price et al. on the effect of transplantation of the liver have indicated that portal perfusion of the liver is necessary for excellent hepatic function in the transplanted liver. Although it was originally thought that any comparable amount of blood flow would be essentially equal in providing for optimal liver function, this did not prove to be the case. Another complication is that of chronic encephalopathy, a problem of great enough severity to cause the imposition of protein restriction or

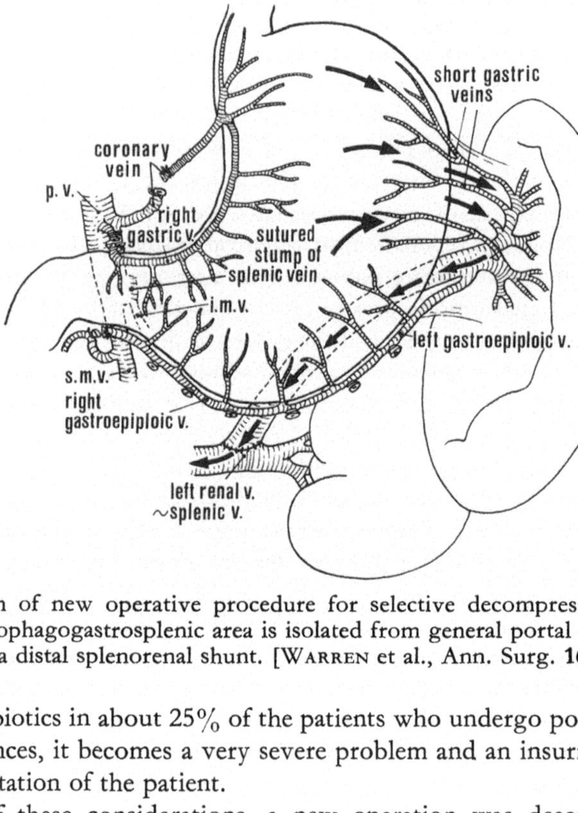

Fig. 5. Diagram of new operative procedure for selective decompression of esophageal varices. The esophagogastrosplenic area is isolated from general portal system and decompressed by a distal splenorenal shunt. [Warren et al., Ann. Surg. **166**, 443, (1967)]

intestinal antibiotics in about 25% of the patients who undergo portacaval shunting. In some instances, it becomes a very severe problem and an insurmountable barrier to the rehabilitation of the patient.

Because of these considerations, a new operation was described recently by Warren et al., in which selective decompression of esophageal varices has been accomplished. In this procedure the primary aim is to convert the organs of the left upper quadrant, encompassing the esophagogastric venous system, into a single unit draining through the spleen into the low pressure renal system. All connecting veins between the general portal circulation and this isolated group of organs are divided insofar as possible. The coronary vein is specifically identified, ligated and oversewn to prevent direct entry of large quantities of blood into the esophagogastric region. The esophagogastric varices are decompressed by draining through the gastrosplenic and diaphragmatic collaterals to the spleen and then through a distal end splenorenal shunt (Fig. 5). By contrast, portal hypertension is deliberately maintained in the portal system of the intestinal tract in order to continue perfusion of the liver.

At the present time there are 6 patients being studied postoperatively following this operation. In all, except 1, in whom anastomosis was disrupted by a technical error at the time of surgery, the shunt has remained patent as demonstrated by splenoportography (Fig. 6). In addition, in 4 of the 6 there is continuing perfusion of the liver by intestinal blood. The clinical results in all of these patients have shown a complete disappearance or marked regression of varices. There has been marked improvement in the handling of protein, evidenced by the protein tolerance test while monitoring peripheral blood ammonia. These patients demonstrate a curve not unlike an unoperated cirrhotic which is in marked contrast to the high peak blood ammonia seen in portacaval shunt patients. In addition, encephalopathy has not

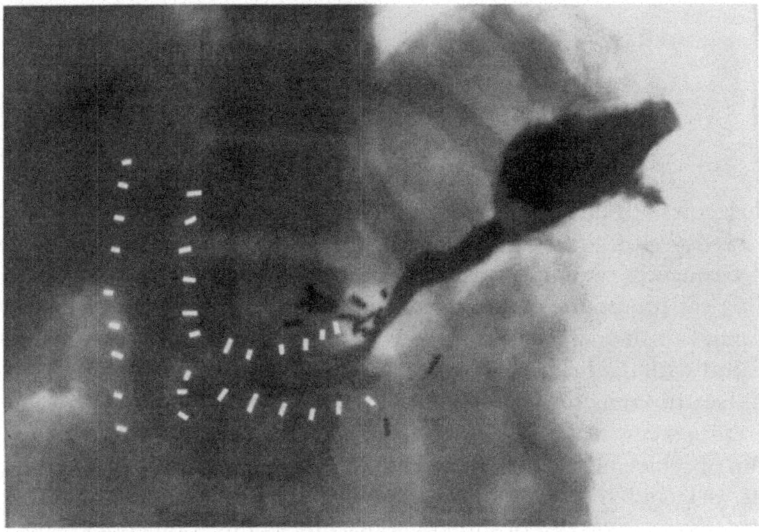

Fig. 6. Patency of a distal splenorenal anastomosis is demonstrated by splenoportography 2 weeks postoperatively

been present and protein restriction and intestinal antibiotics have been unnecessary. Although the number of cases involved is obviously too small for a clinical evaluation, the theoretical aim of the procedure has been accomplished, namely the selective decompression of esophagogastric varices while maintaining a high pressure hepatopetal flow through the intestinal branches of the portal venous bed. This new approach may well allow the successful control of bleeding while avoiding the serious defects of portacaval shunting.

References

Aldrete, J. S., D. G. McIlrath, and G. A. Hallenbeck: Surg. Forum **17**, 363 (1966).

Birtch, A. G., B. H. Casey, and R. M. Zakheim: Surgery **62**, 174 (1967).

Callow, A. D., J. B. Lloyd, A. Ishihara, E. Ponsdomenech, E. T. O'Hara, T. C. Chalmers, and A. J. Garceau: Surgery **57**, 123 (1965).

Chalmers, T. C.: Personal communication.

Conn, H. O., and W. W. Lindenmuth: New Engl. J. Med. **272**, 1255 (1965).

Grace, N. D., H. Muench, and T. C. Chalmers: Gastroenterology **50**, 684 (1966).

Hubbard, T. B., Jr.: Ann. Surg. **147**, 935 (1958).

Johnson, G., Jr., C. H. Dart, R. M. Peters, and J. A. MacFie: Ann. Surg. **163**, 692 (1966).
Mikkelsen, W. P., H. A. Edmondson, R. L. Peters, A. G. Redeker, and T. B. Reynolds: Ann. Surg. **162**, 602 (1965).
Powell, W. J., Jr., and G. Klatskin: Amer. J. Med. **44**, 406 (1968).
Price, J. B., A. B. Voorhees, and R. C. Britton: Surgery **62**, 195 (1967).
Restrepo, J. E., and W. D. Warren: Ann. Surg. **156**, 719 (1962).
Smith, G. W., R. C. Zug, and S. K. Wilson: Amer. J. Surg. **113**, 117 (1967).
Warren, W. D., and W. H. Muller, Jr.: Ann. Surg. **150**, 413 (1959).
—, and W. M. Thompson: Surg. Gynec. Obstet. **110**, 377 (1960).
—, J. E. Restrepo, J. C. Respess, and W. H. Muller, Jr.: Ann. Surg. **158**, 387 (1963).
—, J. J. Fomon, M. Viamonte, and R. Zeppa: (1) Ann. Surg. **165**, 999 (1967).
—, R. Zeppa, and J. J. Fomon: (2) Ann. Surg. **166**, 437 (1967).
—, J. J. Fomon, M. Viamonte, L. O. Martinez, and M. Kalser: Surg. Gynec. Obstet. **126**, 315 (1968).
— — Unpublished data.

Selection and Preparation of Patients for Porto-Caval Shunt Operation

Alfred Gütgemann

The surgeon finds himself in the difficult position of diverting a severe complication, the *impending* or *actual bleeding from varices*, which bears a letality of more than 50% and frequently cannot be managed by internal conservative measures, by an unphysiological procedure — the porto-caval shunt — which basically varies the hemodynamics of the deseased liver. This is carried out despite impaired liver performance and with the risk of causing temporary or further deterioration of the liver functions, hepatic coma or hepato-portal encephalopathy.

It therefore seems reasonable to perform porto-caval shunt procedures only if the desired aim of achieving freedom from bleeding appears obtainable under an agreeable immediate risk and the least disadvantageous consequences. This obliges us to narrow the *selection* to *the time* of surgery upon sufficient liver functions and to enforce *suitable preparations* until sufficient liver reserves appear guaranted.

At the same time appearance and type of a bleeding from varices, degree and development of varicosities and the anatomical and pressure conditions which can be registered by splenoportography and manometry severely determine the *time of intervention* and the *type of the anastomosis*.

The following reflections, as a result of 1000 patients with cirrhosis observed during hospital stay determine the *criteria* according to which we select patients with cirrhosis with danger of bleeding for the porto-caval shunt operation and perform the *preparing measures*.

I. *Etiology and pathogenesis of a cirrhosis*, its special *morphology* already decide on activity, progression and ability to compensate and therefore on the prognosis of each first and following bleeding episodes, also on the tolerance and possible deterioration into hepatic failure as a result of any form of stress combined with anesthesia, surgery and the hemodynamic changes of the portal and liver circulation. The regenerative, postnecrotic and postdystrophic cirrhosis tolerates more than cirrhosis from alcoholism, the latter more than the posthepatitic cirrhosis and the frequent intermediate forms. The longest postoperative survivals after shunt procedures — up to 15 years — we have observed in postdystrophic forms.

II. *Progredient and still active cirrhosis and acute episodes of decompensation* present an increased operative risk. Here a procedure is only justified in view of an enforced indication of abundant bleeding from varices which cannot be managed by conservative measures and with the hope that immediate and permanent interruption of the bleeding may inhibit further anemic-anoxemic damage of liver parenchyma.

If possible one should operate in a *bleeding free interval* and *only after remission* has been obtained. This presupposes a thorough and patient internal-conservative, dietetical-pharmaceutic preparation over weeks and months. Most important principles are:

Measures for preoperative preparation of the cirrhotic patient

1. Bed rest, small walks.
2. Diet, most important no alcohol at all.
3. Drugs, (Levulose, B-vitamins, Xanthinderivates etc.)
   — so called basical therapy —
4. Removal of ascites.
5. Time and patience.

However, longer preparing treatment always bears the risk of an intermediate occuring bleeding episode acute or recurring at short intervals. Then the principles as in any acute bleeding hold valid. If signs of an activation of the cirrhotic process are present, one should indeed wait for stabilisation before operating.

Signs for an activity of cirrhosis are:

1. Development related to time

a) short interval between acute hepatitis and change into chronic hepatitis or cirrhosis,

b) frequent, brief recurrent hepatitic episodes and phases of decompensation.

2. Changes in serum bilirubin over 2 mg-%.

3. Elevation of the serum transaminases SGOT and SGPT over 24 mE (normal up to 12 mE).

4. Inflammatory-cellular infiltrations or fresh necrosis in specimen obtained by liver puncture.

III. In the *elective indication*, that is the operation in the bleeding free interval and with *sufficient* preparation which should always be sought for, we orientate ourselves in the judgement of the actual capability and reserves of the liver parenchyma at an empiric number of chosen limit or low values for the permissability of a porto-caval shunt. More important than minor changes of the individual values appears to us the

Liver partial functions as criteria for surgery of porto-caval shunts

Test	Normal values	Minimum value
Serum-bilirubin	up to 1 mg-%	under 2 mg-%
Takata	80—100 mg-%	over 40 mg-%
Total protein	6—8 g%	over 6 g%
Albumin	4—6 g%	over 3 g%
Prothrombin	80—120%	over 50%
Factor V	80—120%	over 50%
Factor VII	80—120%	over 50%
Cholinesteraseactivity	1900—3800 mE	over 1600 mE
Bromsulfaleinretention	up to 5% i. 45 min	under 25%

cross section of selected liver-partial functions, as much as a recognisable tendency for improvement or stabilisation to be seen in repeated controls and with that reserves for surgery.

IV. In the full picture of cirrhosis ascites must be regarded as a decompensation of liver functions. The large number of hepatic factors which influence the regulation of the intra-extracellular water distribution make it appear advisable to *remove ascites* at first by means of bed rest, low sodium diet, aldosteron antagonists and saluretics and at least in the case of elective indication to *operate in an ascites free interval*. In fact one always succeeds, provided sufficient time and patience are invested by physician and patient.

Little amounts of remaining ascites in a patient with otherwise compensated liver functions do not present hazards as to the success of a shunt procedure. They disappear afterwards. Considerable amounts of ascites, however, always present an increased risk regarding postoperative liver failure. They should only be handled in a case of severe urgency because of untreatable bleeding from varices.

Conservative treatment of ascites in liver cirrhosis

1. Bed rest.
2. Low sodium diet.
3. Daily fluid intake not exceeding one L.
4. Diuretics.
   a) Saluretics (Potassium substitution).
   b) Aldosteron antagonists (Aldactone A up to 300 mg daily or Jatropur up to 200 mg daily).
5. Liver protective therapy.
6. Protein substitution (preferrably by oral intake).

V. *Hepato-portal encephalopathy* in cirrhosis can be observed in an almost equal number of cases spontaneously or following surgical shunt if varices are present. For once and in our opinion most important, this is the result of the limited detoxicating and synthetical functions of the liver parenchymal in other words the underlying liver disease. On the other side this occurs more markedly, however, the more cerebrotoxic protein metabolites remain in the systemic circulation through bypassing the liver filter via spontaneous or operative collaterals and anastomosis. It seems to be the total complex of partly physiological *protein metabolites* which are being filtered and detoxicated slower because of liver disease and hemodynamical changes. By no means does hyperammonemia alone cause the picture of spontaneous or postoperative that is postanastomical hepato-portal encephalopathy.

In two comparable groups of patients consisting of 142 non operated cirrhotics with portal hypertension and 114 patients with porto-caval anastomosis we found a frequency of 27%, taking into consideration any minor signs encountered by psychopathological and electroencephalographical changes often hardly registered by the individual himself, while clinically significant forms only numbered 9%. Spontaneous encephalopathy is of a more chronical character, while in postoperative encephalopathy more acute forms prevail. They are therefore more prominent. This would mean that activity as well as the grade of a hepato-portal encephalopathy are significantly determined by the actual capability of the liver parenchyma or the capability changed by the shunt procedure. Therefore its presence along with *preexisting syndromes* as common slowness, disturbances of registration, restlessness and a possible progression and therapeutical changeability present indirect parameters in judging the condition of the diseased liver. It is certain that the cirrhotic showing signs of encephalopathy has a higher risk in a shunt procedure and will more easily run into postoperative encephalopathy or liver failure. *Spontaneous* hepato-portal encephalopathy therefore in our view represents a *relative contraindication* for a shunt procedure. In any case it will require a most careful preparing treatment.

Treatment of pre- and postoperative hepato-portal encephalopathy

1. Basical therapy, conventional liver therapy.
2. Limitation of protein intake, most of all animal protein.
3. Reduction of resorption of toxic protein metabolites from the intestines
   a) thorough laxation,
   b) reduction of intestinal bacteria by antibiotics (neomycin, chloramphenicol and others),
   c) displacement or change of bacterial flora by lactobacillus acidophilus (bifidus milk).
4. Promotion of body own detoxication by malic acid — arginin-glutamin applications.
5. Elimination of individually damaging factors (alcohol, dietary errors, drugs and others).

We believe we have found that the danger of severe encephalopathy is less in the indirect porto-caval anastomosis, the spleno-renal shunt, showing a more transitory course and can be more easily managed by therapy than in the direct porto-caval shunt. On the other side this is opposed by a lesser degree of hemodynamic improvement and according to the literature a more frequent obstruction of the spleno-renal anastomosis by thrombosis. However, in cases with a large splenic vein free of thrombi we tend today to a spleno-renal anastomosis, this with the idea of achieving sufficient hemodynamic improvement of varices with the danger of bleeding in cases with questionable liver functions and finally of possibly decreasing the danger of hepato-portal encephalopathy and of favourably influencing higher degrees of hypersplenism through a splenectomy which is then always performed. Perhaps the indication can be broadened here.

VI. Along with these *genetal aspects* in the selection and preparation of cirrhotics with the danger of bleeding *further thoughts concerning timing* and *type of surgery* need be added in the individual case:

a) The danger of single or recurrent post splenectomy bleeding following *simple primary splenectomy* without shunt is exceedingly high in the cirrhotic. It runs above 50% and carries a very grave prognosis. Possibilities of a surgical management of further bleeding episodes are then strictly limited because of the always existent far reaching thrombosis of the splenic vein.

The effect of *simple splenectomy* as a palliative measure in the acutely bleeding cirrhotic mainly of the decompensated type is for once limited in time and on the other side bears no less risk than a shunt procedure.

b) The *acute*, *abundant* and not seldom the *first episode of bleeding from varices* truly deserves the attribute "catastrophal" because of the high danger of bleeding to death, also for preparing the path for a lethal liver coma. Its mortality ranges over or about 50%, in conservative and surgical treatment alike. If the patient reaches the surgeon severely bleeding and shows signs of a beginning liver coma, one will only succeed in a rare exemption to divert the lethal outcome. Surgery in such a case will frequently hurt the patient more than help him.

If bleeding has just started and no severe signs or hepatic failure or encephalopathy are present, if bilirubin, enzyme and protein-levels appear sufficient, then the fast decision for a shunt operation may save the patient before a more severe status of bleeding has occurred: Immediate operation.

Generally, however, bleeding has already persisted for a longer time. Massive resorption of liver toxic protein metabolites from decomposed blood masses in the bowel causes an additional, often decisive burden to a liver with anoxemic damage. According to our own favorable experience it appears more favorable in such a case to carry out the porto-caval shunt operation with a delay of 24 to 48 h. In the meantime care must be taken to stabilize circulation by continuous volume- and erythrocyte substitution and compression of the varices by ballons. Most of all the bowel has to be emptied thoroughly. If under such preparations a shunt procedure is carried out with a double ballon probe in place, a so called *delayed* or *postponed emergency operation*, the mortality of the porto-caval anastomosis during acute bleeding from varices could be improved from a former 53% to 20% presently. This experience is based on 235 cases of acute bleeding from varices.

Therapy in acute bleeding from varices

1. Immediate sufficient blood replacement.
2. Double ballon tamponade of the varices.
3. Shunt operation after removal of blood from the bowel
   a) porto-caval anastomosis in cases with good liver functions,
   b) spleno-renal anastomosis in cases with sufficient liver functions.
4. Conservative treatment in cases with bad liver functions
   a) blood transfusion (fast and sufficient),
   b) Hemostyptics (Thrombin p. o. epsilon amino-capronic-acid or AMCHA, Cohns fraction 1, calcium),
   c) ballon tamponade,
   d) bowel effective antibiotics (Neomycin, Chloramphenicol etc.),
   e) Magnesium-sulfate,
   f) Enemas,
   g) pharmacological liver protective therapy,
   h) coma prophylaxis (arginin-malic acid, glutamin acid).
5. If conservative therapy fails: surgical treatment via lymphovenous fistula, extracorporeal umbilicaval shunt or procedure at location of bleeding.
6. No surgery during hepatic coma.

c) Considering the comparatively high frequency of peptic gastro-duodenal ulcers of 5 to 6.9% in the average population and therefore the possible coincidence of cirrhosis and ulcer, cases of severe gastro-intestinal bleeding always require an intermediate radiological information whether cirrhosis or ulcer may be the cause of bleeding before further surgical measures are being taken. X-ray series are done immediately following management of bleeding shock. Emptying the stomach while the ballon probe remains in place and rinsing it cold, which appears necessary for clearing of radiological conditions, has both a relieving and an indirect blood clotting effect.

d) In view of the high spontaneous mortality ranging above 50 to 60% in the first bleeding episode and around 50% in the second and third bleeding episodes and the problem of conservative and operative definitive and palliative measures to stop bleeding, a *prophylactic shunt procedure* seems to us the more justified, the more pronounced present varices appear, the more they seem to develop and the better and equal liver functions are. This holds especially true if prodromas for bleeding exist, psychopathological changes are absent and the general prognosis as judged from little progredience, missing signs of activity and equalized test results may appear favorable. It would be wrong in this case to leave the patient to the uncertain fate of premature bleeding death. 8% among a total of 344 porto-caval shunt procedures in our material were prophylactic shunt operations.

List of shunt procedures
Department of Surgery, University of Bonn, 1953—1. 6. 1968

Patients with cirhosis of the liver — Total number of in-patients —	1056
Cirrhosis of the liver with portal hypertension	711
Shunt procedures *total*	344
porto-caval anastomosis	292
spleno-renal anastomosis	39
coronario-caval anastomosis	8
mesenterico-caval anastomosis	3
omphalico-caval anastomosis	1
epiploica-caval anastomosis	1

Observing strict criteria we believe it to be permissable to carry out prophylactic shunt procedures more frequently, mainly if this is possible via the spleno-renal anastomosis with a hemodynamic effect.

Criteria for prophylactic procedures

A Suppositions

1. Marked varicosis of the esophagus-gastric fornix.
2. Good liver function.
3. No encephalopathy.

B Risk of bleeding

1. Increase of esophageal varices according to controls.
2. Concomitant diseases increasing risk of bleeding (hiatal hernia, gastric volvulus, blood clotting defect).
3. Prodromas for bleeding (nose and tooth-bleeding, positive blood test in feces).

e) There is no doubt that aside from the selection of cirrhotics with a risk for bleeding for a shunt procedure and a thorough preparation, *optimal conditions in carrying out a shunt operation* can minimize the immediate risk of an additional liver damage. I believe this to be a decisive factor of paramount importance. Such optimal conditions consist in:

Surgical conditions for porto-caval shunt operation

1. *Short operating time* — in direct porto-caval anastomosis 1.5 to 2 h.
2. Minimize the total surgical trauma — *abdominal approach* —
3. *Avoid hypotensive phases* — no pharmaceutical, no hyperventilatory lowering of blood pressure —
4. *Avoid anemia and anoxemia* — no heparinisation, adequate blood and volume substitution —
5. *Liver protective anesthesia* (Neurolept analgesia).
6. *Hemodynamic effective anastomosis* (volume- and pressure relieving).

The fate of the patient with cirrhosis is determined as much by the character and the progression of his liver disease as well as in cases of portal hypertension by the occurrence of bleeding from varices. This is always severe and threatens the patient not only by the extent of the bleeding alone but also by the always accompanying further deterioration of reserves of the diseased liver. If we protect the patient from the danger of bleeding from varices by a porto-caval shunt operation and by that offer him a prolonged lifespan, this may not be bargained at the danger of an increased operative risk, especially a further liver damage caused by the surgical procedure, also not at the disadvantage of a therapeutical damage impairing the gained life span, especially a more prominent hepato-portal encephalopathy.

The selection and adequate preparation in this regard are of paramount importance as are the favorable timing of a suitable shunt form and last not least an unobjectionable technique.

References

1. BECKER, K.: Fortschr. Med. **82**, 593 (1964).
2. BURGMANN, W.: Med. Klin. **58**, 1039 (1963).
3. ESSER, G.: Med. Welt (Stuttg.) **1963**, 2388.
4. — Treatment of severe hemorrhage from esophagogastric varices in patients with cirrhosis of the liver. Recent Advances in Gastroenterology, Vol. III. Basel: Karger 1967.
5. — Pfortaderhochdruck und Eiweißstoffwechsel. Berlin: De Gruyter 1968.
6. —, A. GÜTGEMANN, H. HÜNERBEIN, H. W. SCHREIBER und K. H. SCHRIEFERS: Münch. med. Wschr. **108**, 2436 (1966).
7. GÜTGEMANN, A.: Langenbecks Arch. klin. Chir. **319**, 25 (1967).
8. —, G. HENNRICH und W. NAGEL: Dtsch. med. Wschr. **88**, 1082 (1963).
9. — — und H. W. SCHREIBER: Med. Welt (Stuttg.) **1961**, 1815.
10. —, u. H. W. SCHREIBER: Chirurg **33**, 509 (1962).
11. — —, K. H. SCHRIEFERS und H. PENIN: Dtsch. med. Wschr. **86**, 2370 (1961).
12. KALK, H.: Wien. Z. inn. Med. **39**, 1 (1955).
13. PENIN, H.: Fortschr. Neurol. Psychiat. **35**, 173 (1967).
14. SCHREIBER, H. W.: Langenbecks. Arch. klin. Chir. **300**, 187 (1962).
15. —, K. H. SCHRIEFERS, G. ESSER und W. M. BARTSCH: Germ. med. Mthl. **IX**, 457 (1964).
16. SCHRIEFERS, K. H.: Ergebn. Chir. Orthop. **48**, 103 (1966).
17. WÜLFING, D., u. G. ESSER: Langenbecks Arch. klin. Chir. **303**, 404 (1963).

Ausführliche Literatur bei 1, 3, 5, 6, 13, 14, 16.

Porto-Caval Shunt and Ascites*

CARL-AXEL EKMAN

A number of factors have been suggested in the development of ascites in patients with cirrhosis of the liver. How important these mechanisms are particularly in a given patient is, however, difficult to analyze. The factors that appear to play the most pertinent rôle in patients with liver cirrhosis and portal hypertension are

1. Outflow block and portal hypertension.
2. Increased hepatic lymphflow.
3. Decreased effective colloid osmotic pressure.
4. Hormonal influences.
5. Renal factors.

This paper will concentrate on the first three factors.

70 years ago it was generally believed that high pressure in the portal system was the dominant cause of ascites in cirrhosis. With this in mind, the Eck fistula was devised for the purpose of relieving ascites by reducing portal hypertension in patients with cirrhosis. In the succeeding years this concept was looked upon with scepticism.

---

* From the Department of Surgery (Head: PH. SANDBLOM, M. D., Professor of Surgery), Lasarettet, Lund, Sweden.

Porta-caval anastomosis often could not be tolerated by the patient who had cirrhosis severe enough to cause ascites. For many years ascites was therefore looked upon as a contraindication for shunt operation. Studies on the effect of portal pressure on ascitesformation by means of porta-caval anastomosis were delayed.

Some further delay in testing this procedure was caused by doubts of the importance of portal hypertension in the development of ascites in cirrhosis from principally two sets of observations.

1. Portal hypertension secondary to extrahepatic thrombosis of the portal vein is not associated with ascites.

2. Efforts to produce ascites in dogs and monkeys by experimental obstruction of the portal vein alone have been unsuccessful.

On the other hand supradiaphragmatic constriction of the inferior vena cava in dogs thus interfering with hepatic venous outflow, is followed by a rapid and massive ascites formation. This is, however, despite the lack of portal hypertension in some animals. Further evidence that would reduce the rôle of portal hypertension in the genesis of ascites is that no correlation has been found between the height of portal pressure and the presence of peritoneal fluid (HABIF et al., 1953).

An increase in hepatic lymph-flow has been noticed for many years in a hepatic venous outflow block such as in congestive right heart failure, constrictive pericarditis and in the Budd-Chiari-Syndrome. This is now also held as a factor for the development of ascites in cirrhosis of the liver.

In liver cell failure serum albumin, which for the most parts accounts for the *colloid osmotic pressure* of the plasma, is low. The degree of ascites in patients with severe hepatitis is usually only moderate even if the patient has low serum albumin level and leg edema. In cirrhosis ascites is frequently more severe and shows no correlation with colloid osmotic pressure of the serum (GIGES and KUNKEL, 1954). This infers a local intraabdominal active factor which probably is portal hypertension.

Material and Results

In an attempt to find out the rôle of portal hypertension in the genesis of ascites in patients with cirrhosis and portal hypertension, an analysis was made of the cases that have been operated upon with porta-caval shunt by Professor PH. SANDBLOM and myself at Lund. Of our 365 patients operated upon for portal hypertension 355 had undergone shunt operation up until 31. December, 1966. The total operative mortality for shunt operation was 12.4%. Compared with other series, this mortality may appear high. But I should perhaps point out that our series included many poor risks as well as emergency cases.

The main indication for the operation was esophageal hemorrhage. 35 operations were, however, performed on patients with ascites who had not had esophageal hemorrhage. The indication for operation was intractable ascites in 29 of these patients and in 6 it was the risk of such hemorrhage. Most of the patients with ascites have been treated with diuretics before the operation.

Of our 151 patients with ascites, 98 had more than 2 l of intraabdominal fluid found at operation and 53 had between 500 cc and 2 l. The following observations were made on these patients.

Portal pressure did not correlate with the amount of ascites nor with the presence of peritoneal fluid (Fig. 1). The portal pressure in a group of 82 patients with severe ascites was on the average 37.7 $\pm$ 3.6 cm H_2O and in 45 patients with mild ascites

37.0 ± 3.6 cm H_2O. In 125 patients without ascites the portal pressure was 39.2 ± 4.0 cm H_2O. The values for serum protein and serum albumin showed a slight difference. The mean serum albumin for the group of patients with severe ascites was 3.11 g% against 3.61 for the patients with mild ascites.

Comment: Thus no correlation was found between the amount of ascites and the height of portal pressure itself.

The effect of shunt operation on ascites has been a disappearance of ascites in all patients who survived the postoperative period. In all patients but five end-to-side porta-caval anastomosis has been used as the shunting procedure. During the postoperative period reaccumulation of ascites was found in 15 patients. 5 of these patients died from hepatic coma within the first month after the operation. In the remaining cases ascites disappeared spontaneously during the later course. The serum albumin was as low after the operation as before and therefore changes in serum albumin cannot be held as the main reason for the disappearance of the ascites in these patients.

Fig. 1. Portal pressure and ascites

		Portal pressure cm H_2O
Severe ascites	(82 pat.)	37.7 ± 3.6
Mild ascites	(45 pat.)	37.0 ± 3.6
No ascites	(125 pat.)	39.2 ± 4.0

Fig. 2. Effect of end-to-side porta-caval shunt on the splanchnic portal pressure

	Severe ascites (39 pat.)	Mild ascites (29 pat.)
Before shunt	36.4 ± 4.0 cm H_2O	37.7 ± 4.7 cm H_2O
After shunt	19.4 ± 3.3 cm H_2O	19.8 ± 3.9 cm H_2O
Decrease in pressure	17.4 ± 4.7 cm H_2O	18.3 ± 5.5 cm H_2O

The portal pressure, on the other hand, changed significantly after porta-caval shunt (Fig. 2). In the 68 patients in whom pressure measurements were performed before and after end-to-side porta-caval shunt the pressure in the splanchnic part of the portal system dropped on an average from 37 to 19 cm H_2O i.e. a difference of 18 cm. The hepatic portal pressure (Fig. 3) was determined in the portal vein at the hilum of the liver after the portal vein was ligated and divided for anastomosis. Also here a significant fall in pressure was noticed. Before the ligature the hepatic portal pressure was on the average 38 cm and after it dropped to 28 cm i.e. a difference of 10 cm.

The operative mortality rate (Fig. 4) in our series of 300 patients with cirrhosis and portal hypertension who had undergone shunt operation was 14%. In 151 patients with ascites it was 23.5% compared to 4.2% in patients without ascites.

The long term survival rate of our material is seen in Fig. 5. The figures represent number of survivors and the total number of observations. Of our 151 patients with liver cirrhosis and ascites 38 are still alive. The survival rate 1 year after the shunt operation was 62.3%, 3 years after 43.7% and 5 years after 27.5%. 4 patients have lived more than 8 years after the operation and 3 of these are still alive 9, 10, and 11 years after the operation.

Fig. 3. Effect of ligature of the portal vein on portal pressure at the hilum of the liver

	Severe ascites (39 pat.)	Mild ascites (29 pat.)
Before ligature	36.4 ± 4.0 cm H_2O	37.7 ± 4.7 cm H_2O
After ligature	26.8 ± 3.7 cm H_2O	28.0 ± 5.6 cm H_2O
Decrease in pressure	10.1 ± 4.4 cm H_2O	10.0 ± 5.0 cm H_2O

Fig. 4. Operative mortality

300 (42 op. deaths 14%)
cirrhosis

151 (35 op. deaths 23.5%) / \ 149 (7 op. deaths 4.2%)
with ascites — without ascites

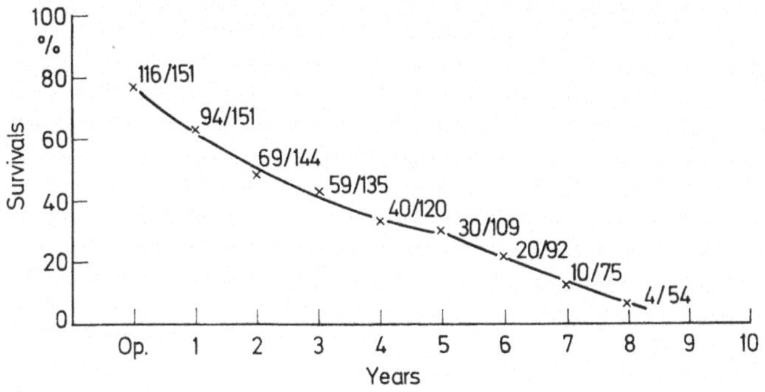

Fig. 5. Survival rate of cirrhotics with ascites after porta-caval shunt

Conclusions

From our present knowledge of the effect of shunt operation on ascites it seems obvious that portal hypertension plays a dominant rôle in the genesis of ascites in patients with cirrhosis of the liver. That ascites disappears after shunt operations is not a new observation. In a relatively large material as this it is interesting to find a relief of ascites after porta-caval shunt in every case despite continuous low serum protein and albumin and despite there being no correlation between portal pressure and the amount of ascites before the operation.

During the last 10 years it has been discussed which type of shunt operation is the best one to give relief of ascites in patients with portal hypertension. Many people have stressed that the side-to-side porta-caval shunt is to be preferred because it gives decompression not only of the splanchnic part of the portal system but also of the liver. McDermott has gone so far that he advises a double barrel shunt to give maximum relief of hypertension in the liver. Our experiences have shown that an end-to-side porta-caval shunt also gives a reduction in portal pressure both in the splanchnic and hepatic part of the portal system. They also show that the procedure has been very effective for ascites.

The most difficult question to answer is whether ascites is an indication for porta-caval shunt operation. The high operative mortality and the rather rapid fall in the curve of survival render it difficult to recommend shunt operation for ascites except in special cases. The modern conservative treatment with a combination of *aldactone* and *diuretics* gives a good relief for ascites in most instances. Patients who have bled from esophageal varices ought to be operated upon but only after their ascites has been treated conservatively. For patients who have not had any episode of esophageal bleeding we recommend conservative treatment during which we follow the course of liver damage. Should be patient begin to bleed during expectant treatment an emergency shunt is recommended. In the event of intractable ascites despite conservative treatment, operation should be considered.

References

EISENMENGER, W. J., and W. F. NICKEL: Amer. J. Med. **20**, 879 (1956).
GIGES, B., and H. G. KUNKEL: J. clin. Invest. **33**, 257 (1954).
HABIF, D. V., H. T. RANDALL, and H. S. SOROFF: Surgery **34**, 580 (1953).

The Late Results of Portacaval Shunts*

ARTHUR B. VOORHEES, JR., JOHN B. PRICE, JR., and RICHARD C. BRITTON

Introduction

WHIPPLE [*4*], BLAKEMORE, ROUSSELOT and LORD began the first systematic approach to the treatment of portal hypertension in 1943 at the Columbia-Presbyterian Medical Center. Over the ensuing 25 years, approximately 1,500 cases of portal hypertension have been treated in this center and of these, 651 patients have undergone 713 portal decompression procedures.

The purpose of this report is to record the long-term results of therapy in the adult patient with portal cirrhosis.

General Description

Among the 651 patients, 58 had more than one portacaval shunting procedure performed which increases the total number of procedures to 713. To bring clarity to the presentation, the term case will refer to an operative procedure rather than to a patient.

This study is composed of 404 cases (390 patients — 1 operation each, 12 patients — 2 operations each, 1 patient — 3 operations). Of these, 45 (11%) died following operation, 238 (59%) died during the follow-up period, and 121 (30%) are living. 60% of the group were males and 40% were females. 96% of the group were of the white race, ranging from 20 to 70 years of age with 40% falling between 50 and 59 years. 99% of the 404 cases were followed to the time of death or to the time of this study. The longest follow-up for any single case was 19 years. 52% of the cases had nutritional cirrhosis, 15% had postnecrotic cirrhosis and 32% had a cirrhosis of unknown etiology. The 404 cases represented 250 (62%) end-to-side portacaval, 67 (17%) side-to-side portacaval, 65 (16%) splenorenal, 16 (4%) mesocaval, and 6 (1%) makeshift shunts.

*From the Surgical Service, Presbyterian Hospital, the A. H. Blakemore Laboratory of Surgical Research and the Department of Surgery, College of Physicians and Surgeons, Columbia University, New York, New York. Supported by the Fund for the Advancement of Blood Vessel Surgery and in part by U.S. Public Health Service grant AM 07646, Research Career Development Award 1-K3-HE-4921 and Health Research Council of New York City Investigatorship I-317.

Recurrent Hemorrhage

It is difficult to determine the exact incidence of shunt failure since not all instances of postshunt bleeding originate from varices and some known instances of shunt thrombosis do not bleed. For instance, in 32 cases with portacaval shunts actively bleeding into the upper gastrointestinal tract immediately prior to death, subsequent postmortem examinations disclosed that 13 (40%) were due to demonstrated shunt closure and the remaining 19 cases (60%) were due to peptic ulceration, hemorrhagic gastroenteritis or clotting dyscrasias. It, therefore, seems clear that estimates of shunt failure must be based on information gathered from multiple sources such as history of recurrent bleeding without other demonstrated sources, portal venography, directly measured persistent portal hypertension, a subsequent surgical exploration and postmortem examination.

Reasonable clinical data bearing on shunt patency was secured from 359 cases out of a total of 404. An estimated incidence of probable shunt occlusion was developed and is set forth in Table 1.

Table 1. *Estimated incidence of shunt occlusion in 359 shunts*

	Total	Occluded	Percentage
End-to-side	217	14	6%
Side-to-side	66	4	6%
Splenorenal	57	17	30%
Mesocaval	13	0	0%
Makeshift	6	3	50%

Ascites Control

117 cases entered the study with overt, severe and persistent ascites preoperatively. 287 cases had no ascites preoperatively. In the preoperative ascites group, 26 (22%) died postoperatively and 91 were followed. In the preoperative ascites-free group, 19 (7%) died postoperatively and 268 were followed. The findings are summarized in Table 2.

Table 2. *Shunt effectiveness in ascites control*

Ascites status	End-to-side case ratio	%	Side-to-side case ratio	%	Splenorenal case ratio	%	Mesocaval case ratio	%	Makeshift case ratio	%
Relieved by shunt	49/61	80	16/16	100	8/9	89	3/3	100	1/2	50
Appeared after shunt	18/155	12	0/50	0	7/50	14	0/10	0	1/3	33

Longevity Following Shunt Surgery

It is evident from the data that the operative mortality, the incidence of postoperative complications, and the longevity of the patient following shunt surgery are directly related to the level of liver function. Therefore, longevity of a group is a reflection of the level of the liver function of the group as a whole. An example of this relationship has been drawn up in Table 3 in which 339 cases (all have died within 5 years postshunt or have lived 5 or more years and have known preoperative serum albumin levels) have been used in a comparison of the preoperative serum albumin levels and the postoperative survival.

A similar comparison was carried out between the type of surgical shunt and longevity. There was no difference in the three major shunt types in the postoperative 5 year follow-up; excluding operative deaths, all three were 51%.

In 24 cases a correlation [3] of direct blood flow with the postoperative course was conducted utilizing direct hepatic artery and portal vein blood flow determinations made immediately prior to and following construction of the shunt. Even though a wide range of final hepatic blood flows (139 to 1400 cm³ per min) were recorded, there was no positive correlation with the subsequent clinical course in each of the 24 cases. A surprising extreme was the case who had an excellent follow-up course and yet had a postshunt flow of only 139 cm per min at operation, a figure later confirmed by indirect flow measurements.

Table 3. *Correlation of survival to preoperative serum albumin concentration*

Time of death	Postop.	Under 1 year	1 to 4 years	5 or more years
No. of cases	43	56	96	144
% of 339 cases	13%	16%	30%	42%
% of 339 cases c̄ serum albumin of 3.5 or more	46%	48%	61%	71%

Table 4. *Principle cause of death in the follow-up period*

	No. of cases	Percentage
Liver failure	104	44%
G.I. hemorrhage (10c̄ proven ulcer)	28	12%
Hepatoma	14	6%
Acute hepatitis	8	3%
Bleeding dyscrasias	5	2%
Cardiac	16	7%
Unrelated causes	47	19%
Unknown	16	7%

The final causes of death listed in Table 4 cannot be thought of as a single mechanism in any instance and only an estimate of the most important factor has been made. Out of the series of 404 cases, 45 (11%) died following operation and 238 have died in the 25 year follow-up period. The percentages which appear on the table are based on a group of 238 deaths.

Complications of Portacaval Shunting

The appearance of portal systemic encephalopathy is dependent on the amount of shunted blood, the degree of liver insufficiency, the amount of "toxins" absorbed from the gastrointestinal tract, and the particular receptiveness of the central nervous system to these "toxins". Since all are variables, meaningful strict correlations are difficult to establish; therefore, our data can no more than suggest trends. Encephalopathy can be conveniently divided into three grades in which *minimal* denotes transient symptoms, clearing spontaneously without specific therapy; *moderate* denotes persistent symptoms which clear on continuous therapy and *severe* denotes persistent symptoms which fail to clear completely on continuous maximum therapy.

The incidence of encephalopathy in 359 (404 minus 45 postoperative deaths) cases averages 44% (minimal 10%, moderate 23%, severe 11%). When the group is subdivided as to shunt type, the end-to-side shunt had a 5% higher average, the side-to-side shunt was average and the splenorenal shunt was 5% below average. These small variations may be explained by the longer period of follow-up in the end-to-side shunt. The incidence of encephalopathy in all shunt cases followed for less than 5 years was 27% and for those followed for more than 5 years it was 57%. In the splenorenal group, the higher thrombosis rate of the shunt correlates almost precisely with the reduced encephalopathy rate.

The same group of 359 cases were studied for possible factors influencing the incidence of encephalopathy. *The etiology* of the cirrhosis seemed to play no part; however, in 67 diabetics in the group, the incidence of encephalopathy was increased twofold. A return to alcohol plays a large rôle for in 192 nutritional cirrhotics, 59 were known to have returned to drink and the incidence of moderate and severe encephalopathy was 66% which is substantially above average. Under 50 years of age, the incidence was 23% and over 50 years, the incidence was 44% for a grouping of both moderate and severe encephalopathy. The incidence of liver function preoperatively compared with postoperative encephalopathy discloses a paradox. When serum albumin concentration is utilized as an index of liver function and is over 3.5 gms percent, 60% of the cases develop moderate or severe encephalopathy. Since these cases also have the greatest life expectancy, the increased incidence of encephalopathy is probably a function of their longer follow-up period.

The incidence of postoperative complications of peptic ulceration (12%), diabetes mellitus (10%), and congestive heart failure secondary to increased cardiac return (undetermined) are often subtle in their manifestations but as indicated in Table 5 these may be significant contributors to follow-up death.

Return of Patient to Social Effectiveness

The socioeconomic status of the 404 cases disclosed that 36% were of low income, 42% were of middle income and 22% were of high income. Of the males, 15% were unskilled workers, 24% were skilled, 30% were office workers, and 31% were executive or professional workers.

100 consecutive cases were selected where the follow-up period was a minimum of 2 years. There were 40 women and 60 men in the group and 84 of these survived their operative experience. 60 survived 2 years and these were subject to close study as to their return to a socially effective state. The appraisal was more accurate in the instance of men and for this reason, the comparative study is limited to them. Of the 60 cases alive at 2 years, 36 were men; 28 of whom had been fully employed prior to operation and of these 28, only 14 returned to full employment postoperatively.

Discussion

The primary therapeutic objective of a portacaval shunt is to control repetitive hemorrhage from esophageal varices in a manner which will not unfavorably alter the course of the underlying cirrhosis. Another objective is to control the formation of ascites in incidences in which conservative control measures have failed or are deemed impractical. A final objective is to introduce as few complications as possible which would diminish the therapeutic value to the patient.

Unfortunately for the analyst, the data covering the natural history of the disease is fragmentary and it is difficult to develop parallel matched studies. BAKER's [1] study asserted that only 33% of all patients with varices bled but that once bleeding occurred, it was almost certain to be repeated and with each hemorrhage there was a 50% chance of death. There is no question in our analysis that an effective shunt does reduce the mortality from hemorrhage. Whether a shunt prolongs life is a point under current debate and awaits alternating therapy studies with matched cases. The life expectancy following shunting in our series is just below but parallel to the survival table developed by GARCEAU [2] from the Boston Inter-Hospital Liver Group study comparing a prophylactically shunted group to a non-shunted group in 93 selected randomized subjects with varices. We infer from this parallel that the shunt performed in our series for proven bleeders does not reduce the life expectancy significantly from those who have not bled.

In assessing the value of shunt therapy, bleeding control and life expectancy are only part of the picture. In our experience, the shunt and specifically a shunt which decompresses the intrahepatic portal bed is being utilized to control the more protracted forms of ascites. On re-evaluating our data, the side-to-side portacaval shunt offers the greatest control for established ascites and is attended by no instance of chronic ascites accumulation in the postoperative period.

During the 25 years of development of portacaval shunts, there has been a wide proliferation of shunt configurations. Resulting from this wide selection, the anatomical possibilities and the hemodynamic needs of a given case present the surgeon with the necessity to make a selection. It has been our experience that the centrally placed shunt, utilizing the portal, superior mesenteric and the splenic veins all offer about the same protection from hemorrhage, have the same incidence of encephalopathy and the same life expectancy. The failure to control ascites or the development of ascites as a troublesome, occasionally lethal, postoperative complication is more common where the hepatic side of the portal vein is ligated or where a distally placed hemodynamically inefficient shunt has been created. Based upon these observations, we performed during the past 4 years far fewer end-to-side portal vein to vena cava shunts and far more side-to-side, central splenorenal and mesocaval shunts.

The problem of encephalopathy is a great one and in our experience, it has been the major reason why many otherwise successfully shunted patients have not been able to re-enter a productive existence. It is readily demonstrated that age, the length of time following the shunt, the presence of diabetes, the return to alcohol, the severity of the hepatic damage, the quantity of blood being shunted and the amount of absorption from the bowel are significant factors in the production of encephalopathy. The main objectives in current investigative work are being directed toward the reduction of this most crippling by-product of shunt therapy.

References

1. BAKER, L. A., C. SMITH, and G. LIEBERMAN: Amer. J. Med. **26**, 228 (1959).
2. GARCEAU, A. J., R. H. RESNICK, H. MUENCH, and T. C. CHALMERS: Progress report of the controlled trial of prophylactic portacaval anastomosis. The Boston Inter-Hospital Liver Group. (in press).
3. PRICE, J. B., A. B. VOORHEES, and R. C. BRITTON: Arch. Surg. **95**, 843 (1967).
4. WHIPPLE, A. O.: Ann. Surg. **122**, 449 (1945).

Surgery of Infants and Children

Anomalies of the Genitourinary Tract

Willard E. Goodwin

Recently I had the opportunity to visit a pediatric hospital in The Hague. There I found 60 surgical beds, and 30 of them were filled with children who had urological problems. This is probably a clear and accurate index of the incidence and importance of Genitourinary anomalies in childhood.

Although the diagnosis and treatment of Genitourinary problems of children is one of the most interesting, satisfying and rewarding parts of urological surgery, time does not permit more than an outline of the problems here.

It is the purpose of this paper to discuss briefly the following general categories of pediatric urogenital anomalies and to describe current methods of management:

Congenital anomalies
Obstructions
Infections
Stones
Foreign bodies
Anomalies of the External Genitalia
Neoplasms.

The commonest important urological symptoms which bring children to the attention of pediatricians and urologists are the following: pyuria, hematuria, unexplained abdominal pain and "failure to thrive". The signs of abdominal mass, anemia and visible hesitancy or difficulty in urination, may also lead to suspicion of disease in the urogenital system.

Basic diagnostic studies which are important are of course the history and physical examination, urinalysis, determination of the blood chemistries and a PSP test to estimate renal function. At this point, an intravenous pyelogram — if there is good renal function — may be an extremely valuable screening test. If there is any suggestion of abnormality in the intravenous pyelogram, a voiding cystogram should be obtained. These studies may then be followed by cystoscopy and retrograde pyelography if indicated. Further studies, such as the renogram and arteriography may follow later if there is a clear indication.

It is our view that the symptoms of pyuria or hematuria and unexplained abdominal pain should never be overlooked. It is my personal feeling that an intravenous urogram is probably the single most valuable screening test and should be used a great deal more frequently than it is commonly employed at present.

Anomalies of the External Genitalia in the Male

Hypospadias and phimosis are the commonest visible external anomalies. Hypospadias should be repaired in a two stage operation, the first stage, release of chordee, usually at about 3 years and the second stage, reconstruction of the urethra, before the age of 6 years when the child approaches school. Phimosis may be treated by simple dilatation of the prepuce, but it is better managed by circumcision. When paraphimosis occurs as an acute problem, it can usually be reduced by manual decompression between the thumb and the first two fingers very much as in the use

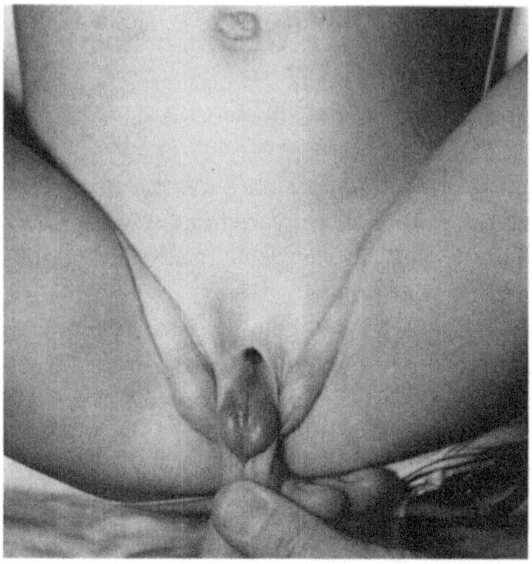

Fig. 1. Epispadias with incontinence

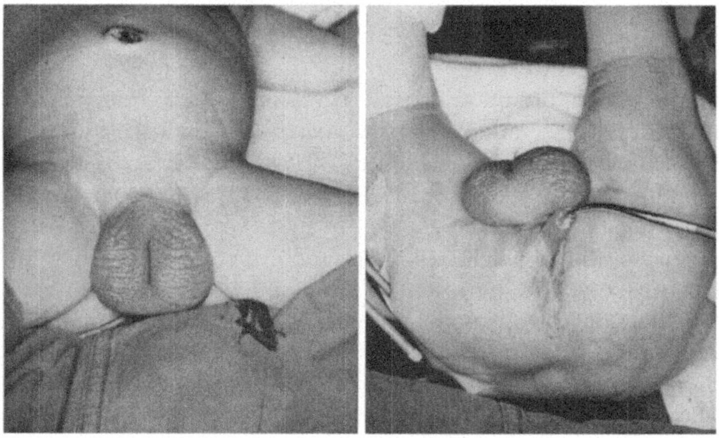

Fig. 2. Congenital absence of the penis. Note perineal dimple marked with clamp (B). This is the urethral meatus

of a syringe. Malrotation of the penis may be corrected by a simple plastic procedure to rotate the glans into its normal position.

Epispadias, which is the opposite of hypospadias is relatively uncommon. It should be repaired. Often it is associated with urinary incontinence, and the repair should include a plastic plication of the bladder neck as described by Hugh Young.

Occasionally a case of cryptophallus is observed. This should be distinguished from congenital absence of the penis by careful physical examination. Usually no treatment is necessary for cryptophallus as mother nature will overcome this problem with time.

On the other hand the problem of congenital absence of the penis is a serious one. Fortunately it is very rare, although I have seen four cases. It has been recommended that a new penis should be constructed, but on the basis of some past experiences we have come to believe that a child born with absence of the penis should be raised as a girl.

Microphallus or micropenis can be a very distressing condition, especially to the parents. In my experience some of these patients have responded well to hormone therapy. Although this has not been generally accepted, I am convinced it should be tried. I have under my care 3 or 4 children with micropenis whom I have treated on various occasions with intermittent, short courses of testosterone and the gonadotropic hormone. Satisfactory growth of the penis was produced.

Anomalies of the External Genitalia in the Female

Although less common than in boys some little girls are born with hypospadias or epispadias. Usually this does not require treatment unless there is associated incontinence. When incontinence is a problem it should be treated the same as epispadias with incontinence in the male.

Absence or atresia of the vagina is a distressing abnormality which does not demand early treatment. It can be satisfactorily treated by careful plastic surgery and creation of a vagina from a skin graft at the age of puberty or later.

Hydrocolpos can be a confusing condition especially when it is associated with urinary obstruction. When properly recognized it is best treated by surgical incision of the imperforate hymen which relieves the condition. Although it is rare, it certainly must be considered in any case of urinary outlet obstruction in a young girl with an abdominal mass.

Intersex States

The varying spectrum of intersex states which comprises male and female pseudohermaphrodites is extremely interesting and can be a challenging problem both for

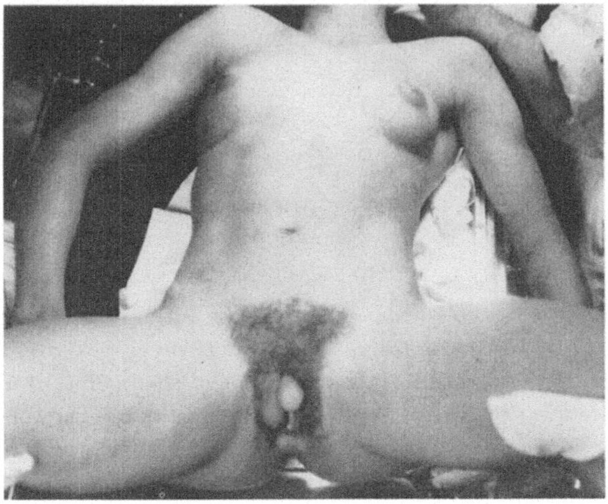

Fig. 3. A true Hermaphrodite [(Goodwin, W. E., P. L. Scardino, and W. W. Scott: J. Urol. (Baltimore) **71**, 748 (1954)]

diagnosis and treatment. Accurate sex determination is possible in most cases by the use of chromosome analysis and sex chromatin studies. However, some doubtful cases may be true hermaphrodites and should have surgical exploration to be certain of the internal genitalia and of the gonads which should be biopsied before definitive surgical treatment is undertaken. Usually males should be made into males and females should be females, though there are some exceptions. Female pseudohermaphrodites with large clitoral growth may require partial amputation. We have for many years employed a method of removing the central portion of the corpora inside the skin of the clitoris thus leaving behind the small glans to achieve a more normal external appearance and sensation. Male pseudohermaphrodites with third degree hypospadias and a vaginal cleft should be carefully studied to look for a concealed vagina which may need to be removed surgically in order to prevent retention of urine after the final plastic construction of the urethra.

Scrotum and Testes

Cryptorchism, "concealed testis", is one of the commonest conditions. The testis is either undescended or may lie in an abnormal position. It can be unilateral or bilateral. It is generally agreed that if the testes are not descended by the 6th year, the condition should be treated surgically, even if they lie high in the abdomen. I

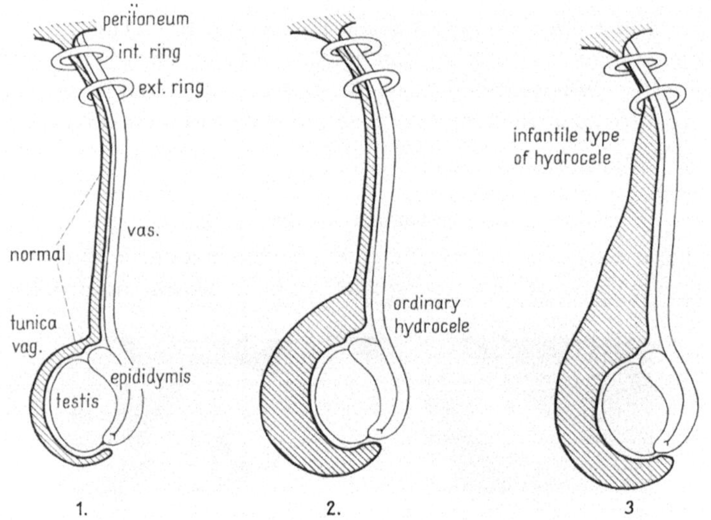

Fig. 4. Infantile type of hydrocele, persistence of "processus vaginalis" with intra peritoneal connection

have treated a few boys who's testes could not be brought lower than the external inguinal ring. It was possible later, in a second stage orchiopexy to get the testis into a normal position in the scrotum. It is important in the operation of orchiopexy to pay particular attention to careful anatomical dissection and careful preservation of the blood supply. There is usually an associated hernia, which must also be repaired. An occasional child with cryptorchism will respond satisfactorily to treatment with the gonadotropic hormone. I see no harm in preliminary hormone treatment, though favorable responses are few.

Occasionally a boy is born with congenital absence of one or both testes, or perhaps they have been destroyed "in utero" by an unrecognized torsion. The presence or absence of the testis can only be determined by very careful abdominal exploration, preferably though a midline incision. The best landmark is to look for the vas deferens and follow it from its emergence behind the bladder. Recently I saw a boy who had a false diagnosis of absent testes on the basis of an incomplete exploration when he was an infant.

There are a few well-documented cases of polyorchism. Probably no surgical treatment is indicated, though exploration may be necessary to be sure that the extra mass does not represent a neoplasm.

Hydrocele in infants is fairly common. It usually does not require surgical treatment because the hydrocele sac usually seals itselfs off from the peritoneal connection with advancing maturity. When however a hydrocele persists and requires repair at a later age, it is a good idea to look for an associated hernia or an incipient hernia.

Torsion of the testis is one of the few acute emergency situations in pediatric urology. It occurs most commonly in preadolescence but is also seen in older boys. It must be distinguished from epididymitis which also produces acute scrotal pain and a swollen testis. When this is suspected, prompt surgical exploration is mandatory because untreated torsion can cause loss of the testis due to loss of its blood supply. The opposite testis should also be explored and "fixed" to prevent the condition from happening on the second side.

Torsion of the appendix testis, which also causes acute pain and swelling, may mimic torsion of the testis. I saw one such patient who had had several attacks of pain. When I finally had the opportunity to explore the scrotum I found the tiny appendix testis lying calcified and floating free in a small amount of hydrocele fluid.

In all conditions involving the testis, the differential diagnosis must include the possibility of epididymitis and orchitis. The history of onset is important here, and epididymitis is usually associated with urinary infection. Orchitis associated with mumps should be treated with cortisone. If this does not afford early relief the testis should be explored and the tunica albuginea incised to relieve pressure and prevent atrophy.

Varicocele, usually seen at puberty and early adolescense, is fairly common. At one time during my military experience I had the opportunity to examine some 2000 young soldiers on their way over seas, and I kept track of the incidence of varicocele. About 15 of every 100 had a varicocele of some magnitude, though most of them had never noticed it. Usually varicocele does not require treatment. If it becomes too large or painful it is easily managed by surgical ligation of the large venous plexus.

Urethra

The commonest and most dangerous anomalies of the urethra cause obstruction. Meatal stenosis is most frequent in both sexes and when recognized should be treated by meatotomy. Some children are born with congenital urethral strictures, which especially in girls, lead to urinary infections due to retained urine. Most of these strictures respond to simple dilatation though internal urethrotomy may be necessary in some cases. Some boys develop urethral strictures after instrumentation. I have used Johansson's operation for urethral stricture in children with good results.

Duplication or absence of the urethra may occur in both sexes but is fortunately rare. I have only seen a few cases. Diverticulum of the urethra may be congenital.

Valves of the urethra occur in both sexes but are more commonly recognized in the male in the prostatic urethra. They can produce anything from mild to complete obstruction and are usually associated with retained urine, urinary infection and severe hydronephrosis. This condition demands early treatment as soon as it is recognized. Most are treated satisfactorily by trans urethral resection, but when recognized in the newborn it may be necessary to perform supra-pubic cystostomy for diversion and to postpone definitive treatment until the child grows older. In some instances I have quite satisfactorily removed valves in the prostatic urethra by a rather radical retropubic approach combined with a Y-V plastic operation on the bladder neck. It is likely that many or most of these boys will have retrograde ejaculation when they reach maturity.

A few cases of enlargement of the verumontanum, large enough to produce urinary obstruction, have been described. Also urethral polyps may produce obstruction. These conditions are best managed transurethrally.

Retained MÜLLERIAN duct with cyst formation may cause obstruction at the bladder neck. This is best treated surgically by a trans-vesical approach.

Occasionally urinary calculi may pass into the prostatic urethra and cause obstruction. This may occur when urethral obstruction already exists and a bladder stone starts to pass into the prostatic urethra and gets stuck so that the stone grows up out of the urethra into the bladder to form a mushroom shaped stone with its "stem" in the prostatic urethra. Stones should be removed, and associated strictures and infections should be treated.

Fistulae between urinary tract and intestine or between urinary tract and vagina in the female are fortunately not very common. Usually they are associated with imperforate anus and may follow surgical repair of this condition. This can be one of the most difficult problems of all and demands extremely careful surgical closure with great attention to anatomical detail and preservation of the spincter. The urine should be diverted by temporary cystostomy in connection with this type of repair.

Anomalies of the Bladder

Congenital extrophy of the bladder associated with epispadias is one of the most fearful of the urogenital anomalies. Often there is associated cryptorchism in little boys. Many attemps have been made to repair the extrophy, and this can be done satisfactorily after iliac osteotomy to allow the separated pubic bones to be brought together. However, very few of these patients obtain true urinary continence with a satisfactory urinary tract and no infection. It is my opinion that this procedure is doomed to failure until someone learns how to make a good sphincter.

In recent years my practice has been to ask the Orthopedists to do an iliac osteotomy so that the pubic bones may be brought more closely together. Then at a second operation about 10 to 14 days later the urinary bladder and prostatic urethra are closed in as near normal a manner as possible. The urine is diverted to the large bowel by ureterosigmoidostomy. This has the advantage of gaining urinary continence and plastic closure of the defect without destroying any of the bladder. It makes the closure of the ventral defect much easier. Those who object to ureterosigmoidostomy could perform cutaneous diversion by BRICKER's operation at a later date if it seems indicated. It can be quite difficult to take care of a small baby with an ileocutaneous diversion, and for this reason we have preferred ureterosigmoidostomy.

Other anomalies of the bladder include such things as duplication, absence, persistent urachus duct etc. Many of these are associated with obstruction which must always be considered and evaluated.

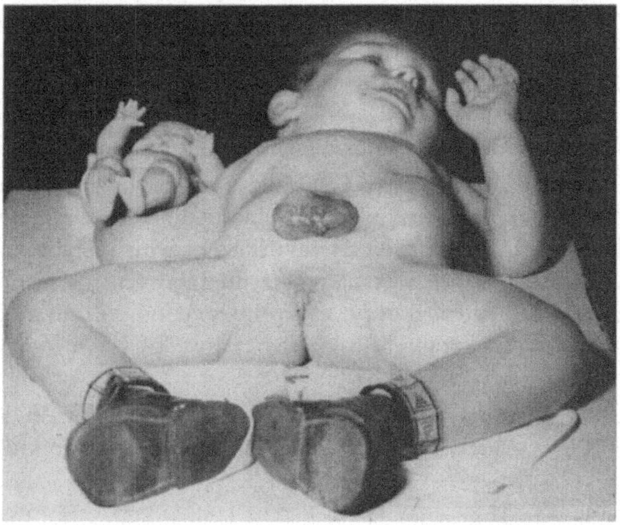

a

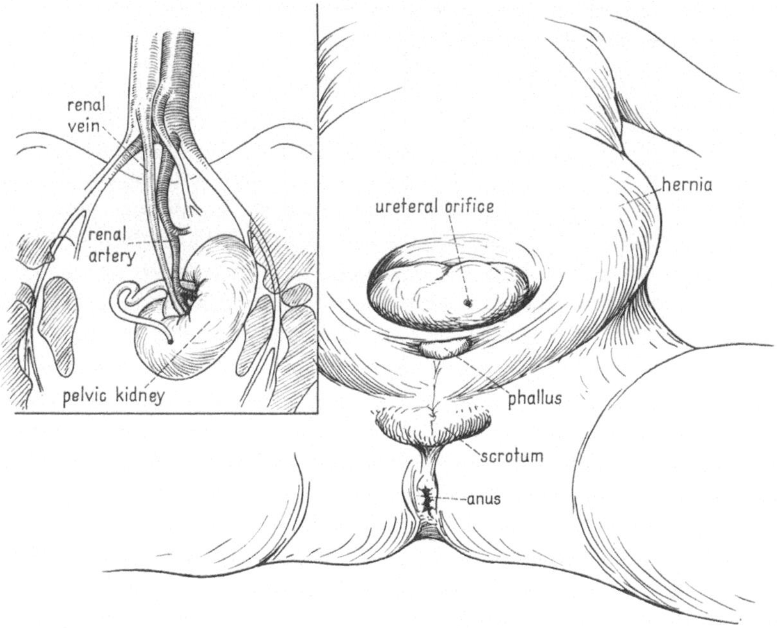

b

Fig. 5. A. Extrophy of urinary bladder with associated multiple anomalies: solitary pelvic kidney, cryptorchism, epispadias, history of imperforate anus treated after birth, left flank hernia, double sacrum and coccyx. B. Diagram of A. Treatment was to place the pelvic kidney in left lumbar area and divert the urine to the skin through an isolated segment of sigmoid colon (1953). Child has grown normally and is now a strong healthy teen-ager

Foreign bodies are not infrequently found in the bladders of children, particularly little girls. They must always be kept in mind and searched for in cases of unexplained, persistent urinary infections.

Outlet obstructions are sometimes difficult to pinpoint as to whether they are in the urethra or at the bladder neck. The decision can usually be made after careful cystoscopy and a voiding cystourethrogram. Sometimes the cystourethrogram is best done by suprapubic puncture, filling the bladder from above and watching the voiding mechanism on a television screen. This dynamic view of urination is of far greater value than individual spot films which may miss a moment of reflux etc.

Associated anomalies which may be found with outlet obstructions are: contracted bladder neck, trabeculated bladder, diverticulum formation which may be congenital and lie just medial to the ureteral orifice or which may be acquired due to obstruction. Megacystis and megacystis with reflux may also be secondary to outlet obstruction, though they can also occur as a primary condition. In all of these conditions a voiding cystourethrogram, followed by cystoscopy is a mandatory part of the investigation.

Like hydrocolpos, which causes bladder outlet obstruction in girls, excessive constipation can cause urinary obstruction and even acute retention in either boys or girls.

Bladder calculi are not a major factor in The United States, but they certainly are elsewhere in the world. Pediatric bladder calculi are endemic in certain parts of South East Asia and elsewhere and are probably related to a dietary insufficiency — most likely a deficit in magnesium, phosphorus, protein and vitamins which occurs at the time the child stops nursing at the mother's breast.

When I was in Indonesia in 1964 I had the opportunity to see a large number of children with bladder stones. I was extremely interested to find that almost all of these children had associated anomalies of the urinary tract such as outlet obstruction, vesicoureteral reflux and infection. A few did not have any infection at all. I came to believe that in most cases these stones had formed in the kidneys near the age of 2 years and that they had then dropped down to the bladder while still very small stones. Those children who had outlet obstruction retained the stones which became lodged in the bladder or urethra and continued to grow. With Indonesian colleagues, hospital records were reviewed as to age incidence of these children who were operated on for bladder calculi. The numbers of cases for both boys and girls peaked just after 2 years, when most of the children stopped nursing. Thus I came to believe that poor nutrition, plus inadequate fluid intake at that time were the contributing factors in stone formation in those children. Most of them had only one operation for stone and did not suffer recurrences.

Children with bladder stones should be studied by intravenous pyelography, voiding cystograms and cystoscopy. Serum calcium, phosphorous and uric acid levels should be determined. The stones should be removed, usually by the suprapubic route. The stones should be analyzed, and metabolic causes of stone formation should be excluded.

Neurological bladders may prove a terrible challenge, first in diagnosis and then in management. When the cause is irremediable and obvious such as in congenital absence of the sacrum, perhaps the simplest and kindest thing is to perform early cutaneous diversion by means of Bricker's operation.

Congenital absence of the abdominal muscles, "prune belly" is another condition in which the bladder is massively enlarged usually with associated dilatation of the ureters, hydronephrosis and reflux. Usually cryptorchism is also found. On the basis of my experience with failure in trying to establish a normal urinary tract in these cases, I would recommend early cutaneous diversion.

The problem of enuresis, "bed wetting", is usually functional and should be handled in that way in perhaps 99% of the cases. However, in my view every child

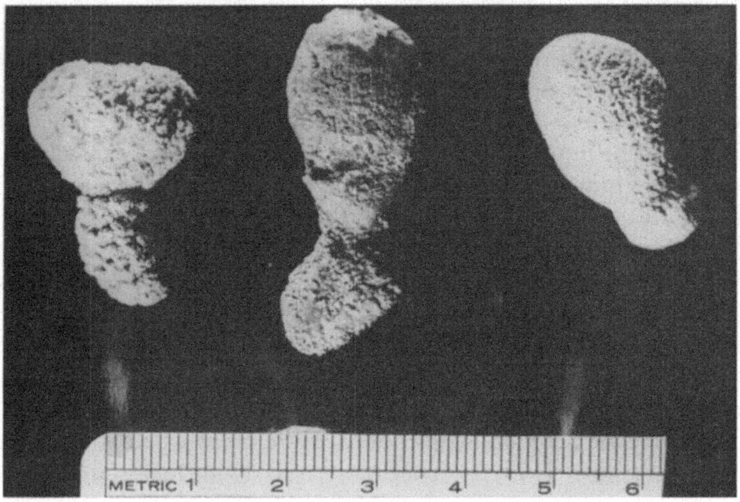

a

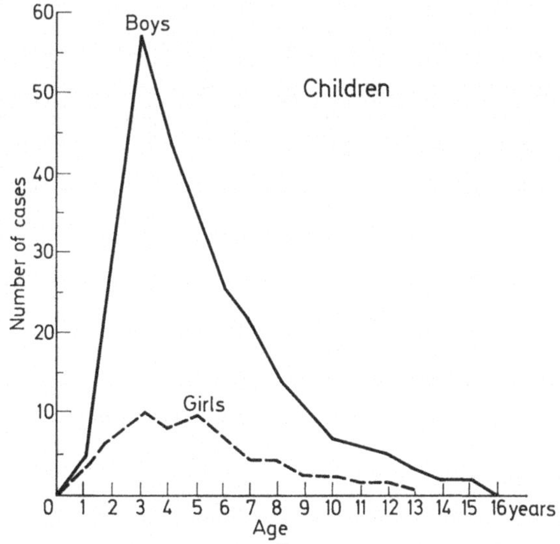

b

Fig. 6. Bladder stones in Indonesian children. *Top*: stones which represent a "cast" of prostatic urethra and bladder. *Bottom*: age and incidence of bladder stones in a children in 1 year in one hospital, "Rumah Sakit Umum Pamum", Surabaja, Java. Note sharp speak at 4 to 5 years which begins shortly after 2 years, when children stopped breast feeding who has enuresis deserves to have a careful urinalysis; and if there are any abnormalities suggesting infection or decreased kidney function the child certainly should have an intravenous pyelogram. I have seen a number of children who were thought to be functional enuretics who in fact had obstructive lesions of the urinary tract which were causing an excessive irritation of the bladder due to associated infection.

Anomalies of the Kidney

Because of its curious embrylogical history of ascent from the pelvic region upward to its normal position, the kidney may have numerous anomalies of structure and of blood supply. Agenesis of the kidney may be unilateral or very rarely bilateral. Unilateral agenesis in females is often associated with anomalies of the genitalia such as atresia of the vagina etc. Hypoplastic kidneys may either be congenital on the basis of a vascular accident in utero or acquired on a basis of multiple infections, usually due to reflux and chronic pyelonephritis from an early age. Hypertension may be associated with this situation. Nephrectomy is indicated in these cases.

Multiple kidneys have been reported, also crossed ectopia in which both kidneys lie on the same side although the ureteral orifices are normally placed. Horseshoe and "pancake" kidneys also occur. In all of these conditions, the mere finding of the anomaly is not usually enough to indicate treatment unless there is associated obstruction, infection, stone or some other disease. The commonest problem is one of obstruction with associated infection. This can happen in cases of horseshoe kidney for instance when the ureteropelvic junction is obstructed at the point where it crosses over the isthmus of the horseshoe. The treatment for this is to divide the isthmus of the kidney and move both kidneys outward to their normal position, thus allowing the ureters to descend medially in a more normal manner. It is often necessary to include some sort of plastic operation on the ureteropelvic junction.

There is a rare condition of unilateral atrophy or agenesis of the kidney in the male, with the ureter emptying into the seminal vesicle. This may cause pelvic and perineal pain in later life in connection with sexual activity.

Various types of cystic kidney formation are encountered. Congenital polycystic kidneys are bilateral and usually not discovered until later life. However, occasionally an infant or young child will die of renal insufficiency due to this condition. This may be one of the indications in the future for consideration of renal transplantation in a newborn child.

Perhaps a more commonly recognized anomaly is congenital unilateral multicystic kidney, which is a well recognized and distinct condition. It is unilateral; there are no cysts on the opposite, normal side; and the diseased kidney is usually discovered as a palpable mass which must be distinguished from a possible neoplasm. The diagnosis can be made when it is found that there is no visualisation on intravenous pyelography and when a retrograde pyelogram shows that the upper ureter terminates in a long thin, filiform narrowed ureter. Characteristically these kidneys have multiple large cysts, "like a bunch of grapes", with an attenuated blood supply and a very tiny, probably completely occluded, ureter in the upper third. I have speculated that this might be due to a vascular accident in utero, which produced atresia of the ureter and also led to cyst formation. The usual treatment is surgical exploration and excision. This is to be differentiated from solitary cysts which should be left alone or simply drained with preservation of the kidney.

Renal vein thrombosis may occur in newborn children who have severe diarrhea and also in older children in association with trauma. When there is an acute onset there may be blood in the urine. In the chronic state it may produce the nephrotic syndrome. The usual treatment in the newborn, when it is unilateral has been nephrectomy. However there are some cases in older children after careful diagnostic studies including renal venography where it has been possible to treat the condition by surgical exploration and removal of the thrombus from the renal vein. My colleagues, CHRISTIANSEN and KAUFMAN have recently described such a case where they successfully removed thrombi from the renal vein and from the vena cava.

Renal stones should be removed, and any associated obstruction or reflux and infection should be treated at the same time. However, it is always important to make an attempt to find out why the stone was formed. Hyperparathyroid disease should be ruled out as well as performing careful analysis of the stone to be sure that it is not uric acid or cystine which are amenable to medical management. Many renal stones seen in children are related to reflux with infected urine, and this should always be considered and ruled out by study with a voiding cystogram before excision of the stone.

Chronic infections and pyelonephritis in children are nearly always related to vesico-ureteral reflux and persistent lower urinary tract infection, most often but not always associated with obstruction. The infecting organisms should be identified and treated appropriately, but always a search should be made for obstruction or another anatomical abnormality as a cause. The first steps are a voiding cystourethrogram and an intravenous pyelogram.

Kidney Pelvis and Ureter

Some of the most difficult problems of the surgical urology of childhood are related to anomalies of the drainage system of the upper urinary tract. Such conditions as hydrocalyx and calyceal diverticulum may be congenital and usually do not demand treatment. Some patients with infundibular stenosis and hydrocalyx should be managed surgically by an intrarenal plastic operation to improve drainage from the calyx. (I have seen one such child who had an obligatory nephrostomy in whom I found it necessary to attach a segment of ileum to the intrarenal calyx in order to obtain satisfactory drainage and get rid of the nephrostomy tubes.)

Hydronephrosis due to ureteropelvic junction obstruction is one of the commonest anomalies. This condition is usually "silent" and uninfected, unlike the hydronephrosis due to reflux. The condition may be discovered either because of a large abdominal mass which can be confused with a neoplasm, — or because of repeated attacks of unexplained abdominal pain. I once saw a child with advanced bilateral hydronephrosis who was on his way to the operating room to have a nephrectomy by a Pediatric Surgeon because of an incorrect suspected diagnosis of Wilm's tumor. This should never happen with informed and intelligent urological evaluation.

Hydronephrosis which is discovered because of unexplained abdominal pain is quite interesting. It probably represents intermittent attacks of acute hydronephrosis. I have seen several such children who had puzzled their pediatricians and their families for a long time before someone finally thought to make an intravenous pyelogram. Once again it should be emphasized that an intravenous pyelogram is an innocuous procedure and can be extremely informative in cases of "failure to thrive", or unexplained abdominal pain.

There is no question that some types of hydronephrosis have a familial tendency. After I had done bilateral pyeloplasties on one brother for hydronephrosis, the mother made the correct diagnosis when a second son developed similar symptoms. — Another mother told me that she was the one who had insisted that the family Pediatrician get a pyelogram when her boy became a bedwetter because she knew that everyone in the family had kidney disease. (The boy had severe bilateral hydronephrosis.)

Anomalies of the ureters are extremely interesting although usually they are secondary to disease elsewhere. However such conditions as duplication of the ureters, multiple ureters, congenital ureteral strictures, ureteral diverticula, and Östling's valves are congenital conditions which may be recognized at the time of pyelography.

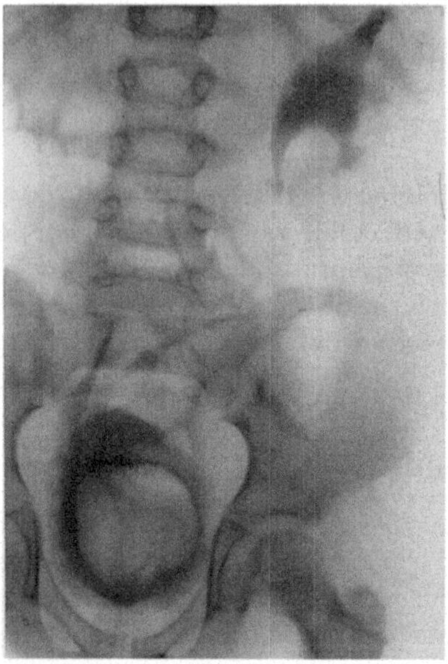

Fig. 7. Ureterocele, left, from upper segment of duplicated left kidney. Note left renal pelvis is pushed laterally due to hydronephrotic segment in upper pole

One of the most interesting conditions is duplication of the upper tract with ureterocele formation. This usually produces obstruction at the bladder neck by a ball-valve type of action, and there is often associated reflux in the other segments of the upper urinary tract. These are some of the most interesting and challenging problems in Pediatric Urology, and all possible skill in diagnosis should be brought to bear before attempting treatment. In some cases it is possible to anastomose the refluxing segment of a double system to the non-refluxing segment and thus produce a relatively normal upper tract. Some patients who have ureterocele increasing from infancy have so much damage to the base of the bladder, where the ureterocele in fact produces a kind of hernia, that the bladder never empties normally even after repair of the defect. In some of these patients a cutaneous diversion may be necessary.

Some ureters seem to have a distal stenosis near the bladder, a so-called Chwalla's valve. If this is the sole cause of the obstruction and the hydroureter above it, the narrowed segment can be excised and the tailored end of the hydronephrotic ureter above it may be reanastomosed, usually with good results, as recommended by Bischoff. If this is not feasible, the ureter may be reimplanted into the bladder by the method of Politano and Leadbetter.

There is a condition of megaureter, which is similar to megacolon and which may also be related to an associated neuromuscular defect caused by absence of the ganglion cells in the ureter. Some of these ureters can never be rehabilitated; and in some cases if they do not respond to reimplantation in the bladder, it may be necessary to do a cutaneous diversion.

Multiple, congenital ureteral diverticula have been observed. They are rare and often do not demand treatment. However when there is associated infection and a trapping residual urine in the diverticulum, it may be necessary to excise the diverticulum surgically.

In some little girls the ureteral orifice empties in an ectopic position outside the urethral sphincter. The history in these cases always suggests the diagnosis, for such a child is *always* slightly wet — never intermittently wet. This condition must be kept in mind when evaluating little girls and when the mother's complaint is that the child has "wet panties".

Ureteral calculi in children are uncommon, but of course when they are found they must be removed. A cause should always be sought.

One of the greatly discussed problems of present day Pediatric Urology has to do with operations aimed at preventing vesico-ureteral reflux. It is accepted that reflux may be congenital due to immaturity of the vesical ureteral valve mechanism. It also may be secondary to outlet obstruction and may also be due to recurrent lower urinary infections. In general it is agreed that such patients should be managed conservatively with long term treatment of infections, and urethral dilatations if indicated. However, a certain number of these children still continue to have reflux and still continue to suffer with recurring infections. These are candidates for an anti-reflux operation. There are numerous techniques for this, each one having its advocates and its advantages. My personal preference at present is either the extravesical method described by Lich and by Gregoire or the transvesical method of reimplantation through a submucosal tunnel described by Politano and Leadbetter. Success rates should be 85 to 90%, depending in large part on how seriously damaged the ureter is at the time of the operation. Some failures lead to nephrectomy and some to cutaneous diversion. It is my belief that this type of "protective surgery" should be attempted before the damage to the lower ureter and to the rest of the urinary tract becomes irreversible.

Neoplasms

Perhaps the commonest and most important neoplasm of childhood is embryonal carcinoma of the kidney, Wilm's Tumor. It is considered by many that these tumors actually start their growth before the child is born. This may be so in some cases but probably is not in all cases. The usual presenting sign is an abdominal mass. The enlarged kidney tumor can usually be differentiated from the equally important neuroblastomas by the fact that the intravenous pyelogram in Wilm's tumor shows a bizarre and abnormal pattern in the calyces. This is also a distinguishing factor from hydronephrosis which also presents as a huge retroperitoneal mass which either appears as an obstructed or as a non-functioning kidney on the intravenous pyelogram.

Current treatment for Wilm's tumor has increased the survival and the optimism of the outlook for these patients considerably. The matter of preoperative radiotherapy is not yet settled except in cases with massive tumors which must be shrunken before definitive therapy is undertaken. However, most American authors at present favour intravenous Actinomycin D, given for 1 or 2 days before operation and also on the day of operation. This is followed by continuation of Actinomycin D therapy after surgical removal of the tumor, plus radiotherapy if indicated. It is known that about 10% of these patients have bilateral tumors, and it is considered proper that most if not all of them should be explored transperitoneally with careful exploration and observation of the "normal", contralateral kidney. SWENSON has described bilateral exploration and bilateral partial nephrectomy on the same day for some of these patients who have bilateral disease.

I saw a young boy who had had the right kidney removed for Wilm's tumor and who returned about 9 months later with a second large tumor in the remaining, solitary left kidney. This was explored, and the area of the tumor was carefully marked off with silver wire sutures whilst the radiotherapist watched. Then he gave "pin point" radiotherapy to the marked area, sparing the rest of the normal kidney. The Wilm's tumor melted away, and the normal kidney substance was not damaged. The patient was alive and well 12 years after that experience.

There are well-documented cases now of children with metastatic Wilm's tumor who have survived and appear to be cured after the combination of Actinomycin D, irradiation and surgical removal of the primary tumor.

Hypernephroma does occur in childhood but is very rare. I saw one 12 year old girl who had a huge hypernephroma, which extended from the xiphoid process to the bony pelvis and had invaded and obstructed the vena cava. There was clear evidence from previous x-rays that the tumor had been present at least 5 years before when she had her first attack of hematuria. Despite pre-operative irradiation and a very radical excision of the kidney, ureter and inferior vena cava, she subsequently died within about 6 months, of metastatic disease.

Tumors of the adrenal gland are of extreme interest, although fairly rare in childhood. Pheochromocytoma occurs occasionally in children. Adrenal cortical tumors, producing the adreno-genital syndrome are more common. They should be removed, whereas adrenal cortical hyperplasia is best managed with cortisone therapy. I saw a young boy with an adrenal cortical tumor which was producing unexpected masculinization. Carcinoma of the adrenal gland is rare in children but is extremely dangerous and nearly always fatal. Surgical treatment is indicated in all of these conditions. We have found preoperative radiographic evaluation with the aid of retroperitoneal oxygen insufflation to be of considerable value in localising the tumor.

Ureteral tumors are almost unknown as primary neoplasms in children. Bladder tumors of the conventional sort seen in adults are extremely rare in children. I have only seen one boy with a papillary tumor of the bladder. However, sarcomas and rhabdomyosarcomas ("hydatid disease") are not so uncommon and are extremely dangerous. Some of them respond to X-ray treatment and possibly to Actinomycin D. All should be treated by radical surgical excision and X-ray therapy, after diversion of the urine. A few cures are reported.

Rhabdomyosarcoma of the prostate has been universally fatal in boys until recently. With MIMS and HUGH YOUNG II, I recently reported the first 5 year cure of a rhabdomyosarcoma of the prostate in a boy. This cure was accomplished by a combination of early diagnosis and radical surgical treatment, plus chemotherapy. The patient was given preoperative irradiation and Actinomycin D, and then a very radical excision was performed, followed by ureterosigmoidostomy for urinary diversion. During the operation which was done under hypothermia, he received intra arterial nitrogen mustard by direct infusion into the hypogastric arteries, which were subsequently ligated. He received further Actinomycin D during the post operative period.

Malignancies of the penis and urethra are very rare in children.

Testis tumors, although rare, are well-recognized. They are usually teratomas or sarcomas in children though other types are known. — An uncommon but extremely interesting type of testis tumor which may occur in childhood is an interstitial cell tumor. These tumors are usually at first benign, and they are discovered because of precocious sexual development in young boys. Some have been bilateral. Treatment is orchiectomy. — Seminomas and embryonal carcinomas of the testis occur in young adults from age 16 years onward and should be managed according to the cell type as they are in adults. Sarcomas and rhabdomyosarcomas of the spermatic cord occur but rarely in children. They should be radically excised. — The general rule concerning scrotal masses at any age applies to children as well. When in doubt, a scrotal mass should be explored. Nothing is lost by exploration, and the penalty of incorrect or late diagnosis of a malignant tumor is severe.

Renal Artery Disease and Hypertension

Inevitably, as renal vascular surgery for hypertension has developed, there have been scattered reports of pediatric cases. There are well-documented cures of hypertension after nephrectomy for unilateral, advanced pyelonephritis. There are also some dramatic reports of cures of hypertension with preservation of the kidney after appropriate surgery for renal artery stenosis. Spleno-renal grafts have been used. There is some question whether it is justified to use prosthetic grafts for the renal artery in children in view of their later expected growth and activity. Recently, my associate, KAUFMAN, successfully employed autotransplantation of a solitary kidney to the iliac fossa in order to treat renal artery stenosis in a young boy. This may become an important usefulness for this procedure in the future. Probably interrupted sutures should be used for the vessels because the anastomosis cannot grow with the child if continuous sutures are used.

Transplantation of the Kidney

One should not close a discussion of the urological surgery and anomalies of children without a brief mention of the fact that the time has come already when some children are definitely candidates for kidney transplantation as treatment for irreversible uremia. In general children are poor subjects for hemodialysis on a long-range basis. The best results in kidney transplantation have been with children of 5 to 6 years and older who have received a transplanted kidney before dialysis is required. Our experience with a few such cases is good, and the results are gratifying. Obviously the donor should be a parent. And the donor should be carefully screened to be certain that he or she is a willing donor and also has an absolutely normal urinary tract and is normal in every other way. Once these criteria have been established and the proper blood match between parent and child has been done, the transplantation may be performed with the expectation of good results. This form of treatment of advanced, incureable renal insufficiency has yet to be worked out completely, but it seems certain that in future years as transplantation becomes an established procedure it will have a definite place. STARZL has perhaps had the most experience in this field and has written most about it. It must be remembered that in children as well as in adults the recipient of a transplanted kidney should have a normal lower urinary tract. MARKLAND described some experiences with kidney transplantation in children where the ureter was anastomosed to a segment of ileum for a cutaneous diversion as in BRICKER's operation. Some of these patients did well, but infection was a serious problem. We described an unsuccessful attempt to place both kidneys of a newborn monster into an infant. The procedure, which was done by the "en bloc" technique of CARRELL and GUTHRIE was technically satisfactory, but the kidneys never functioned due to spasm of the renal arteries. Nonetheless this technique may have some future application.

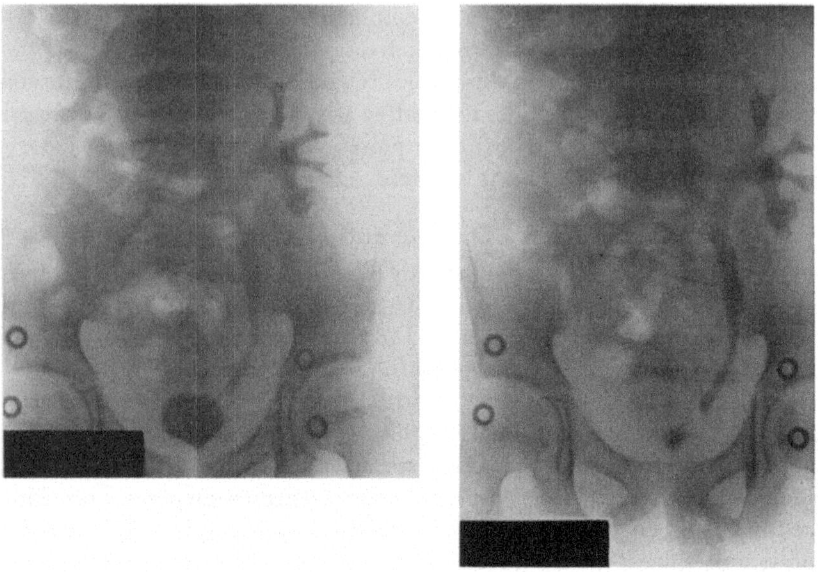

Fig. 8. Kidney transplantation in a 9 year old boy. Note large kidney from father. Patients own kidneys have been removed. He is now rides horseback and remains well more than 2 years after transplantation

References

CAMPBELL, M.: Clinical pediatric urology. Philadelphia and London: W. B. Saunders Company 1951.

HIGGINS, T. T., D. I. WILLIAMS, and D. F. E. NASH: The urology of childhood. London: Butterworth & Co. (Publishers), LTD 1951.

KJELLBERG, S. R., N. O. ERICSSON, and U. RUDHE: The lower urinary tract in childhood. Stockholm: Almquist & Wiksell 1957.

STEPHENS, F. D.: Congenital malformations of the rectum, anus and genito-urinary tracts. Edinburgh—London: E. & S. Livingstone LTD 1963.

BERENS, S. C., L. M. LINDE, and W. E. GOODWIN: Pediatrics **38, I.** (1966).

BURKLAND, C. E., W. E. GOODWIN, and W. F. LEADBETTER: Surgery **28**, 67—70 (1950).

CASEY, W. C., and W. E. GOODWIN: J. Urol. (Baltimore) **74**, 164—173 (1955).

DUNCAN, G., and W. E. GOODWIN: Surgery **25**, 113—116 (1949).

GOODWIN, W. E.: Discussion of „Mageloureter" by ORVAR SWENSON. Surgery **40**, 232—233 (1956).

— Chapter Retroperitoneal causes if abdominal pain. In: The differential diagnosis of abdominal pain, SHERMAN M. MELLINKOFF, Ed. New York: McGraw-Hill Book Co. 1959.

— Urol. int. (Basel) **23**, 135—136 (1968).

— Discussion of paper: Urinary diversion operations, WEYRAUCH, H. M., J. F. PATTON, J. H. MCDONALD, SIR ERIC RICHES, C. V. HODGES, F. HINMAN JR., W. P. HERBST JR., W. LEADBETTER, J. H. KIEFER, J. K. LATTIMER, T. E. GIBSON H. M. SPENCE, J. LAPIDES, J. D. YOUNG, 76th Annual Meeting Royal Orleans Hotel, New Orleans. Transactions of the American Assoc. of GU Surgeons **57**, 37 (1965).

—, and P. B. Hudson: Surg. Gynec. Obstet **93**, 331—342 (1951).
—, and W. W. Scott: J. Urol. (Baltimore) **68**, 903—908 (1952).
—, E. F. Alston, and J. H. Semens: J. Urol. (Baltimore) **63**, 79—96 (1950).
—, J. J. Kaufman, and D. C. Martin: J. Urol. (Baltimore) **99**, 827—828 (1968).
—, M. M. Mims, and H. H. Young II.: J. Urol. (Baltimore) **99**, 651—655 (1968).
—, E. V. Moore, and E. Peirce II.: J. Urol. (Baltimore) **74**, 231—242 (1955).
—, P. L. Scardino, and W. W. Scott: J. Urol. (Baltimore) **71**, 748—758 (1954).
—, A. P. Harris, J. J. Kaufman, and J. M. Beal: Surg. Gynec. Obstet. **97**, 295—300 (1953).
—, E. W. Fonkalsrud, R. Goldman, J. J. Kaufman, D. C. Martin, J. M. Riley, C W Roe, A. E. Schapiro, and J. A. Wilkerson: Ann. intern. Med. **65**, 160—184 (1966).
Grey, D. N., P. Flynn, and W. E. Goodwin: J. Urol. (Baltimore) **77**, 154—163 (1957).
Hodges, C. V., D. E. Pickering, J. E. Murray, and W. E. Goodwin: Kidney transplant between identical twins, J. Urol. (Baltimore) **89**, 115—121 (1963).
Longm re Jr., W. P., D. G. Buckberg, and W. E. Goodwin: Ann. Surg., June 1967.
Martin, D. C., and W. E. Goodwin: Brit. J. Urol. **36**, June (1964).
— — Urol. Dig. **7**, 11—17 (1968).
Mosier, H. D., and W. E. Goodwin: Pediatrics **27**, 1016—1021 (1961).
Stein, J. J., and W. E. Goodwin: Amer. J. Roentgenol. **96**, 626—634 (1966).
Walter, R. C., and W. E. Goodwin: J. Urol. (Baltimore) **77**, 323—328 (1957).
Williams, J. L., and W. E. Goodwin: Brit. J. Urol. **37**, 299 (1965).
Winter, C. C., and W. E. Goodwin: Malformation of the urinary bladder. Walters-Lewis: Practice of surgery, IX, Chapt. **17**, 1959.
Young, H. H., **II.**, and W. E. Goodwin: Brit. J. Urol. **39**, 712—717 (1967).

Treatment of Megacolon

Fritz Rehbein and Heinrich Halsband

It is impossible to cover the whole complex of congenital megacolon (Hirschsprung's disease) with its various aspects in a short lecture. I should therefore like to report only on our own experiences and then try to compare the various operative procedures.

Between 1953 and 1967 we have operated altogether on 231 cases of Hirschsprung's disease. The remarkable factor here is that we had 38 cases without a narrow segment. This is a comparatively high figure. There is, however, no doubt at all that these are true cases of Hirschsprung's disease. In every child symptoms appeared soon after birth and in the majority defects or anomalies of the ganglionic cells or an increase of the nerve fibres in the region of the lower end of the specimen were found. Swenson has described such cases. Duhamel classified them as formes anales. The majority of cases (127) belongs to the group in which the narrow segment is restricted to the rectosigmoid region. In seven cases the entire colon and varying parts of the lower ileum were aganglionic.

All 231 cases were treated in the same way. The intraabdominal anterior resection suggested by State in 1952 has been modified by us and invariably carried out since 1953. Different from the methods employed by Swenson and Duhamel in this operation the rectum is not completely removed or excluded, but remains in connection with the pelvic organs. The upper rectum is divided just beneath the peritoneal floor. The level of the proximal section of the colon is usually in the descending colon or somewhat higher. The narrow segment of the rectosigmoid junction and the dilated sigmoid and descending colon are thus eliminated. An end-to-end anastomosis is carried out between the transverse colon and the rectum followed by energic digital dilatation of the anal sphincter. The distance of the anastomosis from anocutaneal line was 4 cm in infants and 6 to 8 cm in older children.

Table gives a review of the results. We lost 19 children altogether. Of these 6 died shortly after the operation. These deaths occured in the early years of this period. Some children were high risk cases.

We were able to examine personally 131 children and we received exact data on 69. "Very good" results means that the children had daily spontaneous movements of the bowel, needed no laxative or enemas and developed no abdominal distension. The children in the second group need a laxative from time to time but otherwise show no sign of constipation. The children in the third group require a laxative regularly and occasionally show distension of the abdomen.

It must be mentioned that this classification of results is not final, as we have established in our follow-up, but may be subject to changes. Renewed symptoms of constipation have appeared occasionally in children in group one in the early years after the operation. This is due to the fact that following successful operation and dilatation of the anus the sphincter muscle has become rigid again and achalasia has reappeared. This deterioration can occur 2 to 3 years after operation or even later still. This necessitates a renewed dilatation of the sphincter ani. By this means normal bowel habits are immediately restored. In some cases dilatation of the sphincter has to be repeated 2 to 3 times. In difficult individual cases we used sphincterotomy, and for some months now, myectomy as suggested by Lynn. By this means we have achieved results with children in group 2 and 3 which have enabled them to be transfered to group one. No loss of sphincter control has been observed in any child after repeated dilatation, following sphincterotomy or myectomy.

Table. *231 cases of anterior resection in Hirschsprung's disease (1953—1967)*

Follow up until May 1968	Group 1 very good	Group 2 good	Group 3 fair	Fatal cases	Fatal cases independent of operation	No response
200 personally 131 questionnaire 69	158 (= 72,2%)	33 (= 15%)	9 (= 4,1%)	6 (= 2,7%)	13 (= 6%)	12

Long Segment Cases

A very interesting group are the so-called long segment cases. The group includes cases with aganglionosis of the entire colon and cases with aganglionosis of a large part of the colon. There are two survivors of cases with total colectomy. We performed a total colectomy on a girl 16 years ago. Today she is married and has visited us with her healthy little daughter. An other child remained healthy for 4 years after total colectomy and then suddenly died at home from cerebral causes.

Discussion

It has become clear, particularly during the last 10 years, that, in Hirschsprung's disease, completely different methods of treatment can lead to success. Swenson developed in 1948 his surgical technique which was soon very popular; although the mobilisation of the rectum is very tedious, difficult and not without risk, good results have been reported many times.

I am very delighted that in 1966 I had the chance to see this operation in Chicago by SWENSON himself. I was very impressed by the careful and subtile manner of his operative technique. I am convinced that in cases where his suggestions are strictly observed one does not need fear for damage to the innervation of the bladder and the reproductive organs. Especially NIXON was able to state the good results of this procedure.

With the Swenson-method a relatively extensive resection of the rectum is done. According to his communication in 1963, he leaves ventrally 2 cm and dorsally only 1 cm of the rectum in situ. The rectum, however, is mobilized and dissected free to the mucocutaneous line.

In comparison with this procedure the Duhamel-method is much simpler. His retro-rectal approach is characterised by the fact that the rectum remains in the true pelvis and therefore the dangerous and time consuming mobilisation is not necessary; so it remains excluded from the main alimentary canal as a diverticulum. The number of supporters of this technique increased considerably especially after GROB in 1959 published a very useful modification which allowed for better preservation of the sphincter. This excluded the risk that children with liquid stools no longer had control over their sphincter. DUHAMEL himself in 1964 reported uniformly good results. Only in a few cases the blind rectal pouch filled up with faeces which acted as an obstruction for the through-pulled colon. But EHRENPREIS reported that it is easy to overcome these difficulties. With the original technique less is left over and with GROB's modification more is left over at the dorsal side.

SOAVE excises the rectal mucosa, while the muscular wall remains behind.

In our modification of the State-procedure a bigger part of the rectum, with mucosa, is left over.

If it is true, which is undoubtedly the case, that one can achieve good results with completely different methods, then there must be something, which all these methods have in common. I thought it would be interesting to discuss this point of view.

All methods have in common that the rectum is only partially resected. With the Swenson-method less of the rectum remains, with DUHAMEL rather more, and with our method most of all. In the last 14 years we operated upon 231 cases only in this way without any change. In our experience with this procedure it is necessary that the children are carefully supervised by their mothers as regards the daily evacuation for at least 2 to 3 years after the operation. The children must have stools every day spontaneously and if they miss sometimes 1 day they must be brought back. I will come to this point later on.

Now a second point of view. I mentioned already the importance of sphincterachalasia in Hirschsprung's disease. With the first three methods, Swenson, Duhamel and Soave, it is technically necessary to dilate the sphincter. SWENSON has to dilate a little bit, to be able to perform the pull-through of the colon. DUHAMEL must stretch the sphincter to be able to incise and anastomose in the dorsal side of the rectum, and SOAVE dilates while removing the rectal mucosa. Only with the anterior resection dilatation of the sphincter is not necessarily a part of the procedure. With the intraabdominal anastomosis one does not touch the anus at all. The mobilisation of the rectum to the mucocutaneous line, like SWENSON advises it in his last publication leads to a weakening of the anus. Besides that, SWENSON removes since 1963 dorsally partially this internal sphincter. This is done on purpose, and it is called: partial sphincterectomy.

This on purpose or incidential dilatation of the sphincter is in our opinion the most important for success. This weakening seems to us really more important than the extensive resection of the rectum.

When we started, 15 years ago, with our modification of the anterior resection of the State-procedure, we made in one of the first cases the following experience: After a primarily good result, stool-retention and abdominal distension occured again. To our surprise the remained aganglionic portion of the rectum was not contracted but extremely dilated, and there was a strong and spastic sphincter. After dilatation of the anal sphincter, the symptoms subsided.

Since that time, we combine sphincterdilatation with the anterior resection, and our results have become as good as others. We have never observed that the remaining portion of the rectum was the cause of stool-retention. Sometimes, this sphincterachalasia recurs. Then again, stretching of the anus leads to normal function. In some stubborn cases, the dilatation was not sufficient and we had to perform a sphincterotomy, like Bill and Chapman described in cases operated with the Swenson-method.

The fact, that Swenson does a partial sphincterectomy, proves the importance of a weakening of the anal sphincter.

At the Congress of the British Association of Paediatric Surgeons in Edinburgh 1965, Bentley and Duhamel made the importance of the sphincter very clear. The question remains only: is it a true or a Pseudo-Hirschsprung case.

Duhamel found in some of these children without a narrow segment ganglioncell-defects in the internal sphincter. In these children too, partial sphincterectomy alone was leading to success.

One can observe the same principle in the report of Lynn from the Mayo Clinic. He employed a very intensive form of myectomy in an attempt to relieve persistent symptoms of patients who had had — what he calls — inadequate operation of the Swenson pull-through or in patients who had had an intraabdominal resection. Lynn says that the dramatic success of myectomy has led him to its use in similar cases and eventually in cases of aganglionic megacolon in patients who had had no previous operation. This means cases without a narrow segment.

This pseudo-recurrence, which we have seen sometimes after anterior resection looks like such a megacolon without narrow segment. It is caused only by recurrence of the sphincterachalasia and should be treated like this with redilatation, with sphincterotomy or myectomy. The difference in these three procedures is only of degree.

We have now started a strict treatment of cases with insufficient results or with recurring symptoms by redilatation or by myectomy and dilatation. I am convinced that in all these cases which were neglected due to bad social conditions a success can be achieved. The exceptions in our experience are to be found only in children who are mentally retarded.

Leaving aside the operative technical procedure we can state, that anterior resection in combination with treatment of the sphincter achalasia cannot, as has often been done, be described as an inadequate operation. On the contrary this procedure has widened our theoretical knowledge of Hirschsprung's disease. Besides the narrow segment, there exists, in every case, a, from slight to severe varying achalasia of the sphincter, like Callaghan (1964) proved tonometrically. This achalasia becomes more important and obvious after resection of the narrow segment.

A neurogenic disorder is doubtless the cause of the complete picture; of the narrow segment as well as of the achalasia.

There must be some difference between aganglionosis of the recto-sigmoid and of the rectum. They behave differently. In our experience, an aganglionic rectum can, just like a normal rectum, function as a stool-reservoir, and is not contracted like the narrow segment in the recto-sigmoid.

I would not like to give any judgement about the various operative techniques, because I don't have personel experience with all of them. But it is of interest to show the principles which in my opinion these different methods have in common. According to my point of view it is not essential if 2 or 5 cm of the rectum remain. The achalasia of the sphincter ani is the major problem in the treatment of Hirschsprung's disease. This is by this time solved in several ways, partially on purpose, partially incidentally. Just now, the complicated and subtile sphincter mechanism can only be influenced by very rough methods, like dilatation, sphincterotomy or myectomy. In the normal practice this seems to be sufficient. Fortunately, one can weaken the sphincter very much, without, by doing so, loosing the anal control and this in my opinion is the reason why we can be successful in operating Hirschsprung's disease at all.

Surgical Treatment of Endocrine Disorders in Children

W. Hardy Hendren* and John D. Crawford**

The subject about which we have been invited to speak is the surgical treatment of endocrine disorders in children. We shall try to cover some of the more important surgically correctible diseases of the endocrine glands, and their target organs, as they are treated currently on the Children's Service at the Massachusetts General Hospital. The pituitary gland will be omitted from consideration because those disorders requiring operative intervention are cared for by neurosurgeons.

The Thyroid

Thyrotoxicosis

This is one of the more common endocrinopathies in childhood. We treat practically all of these children initially with propylthiouracil or methiamzole to which they respond well. Treatment can be prolonged in those faithful to the demanding schedule and in whom hematologic, dermatologic or other untoward reactions do not occur. Upon discontinuing the drug after 2 years of continous treatment, about half of the patients are observed to maintain prolonged remission (Saxena et al.). Thyroidectomy is recommended for those in whom thyrotoxicity recurs or those in whom medical treatment fails because of idiosyncrasy to the thioamide drugs, irregularity of therapy, or progressive gland enlargement. We have been reluctant to use RAI ablation of the gland in the pediatric age group because we do not yet know

* Clinical Associate in Surgery, Harvard Medical School, Surgical Chairman, Children's Service, and Associate Visiting Surgeon, Massachusetts General Hospital.

** Associate Professor of Pediatrics, Harvard Medical School, Chief, Endocrine-Metabolic Unit, Children's Service, Massachusetts General Hospital.

This investigation was supported in part by a grant from the National Institute of Child Health and Human Development, 5-Tl-HD-00033.

the end result as regards cancer 50 to 60 years later. In one child with recurrent hyperthyroidism following two operations elsewhere and a third in our clinic, we elected to use radioactive iodine rather than undertake the risk of a fourth procedure. In operations for toxic goiter meticulous dissection with preservation of the parathyroid glands and recurrent nerves is mandatory. Some surgeons do a bilateral sub-total thyroidectomy; we prefer a total removal of one side, leaving a remnant of about 4 g on the second side, so that if recurrence should take place reoperation is necessary on only that side. This is important, since at secondary operation the risk of injury to nerves and parathyroids is greater. Recurrent toxicity is very rare; all patients are given replacement doses of thyroid for several months following surgery and the majority prove euthyroid when this is discontinued. Approximately one third are rendered permanently hypothyroid and are treated by replacement therapy which is inexpensive and quite satisfactory. Permanent hypoparathyroidism has been absent in our series and transient postoperative hypocalcemia has been unusual.

Thyroid Cancer

A solitary nodule of the thyroid in a child has a 50% chance of being malignant in contrast to the much lower likelihood in adults. Some may be result from previous X-ray therapy (Hempelman et al.; Uhlmann). We advocate exploration in most cases. RAI scan has not been wholly satisfactory in predicting whether these lumps are benign or malignant. There is controversy as to how extensive surgery should be in the malignant cases, the majority of which are papillary cancers. Even without exstirpative surgery, some adults have been noted to live many years. In children, however, in whom we desire 60 to 70 year survivals, we do not believe that these cancers can be regarded as benign. In a large series of 62 children at Memorial Hospital in New York neck metastases were present in 87% and metastases to lung in 20% (Exelby). Several died of their disease. Some papillary cancers are multifocal (Russell et al.). We therefore favor meticulous total thyroidectomy, preserving nerves and parathyroids, together with a modified radical neck dissection if there are positive nodes on the grossly involved side. Rarely a bilateral neck dissection is required, but we would not remove both internal jugular veins simultaneously.

Neonatal Goiter

Thyroid enlargement with respiratory obstruction is seen occasionally in neonates where there has been maternal ingestion of goitrogens during pregnancy, as well as in certain women who have had prior thyroidectomies for thyrotoxicosis. Both the goitrogens and the long acting thyroid stimulating substance (LATS), a γ-globulin, readily cross the placenta. We have treated one neonate by division of the thyroid isthmus with relief of tracheal compression. Most cases due to the goitrogens, which block thyroid hormone biosynthesis, respond to thyroid medication, those associated with neonatal thyrotoxicosis respond to iodine or the thioamides.

Lingual Thyroid

Ectopic location of the thyroid in the base of the tongue can cause dysphagia or respiratory difficulty (Hung et al.) and may have a slightly increased incidence of cancer (Ward et al.). We favor surgical excision and have employed a high collar incision, transecting the strap and tongue muscles just above the hyoid bone (Fig. 1). This gives easy access to the mass. After excision permanent substitution drug therapy is necessary.

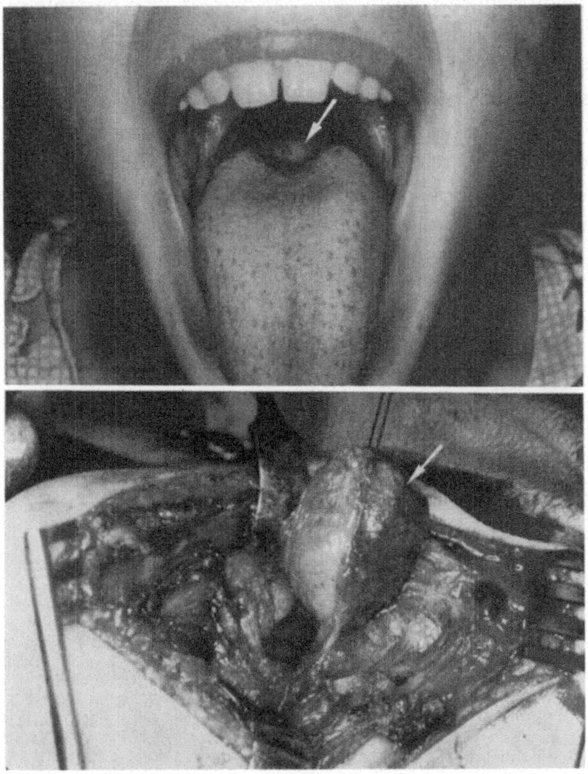

Fig. 1. 12 year old boy with lingual thyroid. Top: Mass evident at base of tongue causing dysphagia. Bottom: As seen during removal through high collar incision, transecting base of tongue above hyoid bone to delivering mass. This is preferred to transoral or lateral pharyngeal approach

Hyperparathyroidism

This is very rare in children and will not be discussed it for it is the subject of a symposium elsewhere on this program.

The Pancreas

Pancreatitis

This problem in children is not so rare as once supposed. We have treated 26 cases in children in the past 12 years, some of whom have been reported previously (Hendren et al.). The disorder has been seen secondary to trauma, mumps, and a variety of obstructions of the ampulla by gallstones, congenital fibrosis and ascaris worms. Several patients have had pseudocysts. The etiology was unknown in some. For certain cases we favor transduodenalsphincterotomy and gentle intraoperative pancreatography to exclude intrapancreatic pathology. Pseudocysts should be drained into the stomach or by a Roux-en-Y jejunal loop; marsupialization has been used on occasion.

Episodic Hypoglycemia

This is a common problem of infancy. In past years exploration was performed on many of these babies to rule out functioning adenomata which is quite rare. In negative explorations subtotal pancreatectomy was performed with variable results (HAMILTON et al.). Since the advent of plasma insulin assay and provocative tests with tolbutamide and leucine, fewer explorations are needed and should be restricted to those infants showing elevated plasma insulin levels (Fig. 2). Thiazide drugs and growth hormone are available to control hypoplycemia in idiopathic cases especially those with low plasma insulin levels (CRAWFORD and SOYKA). It can be difficult to make the differential diagnosis between leucine sensitivity and adenoma. We have encountered two children (CRIGLER), under 1 year of age, with adenomas and so, although rare, if this cannot be excluded by diagnostic tests, exploration should be performed.

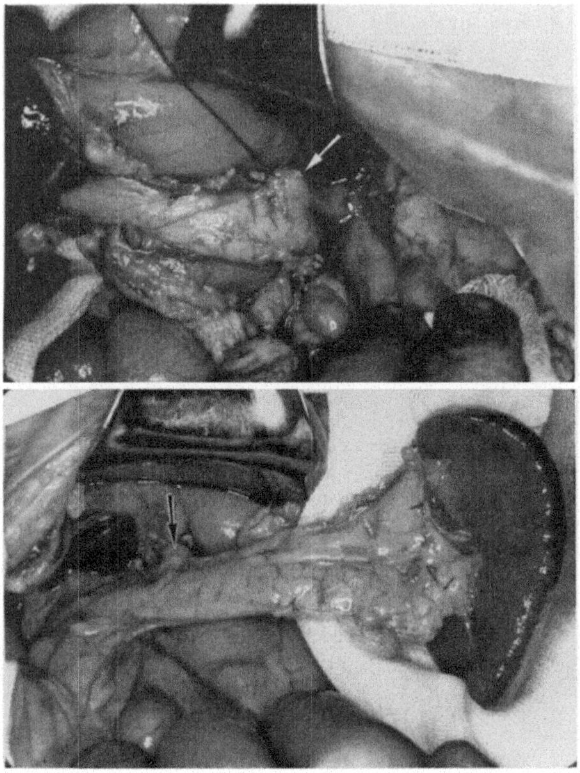

Fig. 2. Functioning adenomas of pancreas causing hypoglycemia; both are on upper border of body of pancreas. Top: In a 6 month old infant. Spleen and tail of pancreas have been reflected toward opposite side. Bottom: In a 4 month old infant. Episodic hypoglycemia disappeared in both infants after removal of these tumors

Pancreatic Tumors

These are rare in children; we have seen 3, 2 adenocarcinomas and 1 lymphoma, all resectable by radical surgery.

The Adrenals

There are several entities of surgical importance in children relating to the adrenal glands, including Cushings disease, virilizing tumors, pheochromocytoma, and genital abnormality associated with congenital adrenalcortical hyperplasia (MURISON).

Cushing's Syndrome

These children have a characteristic picture of stunted growth, poor musculature and marked obesity (Fig. 3). This can result from diffuse nodular hyperplasia or from tumor. These two causes may be discriminated by the dexamethasone suppression test in which the hydroxycorticoid production in tumor cases does not fall. Originally in nodular hyperplasia we did bilateral subtotal adrenalectomy; later we performed total removal of one gland and subtotal of the other. Because of some recurrences even after 95% resections (EGDAHL) we now prefer bilateral total adrenalectomy, followed by cortisone and 9-α-fluorohydrocortisone therapy. In tumor patients the

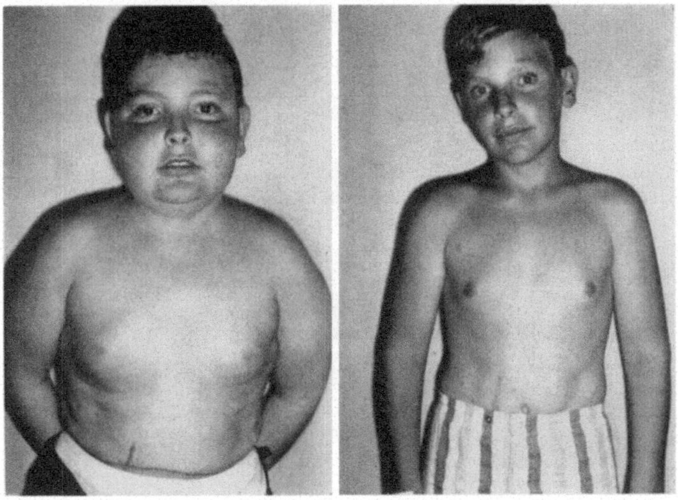

Fig. 3. Cushing's Syndrome in 13 year old boy caused by bilateral nodular adrenal hyperplasia. Left: Immediately after removal of all of left gland and 90% of right gland. Right: 2 years later, Note disappearance of Cushingoid habitus. Later, at 17 years of age, certain features of the syndrome recurred and the right remnant was removed. It had hypertrophied and contained several large adenomas. He is currently well on total replacement therapy

opposite adrenal may be atrophic and temporary cortisone treatment may be required after removal of the autonomously functioning mass.

Pheochromocytoma

Both benign and malignant chromaffin tumors may occur in children with the same manifestations as are seen in adults (Fig. 4) (Clinical Staff Conference, N.I.H.). Various provocative and blocking agents are available to aid in diagnosis. They may be familial and multifocal.

Neuroblastoma

Neuroblastoma is the most common malignant abdominal tumor in children and often arises in the adrenal. The tumor can be very large. An aggressive approach is warranted especially when distant spread is not evident. It is well known that some of these have a high output of catecholamines which may be found in the urine and which may produce hypertension (BILL and KOOP). Elevated urinary levels of cystathionine are usually found when this tumor is present and may be helpful in initial diagnosis as well as in follow-up for recurrence. Occasionally newborn infants

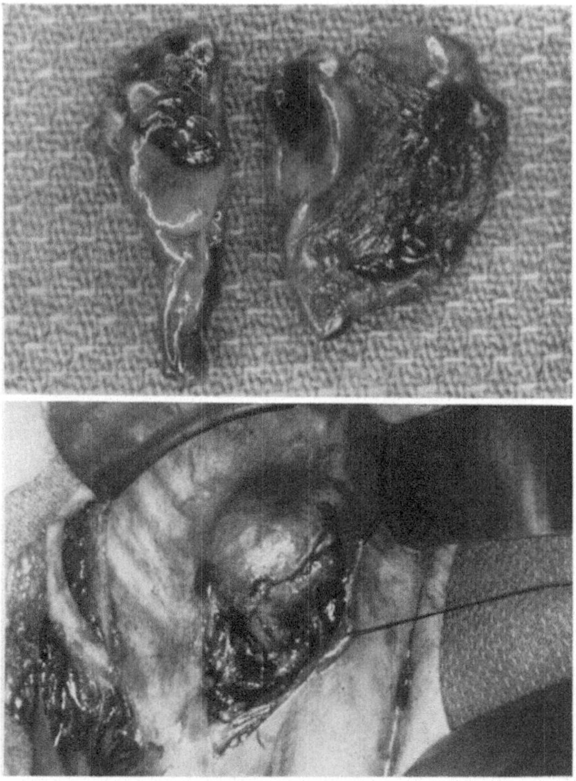

Fig. 4. Two pheochromocytomas from an 8 year old boy in a family with multiple endocrine adenomas. Top: The left adrenal gland containing 1.5 cm tumor. Bottom: 4 cm tumor from left upper chest

are seen with a small primary tumor and extensive liver metastases. Surprisingly, cure may be achieved in 80% of this type of case when removal of the primary tumor is followed by 1,000 R of X-ray treatment to the liver.

Adrenogenital Syndrome

Males with the common form of this disorder have no genital abnormalities at birth. The affected females, however, usually present as neonates with varying degrees of external genital masculinization ranging from slight clitoral enlargement with minimal posterior labial fusion to essentially complete male transformation. In such patients the buccal smear will show 20% or more of cells with nuclear chromatin masses (Barr bodies), and urinary 17-ketosteroid and pregnantriol excretion values will be elevated. Heavy pigmentation of the genitalia and areolae suggest that the infant will manifest the salt losing tendency associated with the complete block of 21-hydroxylation. Diagnostic laparotomy is usually not necessary, in contrast to the situation in certain other intersex cases. In addition to clitorectomy, vaginoplasty is often required. We believe that the anatomy of these cases should be defined carefully by cystourethroscopy, because in seven recent cases the vagina was found to arise from the urethra proximal to the voluntary sphincter (Fig. 5) (Rosenberg et al.). A special operative procedure is required to transfer the opening of these vaginas to

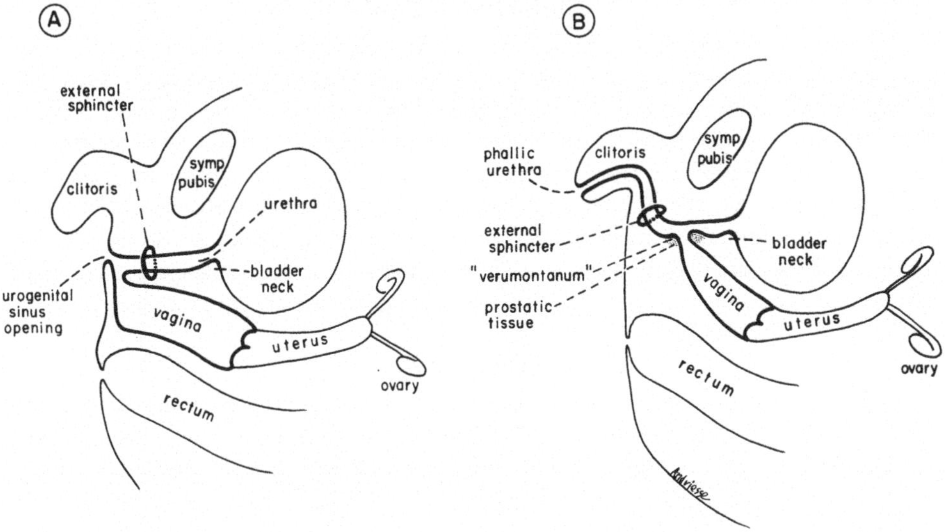

Fig. 5. Anatomy of the lower urinary tract in the adrenogenital syndrome. A The most often encountered type, with a low placed vagina which can be exteriorized by a simple "cut back" perineorrhaphy at the time of clitorectomy. B Marked masculinization of the lower urinary tract with connection of the vagina to the upper urethra requiring a pull-through procedure for its correction

the perineum without injuring the voluntary urinary sphincter (HENDREN and CRAWFORD). Furthermal a simple "cut back" operation will not suffice where the vagina lies as high as it does in these cases.

Genital and Gonadal Abnormalities

Mixed Gonadal Dysgenesis

This should be suspected in a child who looks much like the female with adrenogenital syndrome having clitoral enlargement and posterior labial fusion but no elevation of urinary 17-ketosteroids. The buccal smear is almost uniformly of the male type. The internal anatomy generally includes a testis on one side and a streak ovary on the other. We recommend removal of both gonads because the streak ovary may undergo malignant change (TETER and BOCZKOWSKI) and the testis will cause masculinization at adolescence. Although hypospadias repair and hysterectomy have been accomplished in some of these individuals, the multiple procedures, high morbidity and less than satisfactory end results have led us to prefer to rear them as females. The necessary plastic repairs are readily accomplished in infancy; this leads to prompt acceptance of the assigned gender role, and substitution estrogen and progesterone therapy at adolescence yields a normal feminine appearance with menstrual periods and the capacity for satisfactory marital relations.

Testicular Tumors

Interstitial adenoma of the testis can produce precocious puberty. Occasionally the mass may be so small as to be impalpable. Malignant neoplasms also occur in the testis during childhood. This is most commonly embryonal carcinoma. If distant metastases are not evident radical orchiectomy and abdominal lymphadenectomy offer the best hope for cure (RICHARDSON and LEBLANC; STAVBITZ et al.).

Undescended Testis

In recent years the preferred age for surgical correction of cryptorchidism has gradually become lowered as a result of demonstration of progressive histologic damage to the testis as the child grows older (BONGIOVANNI; HECKER and HIENZ). We believe further that in the small child a very high testis can more often be brought into the scrotum after a retroperitoneal dissection of cord structures than in older boys. Therefore we favor operation during early infancy for the especially high placed cryptorchid. Babies tolerate the operation well and are often discharged the following day. Testicular prostheses are now available in several sizes and are of great psychological benefit for boys where one or both testes are absent at exploration.

The Ovary

Most cases of precocious puberty in girls are due to central pituitary stimulation rather than functioning ovarian tumors (PEPUS et al.; FATHALLA et al.). Occasionally a large follicle cyst is encountered. Treatment is excision of the cyst, not ovariectomy.

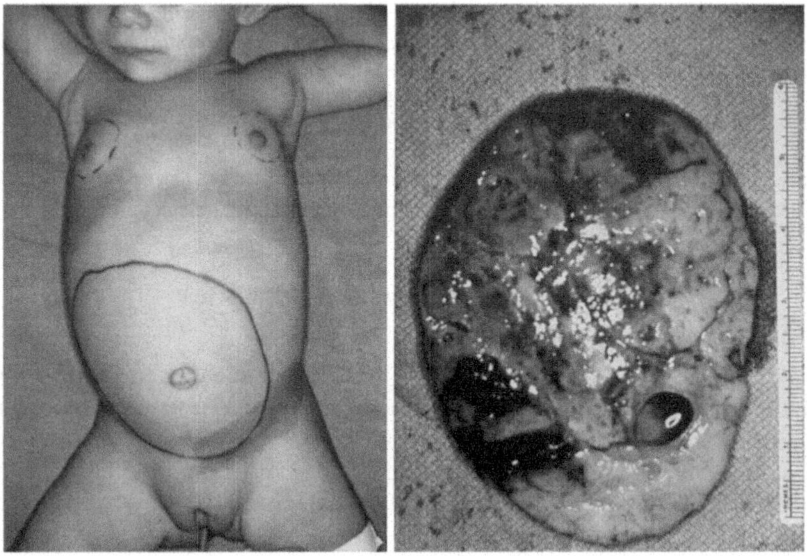

Fig. 6. 1 year old infant with large granuloma cell tumor of right ovary presenting as an abdominal mass in an infant with breast enlargement

Granulosa cell tumor is the most common of the functional ovarian neoplasms in childhood. These may be quite large (Fig. 6). Huge ovarian cysts can be encountered even in the newborn. Dermoid cysts are among the more common nonfunctioning ovarian masses in girls. Occasionally highly malignant and fatal tumors are encountered. Each year, a number of entirely normal ovaries are seen in our pathology department after removal during laparotomy for appendicitis or abdominal pain in adolescent girls. Unfortunately, there is a lack of appreciation for the fact that considerable enlargement of the female gonad takes place at this time, indeed the pathologist is unable to make a diagnosis of Stein-Leventhal ovary unless he knows that the gonad comes from a patient older than 18 years (MERRILL).

The Breast

Non tumorous enlargement of the breasts is common in boys in early adolescence. This is often limited to one side and only reassurance is indicated, not biopsy. In most cases the gynecomastia is transient, persisting for 18 months to 2 years. In certain instances, and, paradoxically, these are often in the otherwise most masculine boys, we do not hesitate to perform simple mastectomy for psychological reasons if the condition persists.

In infant girls, chiefly around the age of 18 months, breast enlargement, often assymetrical or unilateral is quite common. Characteristically, in this syndrome of benign infantile mammoplasia there are no other signs of precocity, the vaginal smear shows negligible estrogen effect and the condition is nonprogressive. We have seen a number of instances where ill-advised breast biopsy has been performed. This is apt to result in regrettable deformity of the breast at maturity and should be avoided (TALBOT et al.).

Lumps in the breast are encountered with significant frequency in adolescent girls. Self induced trauma is an etiology to be borne in mind in the child psychologically unprepared for her adult transformation. By far, the commonest tumor is the fibro-adenoma which is characteristically mobile, firm and painless unless of large size when it may cause discomfort. The intraductal papilloma usually is of small size when attention is drawn to the tumor through a serosanguinous discharge. Cystic mastitis generally results in multiple small nodules. Since carcinoma can occur in the adolescent, persistent masses especially those deforming the breast or adherent to the superficial tissues should be subject to open biopsy, and the benign lesions removed in a conservative operation (McDIVITT and STEWART).

In closing we would like to express our appreciation for being invited to discuss some of these pediatric surgical problems before this meeting of surgeons from our two countries.

References

BILL, A. H., and C. E. KOOP: J. pediat. Surg. **3**, 103—193 (1968).
BONGIOVANNI, A. M.: Pediatrics **36**, 786—788 (1965).
CRAWFORD, J. D., and L. F. SOYKA: Practitioner **195**, 550 (1965).
CRIGLER, J. F.: New Engl. J. Med. **266**, 1269—1276 (1962).
EGDAHL, R. H.: New Engl. J. Med. **278**, 939 (1968).
EXELBY, P.: Carcinoma of the thyroid in children. A review of 62 cases seen at memorial hospital, 1933—1962. Personal Communication.
FATHALLA, M. F., M. N. RASHAD, and M. G. KERR: J. Obstet. Gynaec. Brit. Cwlth. **73**, 810—820 (1966).
HAMILTON, J. P., L. BAKER, R. KAYE, and C. E. KOOP: Pediatrics **39**, 49—67 (1967).
HECKER, W. C., and H. A. HIENZ: J. pediat. Surg. **2**, 513—517 (1967).
HEMPELMAN, L. H., J. W. PIFER, G. J. BURKE, R. TERRY, and W. R. AMES: J. nat. Cancer Inst. **38**, 317 (1967).
HENDREN, W. H., and J. G. CRAWFORD: Adrenogenital syndrome: The anatomy of the anomaly and its repair. J. pediat. Surg. (In Press).
—, J. M. GREEP, and A. S. PATTON: Arch Dis. Childh. **40**, 132—145 (1965).
HUNG, W., J. G. RANDOLPH, D. SABATINI, and T. WINSHIP: Pediatrics **38**, 647—651 (1966).
McDIVITT, R. W., and F. W. STEWART: J. Amer. med. Ass. **195**, 388—390 (1966).
MERRILL, J. A.: Sth. med. J. (Bgham, Ala.) **56**, 225 (1963).
MURISON, P. J.: Med. Clin. N. Amer. **51**, 883—901 (1967).
PEPUS, M., J. B. HUTCHESON, E. H. RUFFOLO, and M. E. SMITH: Obstet. and Gynec. **29**, 828—833 (1967).

Pheochromocytoma: Current concepts of diagnosis and treatment. Combined clinical staff conference at the national institutes of health. Ann. intern. Med. **65**, 1302—1326 (1965).
RICHARDSON, J. F., and G. A. LEBLANC: J. Urol. (Baltimore) **93**, 717—720 (1965).
ROSENBERG, B., W. H. HENDREN, and J. D. CRAWFORD: Posterior urethrovaginal communication in apparent males with congenital adrenocortical hyperplasia. New Engl. J. Med. (In Press).
RUSSELL, W. O., R. L. CLARK, M. L. IBANEZ, and E. C. WHITE: Amer. J. Path. **34**, 552 (1958).
SAXENA, M. K., J. D. CRAWFORD, and N. B. TALBOT: Brit. med. J. **1964 II**, 1153—1158.
STAVBITZ, W. J., T. C. JEWETT, I. V. MAGOSS, W. G. SCHENK, and S. PHALAKORNKULE: J. Urol. (Baltimore) **94**, 683—686 (1965).
TALBOT, N. B., E. H. SOBEL, J. W. MCARTHUR, and J. D. CRAWFORD: Functional endocrinology from birth to adolescence. Cambridge, Mass.: Harvard Univ. Press 1952.
TETER, J., and K. BOCZKOWSKI: Cancer (Philad.) **20**, 1301—1310 (1967).
UHLMANN, E. M.: J. Amer. med. Ass. **161**, 504 (1956).
WARD, G. E., J. R. CANTRELL, and W. B. ALLEN: Ann. Surg. **159**, 536 (1954).
WILKINS, L., R. M. BLIZZARD, and C. J. MIGEON: The diagnosis and treatment of endocrine disorders in childhood and adolescence. 3rd. Ed. Oxford: Blackwell Scientific Publications 1965.

Abdominal Tumours in Infants

M. GROB

The peculiar nature in many aspects of abdominal tumours occurring in infancy, i.e. the first year of life, justifies special consideration of this age group. Errors in embryonal development are, almost without exception, the cause of these early solid or cystic, benign or malignant tumours, which are even seen in neonates, thus making differentiation between genuine neoplasms and tumour-like malformations often arbitrary. This is especially true in the case of cystic changes which may present clinically and radiologically as tumours, for example, reduplication of the intestine or a multilocular aplastic cystic kidney with or without a residual ureter.

Neuroblastoma of the sympathetic nervous system will be considered first. This tumour is occasionally observed in the newborn and is the most frequently seen malignant abdominal tumour in infants (SCHNEIDER et al.).

The biological pattern of these tumours is unique. Their high-grade malignancy and early invasion of regional lymphnodes, liver, skin, orbit and skeleton is in contrast to the successful cures obtained even when extensive metastases are present. Exceptionally, spontaneous maturation of an advanced tumour that is, transformation into a benign ganglioneuroma, has been reported (CUSHING and WOLBACH; BILL; EVERSON; KOOP and HERNANDEZ).

In these abdominal tumours infants are usually detected, often incidentally, by the mother or examining doctor, as palpable, round or nodular masses. Intestinal disorders, failure to gain weight, fever, and anaemia may be present. Often metastatic changes — exophtalmus, hepatomegaly and especially multiple skin metastases — are the first manifestations. Intravenous pyelograms may show downward displacement of the renal pelvis since these tumours originate mostly in the adrenal glands. Differentation from Wilms' tumour is not always possible radiologically. The presence of small calcification is nearly always pathognomic (Fig. 1).

Determination of catecholamine metabolites in 24 h urine specimens (a test which we regularly perform) shows increased excretion of 3-methoxy-4-hydroxymandelic acid (VMA) and homovanillic acid (HVA) (BOHUON; KOOP et al.). The

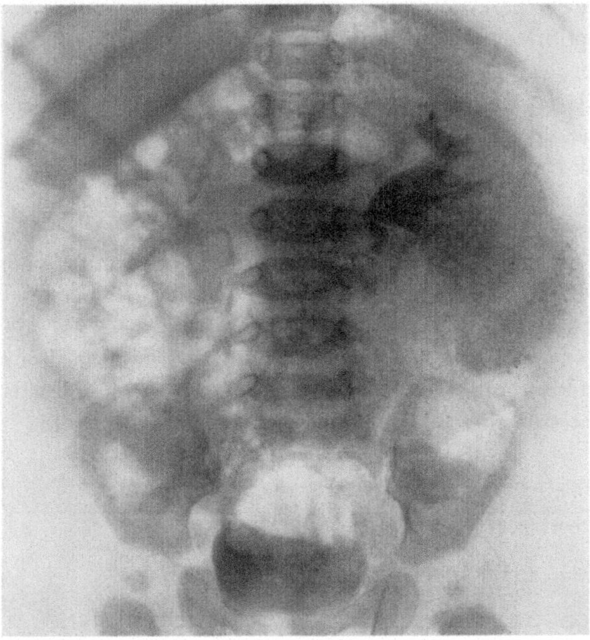

Fig. 1. Ganglioneuroblastoma showing typical calcification. (7-month-old girl)

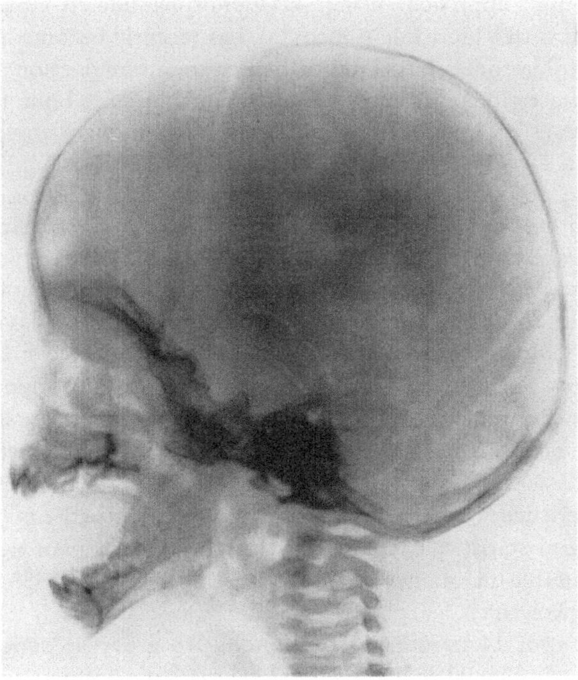

Fig. 2. Skull metastases. (4-month-old boy)

diagnostic value of these determinations is small since tumour excision provides quicker confirmation of diagnosis, but repeated determinations are useful for the post-operative prognosis since the catecholamine level regains normal values in cured cases, while remaining elevated, or even increasing, in presence of metastases or local recurrences.

Treatment of neuroblastoma is primarily surgical, all the more as some cases have been cured by non-radical excision of the tumour (KOOP and HERNANDEZ).

Post-operative radiotherapy is indicated whenever surgical removal of the tumour is impossible or incomplete. Radiotherapy is especially effective where liver metastases are present (GROSS et al.; PRIEBE and CLATWORTHY). We personally observed this in the following case.

Extensive liver metastases developed in an infant 3 months after excision of a left abdominal neuroblastoma, which were confirmed by a second laparotomy. Radiotherapy was successful, the child survived and is now 16 years old.

Table 1. *Age and prognosis*

Age	Neuroblastoma 0—1 year	Thor.	Abd.	> 1 year	total
Cases	17	7	10	20	37
Alive	12 70%	7 100%	5 50%	3 15%	15 40%

Chemotherapeutic approach using cyclophosphamide (Cytoxan, Endoxan), alone or combined with Vincristine (Oncovin), has recently become important in the treatment of neuroblastoma. Not only primary tumour regression but also disappearance of metastases including prognostically unfavourable bone metastases have been reported (JAMES et al., 1965; FARBER and TOCH; SCHWEISGUTH, SUTOW, 1968). Below we report a successful case from our own records:

A 4-month-old boy with multiple skin metastases on admission underwent excision of a left adrenal tumour. At operation, metastases were present in the para-aortic lymphnodes and liver. Tibial marrow puncture showed pathological cell changes. Postoperatively metastases developed in the right testicle and skull (Fig. 2). Treatment with Endoxan 100 mg weekly, alternating with Oncovin 0.5 mg, was continued for 15 months. Skin and bone metastases disappeared in 3 to 4 months. While tibial marrow puncture still showed pathological cells 3.5 months after operation, these had disappeared after the 5th month. Simultaneously the raised VMA level fell to normal. The child is being followed-up and is free from recurrences 2.5 years after operation.

Our own experience with a relatively small number of patients (Table 1) agrees with the known and statistically-based fact that the prognosis of neuroblastoma is much more favourable in infancy than in later life (SUTOW, 1958; GROSS et al.; PRIEBE and CLATWORTHY).

A survival time of 14 months (corresponding to a 5 year period in adults) is prognostically favourable. 90 to 95% of the fatal cases die within a year; 99% in the first 2 post-operative years (GROSS et al.). Among our series of five surviving infants with abdominal tumours, an 8 months old girl with histologically confirmed ganglioneuroblastoma that is, partial maturation of the tumour, which is regarded to carry a more favourable prognosis, is alive 8 years later.

Embryonal mixed tumours of the kidney or malignant embryomas, otherwise called *Birch-Hirschfeld* or *Wilms' tumours*, also occur often in early life. 25% of our patients with Wilms' tumour were infants, including one neonate. In two instances bilateral tumour formation took place at an interval of 5 or 6 months.

As with neuroblastoma, a visible or palpable abdominal mass is usually the first sign of the disease. Haematuria is rarely the main symptom. Pyelography shows displacement or dilatation and elongation of the kidney pelvis and calices, depending on the tumour site.

Every case of Wilms' tumour should be regarded as a surgical emergency. We, therefore, oppose pre-operative radiation. Repeated palpation of the tumour by physicians may increase the danger of metastases and should be avoided (KOOP, 1960).

Table 2. *Age and prognosis*

	Wilms' Tumour		
Age	0—1 year	> 1 year	total
Cases	13	38	51
Alive	7 53%	10 26%	17 33%

Prognosis of Wilms' tumour is also more favourable in infancy than after the first year of life (SUKAROCHANA and KIESEWETTER). This may be connected with the easier recognition of a relatively large abdominal tumour in infants than in an older child and thus it can often be excised before it has penetrated its fibrous capsule (Table 2).

Post-operative radiation of the tumour bed to prevent local recurrences is advisable, although lung metastases are the usual cause of death. Excision of solitary lung metastases may still be successful.

Chemotherapy combined with surgery has also improved the prospects of survival from Wilms' tumour (TAN et al.; PINKEL, SHAW, HOWARD, 1964, 1965; FERNBACH and MARTYN; JAMES et al., 1966; BURGERT and GLIDEWELL). Endoxan and Vincristine are effective and Actinomycin D (Cosmegen), which can even effect dissolution of lung metastases, is particularly valuable. The outlook for infants is again more favourable than for older children, particularly if chemotherapy is begun simultaneously with surgery.

On operating on an 11-month-old child suffering from a left-sided Wilms' tumour of the size of a child's head and a typical left varicocele, the tumour was found to have already invaded the vena cava. Suspicious lung shadows were present in chest radiographs. Two 3-day courses of intravenous Cosmegen 0.5 mg were given and the child is still asymptomatic 2 years after operation.

Compared with Wilms' tumour and neuroblastoma, *other malignant tumours* arising in the pancreas, liver, genitalia, or abdominal wall are less common. Personally we only observed few cases during infancy.

We have seen a 5.5 year old child who underwent operation for removal of a *spindle-cell sarcoma* of the *abdominal wall* at 6 months of age. He was alive 5 years later. 2 infants, 1 with a papillary, mesonephrotic *adenocarcinoma* of the ovary, the other with a *sarcoma* originating in the genital area, died inspite of surgery and radiation. A 7-month-old child suffering from *malignant hepatoma* of the right lobe of the liver (Fig. 3) died 5 months after right lobar resection. Results with these hepatomas are still unsatisfactory, even with the excellent techniques now available for partial hepatectomy (CLATWORTHY et al.; SHORTER et al.; NIXON). We have had better results with *Haemangioma* and *haemangioendothelioma of the liver* (3 cases). These tumours sometimes regress when radiated.

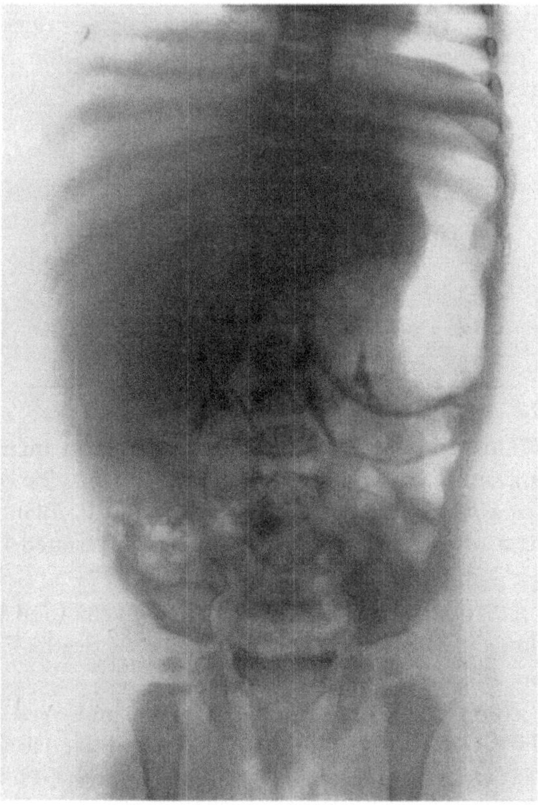

Fig. 3. Malignant hepatoma (7-month-old girl)

Benign cystic abdominal tumours include solitary or multilocular cysts of the kidney, liver, pancreas, and ovary as well as duplications of the gastro-intestinal tract. These tumours usually do not produce clinical symptoms during infancy.

A spherical tumour, detected in the right lower abdominal quadrant of a 5-month-old infant, at operation proved to be a displaced and necrosed left ovarian cyst, which by torsion had become completely detached from the left adnexae and had shifted to the right.

Although cystic duplication of the lower ileum in an 8-month-old patient had caused intestinal intussusception and protruded from anus, successful resection of the cyst and repair were possible.

Retroperitoneal cystic *teratomas* may reach an immense size even in infants (Fig. 4). Fig. 5 shows such a tumour in a 7-month-old girl. Partially filling of the cyst with air showed that the neoplasm extended from pelvis to epigastrium and displaced the descending colon to the right. The tumour was removed through a trans-abdominal incision and was histologically confirmed as cystic neurofibroma originating in the pancreatic region.

Coccygeal teratomas, which are fairly common in neonates, especially females, often spread retroperitoneally into the abdomen. In such cases early resection, preferably by a combined sacral and abdominal procedure, is advisable since the tendency

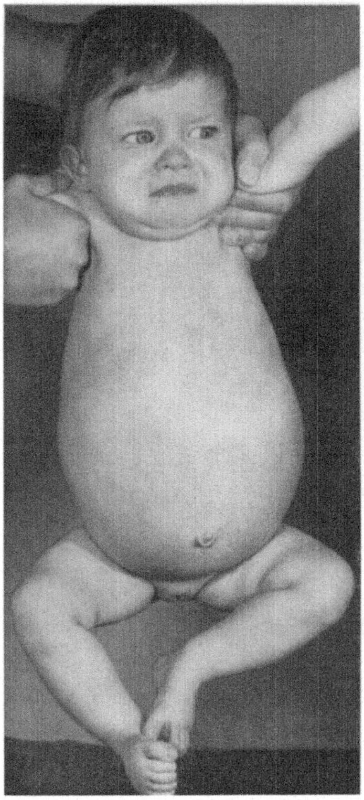

Fig. 4

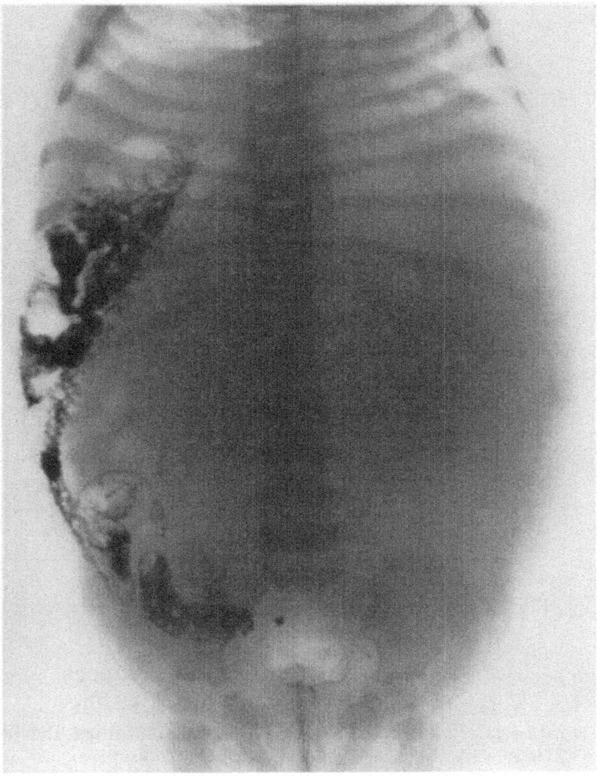

Fig. 5

Fig. 4. Retroperitoneal cystic teratoma (7-month-old girl)

Fig. 5. Right-sided displacement of descending colon. (Same patient as in Fig. 4)

to become malignant increases rapidly after the fourth month with a resultant mortality rate of 40% (Waldhausen et al.).

Rare lymphatic *mesenteric cysts* mostly develop as multilocular, hour-glass, or dumb-bell shaped structures, containing serous, chylous or blood-stained fluid, bilaterally along the small intestine. Of our 10 cases with this tumour 3 were infants.

In one of these infants the symptoms were increasing abdominal distension associated with a soft, moveable mass in the epigastrium. A large omental cyst was found at operation.

In the other two cases, volvulus resulted from extensive cyst formation. In one instance the resulting necrosis of the small intestine was so extensive that only a 26 cm length could be preserved (Fig. 6). The child, however, survived the ensuing malabsorption syndrome although skeletal growth was greatly retarded (80 cm at 3 years of age).

As a clinical curiosity we report the case of a 2-month-old girl with radiological evidence of a partly calcified abdominal tumour. At operation we found a "*Foetus in foetu*" with an umbilical cord connected to the pancreatic vessels.

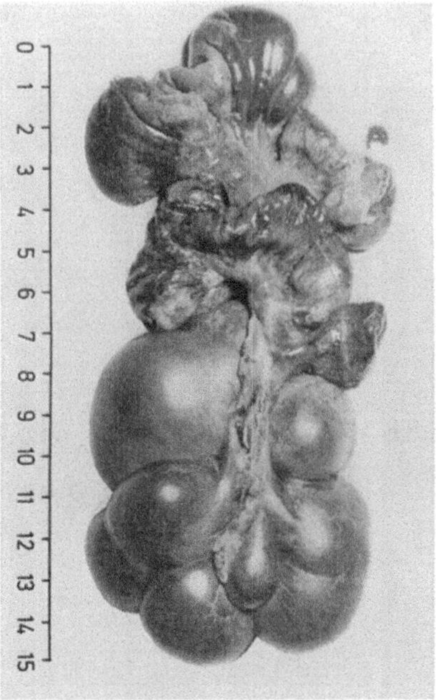

Fig. 6. Mesenteric cyst with volvulus and extensive ileal necrosis (male newborn)

References

BILL, A. H., JR.: J. pediat. Surg. **3**, 103—106 (1968).

BOHUON, C.: Neuroblastomas: biochemical studies. Berlin-Heidelberg-New York: Springer 1966.

BURGERT, E. O., JR., and O. GLIDEWELL: J. Amer. med. Ass. **199**, 464—468 (1967).

CLATWORTHY, H. W., JR., E. TH. BOLES, JR., and W. A. NEWTON: Arch. Dis. Childh. **35**, 22—28 (1960).

CUSHING, H., and S. B. WOLBACH: Amer. J. Path. **3**, 203 (1927).

EVERSON, T. C., and W. H. COLE: Spontaneous regression of cancer. Philadelphia: W. B. Saunders Co. 1966.

FARBER, S., and R. TOCH: Amer. J. Dis. Child. **82**, 239—241 (1951).

FERNBACH, D. J., and D. T. MARTYN: J. Amer. med. Ass. **195**, 1005—1009 (1966).

GROSS, R. E., S. FARBER, and L. W. MARTIN: Pediatrics **23**, 1179—1191 (1959).

HOWARD, R.: Med. J. Aust. **2**, 141—142 (1964).

— Arch. Dis. Childh. **40**, 200—202 (1965).

JAMES, D. H., JR., O. HUSTU, E. L. WRENN, JR., and D. PINKEL: J. Amer. med. Ass. **194**, 123—126 (1965).

— — —, and W. W. JOHNSON: J. Amer. med. Ass. **197**, 1043—1045 (1966).

KOOP, C. E.: Arch. Dis. Childh. **35**, 1—16 (1960).

— J. pediat. Surg. **3**, 103—193 (1968).

—, and J. R. HERNANDEZ: Surgery 56, 726—733 (1964).
NIXON, H. H.: Arch. Dis. Childh. 40, 169—172 (1965).
PINKEL, D.: Pediatrics 23, 342—347 (1959).
PRIEBE, C. J., JR., and H. W. CLATWORTHY: Arch. Surg. 95, 538—545 (1967).
SCHNEIDER, K. M., J. M. BECKER, and I. H. KRASNA: Pediatrics 36, 359—366 (1965).
SCHWEISGUTH, O.: J. pediat. Surg. 3, 183—184 (1968).
SHAW, R. K.: Amer. J. Dis. Child. 99, 628—635 (1960).
SHORTER, R. G., A. J. BAGGENSTOSS, G. B. LOGAN, and G. A. HALLENBECK: Pediatrics 25, 191—203 (1960).
SUKAROCHANA, K., and W. B. KIESEWETTER: J. Pediat. 69, 747—752 (1966).
SUTOW, W. W.: J. Dis. Child. 96, 299—305 (1958).
— J. pediat. Surg. 3, 182—183 (1968).
TAN, C. T. C., M. W. DARGEON, and J. H. BURCHENAL: Pediatrics 24, 544—561 (1959).
WALDHAUSEN, J. A., J. W. KILMAN, F. VELLIOS, and J. S. BATTERSBY: Surgery 54, 933—949 (1963).

Diagnosis and Management of Mediastinal Masses in Children*

J. ALEX HALLER, JR., DAVID O. MAZUR, and WILLIAM W. MORGAN, JR.

Mediastinal masses in children represent a wide variety of conditions and diseases and thus, they present numerous problems in management. Decisions regarding operative and non-operative treatment, including choice of chemotherapy for malignant tumors, continue to be difficult ones. To give some factual, clinical perspective to therapy we have reviewed our experience with mediastinal masses in children at the Johns Hopkins Hospital. The purpose of this paper is to report this clinical experience and to outline our current management of mass lesions of the mediastinum in children.

Clinical Material

Hospital records were reviewed of 80 children who were seen for mediastinal masses in the Johns Hopkins Hospital between July, 1933 and July, 1968. This tabulation of patients includes the cases of mediastinal tumors which were reported by SABISTON and SCOTT in 1952. Patients have been grouped according to ages, infants (0 to 2 years), children (2 to 12 years), and adolescents (12 to 19 years). Using this division, there were 22 masses in infants (28%), 36 in children (44%), and 22 in adolescents (28%). Approximately 70% of the mediastinal masses were neoplasms and of this group 60% were malignant. In other words, 40% of the mediastinal masses in children were malignant tumors. Overall mortality for the series was 33%. Three-fourths of the children who died of tumors had widespread metastases. 65% of children with malignant masses died from them.

Classification of Mediastinal Masses

Masses of the mediastinum in children have a remarkable predeliction for anatomic localization in the mediastinum, roughly according to pathologic types. This segregation is a most helpful feature in the differential diagnosis of mediastinal masses. Several excellent papers have emphasized this tendency for localization of

* From the Division of Pediatric Surgery of the Department of Surgery, The Johns Hopkins Hospital and University School of Medicine, Baltimore, Maryland 21205.

masses within the mediastinum (HOPE et al., 1963; LEYVA, 1962; HEIMBURGER et al., 1963; HEIMBURGER et al., 1965).

For purposes of preliminary diagnosis and management, an arbitrary division of the mediastinum into three compartments has been most useful. These divisions are ourlined on a lateral view of the chest (Fig. 1). They are the *anterior mediastinum*, the *middle mediastinum* and the *posterior mediastinum*.

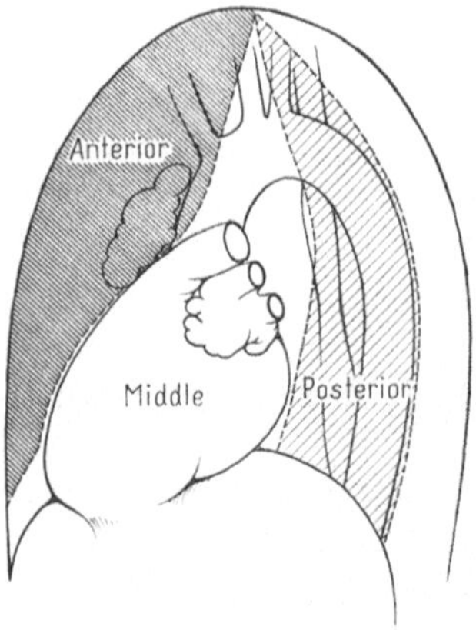

Fig. 1. Division of the mediastinum into three compartments

As emphasized by HOPE and associates (HOPE et al., 1963), it is important to know the normal contents of these three compartments of the mediastinum in any consideration of an abnormal mass in this area. The anterior mediastinum contains the thymus and the anterior portion of pericardium and heart. In addition there are a few anterior mediastinal lymphnodes and a rare substernal extension of the thyroid. The middle mediastinum contains the heart and great vessels, the trachea and the main bulk of mediastinal lymphnodes. The posterior mediastinum contains the esophagus, the thoracic duct, the vagus and splanchnic nerves, and the descending thoracic aorta. As shown in Figs. 2, 3, and 4, mediastinal masses found in our clinical series can be rather precisely fitted into these three compartments.

Our only difficulty with this anatomic classification has been with the proper placement of lymphnode tumors and lymphnode infections because there is naturally some overlap between the anterior and middle mediastinum. However, since the bulk of lymphoid tissue, with the exception of the thymus, lies in the middle mediastinum, we have felt that this compartment is the proper one for these masses.

Anterior Mediastinal Masses

(Fig. 2)

I. Thymic

The commonest mediastinal mass found in infants is an enlarged or hyperplastic thymus. There is a wide range of normal variation in size and shape of the thymus; and in early infancy, it is relatively larger when compared with other structures of the anterior mediastinum. They thymus accounts for typical widening of the upper mediastinum in PA chest films of infants. The most characteristic X-ray feature of thymic enlargement is a "sail shadow" projecting from the right hilum (HOPE et al., 1963). The thymic silhouette may change dramatically with phases of respiration and may actually disappear at times.

There are few if any symptoms related to enlargement of the thymus in spite of older references to thymic compression of the tracheo-bronchial tree. Most recent authors are convinced that a report from the Children's Hospital of Philadelphia in 1963 is correct which said, "There has never been a proven case of tracheal obstruction due to an enlarged thymus gland in this hospital" (HOPE et al., 1963). Primary thymomas within the gland are exceedingly rare in children.

As shown in Table 1, there were 8 thymic masses in our series, only 2 were diagnosed by biopsy or excision. The hyperplastic thymus of infancy will ultimately undergo involutional atrophy. The primary problem in management is in excluding the possibility that a thymic mass might represent some other neoplasm. The recent report by CAFFEY (CAFFEY, 1961) that a brief course of steriod therapy causes rapid decrease in size of the thymus has prompted us to use a therapeutic trial of steriods in

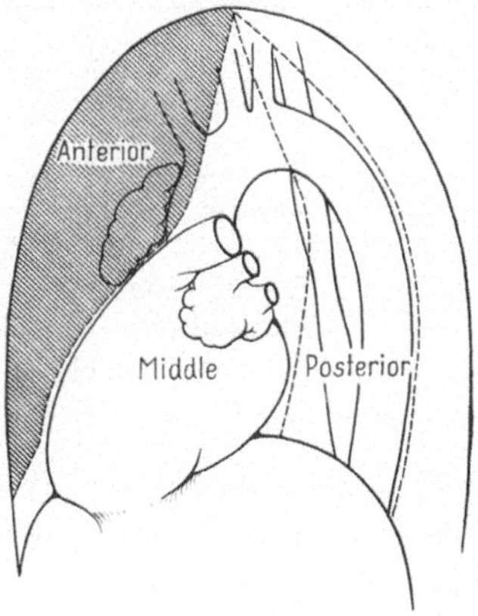

Thymic	8 (10%)
Teratoma	8 (10%)
Lymphohemangioma	4 (5%)
Pericardial cyst	1 (1%)
	21 (26%)

Fig. 2. Anterior mediastinal masses

Table 1. *Thymic*

Type	No. cases	Surgical therapy	Other therapy	Results
Hyperplasia (newborn)	4	None	Steriods[a]	Regression
Hyperplasia 3 months to 5 yers	4	None (2)	None (1) Irradiation (1)	Regression No regression
		Excisions (2)	None (1) Irradiation (1)	Asymptomatic Asymptomatic

[a] See Text

all infants thought to have thymic hyperplasia. The characteristic X-ray features of thymic enlargement have supported this approach. We have used Prednisone or Prednisolone 1.5 mgm/kg/day for 5 days. Irradiation of the superior mediastinal area has been completely abandoned because of the increased incidence of cancer of the thyroid which has followed even low doses of radiation to this area.

II. Teratoma

The second most frequent mass in the anterior mediastinum of children is a teratoma. In an excellent review of dermoid cysts and teratomas of the mediastinum, RUSBY (RUSBY, 1944) pointed out that young infants often present with pressure effects from mediastinal teratoma, but older children and young adults are usually asymptomatic and the teratoma is found on survey chest X-ray. As this is a congenital abnormality, it is not surprising that a large teratoma in the anterior mediastinum in a small infant may produce tracheal or major bronchial compression. HEIMBURGER and associates (HEIMBURGER et al., 1965) reported a similar experience with severe respiratory obstruction in two small infants with teratoid tumors of the anterior mediastinum.

There has been some confusion between the terms dermoid cyst and teratoma, but as pointed out by Hope and associates (Hope et al., 1963) almost all of the teratoid tumors in the anterior mediastinum contain derivatives of all embryonic germ layers and not just the ectodermal derivatives which characterize a dermoid. Accordingly they believe that the terms *benign teratoma* and *malignant teratoma* are preferable for all teratoid tumors of the anterior mediastinum.

Table 2. *Teratoma*

Type	Cases	Surgical therapy	Results
Teratoma	8	Excision (7)	Asymptomatic (6) Expired (1) Autopsy case (1)

Very often a characteristic X-ray finding of calcific areas within the mass is a helpful feature in diagnosis. Otherwise a teratoma may take any form and except for its anterior mediastinal location, it has no definite X-ray characteristics.

In our series (Table 2) all patients were asymptomatic and were treated operatively. Although malignant teratomas are very rare in infancy and childhood, the threat of potential malignant change as well as mechanical problems of a large solid mass in the mediastinum argue strongly for early excision of a teratoma.

III. Lymphohemangioma

Angiomas of the anterior mediastinum are the third commonest mass lesions in this compartment. They may be simple lymphangiomas or hemangiomas but usually there are components of each in this congenital anomaly. Lymphangiomas of the anterior mediastinum commonly represent an extension or component of a larger lymphangioma which originates in the lower part of the neck. Thus it is an extension of a cervical lymphangioma or a substernal cystic hygroma. It is rare for one of these lesions to present as an isolated tumor in the mediastinum. Obviously if it is associated with a neck mass, it poses no difficult differential problem. If the mass is isolated, it cannot be differentiated from other cystic masses in this area.

Table 3. *Lymphohemangioma*

Type	Cases	Surgical therapy	Results
Combined	3	Excision	Asymptomatic
Lymphohemangioma, widespread	1	Partial excision	Expired

In our experience (Table 3) all of the angiomatous masses of the mediastinum were asymptomatic. They were treated operatively. We have not attempted to identify these lesions by angiographic techniques, but as they consist primarily of small vessels and lymphangiomatous tissue, it would probably be difficult to define them using angiographic techniques. It seems logical to leave the substernal component of a proven cervical cystic hygroma alone unless there are symptoms suggestive of compression in the anterior mediastinum.

IV. Pericardial Cysts

Pericardial cysts have rarely been reported in childhood (LEMMON et al., 1965), and there is only one in our series. This is a 2 year old boy who has remained well following surgical excision. As this is a congenital abnormality, it seems likely that such a low frequency of early diagnosis reflects the asymptomatic nature of this lesion which is then detected on chest survey films in later life. The characteristic X-ray feature of pericardial cysts, lying as they do along the right cardio-phrenic angle, usually makes the diagnosis. Proper definitive management is operative excision although a more conservative approach in early infancy is probably wise. Pericardial cysts do not represent pre-malignant lesions and can, therefore, be excised when an infant is older and a little easier to manage.

Middle Mediastinal Masses

(Fig. 3)

Masses in the middle mediastinum are primarily those of lymphnode origin although congenital abnormalities associated with heart and great vessels are properly

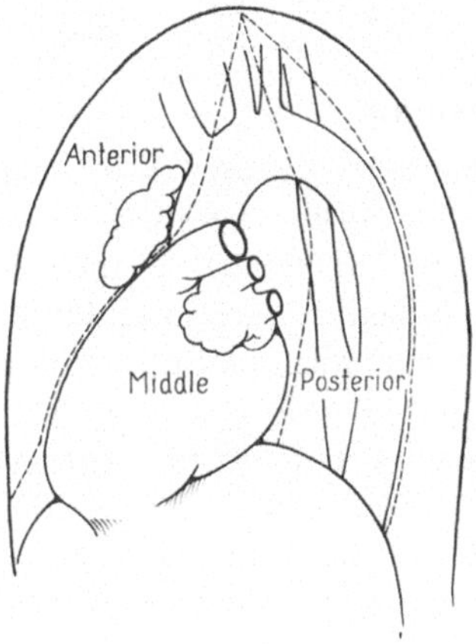

Lymph node neoplasms	9 (11%)
Lymph node infections	9 (11%)
	18 (22%)

Fig. 3. Middle mediastinal masses

included in this compartment. Since cardiovascular lesions rarely represent differential problems in the diagnosis of a mediastinal mass, they are not included in this discussion. The X-ray appearance of lymphnode tumors is variable but characteristically there is a scalloped periphery with vague borders.

I. Lymphnode Neoplasms

Lymphnode tumors include lymphomas, lymphosarcomas, and Hodgkins' disease. The majority of these patients are symptomatic from systemic effects of the malignancy which may present problems in anemia, fatiguability and weakness. A routine chest X-ray then reveals a diffuse middle mediastinal mass. Unless there are peripheral metastatic lesions which can be biopsied, lymphnode tumors are particularly perplexing lesions to diagnose and manage. Without histologic diagnosis no one is willing to embark upon systemic drug therapy in these patients. As seen in

Table 4. *Lymphnode neoplasms*

Type	No. cases	Surgical therapy	Other therapy	Results
Hodgkins	4	Biopsy	See text	Improved (1) Expired (3)
Lymphosarcoma	4	Biopsy (3)	See text	Asymptomatic (1) Expired (1) Unknown (1)
		Excision (1)	See text	Asymptomatic
Letterer-siwe		Biopsy	See text	Expired

Table 4, there were nine patients with lymphnode tumors in our series. All of them were biopsied; most required thoracotomy because there were no metastatic lesions which could be biopsied.

Management of lymphnode neoplasms is based almost exclusively upon the known radio-sensitivity of these lymphoid tumors. Our current plan of management for lymphomas and lymphosarcomas and Hodgkins' disease consists of Cobalt 60 radiation 3,000 to 4,000 r over 4 weeks to the mass combined with drug therapy consisting of Cytoxan 10 mgm/kg/day for 5 days and Vincristine 0.05 mgm/kg/week for 6 weeks. In follow-up of these patients the drug therapy may be repeated on an individual basis.

II. Lymphnode Infection

In this disease category are included all inflammatory diseases of the mediastinal lymphnodes including tuberculosis, sarcoidosis, and histoplasmosis. As noted in Table 5, there were only a few patients in this group. Tuberculosis of the mediastinal lymphnodes without significant pulmonary involvement is rare in childhood. It is the rule, however, to see much more dramatic lymphadenopathy in children than the parenchymal lesion would suggest. The tuberculin skin test is positive, but it may be necessary to use antigens from atypical bacteria to detect this sensitivity.

Histoplasmosis is also rarely seen primarily in mediastinal lymphnodes and is almost always associated with typical lesions within the pulmonary parenchyema. Sarcoidosis of the mediastinal lymphnodes is practically impossible to differentiate from tuberculosis and histoplasmosis or from lymphoma. Characteristically there is much more striking cervical lymphadenopathy associated with mediastinal node enlargement in sarcoidosis. The definitive diagnosis can usually be made from a cervical lymphnode biopsy.

Management of these inflammatory conditions of the mediastinal lymphnodes is based upon clinical and skin test diagnosis of tuberculosis and histoplasmosis and upon biopsy diagnosis for sarcoidosis. The individual inflammatory or infectious lesions are then handled with their appropriate drug regimens.

Table 5. *Lymphnode infection*

Type	No. Cases	Surgical therapy	Results
Histoplasmosis	1	Biopsy	Asymptomatic
Sarcoid	3	Biopsy	Alive
Tuberculosis	5	None	Asymptomatic

Posterior Mediastinal Masses

(Fig. 4)

I. Neurogenic Tumors

Neurogenic tumors are the second most common masses and occur almost exclusively in the posterior mediastinal compartment (HAMILTON et al., 1965). These congenital tumors originate from vertebral sympathetic nerve trunks and intercostal nerves and are not, therefore, within the true mediastinum. The lesions vary greatly in their degree of malignant growth and mitotic activity; accordingly they may present a wide variety of X-ray configurations. Typically a neuroblastoma has an irregular, nebulous periphery in contrast to the smooth, more definite edges of a

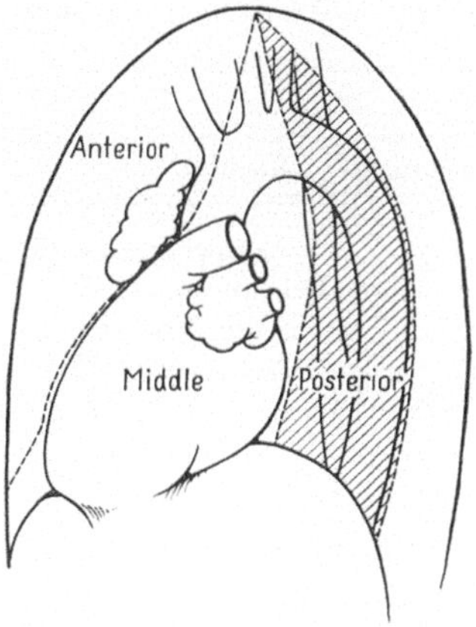

Neurogenic	18 (22%)
Duplication cysts	10 (12%)
Undifferentiated stem cell	13 (16%)
	41 (52%)

Fig. 4. Posterior mediastinal masses

Table 6. *Neurogenic*

Type	No. cases	Surgical therapy	Other therapy	Results
Ganglioneuroma	6	Excision	None	Asymptomatic (5) Surgical death (1)
Neurofibroma	3	Excision	None	Asymptomatic
Neuroblastoma	8	Excision (5)	See text	Asymptomatic (5)
		Biopsy (3)	See text	Expired (3)
Gangliosarcoma	1	Biopsy	See text	Expired

benign ganglioneuroma (HAMILTON et al., 1965). Calcification may be present in malignant and non-malignant lesions; therefore, the presence of calcification is not helpful in a differential diagnosis. Benign neurogenic tumors may become very large before producing any symptoms and indeed neurogenic tumors are usually asymptomatic.

In our series, there were 18 neurogenic tumors half of which were considered histologically malignant (Table 6). In the management of a posterior mediastinal solid mass, it should be considered malignant and operatively removed. If the mass is histologically malignant, appropriate drug therapy can be introduced, as for example, Vincristine, Cytoxan, and Cobalt-60 radiation for neuroblastomas using a similar regiment to that described for malignant lymphnode neoplasms. Because of the high incidence of neuroblastoma in infants with a posterior mediastinal mass, a bone survey and bone marrow studies are an important part of preoperative evaluation.

II. Duplication Cysts

Duplication cysts have been referred to as duplications of the foregut, bronchial cysts, esophageal cysts and enteric cysts. They all constitute embryonic abnormalities which are partial duplications of portions of either the tracheo-bronchial or gastrointestinal systems (OCHSNER et al., 1966). They rarely communicate openly with either the esophagus or the trachea and, therefore, they usually cannot be demonstrated by filling with contrast media. These masses may present with either respiratory or swallowing symptoms due to compression. In such cases distortion of the trachea or esophagus can be demonstrated on either bronchography or esophagography.

Table 7. *Cysts*

Type	No. cases	Surgical therapy	Results
Esophageal duplication	6	Excision (5) Marsupialization (1)	Asymptomatic (5) Expired (1)
Heterotopic lung	2	Excision	Asymptomatic
Bronchogenic	1	Excision	Asymptomatic

Two unusual forms of duplication cysts may create technical difficulties. The first of these is a long extension from the thorax through the diaphragm into the abdominal cavity. This represents a form of thoraco-abdominal enteric or duplication cyst (SHEPHERD, 1965). An upper G. I. series is, therefore, in order in the evaluation of a patient with a suspected duplication anomaly.

The other peculiar form of duplication cyst is associated with the so called split notocord syndrome in which a component of the foregut communicates variably with the neural canal and may actually have a fistulous communication with the skin overlying the vertebral bodies. Duplication cysts of the mediastinum are practically always associated with bony abnormalities of the thoracic spine. This is exclusively true of all split notocord remnants and, therefore, careful X-ray evaluation of the spine is very helpful in a differential diagnosis of this type of mediastinal mass (LE ROUX, 1962; SHEPHERD, 1965).

As seen in Table 7 there were ten duplication cysts in our series and, interestingly enough, all were asymptomatic. The proper management of a duplication cyst is surgical excision. Histologically, these are all benign cysts which are lined either by typical epithelium of the G. I. tract or of the bronchial tree (LUMPKIN, 1966).

III. Undifferentiated Stem Cell Tumors

The least common mass in the posterior mediastinum of children is an undifferentiated stem cell tumor, a highly malignant lesion. They are characteristically rapidly progressive, show undefined borders on X-ray evaluation and are not infrequently associated with peripheral metastases at the time they are first detected. We have included three benign mesenchymal tumors in our group for want of a better classification, but generally these tumors are highly malignant as shown by the ten cases in this group (Table 8). It is rarely possible to excise the malignant lesions completely,

Table 8. *Undifferentiated stem cell tumors*

Type	No. cases	Surgical therapy	Other therapy	Results
Sarcoma	10	Biopsy (5)	See text	Expired (5)
		Excision (2)	See text	Expired (1)
				Asymptomatic (1)
		Unknown (3)	See text	Expired (3)
Lipoma[a]	1	Excision	None	Asymptomatic
Fibroma[a]	1	Excision	None	Asymptomatic
Leiomyoma[a]	1	Excision	None	Asymptomatic

[a] Not malignant

but an operative biopsy will often aid in initiation of irradiation and drug therapy using a regimen similar to the one described for malignant lymphnode tumors.

Conclusions

A 35 year experience with mediastinal masses in infants and children in the Johns Hopkins Hospital reveals thymic masses and teratomas to be the commonest lesions of the anterior mediastinum, lymphnode neoplasms and infection to be the commonest etiology of masses in the middle mediastinum and neurogenic tumors and duplication cysts to constitute the overwhelming majority of posterior mediastinal masses. 40% of all of the mediastinal masses were found to be malignant. Most of the patients were asymptomatic and the mass was detected on routine chest X-ray. The malignant tumors usually produced some systemic and occasionally. Local symptoms due to tumor infiltration. Most of the symptoms in infants were of a respiratory nature. Symptoms in older children were often associated with either bone pain or esophageal compression.

Except in the case of infants with hyperplasia of the thymus, operative intervention was necessary in every case to establish the diagnosis and in most patients, to excise the lesion. Combined post-biopsy irradiation and drug therapy were used for primary lymphnode tumors and for the undifferentiated stem cell tumors of the posterior mediastinum. Neither of these non-operative modalities of management has been particularly effective in decreasing mortality, but they have had significant palliative effect.

References

Caffey, J.: Pediatric X-ray diagnosis, 4th ed. Chicago, Illinois: Yearbook Medical Publishers, Inc. 1961.

Hamilton, J. P., and C. E. Koop: Surg. Gynec. Obstet. **121**, 803—812 (1965).

Heimburger, I., J. S. Battersby, and F. Vellias: Arch. Surg. **86**, 978—984 (1963).

Heimburger, I. L., and J. S. Battersby: J. thorac. cardiovasc. Surg. **50**, 92—103 (1965).

Hope, J. W., P. F. Borns, and C. E. Koop: Radio. Clin. N. Amer. **1**, 17—50 (1963).

Lemmon, W. M., and B. L. Segal: Dis. Chest. **48**, 434—439 (1965).

Le Roux, B. T.: Thorax **17**, 357—362 (1962).

Leyva, F. R., and J. M. Lo Presti: Clin. Proc. Child. Hosp. (Wash.) **18**, 336—343 (1962).

Lumpkin, S. M. M.: Arch. Otolaryng. **84**, 346—348 (1966).

Ochsner, J. L., and S. F. Ochsner: Ann. Surg. **163**, 909—920 (1966).

Rusby, N. L.: J. thorac. Surg. **13**, 169 (1944).

Sabiston, D. C., Jr., and H. W. Scott Jr.: Ann. Surg. **136**, 777 (1952).

Shepherd, M. P.: Thorax **20**, 82—86 (1965).

Plastic and Reconstructive Surgery

Reconstruction Following Facial and Thoracic Burns*

J. B. LYNCH

Burn injuries produce one of the most important and severe forms of trauma. Despite the fact that the majority of these injuries could be prevented, it is estimated that approximately 70,000 patients are hospitalized annually in the United States for the treatment of burns, and burn injuries produce approximately 8,000 deaths annually. The importance of the burn injury lies not only in total numbers, but also because the burn represents such a severe form of trauma. Management of a patient with acute burns requires knowledge of the management of shock with fluid and electrolyte therapy, management of infection, transplantation of tissues, an understanding of metabolic, hematologic, and protein disorders, and a thorough understanding of rehabilitation. The morbidity associated with burn injuries is great because the patients usually require prolonged hospitalization with multiple surgical procedures. After recovery from an acute burn, patients are often faced with months or years of reconstruction to minimize the secondary deformities and disfigurement produced. BLOCKER has presented a comprehensive review of the total impact of a major burn on the patient and his family and analyzed the social, economic, legal, and insurance aspects of burn injuries, in addition to morbidity and mortality.

In the past 20 years there has been an increasing interest in the problem of burn patients, and a number of treatment facilities have been developed specifically for the management of patients with burns. Associated with improved clinical facilities, considerable research effort has been directed toward the basic pathophysiology by a number of qualified investigators around the world, and in recent years national and international meetings devoted to the problem of burns have been held. At the present time many reports in the literature attest the high quality of acute care given to patients in many burn centers. Despite excellent initial care, the subsequent deformities may be quite severe and difficult to correct.

Reconstruction. After deep burns have healed, either spontaneously or with the application of skin grafts, there is a characteristic hypertrophic scarring. This is characterized by thick, elevated, indurated, hypertrophic scar tissue which is usually quite red in color. In the early period spontaneous development of vesicles which rupture leaving a small raw area are characteristic. During this hypertrophic phase, some symptoms in the form of itching, stinging, and mild discomfort are frequently present. These symptoms can be minimized by the regular application of bland lubricating ointments, such as lanolin, although at times the itching may be so severe that specific antipuritic medication may be required. Many patients may also be

* From the Surgery Department, Plastic Surgery Division, University of Texas Medica. Branch, Galveston, Texas.

relieved of itching and discomfort by the periodic injection of triamcinolon directly into the scars at this time. It is important to remember that this hypertrophic scarring is to be anticipated following most burns and does not necessarily represent keloid formation. With the passage of several months, maturation of the scar tissue develops, and regression, softening and improved texture of the scars occurs. The red color fades, and the symptoms of itching and discomfort subside.

In reconstruction it is wise to delay surgical procedures, if possible, until the maturation process of the scars has taken place. This usually requires a minimum of 6 to 12 months, and in most patients spontaneous improvement in the scars continues for an additional year or two and sometimes longer. In certain obvious deformities such as the fingers in children or severe neck contractures which are interfering with development of the mandible, a waiting period of 6 to 12 months may be undesirable, and compromising procedures must be undertaken sooner. Because the thick, indurated, red scar tissue does not lend itself well to technical procedures, the family should be advised that the risk of complications is high, and the result obtained will usually require some further revision in the future. In scar contractures over certain flexion joints, such as the anticubital and popliteal space where the scar is subjected to continual stress and stretch, the maturation process may not take place until the tissue deficiency has been corrected.

Reconstruction of postburn sequelae can be divided into functional deformities and cosmetic disfigurement. In general, we feel that the correction of functional deformities should take precedence over elective cosmetic procedures. Obviously, reconstructive procedures must be individualized for each patient; for example some ladies would prefer correction of a loss of the eyebrow prior to repair of a minor contracture of the elbow. Functional deformities resulting from burns of the face and thorax include: 1) contracture of the neck; 2) circumferential scarring around the mouth with a resulting pursestring effect, with or without severe ectropion of the lips; 3) ectropion of the eyelids; 4) stenosis of the external auditory canal and nares; 5) contracture of the axilla; 6) and scar limitation of the chest wall which prevents the development of breasts in young girls. Cosmetic deformities include: 1) irregular scarring with uneven pigmentation over the broad surfaces of the forehead, cheek, chin, neck, and chest; 2) loss of eyebrows and eyelids; 3) loss of portions of the external ear; 4) loss of portions of the nose; 5) loss of the hair and scalp which destroys the hairline and may produce irregular, unsightly bald areas; 6) deformities of the breast and loss of the nipple. It must be remembered that when these defects are corrected in children subsequent growth may result in secondary deformities requiring additional operations at a later date. For this reason cosmetic reconstruction in children is usually limited to obvious severe defects with delay of many definitive resurfacing procedures and scar revisions until growth is more complete. Many of the above deformities may coexist in a given patient. Following severe burns of the face and thorax, it is not uncommon for a contracture to result in a pull on the lips, cheek, neck, and eyelids to produce a continuous deformity from the forehead to the sternum. Nevertheless, many of these anatomic areas are fairly separate and lend themselves to individual reconstructive efforts.

Contractures of the Neck. The loose, elastic tissue of the neck is particularly prone to develop contractures following extensive burns. The deformity may vary from limited vertical bands which can be corrected by z-plasty to more extensive involvement of localized areas of the neck which can be corrected by local rotational flaps. In many cases the extensive involvement of the anterior surface of the neck, often including the earlobes and lower lip, can only be alleviated by correcting the soft tissue deficiency. Although pedicle flaps from a distance have been advocated from time to time, the ultimate result is usually unsatisfactory. The subcutaneous fat does not allow good attachment of the flap to the underlying tissue, and the flap tends to become loose and sag as time goes by with a very undesirable appearance. Our preference for neck reconstruction is wide release of the scar tissue which often extends from the level of the ear on one side to the level of the ear on the opposite side. The lateral ends of the incision are designed to include "W's" or triangular areas to avoid straight line closure. Thick split-thickness skin grafts are utilized for coverage of the defect, and triangular interdigitations are usually used along the

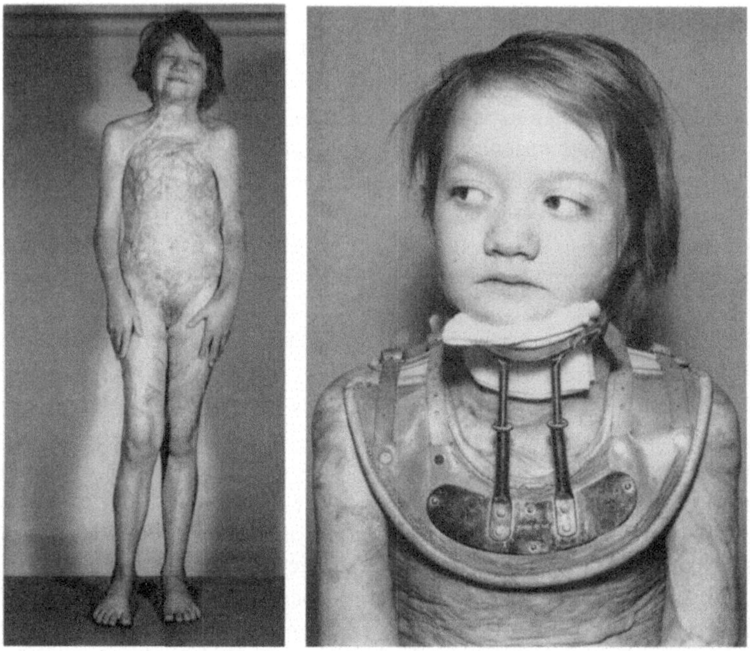

a b

Fig. 1. a Neck and axillary contractures following extensive burns. b The use of a neck splint following release and graft of the neck minimizes recurrence of the deformity

medial limbs as well as at the ends. The notorious tendency for recurrence of contractures of the neck is well known, and we have used neck splints as advocated by CRONIN continuously for the first few weeks after operation and as a night splint for several months. By this technique recurrent contractures can be minimized, and secondary corrections required are usually more limited in scope (Fig. 1). The most frequent technical deficiency we have observed is an inadequate release with a resulting skin graft that is too small and often located on a limited area of the anterior neck which is invariably followed by secondary deformities.

Mouth. Contractures about the mouth may present as ectropion of the lips or bands around the commissure and nasolabial angle which compromise the oral aperture. Some contracture from second degree burns which heal spontaneously without grafts can result in tightness when the mouth is fully opened. Minor deformities can often be eliminated by the use of multiple z-plasties. In more severe deformities from third degree burns where the entire circumference of the mouth may be compromised, release at the commissure and along the upper or lower lip may be required with the application of thick split-thickness skin grafts. It is usually desirable to replace the upper lip as a complete unit from one nasolabial fold to the other with interdigitations into the floor of the nostril to prevent straight line closures. The cosmetic result will often be better if the entire lower lip and chin are also resurfaced as one unit.

Eyelids. Contractures of the eyelid resulting from full-thickness burns may involve only the upper or lower lids or at times may involve all the tissue of the eyelid, adjacent cheek, and forehead and well. In severe contractures with ectropion, corneal

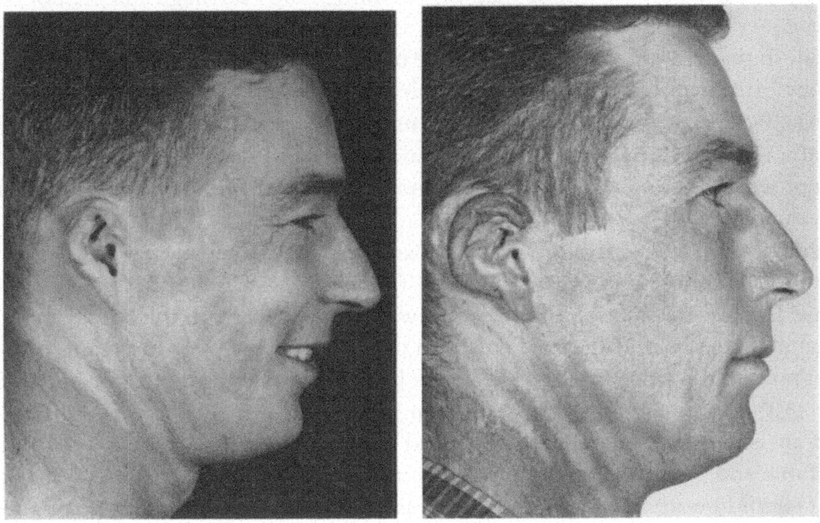

a b

Fig. 2. a Loss of a major portion of cartilage and soft tissue. b Appearance following transfer of a cervical tube and silastic implant

drying and ulceration is a possibility, and early correction of eyelid ectropion is indicated. In localized, vertical contractures z-plasty may often be adequate for correction, though in more extensive contractures excision of scar tissue and application of skin grafts is necessary. When the deformity is severe involving both upper and lower lids, it is desirable to correct the lower lids at one operative procedure and the upper lids at a separate time. This allows maximum overcorrection of the lid being treated and application of as large a skin graft as possible. It must be remembered in treating contractures of lid that the relaxing incision must extend from beyond the lateral canthal area to beyond the medial canthal area. A thick split-thickness skin graft is most often utilized, although from time to time full thickness grafts or adjacent flaps from the opposite eyelid may be utilized. When the burn involves the medial portion of the eyelid, the tear duct may be destroyed, and in these cases reconstruction of the lid should be completed prior to attempting a dacryocystorhinostomy.

Ears. Although not commonly seen, cicatricial stenosis of the external auditory canal can result from burns. When present this should be corrected early since the ear canal is inaccessible for cleaning, and accumulation of moisture and secretion often results in external otitis. The scarring is usually limited to the surface and enlarging the opening to the canal with the use of a skin graft or interdigitating local flaps usually suffice. Partial or complete loss of the external ear with distortion of the remaining fragments is common complication of burns. When the loss is limited to a portion of the helix and conchal cartilage, reconstructing utilizing retroauricular flap followed by implants of autogenous cartilage or inert material such as silastic results in significant improvement. If the scarring locally is so extensive that retroauricular flaps are not available, the use of cervical tubes for transfer of additional soft tissue is frequently utilized (Fig. 2). In complete loss of the external ear, surgical reconstruction requires multiple stages and because the tissue is of poor quality the final result obtained is never perfect. The silastic implants as a supportive material for the ear provide a better contour than carved autogenous cartilage and are not subject to subsequent resorption and distortion. Because of the poor soft tissue covering available in many of these patients, the rate of complication is high in silastic implants, and they often will become exposed requiring removal even after a period of many months. Because surgical reconstruction usually leaves something to be desired, in general a reconstructed postburn ear should be kept somewhat smaller than normal and kept set in close to the head in order not to attract the observers undue attention to the ear.

Eyebrows and Eyelids. The loss of an eyebrow, either partial or complete, is common following extensive burns. Less frequently, the lashes themselves may be destroyed. In reconstruction of the eyebrow, the use of free full thickness grafts from the occipital area behind the ear have been used extensively over the years. Although a good take of the skin usually results, the hair growth is unpredictable and at times sparse. Although many patients have been satisfactorily treated by this method, the use of an island flap of scalp tissue based on the temporal artery is usually more predictable and results in more uniform hair growth in the majority of patients. The patient should be advised that the hair tends to become long and unruly and must be kept clipped to the desired length. Many times in elderly female patients or poor risk surgical patients, the loss of a portion of the eyebrow can be more easily and satisfactorily replaced by the use of cosmetic pencils or false eyebrows. Loss of eyelashes can also be corrected by transplantation of full thickness hairbearing grafts. Because these transplants are so narrow, tilting of the lashes is difficult to control and in the majority of patients we believe that reconstruction of the eyelashes is not required.

Resurfacing of the Face and Scalp. Many patients are encountered following extensive burns with broad areas of irregular scarring over the face, forehead, or scalp. Spotty, irregular pigmentation is commonly encountered, particularly in the darker skinned individuals. Although dermabrasion has been recommended from time to time for smoothing of these irregular scars, our experience has convinced us that the benefit to be derived is so limited and the pigment changes so unpredictable that this procedure has little value in correction of postburn scars about the face. If the scarred area is fairly well localized, it is often possible to perform a serial excision of the scar in an attempt to obtain a thin linear scar which may be broken up with z-plasties. In larger scars where direct excision is not feasible, replacement with rotational flaps may be possible. In the majority of patients with extensive facial scarring, the replacement of the irregular scar tissue with a thick split-thickness skin graft is the procedure of choice. The result obtained is usually a great improvement, although some imperfection in color match may remain. Some secondary irregulari-

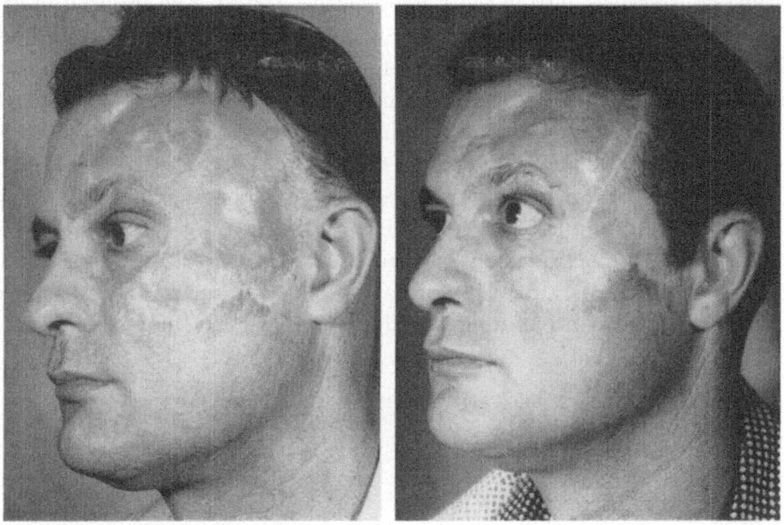

a b

Fig. 3. a Loss of hairbearing scalp from deep facial burns. b Appearance following rotation scalp flap to re-create the hairline anteriorly

ties often develop at the junction of skin grafts to normal skin, but these are amenable to secondary revision with incorporation of z-plasty in the majority of patients.

Extensive loss of the hairbearing portion of the scalp results in unsightly, irregular bald spots. If the loss is complete, the use of a toupee is the only practical answer. When smaller bald areas are at the border of the normal hairline anteriorly, attempts are usually made to rotate scalp flaps for the re-creation of an anterior hairline (Fig. 3). If the anterior hairline can be re-created, most patients do a remarkably good job of camouflaging residual skin grafts over the scalp with this available hair.

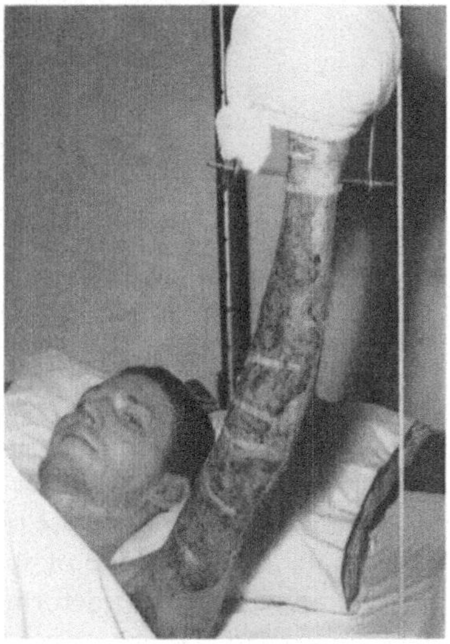

Fig. 4. The use of skeletal traction to maintain joints at full extension facilitates the open method of skin grafting and minimizes subsequent deformity

Axillary Contractures. Burns involving the lateral aspect of the chest, axillary area and inner surface of the arm are quite common from clothes burning. The resulting axillary contractures may be limited linear bands or webs which respond well to z-plasty or local rotation flaps. In more extensive involvement of the axilla in two dimensions, adequate release with correction of the tissue deficit with thick split-thickness skin grafts will be required. In order to be fully effective, the release must extend more than 50% of the circumference of the shoulder with triangular interdigitations at the ends and along the limbs of the relaxing incision to minimize straight line contractures during the postoperative period. The application of splints for several months postoperatively is very helpful in minimizing the development of secondary abnormalities. In fact, the use of skeletal traction for maximum expansion of flexion areas during the pregrafting phase of the acute burn is being extensively utilized on our service in an attempt to minimize contractures of the axilla and other flexion joints (Fig. 4). The use of skeletal traction for forced extension is very effective in minimizing the contractures, although it does not prevent them completely. The difficulty with complete prevention is that following a burn a period of 3 or 4 weeks of progressive debridement is required to obtain a surface that is suitable for skin grafting. During this time the normal physiological attempt at wound closure results in considerable contracture in the size of the original wound. In addition, the

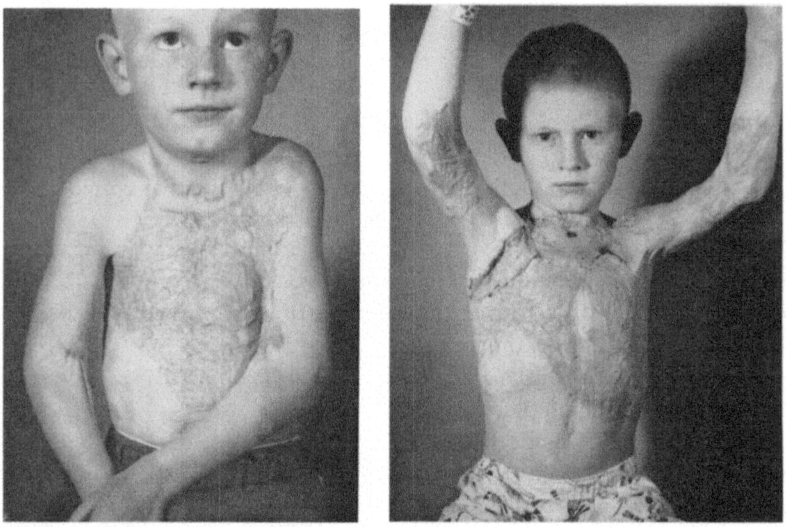

a b

Fig. 5. a Chest and bilateral axillary contracture. b Appearance immediately following simultaneous axillary and upper thoracic release with skin graft

application of skin grafts to the burn wound effects healing, but the skin grafts themselves have an inherent tendency for shrinkage and contracture during the healing phase. These two factors make the complete prevention of subsequent deformities unlikely; but by the combined use of skeletal traction for forced extension during the pregrafting phase and the use of splinting during the postoperative phase, one can minimize the severity of the deformity that results.

Thorax and Breasts. The contracture forces that produce flexion deformities of the neck and axilla can produce similar deformities on the thorax. Many patients are seen after circumferential burn wounds of the thorax who require multiple z-plasties to eliminate linear scar contraction. In some patients the contracture can extend from one axilla across the anterior chest and into the opposite axilla. We will occasionally utilize a single release extending from one axilla across the upper sternum and through the other axilla to correct the tissue deficiency present in two planes (Fig. 5).

It must be remembered that when third degree burns of the upper chest are sustained in female children that the breast bud may be destroyed and will subsequently not develop. More often, however, the third degree burn wounds will result in loss of skin and nipple and at the age of puberty when breast development begins, the constricting effect of the overlying scar must be released. The use of a contracture release in the inframammary fold with application of thick split-thickness skin grafts will provide adequate relaxation for subsequent breast development. The absence of the nipple can be camouflaged with the use of free labium minora grafts which cosmetically simulate the nipple well (Fig. 6). The patient should be advised, however, as she becomes older that nursing during the childbearing period will not be practical.

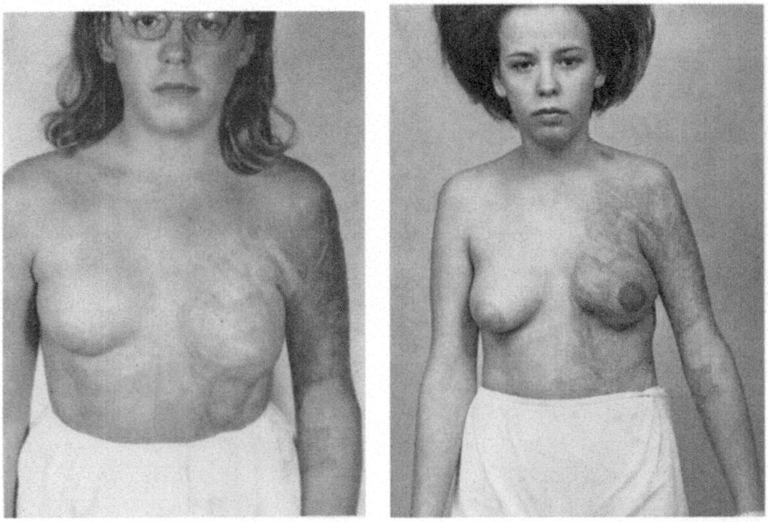

a b

Fig. 6. a Loss of nipple and distortion of breast from old burn scars. b Appearance following revision of breast and graft from labia to simulate the nipple

References

BLOCKER, T. G., JR.: Bull. Amer. Coll. Surg. **50**, 141—145 (1965).
CRONIN, T.: Plast. reconstr. Surg. **27**, 7—18 (1961).

Surgery Following Facial and Thoracic Burns

EDUARD SCHMID

In patients with extensive burns all attention must initially be directed at the treatment of burn shock as well as at prevention of infection. When the patient has recovered to the extent that he can tolerate surgery and the necrotic tissue is beginning to delineate, we start with its debridement. It depends on the extent and the severity of the burn and the general condition of the patient whether we decide on preliminary reconstruction or whether we immediately decide on a final reconstructive procedure. However, in every case it is of importance whether and to what extent the face, neck and fingers are affected as well as where and to what extent and in what quality we can obtain autologous transplants.

With extensive burns it is possible that initially any autologous graft removal is contraindicated. In such cases we use, in steps, the heterologous skin of various donors, mainly from the mother and from relatives. Stored skin and synthetic skin replacement must also be taken into consideration at the present time. To the extent to which the condition of the patient permits it, we attempt, in patients with most severe burns, to achieve provisional skin healing by introduction of smallest, thin autologous islets of skin according to THIERSCH which, as is well known, can be removed several times from the same location. In such cases the Meschgraf-dermatome may be of considerable value. During the removal of epithelium we attempt to preserve the areas of the body which are suitable for subsequent removal of full-

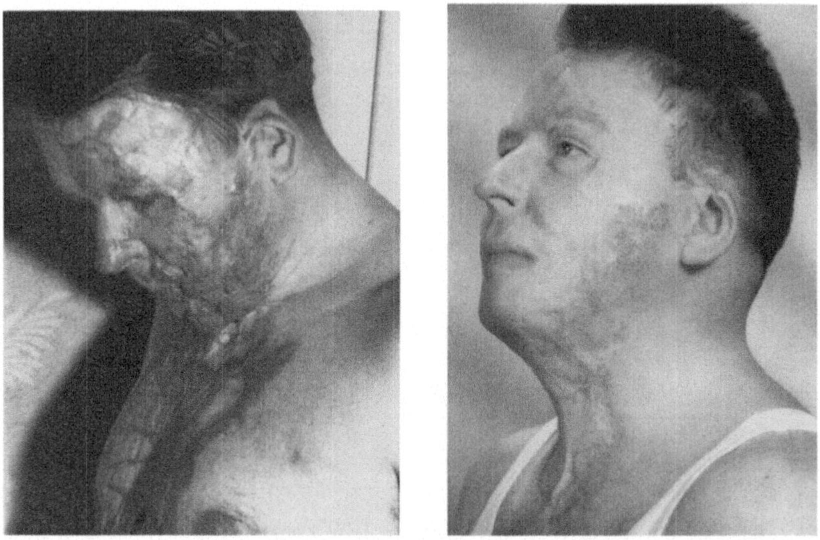

a b

Fig. 1. a A burn case with a definite tendency to pronounced keloid formation. b The result of facial reconstruction and of a freely mobile neck with the aid of full-thickness skin grafts

thickness grafts. From this point of view we prefer to remove thin skin flaps from the lumbosacral region as well as from the areas of the lateral aspects of the thighs. We wish to point out that the surgical plan is also determined by the age and the sex of the patients.

To the extent to which it is possible we cover all cosmetic, functionally important areas of the patient with full-thickness grafts. For this reason we use the dermatome as little as possible in order to preserve the skin which is required for reconstructive purposes, but which is in limited supply from a qualitative and functional point of view.

Infected granulation areas are unsuitable for the application of skin-grafts. They are principally removed. The deeper, well-vascularized wound-bed must be dry before the skin grafts are applied. They are sutured in place without tension, sometimes, however, also under minimal tension. The wound-bed is immobilized and a very careful pressure dressing is applied. If the skin grafts are not tied in and only a careful pressure dressing is applied, they can be checked on the evening of the second or on the morning of the third day and a pressure revision can be carried out in regions of excessive or inadequate compression, i.e., in areas which look blue and pale or dark and blue-livid. If necessary, it is also possible to evacuate hematomas.

Full-thickness skin should not be directly transplanted onto large globular fatty tissue, instead one should rather wait until a granulation surface has formed before the transplant is applied. Frequently keloid scar fields, if they are not too extensive, can be excised or diminished in one operation or in several operations. In this context we found it to be of considerable value to enucleate subepidermally adjacent massive keloids up to the width of a thumb and more. The residual scar tissue cover must not become necrotic (Fig. 1a).

By the way, despite follow-up treatment with Volon A and possible also with Thorium X-lacquer, formation of crayon to pencil-sized hypertrophic suture and margin scars frequently occurs after skin-grafts and revision. After weeks or months they sink into the skin pattern, however, deep down fibrous non-elastic bands remain and these can be very bothersome and restricting. Without fear of recurrences these can be subepithelialy removed through micro-incisions into the scar.

If massive scar contractures have formed between the chin and the chest, a somewhat irregular wound-bed with fresh and hydatidiform fat usually develops after incision and debridement. On such a wound-bed the skin flaps which were removed with the dermatome still take but the cosmetic results are always unfavourable and the patient is faced with a difficult and bothersome period of follow-up treatment which lasts months. We permit such wound surfaces to granulate mildly and then we even transplant full-thickness skin on the neck (Fig. 1b).

Due to the inherent minimal contraction tendency of the skin of the dorsum of the foot and its relative simple nourishment demands as well as its lack of skin and its usually good color appearance, we prefer it at the present time for serious burns of the neck which have a strong tendency to keloid formation. The defects on the dorsum of the foot are in turn covered with another skin-graft.

Conservely the gluteal skin of children is suitable for grafting to the thoracic and arm areas, particularly in girls. With increasing age the character of the gluteal skin changes. It deteriorates from a color and structural point of view. The skin of the abdominal and inguinal areas is usually unsuitable for use in the face and on the thorax.

Particularly careful planning is required for the structure of skin-grafts for total facial skin replacement. For example, in a severely burnt young man we decided to subdivide and use the entire skin of both dorsi for favourable and uniform facial skin replacement. With the aid of patterns of the skin areas the limited supply of skin which was available was optimally distributed (Fig. 2).

In the order of urgency the care of the finger-joints should take first place. The skin from the dorsum of the foot is also particularly well suited for this purpose. Next comes the, possibly even only provisional, reconstruction of lid closure. To the extent to which it is possible the skin of the lid of the opposite side or skin from the region of the ear is used for the replacement of eyelid skin. The skin from the upper arm, from the dorsum of the foot and, in males, the prepuce, are also still acceptable for this purpose. Contracted lids are released from the scar tissues and they are somewhat overstretched by wire mattress sutures which were inserted. Next a full thickness skin-graft which has been cut according to the size of the wound, is sutured

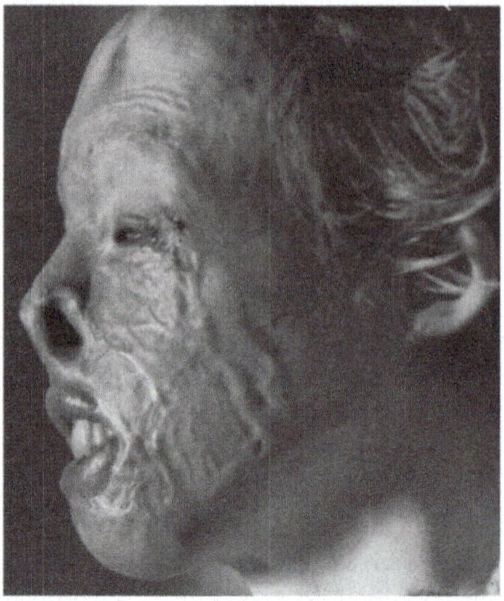

a

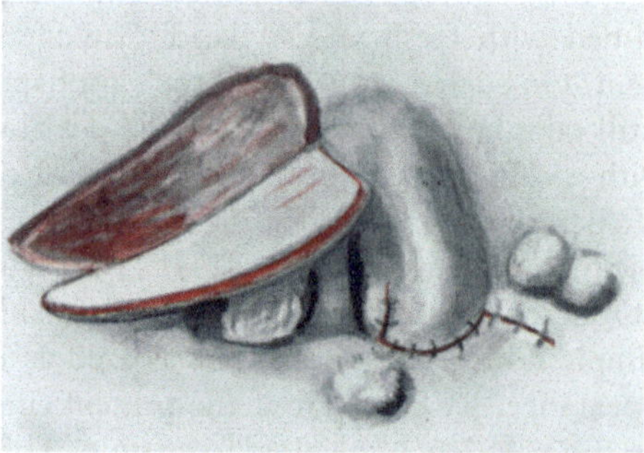

b

Fig. 2. a Condition on admission (the skin of the left upper lip has already been replaced by a graft from the dorsum of the foot). b Schematic drawing of the reconstructive procedure. After the scar tissue on the stump of the nose had been replaced by full-thickness grafts, it was underlined with ear cartilage and subsequently the cartilage and the covering skin were rotated in a doorlike manner by 180° in a caudal direction. The shortened nasal septum was lengthened. The upper lip was reconstructed with a full-thickness skin graft from the dorsum of the foot. c The tension on the lower lip was released by a temporary full-thickness skin graft from the gluteal area. At the present time the red color of the upper and lower lip is being reconstructed with the aid of mucosa from the tongue. Subsequent to this, we are planning to complete the reconstruction of the chin with skin from the dorsum of the foot

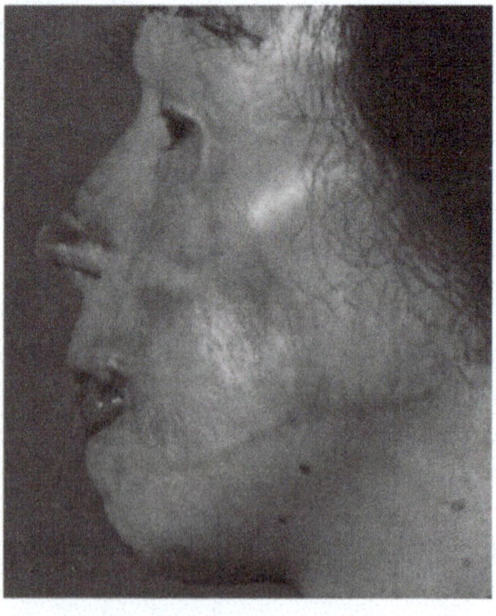

c

on and a light pressure dressing is applied. The transplanted skin with the exception of the available lid skin, as is also the case in the lip region, should overlap the respective commissures in a lateral direction since otherwise bothersome scar tissue band formation may occur. In the lip-cheek area, since we do not tie in the skin-graft as usually, a counterpoint is necessary in order to effect compression. This counterpoint we manufacture from elastic plastic material. Similar to the eyelids, mattress sutures are also inserted into the lips and these, after excision of all scars, stretch them in the direction of the oral orifice until the skin grafts, which have been selected somewhat larger according to the overstretching, have healed in. If the width of the oral orifice is limited, it is advisable to insert a bite prosthesis and to allow the skin-graft to heal in the open mouth position. The skin of the inferior aspect of the mandible and also still the skin of the chest are suitable skin-grafts.

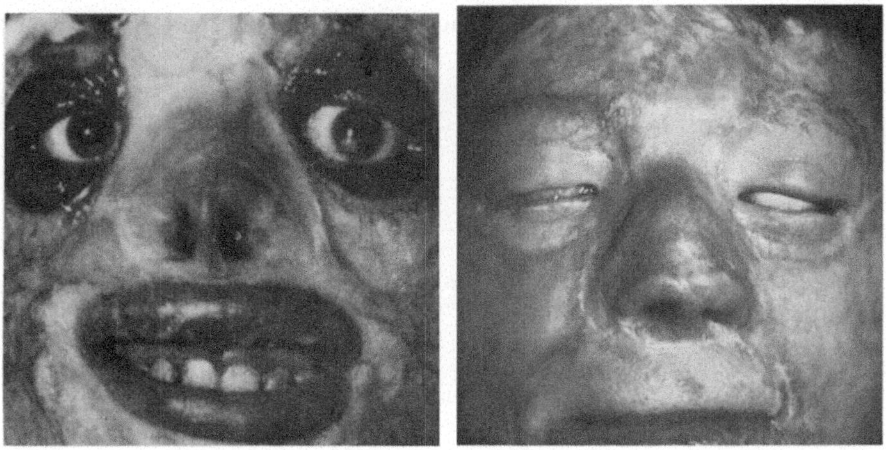

a b

Fig. 3. a This is a picture of a severe burn on admission. b Preliminary result of the reconstruction (replacement of the scarred skin of the forehead and of the left eyebrow are still planned). Reconstruction of the nostrils similar to the method shown in Fig. 2. Lengthening of the nasal septum for which the mucosa of the septum which had previously been underlined with ear cartilage in order to procedure a lengthening of the septum, was used

If, in patients with extensive facial burns the alae nasae are also destroyed, round-pedicle flaps were formally used for reconstruction. Since the end of the war we have adopted the method of cartilage supported nostril pre-formation which was developed by us for total reconstruction of the nose, in an analogous manner, sometimes also in combination with the transplantation of ear particles according to König. If the scar tissue of the nose remnant is unsuitable for plastic purpose, it is previously replaced by full thickness grafts. This, in turn, is underlined with a piece of ear cartilage and, finally, it is rotated with this in a doorlike manner by 180° towards the defect. The residual wound surface is covered with a temporary full thickness graft. In the presence of more favourable conditions one can forego the cartilage graft and an inverted skin flap can be directly covered with a transplant according to König. The bridge of the nose is reconstructed in a similar manner (Fig. 3).

Absent eyebrows are reconstructed by islet flaps or also possibly by a free plasty. In a severely burnt patient, after reconstruction of the other face areas, we were able in 1950 to reconstruct the ear with the aid of an ear scaffold which was shaped from the synchondrosis of two ribs. At that time a pectoral round-pedicle flap was still used for the embedding of the cartilage scaffolding. A photograph which was taken last year shows that the structures have an unchanged good appearance 17 years later. Subsequent to this, only unattached full-thickness skin grafts were used for the replacement of the skin of the ear. With unilateral ear-loss the technique of ear construction has in the meantime been perfected to such an extent that the reconstructioned ear is not only similar to the remaining ear as far as the color of the skin is concerned, but also as far as the structure is concerned.

Late Repair of Facial Injuries

Karl Schuchardt

The method and the extent of secondary operations after facial injuries depend on the primary care: whether it has been carried out at all and — if it had — how far it was successful in preventing functional and esthetical disturbances, respectively in eliminating them.

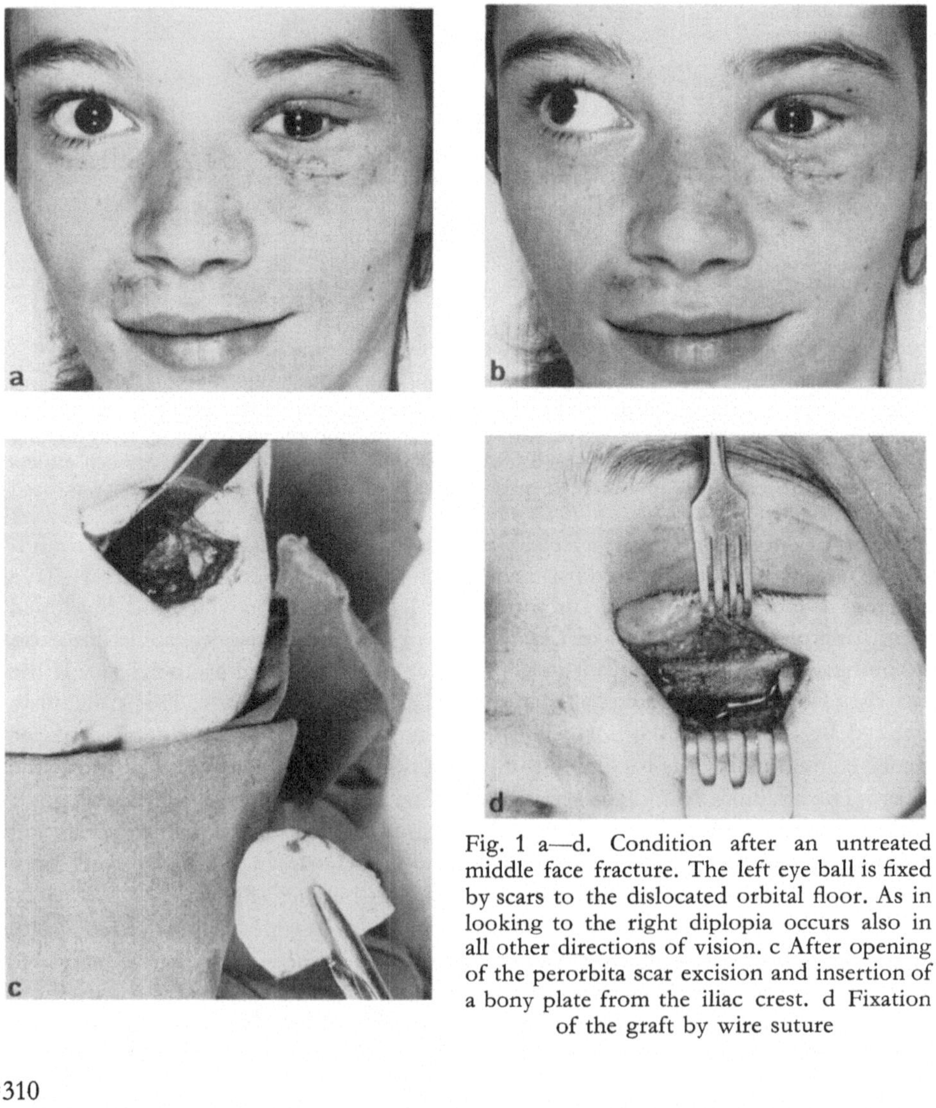

Fig. 1 a—d. Condition after an untreated middle face fracture. The left eye ball is fixed by scars to the dislocated orbital floor. As in looking to the right diplopia occurs also in all other directions of vision. c After opening of the perorbita scar excision and insertion of a bony plate from the iliac crest. d Fixation of the graft by wire suture

In each single case secondary operations will be required for one or more of the following reasons:

1 if, because of the critical general condition, a proper care for the wound was not possible,

2 if, in case of multiple injuries, preference had to be given to those which were of foremost or even vital importance, such as injuries to the chest, the abdomen or the skull,

3 if the primary care of the facial injury was unnecessarily delayed,

4 if not all possibilities of modern accidental care in all fields, especially in the care for facio-maxillary injuries, have been exhausted.

Because of the complicated and differentiated structure of the face and the facial skull a great many possibilities of secondary functional or esthetical disturbances may arise which require correction.

Whoever undertakes this task must have not only a good general surgical training but also special experience in plastic and reconstructive surgery of the face.

The scale of late plastic-surgical measures for the correction of facial injuries comprises anything from smoothing of scar areas by dermabrasion to scar excision, use of the various methods of skin flap plasties, free transplantation of skin, cartilage or bone and also of nerves, to partial or total reconstruction of whole facial parts, such as the lips, the cheek, the jaws, nose, auricle or lids.

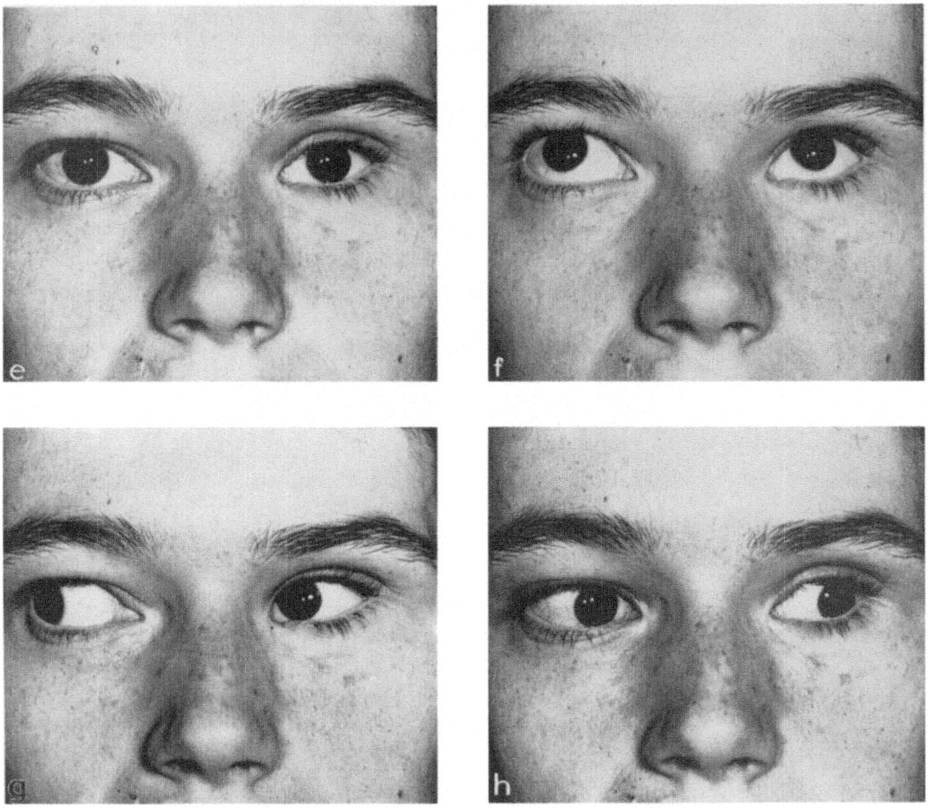

Fig. 1 e—h. Through scar excision and bone grafting free motility of the left eye ball and undisturbed binocular vision was achieved

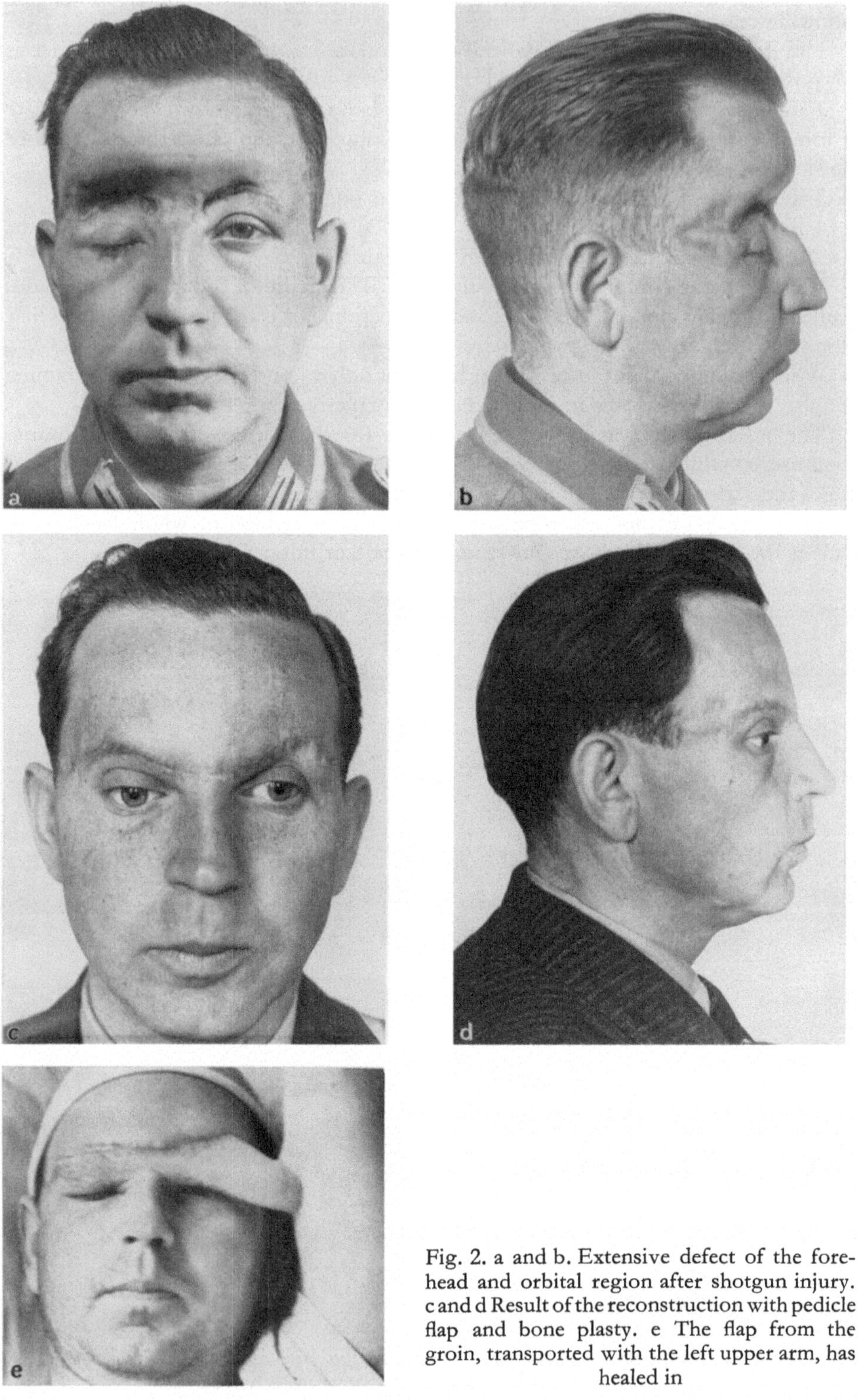

Fig. 2. a and b. Extensive defect of the forehead and orbital region after shotgun injury. c and d Result of the reconstruction with pedicle flap and bone plasty. e The flap from the groin, transported with the left upper arm, has healed in

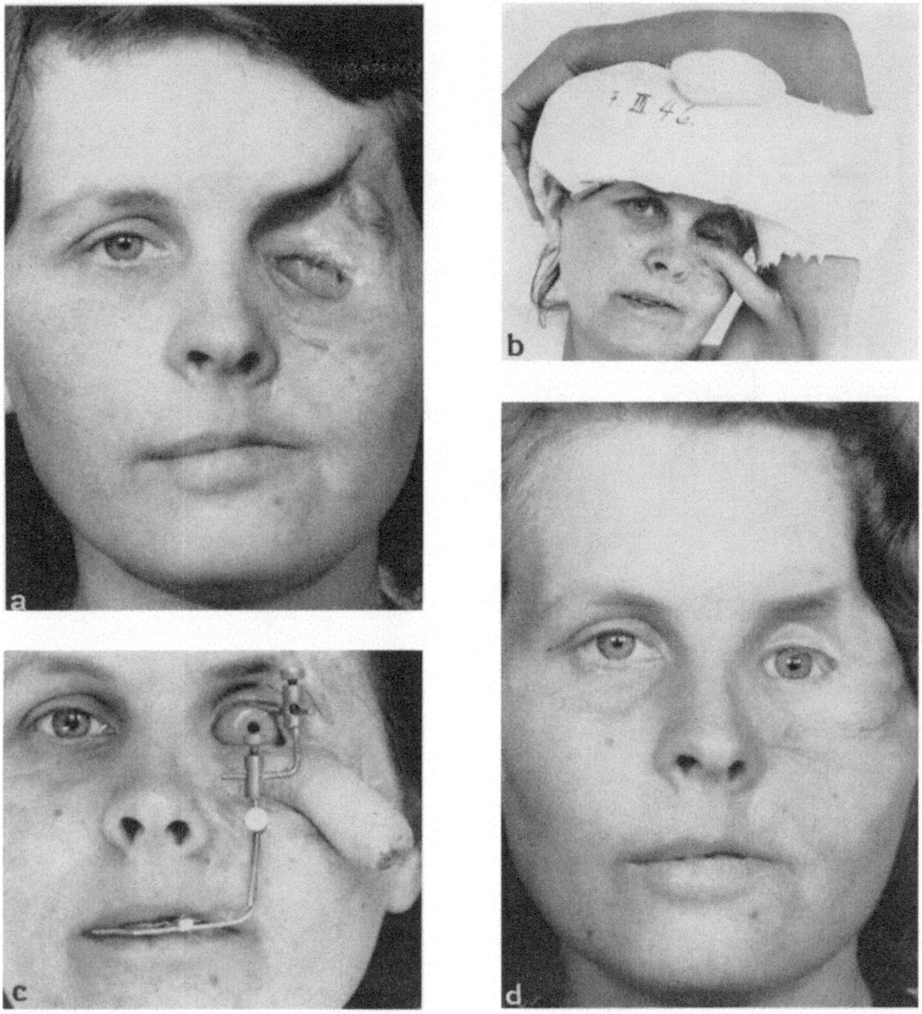

Fig. 3. a Defect of the left eye-socket with loss of the eye ball (shell-splinter injury). b The tubed flap from the arm attached to the infraorbital region. c Shaping of the eye-socket by means of an adjustable acrylic pad fixed to the upper teeth. d Result of the reconstruction

Certain facial injuries are typical and occur — with minor deviations — frequently. I have in mind the middle-face injuries which occur through car accidents. The person who sits next to the driver hits the dashboard with his middle-face, when the car stops abruptly.

These injuries are characterized not only by a conspicuous disturbance of occlusion but by a fracture of the orbital wall, causing the dreaded diplopia through sinking down of the orbital floor. In fresh injuries of this type we reset the orbital floor through the opened maxillary sinus by means of digital pressure and retain it by packing.

If the resetting of the eyeball in this way, or by Freeman's method by means of a Teflon implant, has not been done, the bulb will be fixed in a faulty position through scar formation. Then it will be extremely difficult to free it of its scarry fetters. The

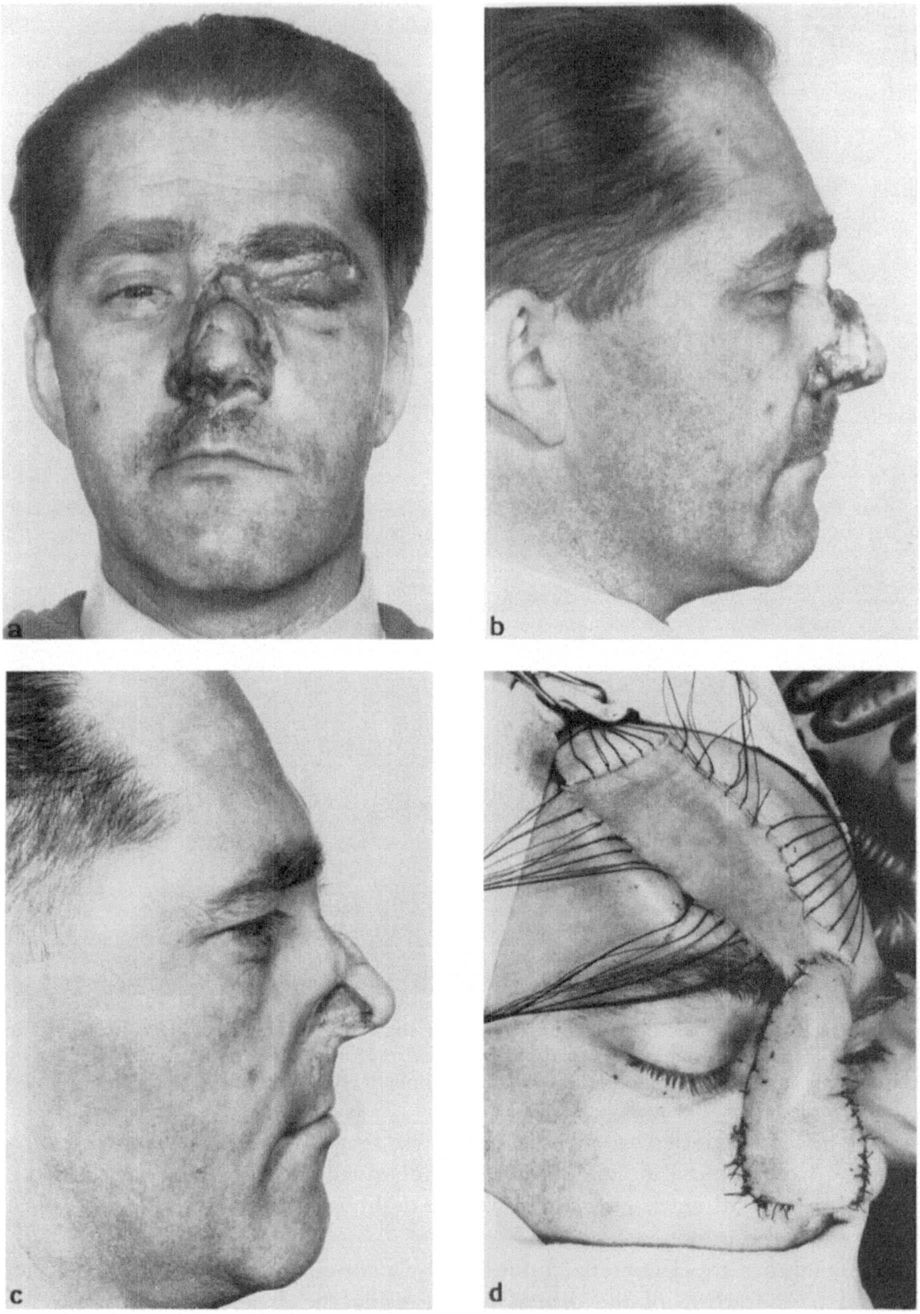

Fig. 4 a—d. High tension current injury of the nose and left upper lid. c Condition 3 months after the injury. d Condition after defect closure by a forehead flap under the end of which a skin-cartilage graft from the auricle was inserted. Secondary defect on the forehead covered with the pedicle and a skin graft

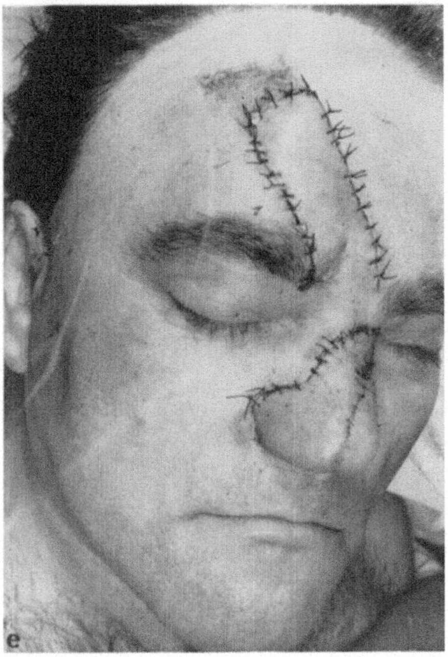

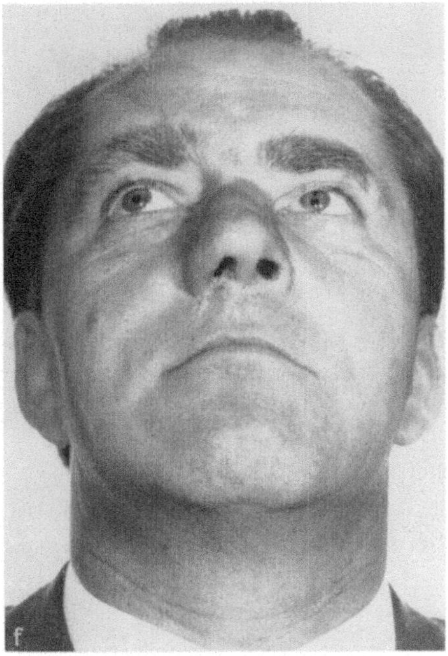

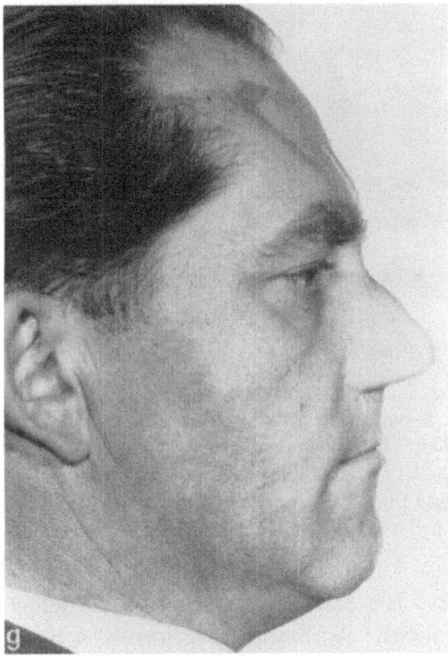

Fig. 4 e—g. e Condition after reposition of the pedicle. f and g Result of the reconstruction

method of choice for the correction of the downward displacement is the implantation of cartilage or bone. This was quite successful in the following case of a middleface injury (Fig. 1).

External wounds are rare in this kind of injury, and, if present, are limited to relatively small cuts.

Extensive wounds with tissue loss occur more often in industrial injuries and are comparable to those known as shotgun and shell splinter injuries during a war.

Primary care for the wound in cases of tissue loss can often not be carried out with final satisfactory success.

More often a correction will be required after an interval of several months. A typical corrective operation is indicated when the anterior wall of the frontal sinus had to be removed in a primary operation after the injury. The correction is relatively easy by implanting a plate of acrylic material, if the skin covering is well preserved. In fronto-basal injuries this simple procedure was often not sufficient.

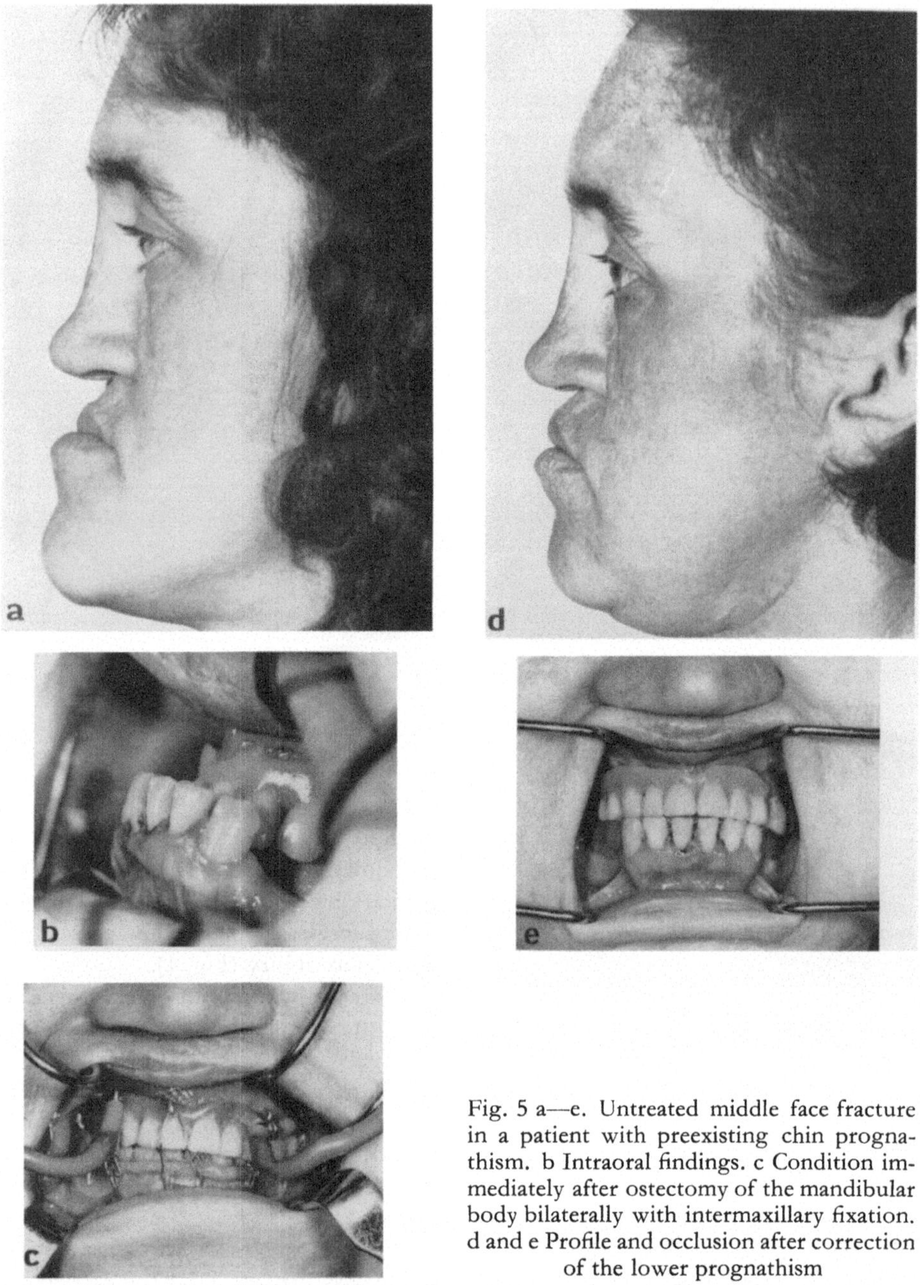

Fig. 5 a—e. Untreated middle face fracture in a patient with preexisting chin prognathism. b Intraoral findings. c Condition immediately after ostectomy of the mandibular body bilaterally with intermaxillary fixation. d and e Profile and occlusion after correction of the lower prognathism

In the case (Fig. 2) of a shotgun injury, for instance, covering the defect of the forehead and the orbit with a flap from the flank and insertion of a bone graft seemed to be the appropriate means to achieve an esthetically satisfactory result.

If an osteotomy and resetting did not have the desired effect in the reconstruction of a deformed orbit, rib-cartilage is especially suitable.

Formerly I always used autogenous cartilage. Since, however, we have gained experience with bank-cartilage at our clinic, I prefer fresh preserved homologenous

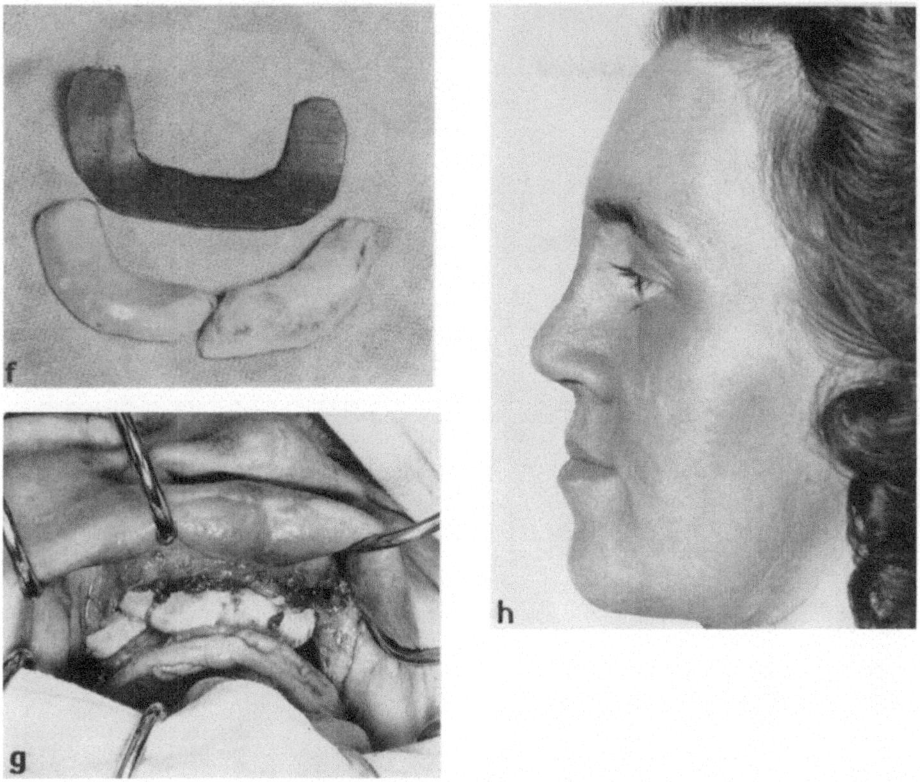

Fig. 5 f—h. f Cartilage grafts formed after lead stencil. g The cartilage grafts for the moulding of the middle face are inserted onto the maxilla. Wound in the oral vestibule not yet closed. h Result of the reconstructive treatment, including the correction of the nose by an L-shaped cartilagenous transplant

cartilage. Certainly, the cartilage is only then sufficient when the skin over the orbital region is intact. If there are extensive defects — as in the orbital injury of the left eye — as shown in the case of this woman, the total reconstruction can be best carried out with a tubed pedicled flap (Fig. 3). Defects of the nose should, if at all possible, be repaired with a flap from the forehead, since this can lead to a satisfactory result within the shortest time. An example for this shows the late repair of the following case (Fig. 4).

The patient had sustained an injury by high tension current and was transferred to us in the condition seen on the two upper pictures. For special reasons the late repair had to be postponed by 3 months. At the end of the planned forehead flap a skin-cartilage graft from the auricle for the internal lining of the nostril was inserted. 4 weeks later the pedicled flap from the forehead was raised and sutured into the nasal defect, and the donor site was covered with a skin graft. After healing of the flap into the nose it was, in part, replaced to the forehead. The result of the nasal reconstruction can be seen on the two lower pictures.

Recently the forehead graft is preferred in the form of the so-called "skalping forehead flap". This method was developed by CONVERSE and has found widespread

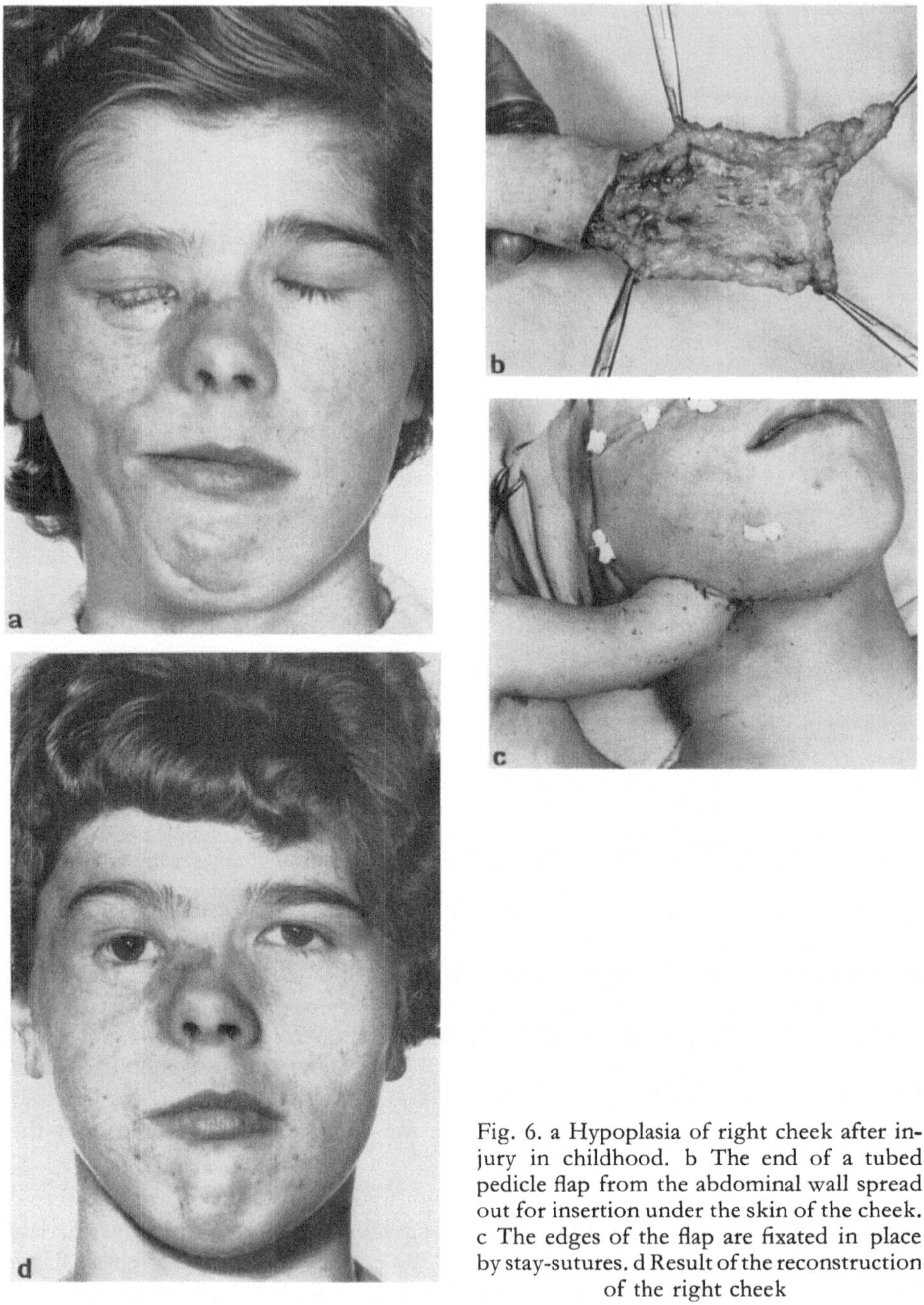

Fig. 6. a Hypoplasia of right cheek after injury in childhood. b The end of a tubed pedicle flap from the abdominal wall spread out for insertion under the skin of the cheek. c The edges of the flap are fixated in place by stay-sutures. d Result of the reconstruction of the right cheek

recognition. There is no method by which a nostril, the tip of the nose and the columella can be replaced at the same time with better result.

In middle-face fractures, which I have mentioned before in connection with the correction of double vision, a backwards displacement of the maxilla may occur and lead to the so-called "dish-face".

In the following I wish to discuss two possibilities to correct this deformity by way of plastic surgery:

The result of a fracture of the middle-face, which so often happens through car-accidents, is the retrusion of the upper jaw. The occlusion in these cases is disturbed in the sense of a so-called pseudo prognatism. A good and also easy way of correcting it is the mobilisation of the maxilla comparable to a Le Fort I fracture. We often employ this procedure even in cases of malocclusion which is the result of an untreated case of Le Fort III fracture of the middle-face.

In the case shown (Fig. 5) a patient with a prognatism of the mandible sustained a fracture of the middle-face. Since an unsatisfactory esthetical result had to be expected by only the retroposition of the mandible, two operations had been performed in order to correct the prognatism together with the correction of the middle-face fracture. At first the mandibular body was shortened by an ostectomy to correct the faulty occlusion. The not very marked dish-face improved after implantation of two L-shaped cartilage grafts which were attached to the maxilla in the region of the naso-labial fold. The nose, too, was — as in the preceding case — corrected by implanting an L-shaped cartilage graft. The functional as well as the esthetical results were satisfactory.

In this patient, demonstrated on Fig. 6, a hypoplasia of the right facial half had developed as result of a childhood trauma. Mandible and zygomatic bone, also muscle and fatty tissues were hypoplastic. The cutaneous covering was merely contracted but not scarred. To round the cheek the fatty tissue of a pedicled flap from the flank was used. This principle, of pedicled flaps of fat — published by me as early as in 1944 — has recently been used in many cases of congenital hypoplasia (Romberg-Syndrome) also in the USA.

In the preceding cases we were dealing with injuries which had caused extensive defects with involvement of skin, muscles, bone or mucous membranes. Such injuries are frequently caused by shotgun or shell splinter lesions. I should like to show you some typical examples from my experience during World War II. They relate to the chin region and the lower lip.

Quite difficult was the repair of a shell-splinter injury involving the lower lip, the chin and the cheek. This patient (Fig. 7) was brought to the military hospital 3 weeks after sustaining the injury. The fragments of the mandible were still attached to the periosteum in the depth but looked necrotic on the surface. Even in such extensive lip and chin defects one can successfully obtain a reconstruction by flaps from the neighborhood.

Under careful conservative treatment granulations over the bony surfaces grew up, and a solid bone span developed. Later a new oral vestibule could be made by skin grafting, and the lower lip was made of two rotation flaps from the neck-cheek area with an additional Abbé-flap from the upper lip. The condition of the patient, about 23 years after the reconstruction is quite satisfactory.

Very extensive defects of the chin with loss of the middle portion of the mandible can best be covered by means of a tubed pedicle flap. Excellently suitable is a flap from the flank which, in my opinion based on a 30 year's experience, is much better transported by the upper arm than by the forearm. After a method which I have tried repeatedly during the war I have used the pedicled flap for the inner lining of the missing lower lip as well as for its skin and the skin of the chin. Herewith it is possible

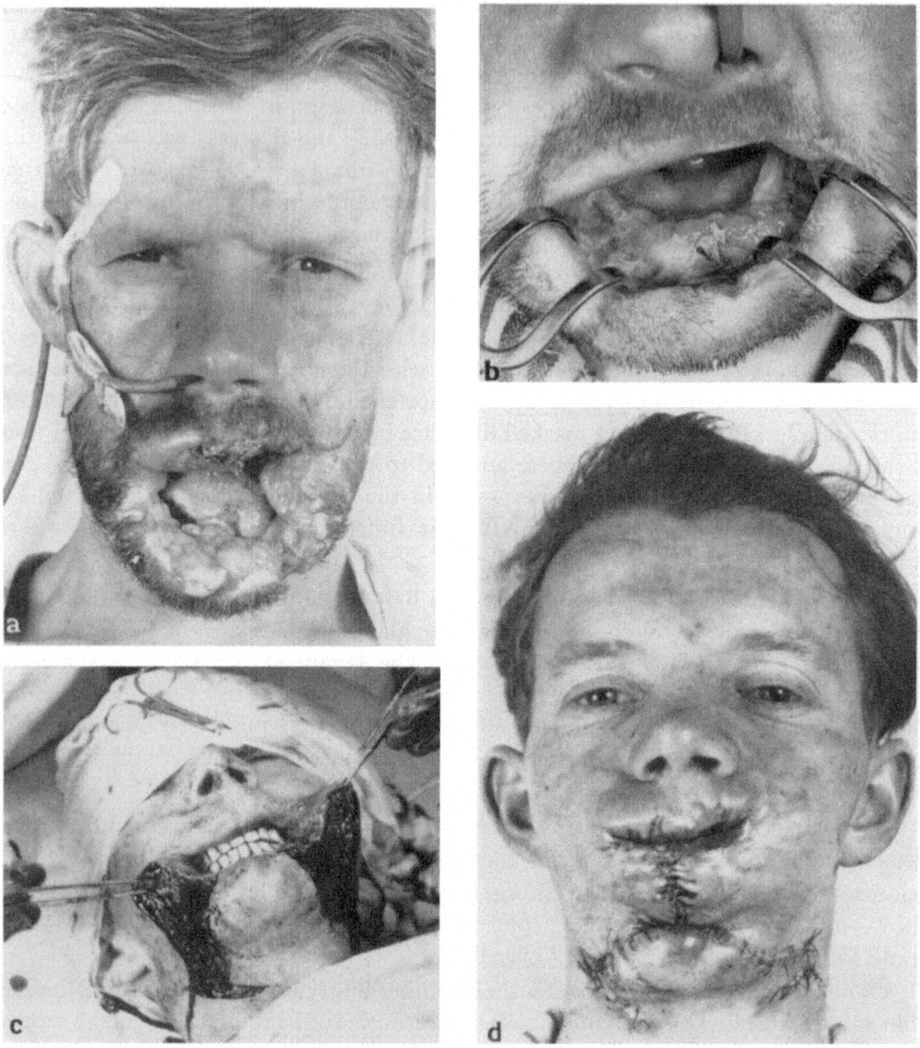

Fig. 7 a—d. a Shell-splinter injury of the chin. The front part of the mandible is comminuted. b After secondary healing and consolidation of the mandibular bone, the vestibulum is reconstructed by free skin graft. c and d Two flaps raised from the cheek and the submandibular region are sutured together above the chin

to form a massive soft tissue bed by which the osteoplasty for the reconstruction of the mandible is favored. The procedure is illustrated in Fig. 8.

Before coming to an end, I want to say a few words about the reconstruction of an injured or missing external ear. As it is well known, this is a difficult task, since the result of much effort and time spent is relatively unsatisfactory. The reconstruction of the helix with a pedicled flap from the neck is rejected by many experienced surgeons as being too complicated and time consuming. However, it cannot be denied that one can obtain quite a natural appearing shape of the auricle with the help of a thin pedicle flap.

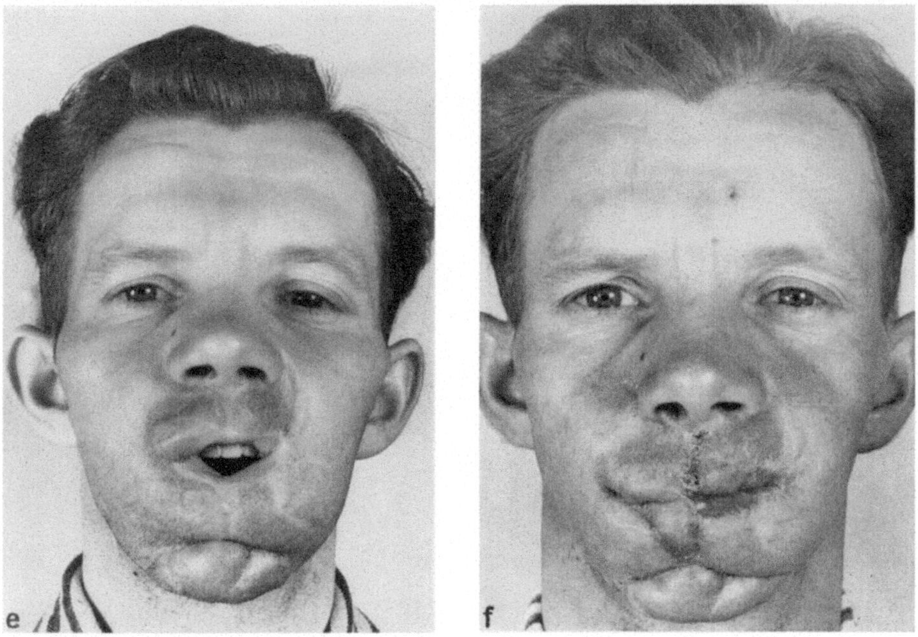

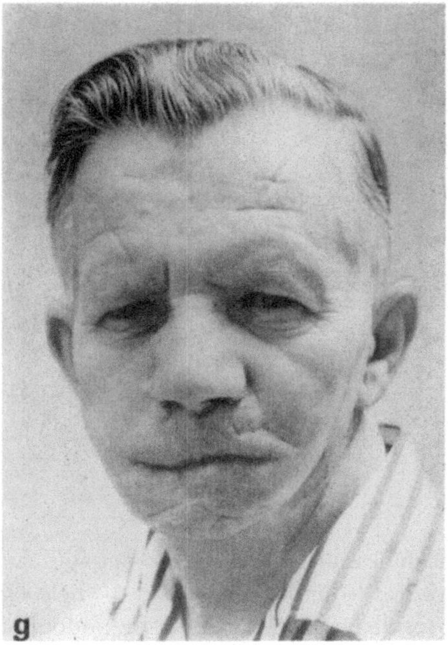

Fig. 7 e—g. e Mouth opening is still unsatisfactory (the aperture is too narrow). f Widening of the oral aperture by Z-plasty and Abbé flap from the upper lip. g Patient 23 years after the completion of treatment

To illustrate this I will show you an example of subtotal replacement of the right auricle after loss through a bycicle accident (Fig. 9). At first a cartilage shell was placed under the skin as substitute for the middle part of the auricle. The transplanted cartilage was detached from the skull, covered with a skin graft, and finally the helix was reconstructed with a pedicled flap from the neck.

The result of this plasty is shown on the lower right illustration.

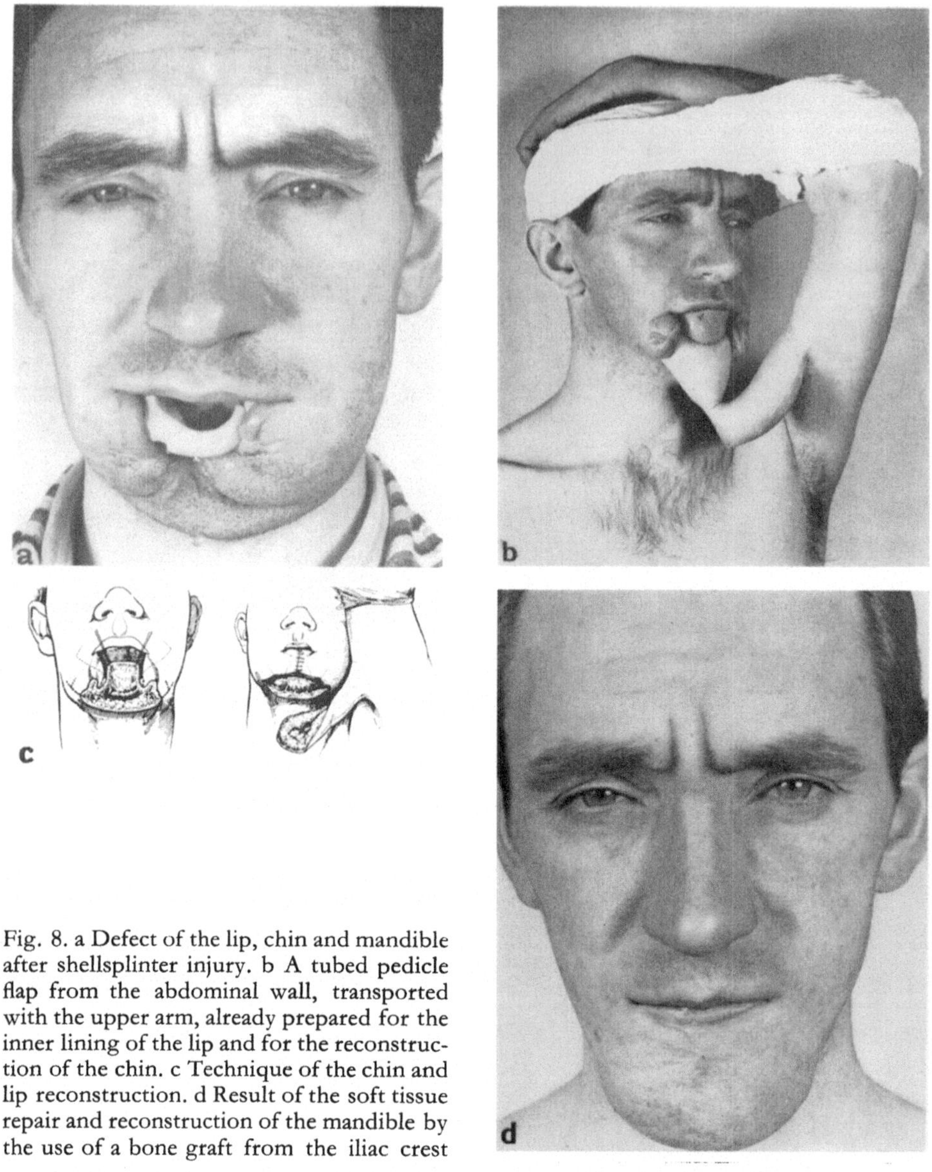

Fig. 8. a Defect of the lip, chin and mandible after shellsplinter injury. b A tubed pedicle flap from the abdominal wall, transported with the upper arm, already prepared for the inner lining of the lip and for the reconstruction of the chin. c Technique of the chin and lip reconstruction. d Result of the soft tissue repair and reconstruction of the mandible by the use of a bone graft from the iliac crest

In cases of total loss of the auricle teflon-frames in the area of the missing ear have recently been inserted. They are later detached from their base with the help of skin transplants to the posterior surface. The results with this method are undoubtedly good.

Another possibility, advocated by RANK, is to provide the patient with an ear prosthesis. For the attachment mastic solution was used, but could — understandibly — not satisfy the patient permanently. But it is easy to form little loops of skin in the surrounding of the ear channel, as RANK recommended. With the help of a long hook on the inner surface of the prosthesis it is fastened to the cutaneous loops by being tucked into them. Modifying the method of Rank I have used the local skin for

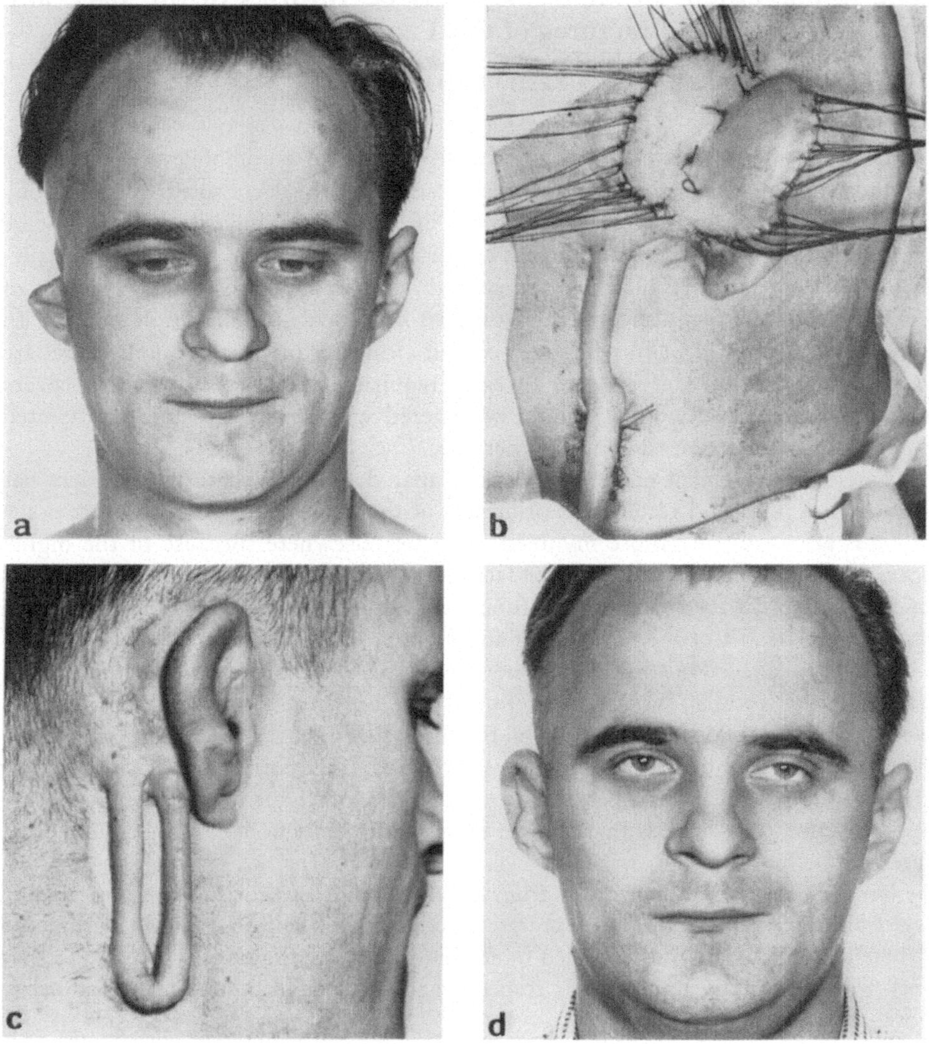

Fig. 9. a Subtotal defect of the right auricle. b A decisive step of the reconstruction: a plate of autogenous cartilage has been placed beneath the postauricular skin, later to be raised and covered by free skin graft. A small tubed pedicle flap from the neck is raised and lengthened in steps. c The tubed pedicle flap for the formation of the helix is always left in a bridge-flap condition. d Result of the subtotal reconstruction of the auricle

the lining of the inner surface and have covered the outer wound surface with a skin graft. In this way the part of the loop that has contact with the synthetic material is better protected and more resistant.

Mister President, Ladies and Gentlemen,

I have made an attempt to give a resumé of certain problems within a short time, of problems connected with the late repair of facial injuries on the basis of experience which I have gathered during the last 30 years as head of a military hospital and later as director of the Nordwestdeutschen Kieferklinik at the University of Hamburg.

The Management of Acute Soft Tissue Injuries of the Face and Fractures of the Facial Bones

Reed O. Dingman

In the United States, 72% of all patients injured in automobile accidents have wounds and injuries of the head and neck. Patients with severe soft tissue and bony injuries of the facial areas often have other life threatening injuries which must be treated first. Some of the more serious associated injuries cause respiratory obstruction, shock, intracranial bleeding and central nervous system damage. A system of priorities must be established in the treatment of patients with multiple injuries. In general, after control of bleeding and careful cleansing of facial wounds, these are never acute surgical emergencies. In cases requiring management of more severe conditions, the facial wounds should be covered with sterile dressings and treated when the patient's general condition permits.

Careful management of the early wound may determine whether the patient has a good or a poor end result. The principles of the management of facial soft tissue wounds are essentially those involved in tissues elsewhere. Because of the highly specialized anatomical features in the facial area, and because of the necessity of obtaining a satisfactory cosmetic and functional result, great attention must be paid to technical details of wound closure and postoperative wound management.

The old adage "Bone first, soft tissue second" pertains in most all cases of management of facial wounds. Whenever fractured bones are associated with extensive facial lacerations, reduction and fixation of fractures through the lacerations should be done when possible before the soft tissues are closed. If the patient is not in satisfactory condition to permit a long operative procedure, the soft tissue wounds can be loosely approximated and held with adhesive strips until reduction of bone fractures is feasible.

To provide the optimal result from the standpoint of function and appearance, facial bone fractures should be accurately reduced and held in position during the course of repair. Care must be used to accurately replace the bone structures so that they will adequately support their respective soft tissues in the region of the orbit, nose, maxilla and mandible.

Careful minimal debridement of facial tissues, cleansing of the wound, approximation in layers with obliteration of dead spaces in the depth of the wound by utilizing fine sutures and needles and accurate approximation of the soft tissues will give adequate results with minimal scarring. Sutures that are too large, left in too long, and tied too tightly invariably result in permanent suture marks along the line of wound healing. The subcuticular suture is the one recommended for approximation of skin margins in the facial area. A minimal number of sutures may be used if the wound is supported with steri-strips or adhesive strips.

The principle of primary wound closure should be observed in management of all facial injuries. If it is not possible to close the wound because of tissue loss, a dressing of a split thickness skin graft or closure by local flap approximation should be done. Early closure will permit healing with a minimal amount of scar tissue contracture and provide an opportunity for a successful secondary operation. Lacerated eyebrows, lid margins and lip structures should be carefully studied to identify normal anatomical structures and to permit approximating them carefully. Lacerations to the major branches of the seventh nerve respond well to identification and suture of the severed portions with fine silk sutures. Lacerations of the parotid duct should be closed primarily over a fine polyethylene catheter passed into the Stenson's duct. Careful attention to these details will prevent a troublesome parotid fistula. Lacerations of the lacrimal system should also be repaired early by means of suturing the severed tissues over small polyethylene catheters or over fine nylon sutures passed through the lumen of the ducts. Tubing used to splint the lacrimal duct system and salivary ducts should remain in place for 1 week to 10 days.

All injured fine anatomical structures whenever possible should be preserved and debridement should be minimal in order to give the best end result. Small segments of the lips, eyelids, ears and nasal structures often will survive with only a minimal attachment. In some, small fragments of tissue, although actually completely severed, may survive as free grafts. Usually these severed tissues will not survive if any part of the tissue is more than 1 cm away from a good blood supply. In most cases of avulsed tissue, it is inadvisable to rely upon survival of the replaced tissue, but to repair the defect with skin grafts or rotated flaps from the immediate area rather than to expect a survival of badly macerated tissues.

Careful wound care from day to day will decrease the incidence of infection. Removal of sutures on the second or third day and support of the wound with adhesive strips will in most cases prevent suture marks along the line of the healed wound. Suture scars may become very distressing and difficult to manage. Sutures tied too tightly, will cut as a result of swelling of the wound margins and even though they appear to be tied loosely, may cause damage resulting in suture scars.

Management of Facial Bone Fractures

Facial bone fractures are significant because of the possibility of extension into the cranium, orbit, the sinuses, the nasal cavities, the external auditory canal and the oral cavity. In the management of fractured facial bones it is our objective to obtain the best possible function, to provide the patient with normal vision, normal airway and normal occlusion for the mastication of food. This presupposes careful replacement of all bone structures and restoration of adequate and satisfactory dental occlusion. To get the best results, this treatment program should be an aggressive one, designed to get the patient rehabilitated and back into society in the shortest possible time with the maximal functional result. It is also the obligation of the physician to restore his patient to the best possible condition from the standpoint of appearance.

The principles of the management of facial fractures are 1) the reduction of the bones to normal position, 2) fixation of the bones during the course of healing, and 3) the prevention and control of infection during the course of repair. The methods of obtaining these objectives are numerous and vary depending upon the background training and ability of the surgeon. Management of facial fractures varies from closed manipulation of fractures with fixation by Barton bandage-type dressings, to open reduction and multiple wiring techniques, and in some cases extracranial appliances for fixation. Generally speaking, the simplest method is the best method. Methods that will permit early ambulation and return to a productive life are advisable. Cumbersome, unstable, unsightly appliances that can easily get out of adjustment should be avoided.

In our clinics we rely heavily upon internal wire fixation and intermaxillary fixation in the management of practically all of our facial bone injuries. Occasionally we resort to extracranial appliances and the various types of splints.

Fractures of the Mandible

Fractures of the mandibular condyle with or without displacement usually are treated by intermaxillary fixation with the teeth in occlusion. Occasionally fractures which extend from the mandibular notch toward the angle of the mandible may be wired if the fragments are large enough to be easily exposed, identified and wired into position. Fractures of the condyle will heal in satisfactory position with good function when treated by simple intermaxillary fixation for a period of about 4 weeks. Fractures of the body of the mandible that will not remain in position by simple intermaxillary fixation are treated by open reduction and direct wiring. Fractures of the edentulous mandible may be treated by use of splints and circumferential wiring or by using the patient's own lower denture as a splint with fixation by circumferential wiring. Intraoral fixation, open reduction and fixation of edentulous fractures is effective.

Maxillary fractures without extensive displacement often can be treated with or without intermaxillary fixation and the use of a Barton type head bandage. We most always use, intermaxillary fixation and cranial suspension from the zygomatico-frontal area for a period of about 4 weeks.

Simple fractures of the zygoma often can be treated by elevation of the zygoma through the Gillies approach, through the temporal fossa or through the mouth by passing an instrument upward behind the zygomatico-maxillary attachment and elevating the bone upward and forward. Because of the possibility of displacement by the heavy masseter muscle attachments, we most often do an open operation with direct wiring of the fragments at the zygomatico-frontal and zygomatico-maxillary suture areas. This approach provides an opportunity for exploration of the floor of the orbit to search for blow-out fractures. Blow-out fractures are managed by replacement of orbital contents and repair of the orbital floor utilizing bone, cartilage or silastic. Zygomatic fractures are frequently associated with fractures of the maxilla and orbital floor and may require packing of the maxillary sinus to hold the orbital floor bone fragments in adequate position for healing.

Nasal bone fractures usually can be reduced by intranasal manipulation with an instrument. Intranasal packing and immobilization with a plaster splint externally for 1 week to 10 days usually results in a satisfactory end result. Attention must be directed to the nasal septum which should be replaced if it is dislocated.

A frequently overlooked and little understood injury is a fracture of the frontal nasal lacrimal ethmoid bone complex. These fractures generally occur as a result of a direct blow to the dorsum of the nose. The nasal structures are driven back and into the interorbital space normally occupied by the ethmoid sinuses. This injury often results in extensive damage to the lacrimal duct system which may be lacerated by small bone fragments or by severing the medial palpebral ligament or detaching it from its position on the lacrimal crest. Often these injuries are associated with cerebral spinal rhinorrhea and with fractures of the anterior cranial fossa. Clinical examination usually demonstrates a wide interpalpebral distance, a blunting of the medial palpebral angle, a narrow palpebral fissure, excess exposure of the sclera below the limbus, and flattening of the nasal dorsum. There is usually severe intranasal obstruction and buckling of the septal quadrilateral cartilage. Failure to recognize and treat these injuries results in interference with function of the lacrimal duct system, the passage of air through the nose, frequently result in diplopia and in severe cosmetic disability. The early treatment consists of open operation through a transverse incision at the root of the nose. This is connected with vertical incisions which run on the lateral aspect of the nose. Through this incision the naso-frontal area can be opened and exposed. This will permit inspection of the medial orbital walls and replacement of bone tissues into normal position. This also provides an opportunity for inspection of the medial palpebral ligaments and their replacement if indicated. Lacerations of the duct system can be approached through these incisions if the original wound has healed. Fixation of bone fragments can be done by plating with wires passed from one canthal area to the opposite one and tied over small acrylic plates on the lateral aspect of the nose and medial palpebral areas. Elevation of the nasal structures and support with intranasal packing also may be necessary in addition to direct wiring techniques. An external plaster splint gives protection for 1 week at which time the fragments are quite well organized.

References

Crikelair, G. F.: Amer. J. Surg. **96**, 631 (1958).

Dingman, R. O.: Chapter on Facial injuries and repair. Ed. by Converse and Littler, Reconstructive surgery, Vol. 2, Chapter 17, pp. 397—548. Philadelphia: W. B. Saunders 1963.

—, and P. Natvig: Surgery of facial fractures. Philadelphia: W. B. Saunders Co. 1964.

Mustarde, J. C.: Repair and reconstruction in the orbital region. Baltimore: Williams & Wilkins Co. 1966.

Kazanjian, V. H., and J. M. Converse: The surgical treatment of facial injuries. Baltimore: Williams & Wilkins Co. 1959.

Early Management of Injured Hands*

Erle E. Peacock, Jr.

More has been written about the early management of injured hands than any other aspect of reconstructive surgery. Yet the increasing demand for experienced hand surgeons to discuss principles of early management testifies to the insecurity which most physicians and surgeons have about early management of a serious injury of the upper extremity. In my judgment, much of this insecurity is the result of unnecessary complexity and ambiguity; the purpose of this paper is to present a simple scheme for the early management of all types of hand injuries.

In simplifying the early management of hand injuries it is helpful to state a single objective which will be universally applicable to all types of injuries. Because the most serious complication of an injured hand is stiffness of the proximal interphalangeal joints, it follows that the single most important objective in the management of injured hands is to prevent joint stiffness from occurring. When one considers that joint stiffness is really a complication of medical treatment and seldom a direct result of injury, the implications of such a universal objective are readily apparent.

* From the Department of Surgery, University of North Carolina School of Medicine, Chapel Hill, North Carolina, 27514.

The agent which inflicts injury to the hand does not, in itself, produce joint stiffness unless it interrupts the integrity of joint structures. Only if an object actually penetrates the joint capsule or divides the collateral ligaments can the inciting injury be held directly responsible for the production of joint stiffness. In most patients, joint stiffness develops secondary to treatment and is a complication which the physician must assume responsibility for. It follows, therefore, that because joint stiffness is the worst complication which can develop in an injured hand and because it is a complication which the physician should be able to control, development of a universally applicable method for preventing joint stiffness is the essence of successful early management of injured hands. Perhaps the single most important step in this direction is to help physicians realize that prevention of joint stiffness is their most important responsibility.

Most physicians and surgeons taking care of an injured hand view care of the wound as their primary responsibility. Of course, good wound care is the essence of good surgical care for any type of injury. Complete concentration on the progress of the wound, however, often is responsible for neglecting changes which are occurring in small joints some distance away. Even the worst complications of a fracture such as malunion, non-union, or osteomyelitis are amenable to good surgical care; stiff proximal interphalangeal joints developing during treatment of these conditions, however, are not amenable to surgery and respond very poorly to physical medicine measures. It would seem obvious, therefore, that if one had the choice between the worst possible complication of a fracture and proximal interphalangeal joint stiffness, the fracture should be neglected, if necessary, to preserve interphalangeal joint mobility. The same reasoning holds for injuries to skin, nerves, and tendons. An unhealed wound or unsatisfactory scar, a dehisced tendon, or a nerve anastomosis which does not transmit stimuli are all amenable to secondary reconstructive surgery. In fact, such injuries often can be reconstructed by secondary procedures more effectively than during repair of the primary wound. Thus if there is any doubt about the proper treatment of nerves, tendons, or bones, the surgeon who only occasionally treats severely injured hands will always be following sound principles to close the wound only and not attempt reconstruction of deep structures. A second chance for proximal interphalangeal joints usually is not possible, however, and if mistakes are made during the first few weeks which lead to joint stiffness, permanent disability usually is produced.

The first serious attempt to reduce the terrible disability of joint stiffness was describing the position of function and recommending use of such splints as the Mason-Allen universal hand splint to assure that joints would be immobilized in a mid-range position. If a joint becomes stiff, it is better to have it stiff in a mid-range position than in an extreme position. Until the concept of assuring that joints become stiff in optimum positions is replaced by similar concern that a full range of motion be preserved, no real progress will have been realized. The wrist joint, metacarpophalangeal joints, and the carpometacarpal joint of the thumb are joints in which a neutral position is extremely valuable when range of motion is decreased. Thus emphasis on the position of function makes the greatest difference upon disability of these joints. The most important joints in hands, however — the proximal interphalangeal joints — are not affected significantly by the position in which stiffness develops. Occupational demands and even general use of these joints is so variable that stiffness in an extreme position may be better or worse than a mid-position arthrodesis. Expressed simply, regardless of the status of the other tissues in the hand, if a hand reaches the stage of secondary reconstructive surgery with supple proximal interphalangeal joints, primary treatment has been superb. Conversely, regardless of the excellence of reparative surgery in other tissues, if a hand reaches the stage of secondary reconstruction with stiff proximal interphalangeal joints, reconstructive surgery usually does not change final disability significantly. We have reasoned, therefore, that the most important objective in primary care of all injured hands is to preserve motion in the proximal interphalangeal joints.

The most damaging influences on interphalangeal joint motion are edema and immobilization. Immobilization is the more serious of the two, although it is possible to immobilize a non-edematous hand for a longer period of time without producing joint stiffness than when edema is present. The single most important factor in preserving motion and eliminating edema is early closure of wounds. It is almost impossible to keep a hand from being edematous as long as there is an open wound and, in addition, pain or fear of moving the injured portion exerts an unsurmountable splinting effect.

The principle of early successful wound closure is so important in the early care of hand injuries that we have taken the position that the most experienced people on our service should be called for consultation when a hand wound is not healed within 7 days. This principle applies to all types of hand injuries, including burns, fractures, complicated tendon and nerve injuries, and compound injuries. Even a badly infected wound, if treated properly, usually can be converted to a wound which can receive a split thickness skin graft by the end of 5 days.

Wounds caused by mechanical agents, regardless of the amount of contused and devitalized tissue, can be converted into surgically clean wounds by meticulous debridement. The frequently expressed concept that a crushing or blast injury which creates a lot of partially or completely devitalized tissue should be closed secondarily is responsible for serious delays in obtaining a healed wound. Under general anesthesia and tourniquet hemostasis, a surgeon who knows the anatomy of the hand should be able to convert any fresh wound into a surgically clean one. Perhaps the most difficult soft tissue injury to treat in this manner is a grease gun or paint spray injury in which a foreign substance has been injected under high pressure through the various connective tissue planes beneath the skin. Although we have not had a great deal of experience with these injuries, the combined experience of many hand surgeons strongly suggests that meticulous debridement of damaged tissue and removal of all foreign material so that primary wound healing can occur is essential to an acceptable final result. Although even a mutilated hand should be so perfectly debrided during the first operation that an abdominal pedicle or local flap can be applied with safety, the concept of a dressing split thickness skin graft should not be forgotten. In wounds elsewhere in the body, it is common practice to insert a gauze pack when the surgeon is doubtful about the completeness of debridement. In the hand there should not be any doubt about the effectiveness of debridement but, if there is, a split thickness skin graft should be used as a dressing instead of a foreign substance such as gauze. A split thickness skin graft does not add additional hazard as far as infection is concerned and it is a much better dressing than a piece of gauze. Even if inadequate debridement was carried out so that devitalized tissue and bacteria produced serious infection, a split thickness skin graft does not close the wound any more dangerously than a gauze dressing. Usually, little or no trace of the graft can be found over a suppurative infection.

In addition to the beneficial effect on prevention of joint stiffness, early wound closure has another significant role in the early management of hand injuries. It is very important that the mechanics of wound contracture not be allowed to progress before a flap or graft is applied. Even a few days delay in closing a wound results in division and migration of cells which ultimately will be responsible for wound contraction. Wound contraction is neither prevented nor stopped by applying a skin graft or pedicle flap after cellular activity has started. Wound contraction can be prevented only by closing a wound primarily or excising the wound edges and wound base entirely. Because wound contraction is so devastating in the hand, this is an additional important reason for not leaving a wound open even a few days when early closure can be accomplished.

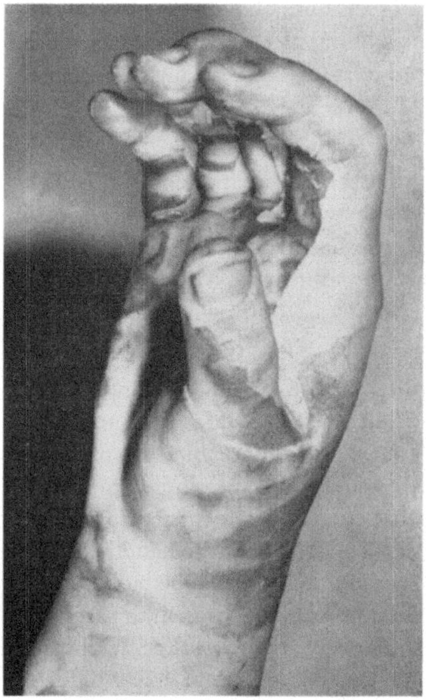

Fig. 1. Circumferential third degree burn of hand, wrist and forearm

An infected wound cannot be closed, thus the difference between contamination and infection becomes pivotal in the planning of primary care. A contaminated wound can always be converted into a surgically clean wound so that some type of closure is possible but an infected wound must be drained and only closed secondarily. The signs of inflammation are the most reliable guidelines to determine when contamination has resulted in infection. Blood supply, length of time between injury and surgical care, strength and type of inoculum, and the care which was administered between the time of injury and definitive surgical treatment all influence the judgment of the surgeon. None of these criteria should be used alone, however, when making a decision about early wound closure.

Radiation induced injuries of the hand are the most difficult to assess especially when electricity has produced the tissue damage. Even the most enthusiastic proponents of the exposure method of treating burns agree that an obvious third degree burn of the skin of the hand should be excised and the hand resurfaced as soon as possible (see Figs. 1 to 5). The difficulty arises when it is not obvious whether a surface burn is a uniform third degree one or a mixture of deep second and third degree damage. It is true that a deep second degree burn or a third degree burn which is not uniformly destructive to all elements of the skin will heal without addition of new skin provided further complications do not develop. Moreover, use of topical agents such as silver nitrate and Sulfamylon has seemed to encourage conservative treatment of such injuries. Such treatment is justifiable only if the condition of the proximal interphalangeal joints is monitored continually during the relatively long periods of secondary healing; treatment should include intensive physical and occupational therapy to maintain or improve active and passive motion. Enthusiasm for such treatment is somewhat diminished, however, by the realization that most burns (particularly on the dorsum of the hand) which are so deep that it is impossible to be certain whether they are deep second degree or partial third degree burns ultimately will require grafting even though epithelization and scar formation produce a healed wound. Although the way hands heal is variable, particularly regarding the amount of scar tissue which develops, most deep second degree burns will not have acceptable cover after primary healing has occurred. Neither appearance nor function of either a hypertrophic or extremely thin, atrophic scar is suitable for most patients. The only treatment for these complications of conservative therapy is to excise the damaged and scarred skin and replace it with a thick split or full thickness graft. The notion

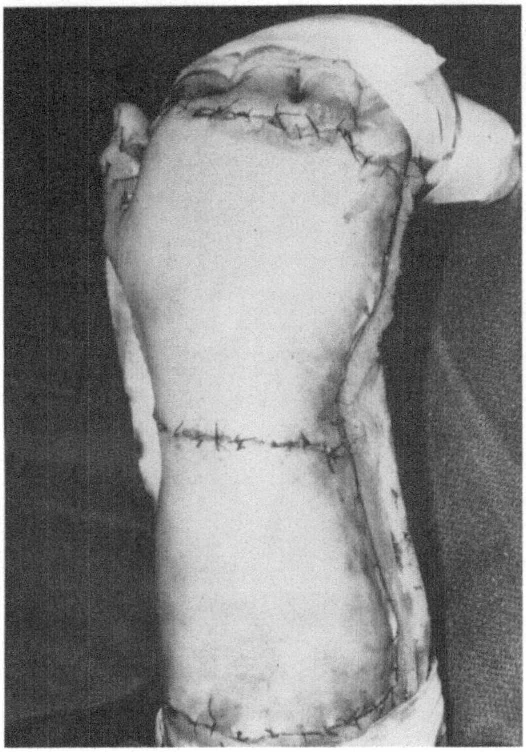

Fig. 2. Split thickness skin grafts applied immediately after excision of dorsal skin

that this can be done more effectively as a secondary than a primary procedure is correct. Certainly there is less edema and less opportunity for infection to occur if final resurfacing is performed after wound healing is complete. On the other hand, conservative therapy is also beset with complications and if the surgeon's judgment was wrong in the depth of the burn or if a subsequent infection or other complication converted a second degree burn into a third degree one, the surgeon will be required to graft a hand which is well along the way toward serious wound contraction and has joints which may have been immobilized for several weeks before grafting is attempted. The poor results of grafting a hand which has been treated conservatively for several weeks and which has granulation tissue and early wound contracture have caused many surgeons to become disenchanted with early excision and grafting of burned skin. This is understandable but unnecessary!

Early excision of burns does not refer so much to the length of time between injury and excision as it does biological changes in the tissues. Because some of the cellular changes involved in wound contraction, collagen synthesis, and epithelization occur in the presence of an eschar, excision of burned tissue and application of a skin graft after several days of conservative therapy may be, biologically speaking, secondary closure of a wound. The objective of successful early excision and grafting is to provide some thickness of normal dermis and epithelium over the entire wound

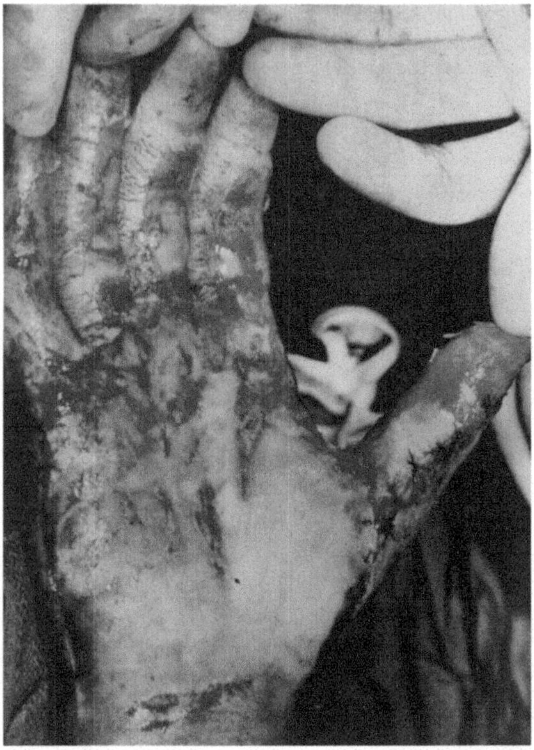

Fig. 3. Volar surface of hand debrided and resurfaced with split thickness skin graft 5 days after dorsal skin applied

before any of the biochemical or biological changes associated with wound contracture and wound healing have started. Poor results which many surgeons have encountered following early excision of eschar and application of split thickness skin grafts are, in our opinion, the results of waiting until cellular changes and prolonged edema have created a wound which is, from a biological standpoint, a secondary wound.

One of the most difficult hand injuries to apply the principle of early wound closure to is the deep electrical burn. It is generally assumed that electrical energy is transmitted along blood vessels which causes a secondary slough several days after the original injury. Because this explanation does not fit other bioelectric data, we have preferred to assume that electrical energy produced more extensive cell death at a greater distance from the point of contact than could be appreciated at the initial examination. Regardless of the mechanism by which excess scar tissue and joint immobilization is produced, however, early excision and grafting of electrical burns frequently is disappointing because necrotic tissue which was not appreciated at the initial debridement results in loss of portions of the graft. Such observations have discouraged many surgeons from being as aggressive about primary wound excision and grafting following electrical burns as following other injuries.

We do not agree that the principle of early excision and grafting is less applicable to electrical injuries than to thermal ones. Although loss of some areas of a graft is

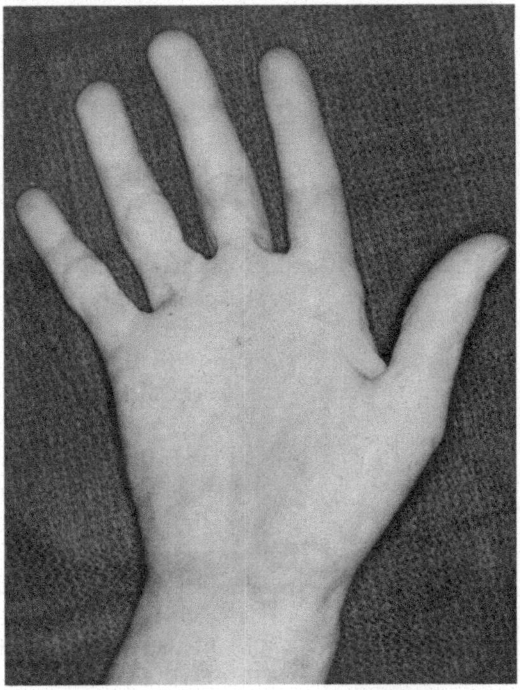

Fig. 4. Extension view of hand shown in Figs. 1, 2, and 3 two months following surgery

frequent, excising recognizable non-viable tissue and replacing as much of the wound surface with a split thickness skin graft as possible should not be denied the patient because the entire wound may not be covered successfully in one operation. The importance of debriding and covering even a portion of the wound as early as possible cannot be overestimated. Even if more than one secondary debridement and grafting is needed, the overall effect measured in reduction of edema and preservation of joint motion is significant with each procedure.

Another difficult problem to apply the principle of early excision and grafting to is dorsal burns which involve more than skin and subcutaneous tissue. The principle of excising all devitalized tissue and applying a graft before severe edema and joint stiffness occur may cause the surgeon to be confronted with exposed and devitalized extensor tendons. Of course, a free graft will not survive on such damaged structures and, if allowed to remain in an open wound, they will have to be mechanically debrided or many weeks may be required for them to slough or be covered by granulation tissue. Actually, granulation tissue does not grow well over dead collagen and inexorably, excision of the extensor mechanism will be required. In our judgment, excision of a damaged but mechanically intact extensor mechanism should not be done during primary care of the wound. It is very difficult to replace multiple extensor tendons so that simultaneous flexion of all joints of the fingers is possible. Reconstruction of the ectensor mechanism so that gross extension and flexion of a few of the interphalangeal joints is not difficult but when the entire extensor mechanism must be replaced, simultaneous flexion of all interphalangeal and metacarpal phalangeal joints seldom is possible. More often a tenodesis effect is produced and considerable function is lost.

Even when the extensor tendons have been badly damaged, if they are mechanically intact, they should be preserved by application of a pedicle flap. A thin abdominal pedicle flap is satisfactory and should be used to cover the extensor mechanism when the tendons are not viable. Passive and active range of motion in the fingers can be maintained through the 14 to 20 days a flap remains attached to the donor area. The biological basis for this approach is that even heat damaged collagen remains mechanically intact for many weeks or months. During this time it can serve as an excellent framework for cells which will later synthesize collagen and ground substance. Particularly when adequate soft tissue coverage has been accomplished and, if passive and active joint motion is preserved, a biologically reconstituted extensor mechanism is far superior to one restored by multiple free tendon grafts. It should be emphasized, however, that full thickness coverage with an abdominal pedical flap must be accomplished before granulation tissue develops or the biological machinery for wound contracture is activated. An abdominal pedicle flap placed on an intact extensor mechanism after wound contracture or collagen synthesis has started or after granulation tissue has appeared will be cosmetically unacceptable and functionally inadequate. Wound contracture beneath the flap will cause it to become an unsightly mound and fixation of the extensor mechanism by newly synthesized collagen will check the metacarpophalangeal joints in extension and tenodese the distal interphalangeal joints so severely that excision of the extensor mechanism ultimately may be needed to permit full passive motion of joints.

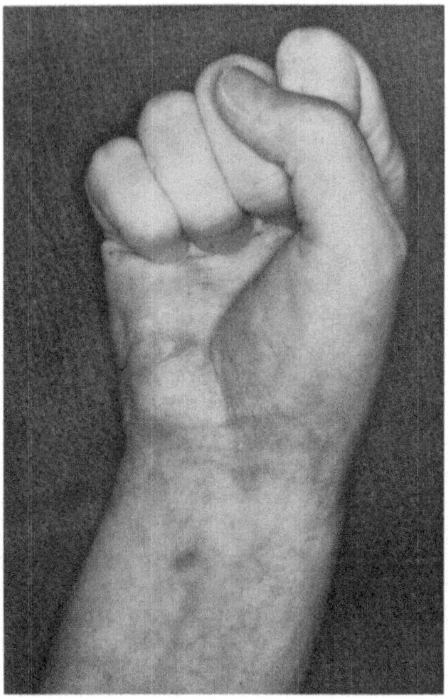

Fig. 5. Flexion view showing normal range of motion of interphalangeal joints 6 weeks after surgery outlined in Figs. 1, 2, and 3

Volar burns in infants and young children are a type of injury which provide an exception to the principle of early excision and replacement of skin. There are two reasons why this is true. The most important is that infants and young children do not develop permanently stiff proximal interphalangeal joints. Actually, the interphalangeal joints in youngsters can be immobilized in extreme positions for months without serious loss of motion. Thus conservative treatment of burns in children does not involve a risk of permanent joint restriction. A second reason why a conservative attitude in the management of volar burns in children is advisable is that free skin grafts are never as serviceable from the standpoint of sensation reception as the highly specialized skin on the volar surface of the hand and fingers. Even small islands of volar skin can provide extremely important sensory reception and, if any of these islands can be preserved by conservative treatment, it is worthwhile to do so.

In summary, most burns in adults involve the dorsum of the hand and the principle of early excision and replacement of damaged skin is pivotal to the concept that prevention of edema and joint stiffness should be the major objectives of early treatment. Most hand burns in children are caused by grasping or crawling upon a hot object; consequently, the burn is located primarily on the volar surface. Such burns usually are not uniformly full thickness and a conservative approach so that every island of sensitive skin can be preserved is indicated.

Although adequate wound closure stands as the most important principle in the primary care of injured hands, a paper on this subject would not be complete without mentioning a few other principles which have seemed to make a difference in special circumstances. Although the subject of fractures is so large that individual methods of treating fractures cannot be covered, the principle that internal fixation should be used wherever possible has made a great difference in the prevention of joint stiffness. Longitudinal Kirschner wires in metacarpals and oblique Kirschner wires in phalanges can provide sufficient stabilization so that an external splint need be worn only for comport. Such a splint can be removed daily to put small joints through a passive range of motion. External traction and elaborate external splinting should be reserved for badly comminuted fractures or fractures involving a joint surface. Even under these circumstances, traction should be applied only to the involved area; traction directed across a number of joints on either side of a fracture is not necessary in most instances.

Divided tendons and nerves should not be repaired as part of the primary care of a hand injury if the surgeon has any question about how to preserve interphalangeal joint motion during the postoperative period. Secondary repair of these structures can be performed with equally good and, in some instances, even superior results than when they are repaired primarily. If here is any question about the technique of repair or postoperative care, nerves and tendons should not be repaired until the patient has a healed wound and the joints no longer are in jeopardy. An exception to this rule is division of flexor tendons in the proximal wrist where there are no restraining forces to prevent severe retraction of the proximal motor unit. If lacerated tendons at this level are not repaired primarily, it is usually impossible to repair them at a future date. Thus, in the proximal wrist, repair of tendons takes precedence over nerves.

Pain and edema syndromes such as Sudeck's atrophy are usually seen following injuries of the midpalm and wrist — particularly a fracture of the distal radius. A salient point in the history of most patients is that severe pain was present following reduction and for as long as a week after application of a cast. We have thought it wise, therefore, to remove all dressings or a cast from any patient who complains of severe pain for longer than 24 h after reduction of a fracture or primary surgical care of an injury. The reasoning behind such a recommendation is that even the worst complication of a fracture or soft tissue restoration is less of a problem than the chronically painful and immobile hand of a patient with a postinjury dystrophy. Although we do not have specific data necessary to understand the pathogenesis of these dystrophies, the observation that they almost always occur after an injury marked by an inordinately painful postoperative course has suggested that relief of pain by change in position and removal of all restricting materials is mandatory.

Conclusions

1. Because proximal interphalangeal joint stiffness is the most difficult complication of hand injuries to treat, the objective of early treatment of all injured hands is to preserve a normal range of motion in small joints.

2. The combination of edema and immobilization should be prevented by early closure of wounds.

3. Where early closure of wounds is impossible because of infection, immobilization should not be permitted.

4. Repair of divided nerves and tendons should be delayed until after wound healing has occurred and edema has subsided, if there is any question about obtaining adequate soft tissue coverage and being able to prevent edema during the healing phase.

5. Fractures should be stabilized by internal fixation where possible; external traction should be reserved for badly comminuted fractures and fractures involving joint surfaces directly. Traction should not be directed through undamaged small joints.

6. The biological basis for early excision of devitalized tissue including burns is presented.

References

Allen, H. S., and M. L. Mason: Quart. Bull. Northw. Univ. med. Sch. **21**, 218—227 (1947).

Boyes, J. H.: Tex. St. J. Med. **52**, 845—848 (1956).

Cannon, B., and J. E. Murray: J. Amer. med. Ass. **200**, 663—668 (1967).

Flynn, J. E.: Ann. Surg. **135**, 500—507 (1952).

Grillo, H. C., G. T. Watts, and J. Gross: Ann. Surg. **148**, 145—152 (1958).

Luccioli, G. M., D. S. Kahn, and H. R. Robertson: Ann. Surg. **160**, 1030—1040 (1964).

Peacock, E. E.: (1) Surg. Clin. N. Amer. **33**, 1297—1309 (1953).

— (2) Ann. Surg. **164**, 1—12 (1966).

—, and C. R. Hartrampf: Surg. Gynec. Obstet. **113**, 411—432 (1961).

Stark, H. H., C. R. Ashworth, and J. H. Boyes: J. Bone Jt Surg. **49**, 637—647 (1967).

Watts, G. T., H. C. Grillo, and J. Gross: Ann. Surg. **148**, 153—160 (1958).

Surgery Following Burns of the Hand

W. Schink

This report is dealing with reconstructive surgery following burns of the hands.

Sequelae of Burns

Following deep thermal injury the scar tissue, especially keloids and cicatricial bands, will impair the function of the hand. In the ungual phalanxes distorsions of the nail matrix and deformities of the finger nails occur. On the knuckle of the fingers loss of elasticity of the skin will cause its easy vulnerability. Here, a concomitant destruction of the intermediate tract and, consequently, of the dorsal joint capsule of the proximal interphalangeal joint leads to ankylosis in maximal flexion. If extension contracture is acting upon the proximal phalanx, dorsal dislocation in the metacarpophalangeal joint with grotesque joint position may develop. Dorsal cicatrices between the proximal phalanxes do not permit the fingers to be spread. Cicatricial strangulations of vessels and nerves lead to vascular disturbance with increased cold-sensitivity and sensory disturbance. Following electrical burns tendons, joints and bones may also be damaged to a greater extent.

Remarks Concerning the Treatment

Goal of the treatment is a rather extensive excision of scar tissue with subsequent skin replacement. In most instances free skin transplants are sufficient; on the palmar surface a defatted full-thickness skin graft is preferred, whereas a thick split-thickness skin transplant is advocated for coverage of the dorsum. A pedicle skin plasty is necessary only over unprotected tendons, ligaments, joints or bones, so that the transplanted subcutaneous fat tissue serves as a slip surface and cushion. Usually pedicle plasty from adjacent skin will be preferred. However, in a widely burned hand this is not always technically feasible. In older patients we are not too eager about pedicle plasty from distant skin areas because of the imminent danger of additional joint stiffening. Following pedicle plasty from distant skin areas a volume increase may occur in the transplanted fat cushion making a reduction of tissue necessary. In pedicle plasty donor sites and pedicle tubes are to be covered by free skin grafts because any exposed wound area invariably becomes contaminated.

Operative Technique

Observing the principles of the atraumatic technique of Bunnell the excision of scar tissue in a bloodless field is always started at the central edge and continued in peripheral direction. This approach provides the best protection against injuries to the vessels, nerves and tendons. Occasionally smaller areas of intact skin must be sacrificed in order to keep the scar tissue at a proper site without impairment of function. To obtain a dry wound surface for the skin graft without the risk of delayed bleeding, a Purantix-soaked pad containing 10 units in 50 ml saline solution is put on the wound for 5 min after the tourniquet has been released. Chemically Purantix is an octapeptid, which in turn is an octapressine-derivative. The transplanted skin grafts are sutured into place, in smaller infants thin catgut material is used. The long ends of the ties are utilized for the fixation of a wet pad or foam rubber, thereby exercising an evenly distributed pressure of the transplant against the granulation surface. Until wound healing is completed an elastic pressure dressing with precast plaster splint provides for adequate immobilisation.

Plasties over the Palm and Dorsum of the Hand

For the correction of contractures over the palmar surface I have listed some therapeutic measures (Fig. 1):

a) Defatted full-thickness skin graft. Here, the incisional edges should run in a curved line to counteract keloid formation due to pressure or tension effects.

b) Pedicle plasty from the adjacent dorsal skin for the palmar surface of the thumb.

c) Pedicle plasty from distant skin area for the palm.

d) Pedicle plasty from the adjacent dorsal skin of the fingers used in amputations at the metacarpophalangeal joint level.

e) Lateral finger-flaps for a palmar wound surface.

f) Narrow band-like cicatrices are corrected by Z-plasty.

g) The Bunnell plasty comprises lateral releasing-incisions for digital erection and closure of the defect by a free skin graft.

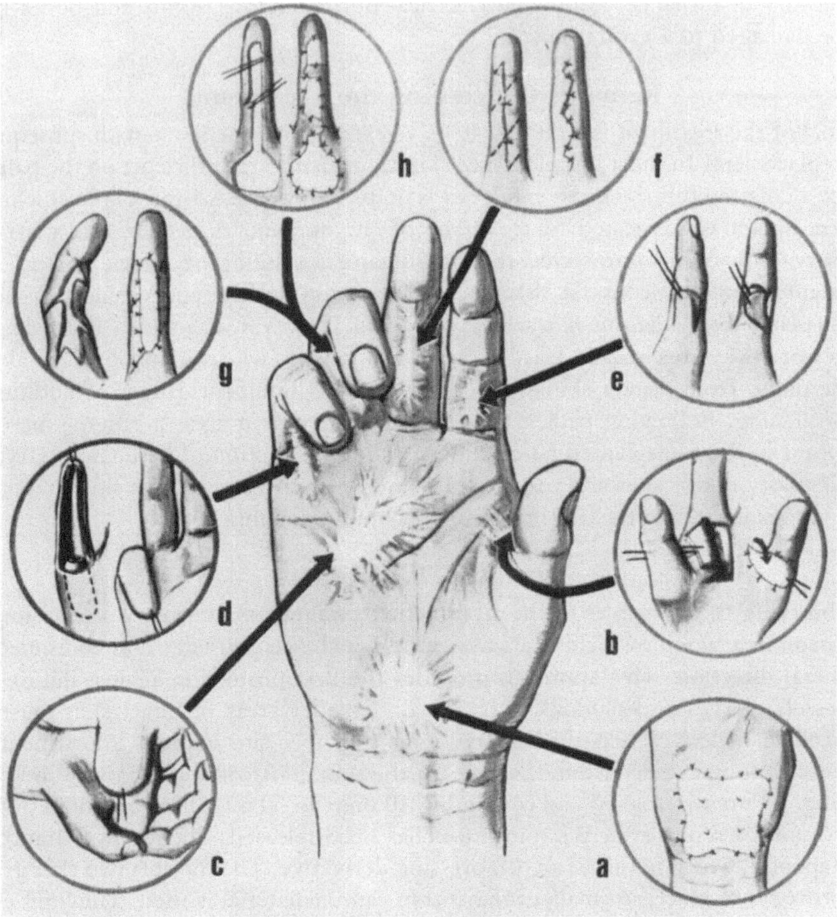

Fig. 1a—h. Correction of thermal keloids on the palmar area. a Defatted full-thickness skin graft, b Pedicle dorsal plasty from adjacent tissue for the palmar surface of the thumb, c Pedicle plasty from distant tissue, d Utilization of the dorsal skin of fingers in amputations, e Lateral finger flaps, f Z-plasty, g Bunnell-plasty (lateral releasing-incisions and free skin transplant), h Iselin-plasty (two lateral finger flaps and free skin transplants). [W. Schink: Sofort- und Spätbehandlung thermischer Schäden der Hände, Münch. med. Wschr. **105**, 1452—1458 (1963)]

h) In the Iselin-plasty 2 lateral finger-flaps are dividing up the wound area, the remaining defects are covered with free skin transplants.

Some measures for removal of contractures on the dorsum of the hand are illustrated in the following table (Fig. 2):

a) For the extensor surface of the fingers a split-thickness skin transplant is suitable, the incision lines are carried over the midlateral aspect.

b) Contracted proximal interphalangeal joints are arthrodesed in a position of function thus improving the prehensile ability.

c) Dorsal rotation flap. This type of plasty from adjacent tissue is only rarely applicable in burn injuries of the hand.

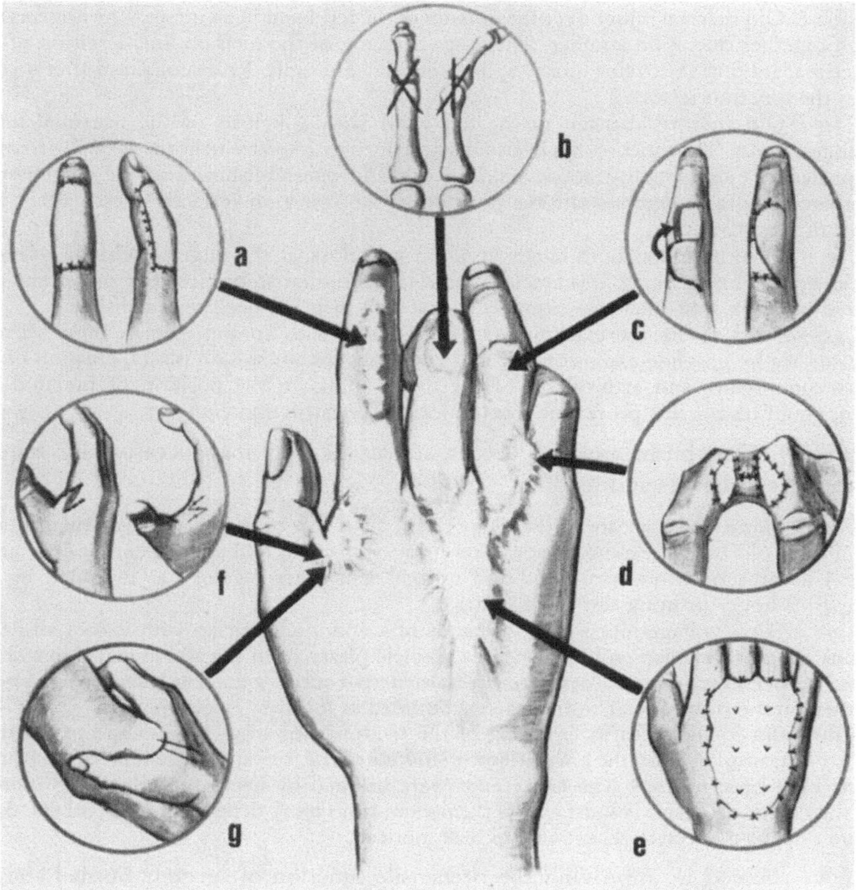

Fig. 2a—g. Correction of thermal keloids on the dorsum of the hand. a Split-thickness skin transplant, b) Arthrodesis in the position of function due to ankylosis in faulty position, c Dorsal rotation flap, d Iselin-plasty to create a commissure, e Split-thickness skin transplant with tongue-shaped flaps to the palmar surface, f Z-plasty, g Pedicle plasty from the contralateral forearm. [W. Schink: Sofort- und Spätbehandlung thermischer Schäden der Hände. Münch. med. Wschr. **105**, 1452—1458 (1963)]

d) In the Iselin plasty a web is formed of a palmar and a dorsal trapezoid skin flap. The remaining lateral triangular wound defects are closed by means of split-thickness grafts.

e) Split-thickness skin grafts with tongue-shaped flaps towards the palmar surface to deepen the commissures of the fingers.

f) Z-plasty in the first commissure is considered only in narrow cicatricial bands.

g) Pedicle plasty from the contralateral forearm is indicated in extensive keloids of the first commissure.

Case reports

Case 1. Gasoline-burn of a doctor's left hand. Considerable impairment of function. 6 months later the keloids are excised and a split-thickness skin graft for the five fingers and the dorsum of the hand is sutured in place. Re-examination after 3 years shows an unimpaired function, the skin is freely movable again.

Case 2. Old thermal injury over the dorsum of the left hand in an infant. The fingers have grown together one upon another. There is a drawing of the incision line. Excision of the surface scar leaving skin veins intact. Split-thickness skin graft. Re-examination after 4 years shows the function restored.

Case 3. Old thermal damage to the left hand with ankylosis of the proximal interphalangeal joints. The function has been substantially improved by arthrodesis of all proximal interphalangeal joints, split-thickness skin plasty and re-establishment of the commissure. The roentgenograms demonstrate the position of the resection-surfaces to each other and the fixation by K-wires.

Case 4. Burn injury of both hands at age 3 with loss of the fingers. With 11 years of age the crippled ring finger was erected, the residual digital stump lysed of scar tissue and covered by thick split-thickness skin graft. A strong grip has been re-established.

Case 5. Most severe thermal injury to both hands with an approximate 50% burn of body surface by gasoline explosion. By means of split-thickness skin plasty, creation of the digital commissure and arthrodeses of the finger joints in the position of function the patient could resume his professional activities as a construction-engineer.

High voltage burns involve deeper structures and may occasionally require replacement of nerves and tendons.

Case 6. Palmar contracture of the index finger with loss of the 3rd neurovascular bundle in a 10 year-old boy. Free autoplastic sural nerve transplant and split-thickness skin graft. After 4 months function is restored and normal sensitivity regained as indicated by the Ninhydrine finger printing test of MOBERG.

Case 7. High voltage-injury to both hands of a young electrician with loss of all flexor tendons and both median and ulnar nerves. Pedicle plasty from the abdominal skin to both wrists had been carried out elsewhere. Reconstructive surgery 2 years later — first on the left, then on the right side. The approach is outlined as follows: Excision of scars extending from the palm to the forearm, bridging of the tendon gaps of all fingers and opposition-plasty. For transplantation the long extensor tendons of the toes and the tendon of the plantar muscle have been utilized. The nerve gaps were bridged by nerve transplants. 15 months later the functional result is satisfactory, the patient is no more dependent upon others. After 3 years a slight protective sensation had been noticed.

If we succeed in improving the prehensile function of severely burned and incapacitated hands it will mean a great gain to the patient; for, as Sterling BUNNELL put it, "When you have nothing, a little is a lot."

Delayed Primary Suture After Severe Injuries of the Hand

H. GEORG

The aim of the treatment of wounds is to achieve uncomplicated healing and restitution of function. In the case of compound injuries to tendons, bones, joints, and nerves, as frequently seen in injuries of the hand, primary repair of all injured parts is generally not indicated in view of the risk of infection. In deep, grossly lacerated, and dirty wounds with exposed bone, crushed muscle, pockets and gaps, the kind of mechanical cleansing, suggested by FRIEDRICH as primary wound toilet, will always be incomplete, if only for purely technical reasons: It is impossible to extirpate the whole wound surface of these compound injuries, and numerous micro-organisms, foreign bodies, and devitalized tissue will necessarily remain and will initiate infection after primary suture.

Secondary reconstruction after the wound has healed aseptically hardly ever gives a good functional result. Everyone who has tried it knows what will happen: extensive scar formation, shrunk and degenerated tendons and muscles, stiff joints, and an altogether unsatisfactory functional result are the usual outcome.

Delayed primary suture is a compromise that was first proposed and used by ISELIN.

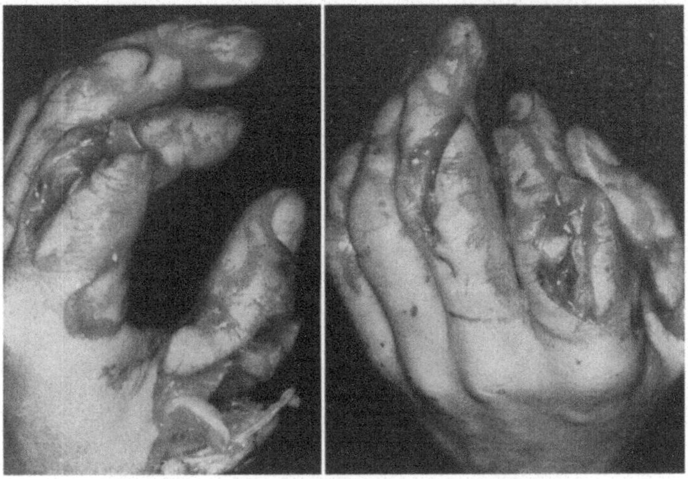

Fig. 1a

Fig. 1. a Injury by machine tool of the left thumb, index and middle fingers with laceration of the ligamental apparatus of all three fingers and crush injury of the 2nd and 3rd middle joints, of the proximal joint of the thumb, the proximal phalanges of the thumb and index finger. b Findings after 46 h. The crushed joints are clearly visible. c X-ray findings of the fresh injury (a), after suturing (b), and 2.5 months later (c). d Primary healing: satisfactory function after 2.5 months. Return to work after 3 months

He called his procedure at first "urgence differée" and now calls it "urgence avec opération differée". He first mechanically cleanses the wound, if it is grossly contaminated, ties spurting vessels, and removes foreign bodies and debris. The wound remains open and is covered with a moist antiseptic dressing. ISELIN suggested a 1% solution of a quarternary ammonium base as antiseptic dressing. Systemic antibiotics are administered, the dressing is changed daily, the wound is washed and dressed with the antiseptic solution.

According to ISELIN it is possible to disinfect any wound within a few days or at least to reduce considerably the number of micro-organisms by leaving the wound open, by local application of a mild antiseptic, and administration of an antibiotic. It is possible then to carry out delayed surgery under practically aseptic conditions and to reconstruct all injured parts without increasing the risk of infection.

At the Clinic at Heidelberg I have used this procedure for injuries of the hand, and I have been able to convince myself of its advantages. It is indeed possible to carry out complete repair in one session without any fear of infection. This is the greatest advantage of the procedure.

Two examples are:

(Fig. 1) a) Injury by a machine tool of the left thumb, index and middle fingers with rupture of extensor tendons of the three fingers and crushing of the 2nd and 3rd medial phalanges, of the proximal joint of the thumb, and of the proximal phalanges of thumb and index finger.

b) Findings after 46 h: the crushed joints are clearly visible.

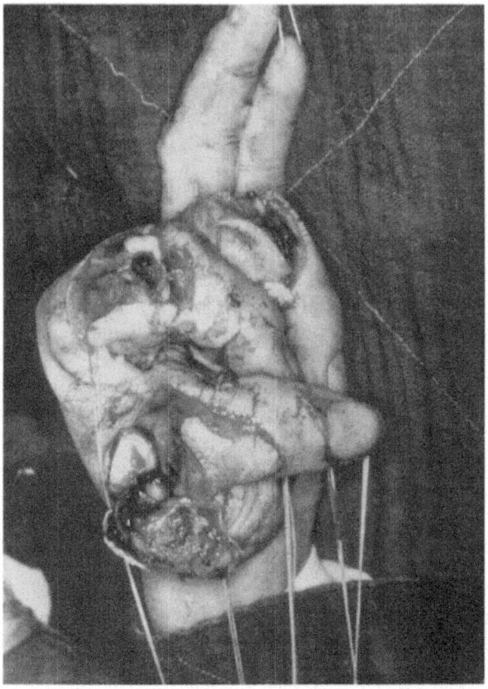

Fig. 1b

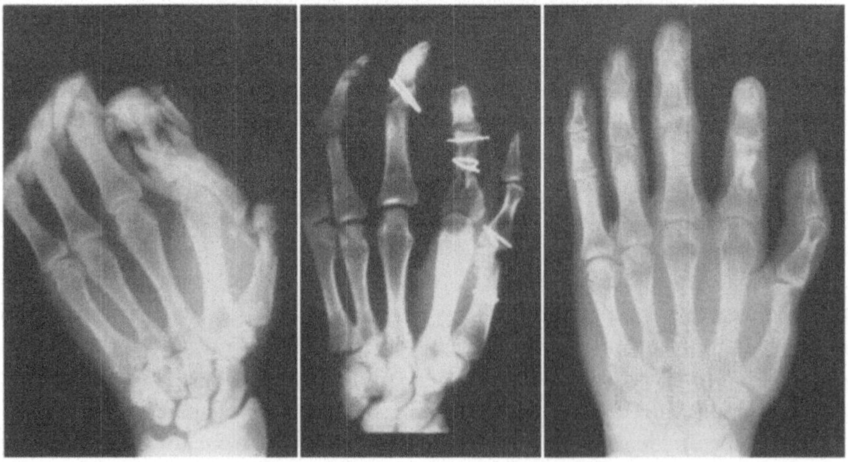

Fig. 1c

c) X-ray findings of the fresh injury (left), after suturing (middle), and 2.5 months later (right).

d) Primary healing: satisfactory function after 2.5 months; return to work after 3 months.

(Fig. 2) Delayed suture is justified not only in injuries of the hand, but also in other injuries, which by reason of their origin may be particularly exposed to infection.

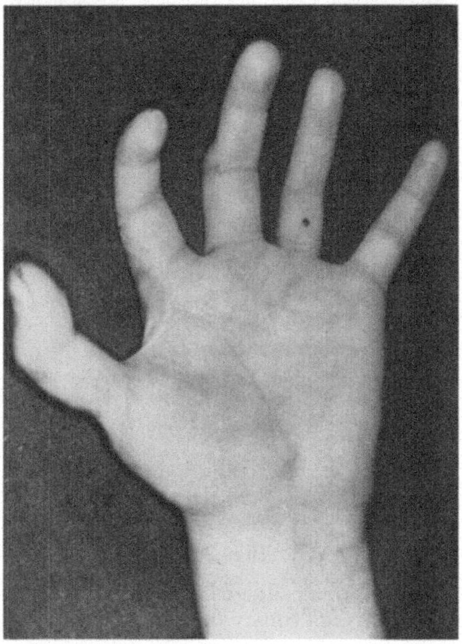

Fig. 1d

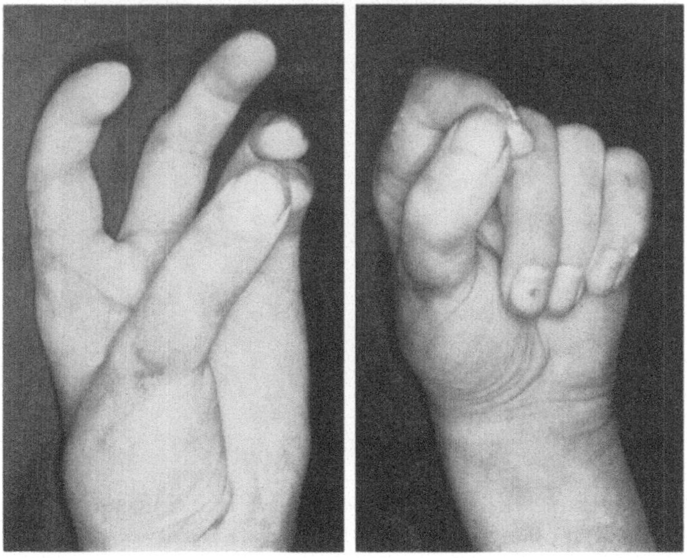

Fig. 1e

a) Dog bite of the face of a 2-year-old girl.
b) Laceration of the right cheek down to the gums. Suture after 4 days.
c) Primary healing: findings 7 days after suture and
d) 1 year later.

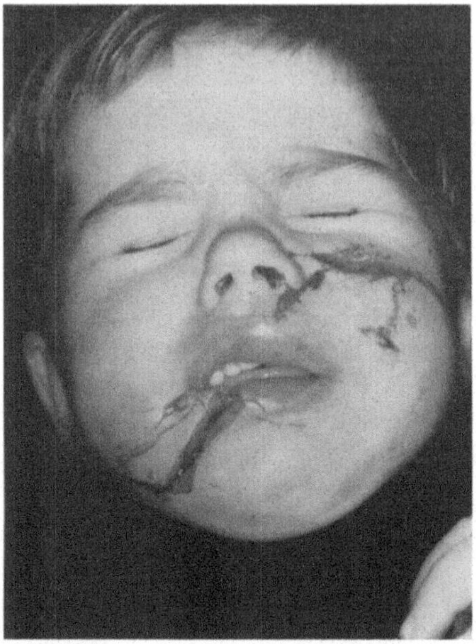

Fig. 2a

Fig. 2. a Dog bite of the face of a 2 year-old girl. b Laceration of right lower lip down to the gums. Sature after 4 days. c Primary healing: findings 7 days after suture

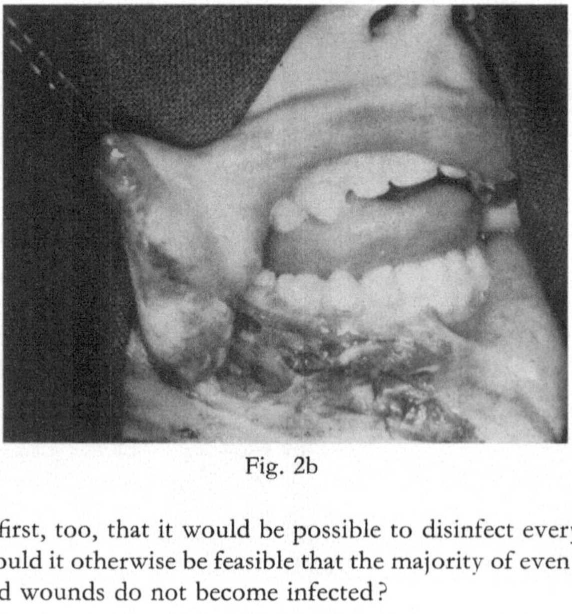

Fig. 2b

I thought at first, too, that it would be possible to disinfect every wound in this manner. How would it otherwise be feasible that the majority of even the most severe and contaminated wounds do not become infected?

At first I tried to prove my point by bacteriological examinations. The results were disappointing. Smears showed numerous micro-organisms at the time of the delayed primary suture, even more than during the first few hours after the injury.

I became convinced that there was no question of wound disinfection and that my experiences of the method did not confirm ISELIN's theory.

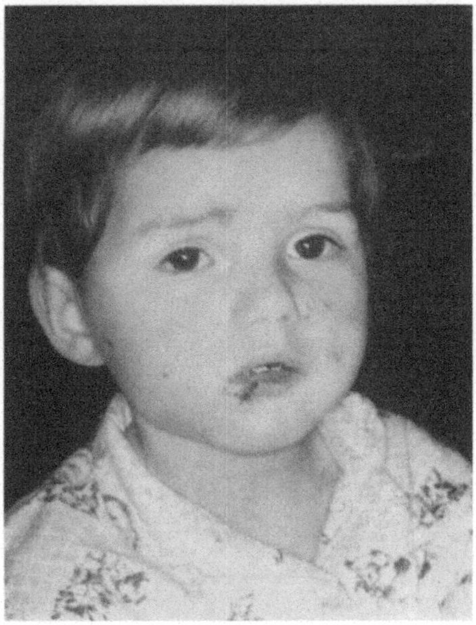

Fig. 2c

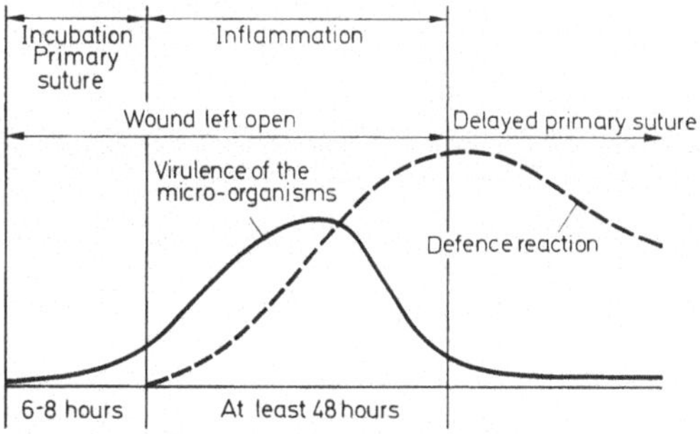

Fig. 3. The defence reactions of the body begin to increase with the increasing virulence of the micro-organisms following the incubation period. As the defensive forces increase, virulence decreases. Once the inflammation has subsided, delayed primary suture may be carried out

Why does infection only rarely happen after delayed primary suture (Fig. 3)? On the basis of my clinical observations and of bacteriological investigations I concluded that infection will have to take its course in every case, but that it would be preferable if favourable conditions could be created, by leaving the wound open and preventing superinfection.

The defence reactions of the body increased as the virulence of the micro-organisms rose after the incubation period. As the defences became more powerful,

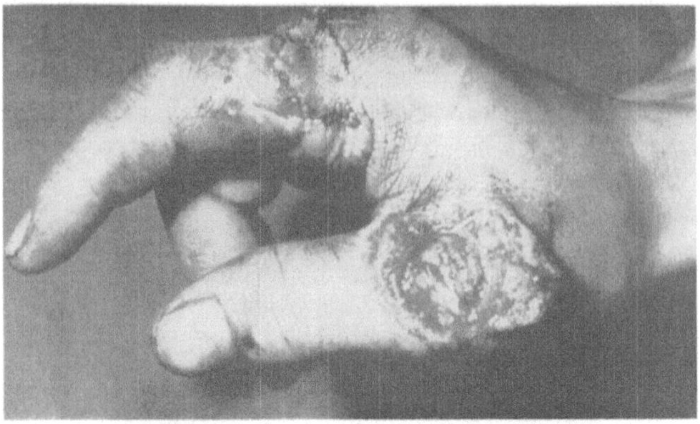

a

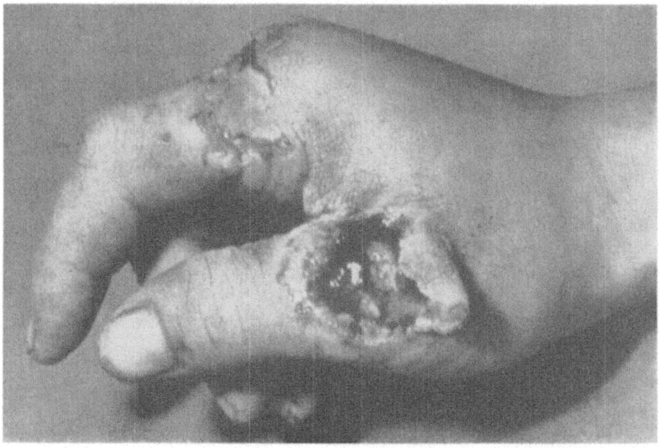

b

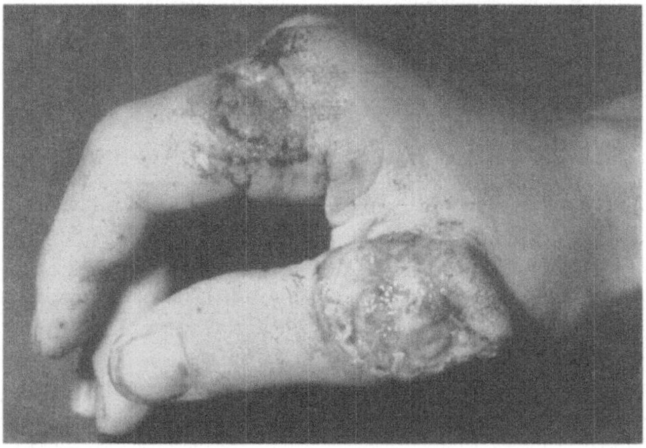

c

Fig. 4. a Injury by machine tool of the right hand with separation of the extensor apparatus of thumb and index finger. b 3 days after injury: edema of the middle of the hand and of the wrist. c 7 days after injury: edema absorbed, no secretion, wounds no longer irritating, patient free from pain virulence decreased (Fig. 4a). Edema and rubor appeared, and secretion increased. (b) Clinical observations confirmed this. (c) Once the edema had drained off and the inflammatory rubor had subsided, and once the wound no longer irritated and the patient was free from pain, then the time for delayed primary suture had come (Fig. 3). The micro-organisms would still grow in vitro, but were no longer sufficiently pathogenic to cause inflammation that was clinically demonstrable.

I therefore tried to test clinically, bacteriologically, and histologically in animal experiments my ideas about the biological cleansing of wounds by inflammation.

It is not possible to communicate the results here in detail. My assumptions were, however, largely confirmed by the results of my experiments:

1. It is not possible to disinfect within a few days a wound by local antiseptic and general antibiotic treatment.
2. In every case there will be a considerable inflammatory reaction.
3. Even after subsidence of the inflammatory symptoms numerous micro-organisms are still present.
4. When primary suture is carried out within 6 to 8 h the conditions under which the ever-present inflammatory process occurs are much more unfavourable than when the wound has been left open, although at the time of delayed primary suture more micro-organisms may be present than immediately after the injury.

My clinical findings and the results of animal experiments indicated that the inflammation, which is really a biological cleansing, is in fact the precondition for delayed suture. It makes it possible for the defensive forces of the organism to act under more favourable conditions, as constituted by the wound being kept open and by avoidance of secondary infection.

The good old rule of primary excision of a wound with immediate closure is still valid, provided the wound is such that there is no increased danger of infection. Although delayed primary suture has great advantages, it also has strict indications. In my experience it is only indicated:

1. in severe contusions, lacerations, and crush injuries;
2. in grossly contaminated wounds and such injuries which by the nature of their origin are in danger of being grossly infected;
3. in compound injuries of skin, tendons, bones, joints, and other functionally important organs, and
4. in multiple injuries of the tendons, especially those of the hand.

There is no doubt that the advantages of the procedure have been fully proven clinically. Delay is only justified, if it is necessary and if it will guarantee better healing of the wound and restitution of function in injuries that are particularly prone to infection. The indication is limited to those injuries in which functional and cosmetic complications due to infection may be expected after primary suture.

The Basic Principles of Tendon Transfers

J. H. Boyes

The operation of tendon transfer to provide essential motion to the hand has a long and interesting history. In the upper extremity, the earliest operations were designed to overcome the palsies which followed radial nerve damage, but through the years a multitude of procedures have become familiar to all surgeons. Operations are now being done for ulnar paralysis, combined median and ulnar paralysis such as is seen in leprosy, and for loss of thenar muscle activity which follows damage to the median nerve at the wrist. In the lower extremity, transfers were done for foot drop and other deformities such as poliomyelitis. Tendon transfer operations have a place; however, not only after injury to the major nerves, but also in instances where loss of motion has been the result of direct muscle or tendon damage.

Many attempts have been made to define a set of common principles. It is often stated that "synergists" must be used as donor muscles. True, perhaps, in the lower extremity where automatic reflex action is so important, but it was STEINDLER and then BUNNELL who showed that in the upper extremity this requirement was not necessary. Both agreed that the basic principles included the need for supple joints and good soft tissues, a donor muscle of adequate power and amplitude and a motor tendon unit passed through the tissues in a direct line with minimum interference with its gliding quality. Neither felt that the donor muscle must be a "synergist" of the intended action. In fact, both denied the importance of such a quality in the donor muscle. STEINDLER expressed his disbelief by saying that when a motor tendon unit is transferred in the forearm or hand, it never enters into a motion with which it is not already familiar or, in other words, every muscle is a synergist of every motion. BUNNELL was fond of pointing out that motions of the hand are determined in the cortex as movements, not as isolated muscle activities. In other words, when an impulse from the cortical area of the thumb is elaborated, any muscle capable of so doing by its power and position, will carry out the motion.

It is, therefore, rather disconcerting to see in current texts and articles that one of the essential requirements for tendon transfer in the hand is that the donor muscle must be a "synergist" of the intended action. Such a belief that if it is true in the lower extremity, it must be true in the upper, is false and experience proves it so.

If one observes the homunculus of the human cortex, it is apparent that the area for the hand is greater than that for the whole lower extremity. The latter is a static mechanism. Its activities are reflex in character to a major degree and its motions are carried out by many muscles working in groups, and in the gait mechanism particularly, working in reflex controlled phases. By contrast, in the upper extremity we have the innumerable variations of position and movement; some reflex activity, true, but a minor part compared to the foot and leg.

A transfer to give motion to the digits is seldom required in the foot; whereas, it is one of the difficult problems in the hand. To move the digits, one must have a wrist joint capable of being stabilized in various positions. Arthrodesis of the wrist is a last resort and all attempts to preserve wrist motion under active muscle control is essential. Many years ago, ZACHARY, studying the results of transfers for radial palsy, pointed out the necessity of maintaining a flexor of the wrist. He found that when both flexors of the wrist were used as motors for the extensors of the digits that the lack of control of palmar flexion was a detrimental factor in the results. Since at that time the flexor carpi ulnaris was the choice of motor for digital extension, he concluded that the flexor carpi radialis function should be preserved, but the flexor carpi ulnaris function is of far greater importance to proper wrist action and it should be preserved. This is possible, for with current technics we can use the sublimis tendons as motors for the digital extensors, and use the flexor carpi radialis for the thumb abductor.

If one views a diagram of the motors acting on the wrist, it is obvious that the major plane of activity is from the radio-dorsal to the ulno-volar position. In fact, there is no motor on the dorsum which truly dorsiflexes the wrist in a straight line, and on the volar surface only the weak palmaris longus acts in this vertical plane. With normal wrist action, transfers of forearm motors to act as digital movers are successful because of this intercalated controlled joint. The effective amplitude of a motor is increased and full extension and full flexion of a digit may be accomplished with a motor of deficient absolute amplitude. To maintain this proper plane of wrist action, it is therefore essential to preserve or, if lacking, to restore activity to the extensor carpi radialis and the flexor carpi ulnaris muscles. With these motions intact, digital motions can be restored by using any other motor unit in the forearm.

Using this principle of maintaining or restoring wrist action in the proper plane and utilizing various motors, the results show that contrary to the belief that the donor must be a synergist, one can say that if the chosen motor tendon unit has adequate amplitude and power, and that if it is transferred in a satisfactory technical manner to maintain its gliding mechanism, that any muscle tendon unit may be carried out to perform any motion in the hand.

As examples, flexor carpi radialis can be used as an abductor of the thumb or as a motor for opposition when rerouted through a pulley mechanism; the pronator teres has been used as a flexor of the thumb or fingers, as extensor of the wrist, or for opposition of the thumb. The brachioradialis has been most useful as a digital flexor, for when its absolute amplitude is increased by freeing it of the overlying antebrachial fascia thus converting it to a pluriarticular muscle, its effective amplitude is sufficient to provide full flexion of the digits. The sublimis muscles can function as extrinsic or intrinsic finger extensors, as flexors or opposers or adductors of the thumb.

It is thus apparent that the question of synergism and antagonism does not enter into the problem of tendon transfers in the hand. If one satisfies the requirement of supple joints and soft tissues, uses a donor muscle of adequate power and amplitude, transplants it in the tissues so that it passes in a straight line or through a pulley mechanism, and maintains or restores the essential controlled motions of the wrist, it is not necessary to consider whether the donor muscle is a synergist or antagonist of the desired action.

References

Boyes, J. H.: Bunnell's surgery of the hand, 4th Ed. Philadelphia: Lippincott 1964.

Dupuytren's Contracture

The Abductor Minimi Digiti Band

J. H. Boyes

The pathological changes in the fascia characteristic of Dupuytren's disease are not limited to the pretendinous bands of the palmar aponeurosis. Involvement of the fingers has long been noted and the relative frequency of digital lesions, including the thumb, was previously reported [*1*]. The presence of knuckle pads and the lesions of the plantar fascia indicate the systemic character of the disease. Recently we reported the unusual involvement of the volar aspect of the wrist in two patients [*2*].

Hueston [3], in his monograph on Dupuytren's disease, has brought our attention to the peculiar involvement of the little finger by a band of fascia from the abductor minimi digiti. Certain characteristics of this involvement of the little finger, if recognized, may aid in a more successful treatment.

If the disease process involves only the pretendinous band of the palmar aponeurosis, the metacarpo-phalangeal (MP) joint of the little finger will be limited in

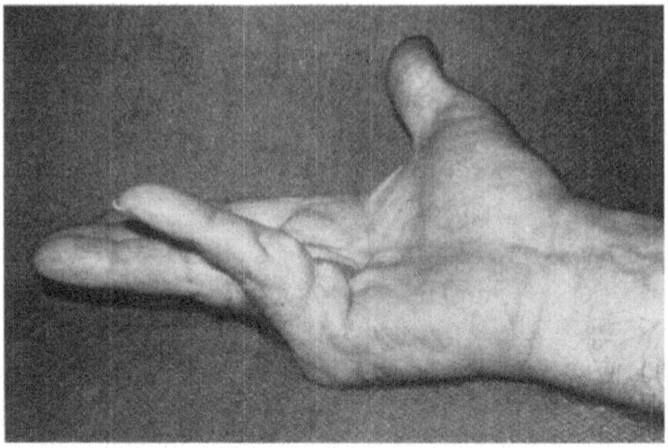

Fig. 1. Dupuytren's contracture involving only the pretendinous band to the little finger. Only the metacarpophalangeal joint is flexed

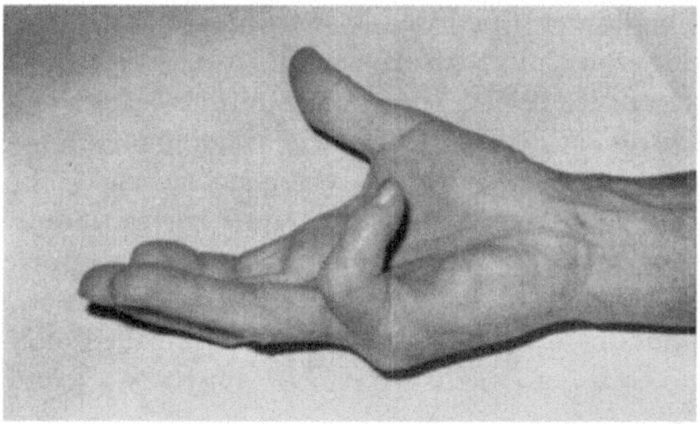

Fig. 2. When the pathological lesion involves the proximal segment of the finger, as well as the palm, both the metacarpophalangeal and the proximal interphalangeal joints are in flexion, the distal interphalangeal joint is in neutral position

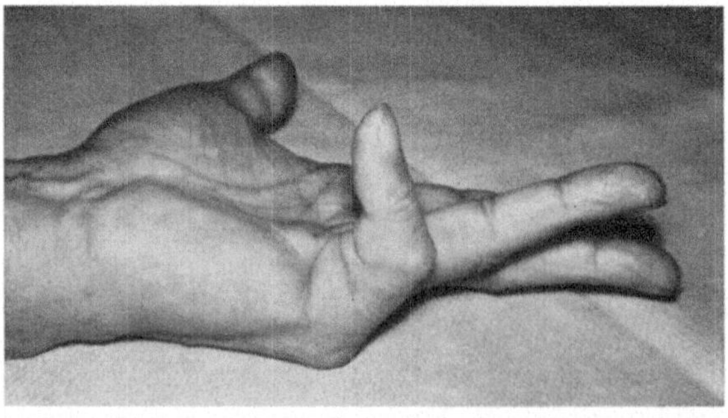

Fig. 3. Involvement of the pretendinous band of fascia and the digital fascia by an extension of the band from the abductor minimi results in flexion of the metacarpophalangeal and proximal interphalangeal joints but extension or hyperextension of the distal joint

extension (Fig. 1), but the proximal interphalangeal joint (PIP) and distal interphalangeal joint (DIP) joints will still extend completely. Such lesions are common, easily recognized and treated; however, if in addition to the MP joint (Fig. 2), there is contracture of the PIP joint, it indicates that the fascia in the finger itself is involved and usually by a thick band of pathological tissue extending across the middle flexion crease to the base of the middle phalanx, inserting along one or both sides and into the tendon sheath over the middle segment pulley. If this is the only lesion; that is, an extension of the pretendinous palmar band into the finger, then the DIP joint will be extensible, freely flexible and without involvement. But if, and not uncommonly, one sees the MP joint and the PIP joint in flexion and the distal joint in hyperextension (Fig. 3), a position resembling that known as the boutonniere lesion, then the lateral bands of fascia and especially that extending along the abductor minimi tendon, are involved. Shortening and contracture of this fascia, known variously as the digital or link ligament or part of the retinacular system of LANDSMEER, bring the PIP joint into flexion and through the resultant shortening, hyperextend the distal joint. Simple removal of the pretendinous band and the nodular thickening over the volar surface of the finger will not completely relieve the contracture. The exposure,

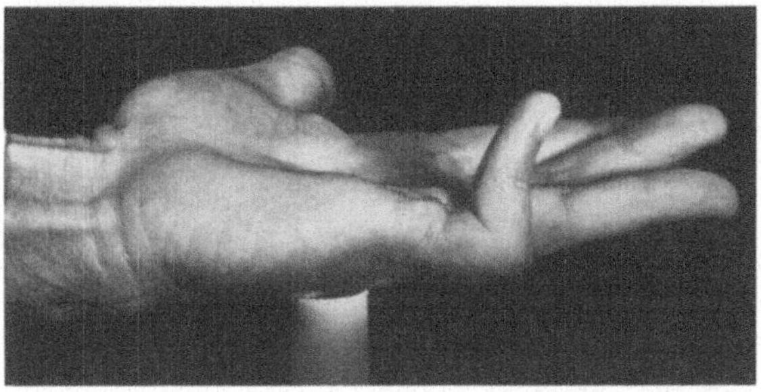

Fig. 4. Isolated Dupuytren's disease in the abductor minimi band allows extension of the metacarpophalangeal joint but the proximal interphalangeal joint is in flexion and the distal interphalangeal joint in hyperextension. The whole fifth ray is abducted from the ring finger

at operation, must include the ulnar side of the palm and finger and complete excision must be accomplished of the thickened fascia from the abductor minimi tendon.

This band of fascia extending from the perimuscular covering along the tendon and into the aponeurosis may occur as an isolated lesion, with no evidence of involvement of the pretendinous band. If so, the finger is not restricted in motion in the MP joint, but only in the PIP and DIP joints. Extension of the disease to the fascia over the hypothenar muscles more proximally results in a slight abduction contracture at the MP joint level with a flexed position of the PIP joint and a hyperextended position of the DIP joint (Fig. 4).

It is more common to find, however, that the thickening of the fascia involves both the pretendinous and the abductor minimi bands and thus a complete resection is usually necessary. This makes the operative exposure and removal of the involved tissues an intricate and delicate procedure, for the neurovascular bundle to the ulnar side of the finger may take a devious course, spiralling around or between the two bands. Here a longitudinal incision followed by Z-plasties, originally credited to MCINDOE and described by SKOOG, is useful providing there is adequate skin. If not, a zigzag incision can be used. When scarring is already present, such as from a previous operation, free or pedicled skin grafts may be necessary.

Many so-called recurrences of Dupuytren's disease in the little finger are probably the result of an unrecognized lesion in the abductor minimi band. For this reason, it is now considered advisable that in any involvement of the little finger one should expose this tendon of insertion of the abductor minimi. In many instances, a thickened band will be found extending into the extensor aponeurotic system, in addition to the more usual preflexor tendon band. Its removal, easily accomplished then, has improved our results of treatment of this most aggravating disease.

References

1. Boyes, J. H.: Amer. J. Surg. **88**, 147—154 (1954).
2. —, and F. E. Jones: Plast. reconstr. Surg. **41**, 203—207 (1968).
3. Hueston, J. T.: Dupuytren's contracture. Baltimore: Williams and Wilkins 1963.

Dupuytren's Contracture

Dieter Buck-Gramcko

The clinical picture of Dupuytren's contracture has aroused the interest of physicians for more than 100 years. The etiology and pathogenesis of this disorder have been discussed in numerous publications, although they have not been clarified yet. Treatment, too, has not been assessed uniformly. Whilst most authors agree that conservative treatment may be successful — if at all — in the initial stages, there is no agreement about the kind and extent of surgical treatment. Especially during the last few years discussion about the advantages and disadvantages of partial and complete removal of the palmar aponeurosis has been passionate.

Depending upon the extent of surgical intervention the following procedures may be distinguished:

a) fasciotomy: division of the indurated fibrous cord-like structure only;

b) limited excision, with removal of the fibrous cord and the diseased tissue in its vicinity;

c) partial fasciectomy with removal of the fibrous cord and its immediate environment in the palm, and

d) complete fasciectomy with removal of the whole palmar aponeurosis, including macroscopically healthy tissue.

The interventions increase the strain on the hand in the above order, whilst the prospect of recurrence decreases reversely. There is no doubt that the hand will regain full function much quicker after a limited or partial fasciectomy than after complete removal of the palmar aponeurosis.

The adherents of the minor and simpler operations stress this point particularly. They do not take into consideration, however, that the quality of a procedure should be assessed not only by its early, but also by its later results. These are best after complete fasciectomy, which is at first much more troublesome. Nevertheless, compared with the other procedures complete removal of the palmar aponeurosis, including its healthy parts, doubtlessly reduces the number of recurrences. Surgeons should therefore not stick rigidly to one single procedure, but should adapt the type of operation to the extent of the disorder, the general state of the patient's health, his age, and his expectation of life.

To assess late and eventual functional results properly a number of factors have to be taken into account, all of which will influence the results (MILLESI). Postoperative contractures due to scars and joint stiffness and limitation of movement due to such complications as hematoma, delayed wound healing, and edema, appear early, whilst recurrences in the operation site or extension of the disorder into healthy tissue, will be discovered only much later. Total assessment is therefore only possible years after operation.

Dupuytren's contracture presents as a variety of clinical pictures. Most common are isolated fibrous cords, which flex one or two fingers, whilst the remainder of the palmar aponeurosis is not or only slightly thickened. This variety is not difficult to treat surgically, except when the contracture has existed for a number of years and has given rise to changes in the joints, so that complete extension is no longer possible. The nodular type of contracture has quite different features. It is much more difficult to treat, because the nodules are wider distributed within the palmar aponeurosis and thus need a greatly extended surgical approach. Moreover, it is not so easy to free the nodules from the skin, as may be done with fibrous cords, as they are usually fused together. Thus removal of diseased tissue is more difficult, and the danger of recurrences due to pieces left behind is greater. CONWAY and HUESTON have therefore recommended the removal of all overlying skin and its replacement by full-thickness skin grafts, especially at the fingers, where the thin skin that would remain after excision often is not sufficiently supplied with blood.

A multitude of mixed forms, in which nodules and fibrous cords occur together, exists between these two extremes. The range of variations of the clinical picture of Dupuytren's disease is large, although there are several types that are seen over and over again. There is no need here to recount these. I shall mention only two relatively rare types. The first is a typical involvement of the thumb: this arises on the ulnar side from the first interdigital fold and on the radial side by a fibrous cord that extends from the thenar eminence to the proximal phalanx. The ulnar fibrous cord is particularly troublesome as it causes an adduction contracture, whilst the radial fibrous cord usually does not cause much impediment.

The second type is a Y-shaped cord to two neighbouring fingers by a fibrous cord from the palm, which divides in the interdigital fold. This also causes an adduction contracture. The contracture may be so severe, that the skin, where the fingers are pressed together, may become macerated.

The fibrous cords terminate distally either at the proximal phalanx or at the base of the middle phalanx. Here they insert laterally of the flexor tendons at the bone and occasionally may cause a small exostosis. A fibrous cord will hardly ever reach the distal phalanx and cause a flexion contracture of the DIP-joint. If the clinical picture shows that the distal interphalangeal joint is hyperextended, obviously an extension of the fibrous cord is running along the dorsum of the finger and terminates at the extensor aponeurosis. This will necessarily hyperextend the distal phalanx and can only be remedied by division and excision of the fibrous cord.

Occasionally digital forms of Dupuytren's contracture will cause diagnostic difficulties. The palm is not involved, and the fibrous cord lies in the finger only. It rises from the proximal to the middle phalanx either on the ulnar or the radial side. When this fibrous cord is going to be removed special attention will have to be paid to the neurovascular bundles, as these often are twisted around the fibrous cord or run between its ramifications.

In the palm the relationship between blood-vessels, nerves, and fibrous cords is occasionally very close. A nerve with or without its accompanying blood-vessel may be twisted around the fibrous cord (Fig. 1). Great care must be taken at dissection, so that the first incision does not sever the nerve that lies directly under the skin. It is rare for both neurovascular bundles of a finger to be included in the ramifications of the cord. The surgeon who has seen these changes several times will never carry out percutaneous discission as recommended by several authors: it is only too easy to sever a nerve, unless there is visual control and careful dissection in a bloodless operation field.

A few remarks as regards incisions: transverse incision of the palm with Z-plasty in the fingers, so popular a few years ago, is used less and less, because it demands extensive undermining of the skin of the palm and because necroses of the border of

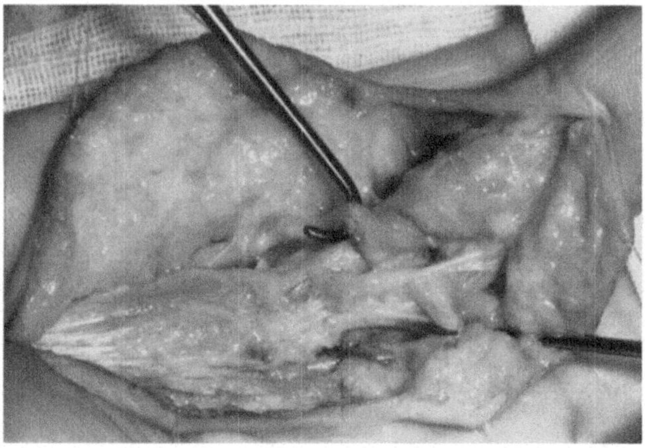

Fig. 1. A nerve (in the hook) has twisted itself around the fibrous cord and runs between skin and cord

the wound are common. It was never possible to have a proper idea how much palmar aponeurosis of the proximal part of the palm was removed. Nowadays, longitudinal incisions are in vogue. These may be wavy, if there is no shortening of the skin, or straight. Such a longitudinal incision should, however, not be sutured longitudinally, because it crosses one or more flexor creases of the joints, so that the scar would later on cause a flexion contracture. In spite of all warnings of plastic surgeons this is a recurrent mistake, so that considerable scar contractures a few months after operation are still being seen. One or two Z-plasties should be interposed in the long longitudinal incision to interrupt the straight course of the wound. The scars are then tension-free and will be hardly visible later on.

The Y-incision, as described by Millesi, has proved its value for the palm. Conway and Stark demonstrated in injection preparations that the blood flow in the middle of the palm was poor. If this area at risk is divided by the Y-incision into three skin flaps, the danger of necroses of the border of the wound is much less than with transverse incisions and extensive undermining. This approach allows a careful treatment of the small blood-vessels, which enter the skin, so that there is less danger of disorders of the blood flow of the skin (Fig. 2). To remove all parts of the palmar aponeurosis around these small vessels needs painstaking effort and takes time. A postoperative course without any complications justifies this careful procedure.

Incisions are particularly difficult when there are multiple fibrous cords, such as Y-shaped, branched cords of two neighbouring fingers. Longitudinal incision above the fibrous cords produces a skin flap that is long, narrow, and has a distal pedicle; its nourishment can only be secured by the conservation of a vessel from the ulnar part of the palm. This vessel travels above the fibrous cord to the little finger, and the cord has to be dissected very carefully beneath it. The first change of dressing will show no disorders of the blood flow of the skin. The Z-plasties of the proximal phalanges and of the palm are then clearly recognizable in the slides.

It is obvious from these few remarks that the treatment of Dupuytren's contractures demands a great deal of detailed attention. The fundamental rules of the surgery of the hand and of plastic surgery have to be observed, for good results to be obtained, which will secure a fully functioning hand even after many years.

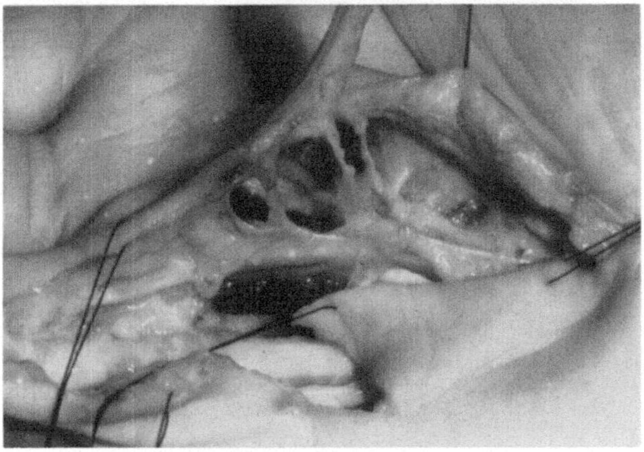

Fig. 2. Wound of the palm with Z-plasty in operation for Dupuytren's contracture. The conservation of the blood-vessels entering the skin should be noted (the palmar aponeurosis has already been removed)

Plastic Surgery of the Hip Following Trauma

Th. C. Reimers

The present heavy accident toll confronts us with many problems in plastic and reconstructive surgery of the hip.

We must deal with injuries of the great vessels and soft tissue, but the main problem are late results of different kinds of injuries to the hip joint. Even if a restoration of the anatomical situation was possible the function often remains impaired.

In this regard I would like to present our operative possibilities.

In Russia during World War II, I made use of the standard methods of plastic reconstruction as advocated by Payr, mainly with interposition of fat tissue as described by Lexer.

In special situations these methods may give good results even today. In comparison, however, reconstruction with Endoprostheses produces better long term results.

Since 1947 — that is for about 20 years — I have dealt with these problems. My experience covers more than 240 operations of this kind.

The uncertainty of the future of a foreign body had lead nearly all authors in this field — from the beginning to the present — to the opinion that these methods should be limited to old patients only.

According to my experience this rule should no longer be valid — as today's injuries involve the adolescent as well.

As an example see a 17-year old boy with severe trauma to the hip. In this case I performed a reconstruction with a Moore-prosthesis in August 1961. Note the

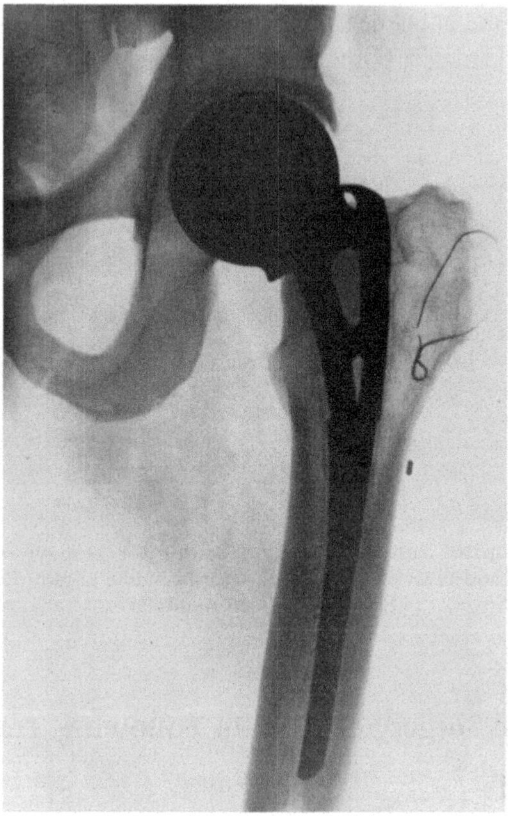

Fig. 1. Male, 24 years; was 17 years, when operated on. Breakage of the stem occured 2 months after insertion without any consequences. X-ray shows the situation 7 years after operation. Walking ability without limit

fracture of the prosthesis, which occurred 2 months after the operation — without any sensation to the patient.

Fig. 1 shows his condition in 1968 — 7 years after operation — he is now 24 years old.

The table gives the age of 140 injured persons we operated upon. The youngest was 15 years old.

In our study over a period of 10 years we sometimes saw slight but never severe or abnormal reactions in the area between bone and foreign body, even when a severe degree of osteoporosis was present.

In three women over 60 years of age we saw, however, a slow penetration of the metallic head through the acetabulum, as shown in Fig. 2. This process required 6 years.

In all three cases the bottom of the acetabulum had suffered previous damage. In this case, for example, by radiation.

There seems to be, however, no reason to exclude adolescents from the use of an Endoprosthesis if the situation makes it necessary.

Studying the relevant, mainly foreign literature on this matter you will be convinced that with an easy technique you should be able to gain good results in roughly 70% of these cases.

With regard to the extended literature on this subject I may refer to my article in the „Handbuch der Unfallheilkunde, Vol. III", Edition Enke, Stuttgart.

Table

10—19 years	3
20—29 years	7
30—39 years	10
40—49 years	15
50—59 years	25
60—69 years	45
70—79 years	32
80—89 years	3
	140

In the evaluation of the results of these methods the opinion on the European continent differs widely. In contrast to the optimistic statistics of the American literature a critical point of view dominates here. The opinion prevails that none of these patients with an Endoprosthesis has a normal ability to walk. Most of them have a painful hip. "None of them is walking without a cane" Jörg Böhler, for instance, pointed out at the Austrian Society for Traumatology in Salzburg in 1967 and the same opinion dominated

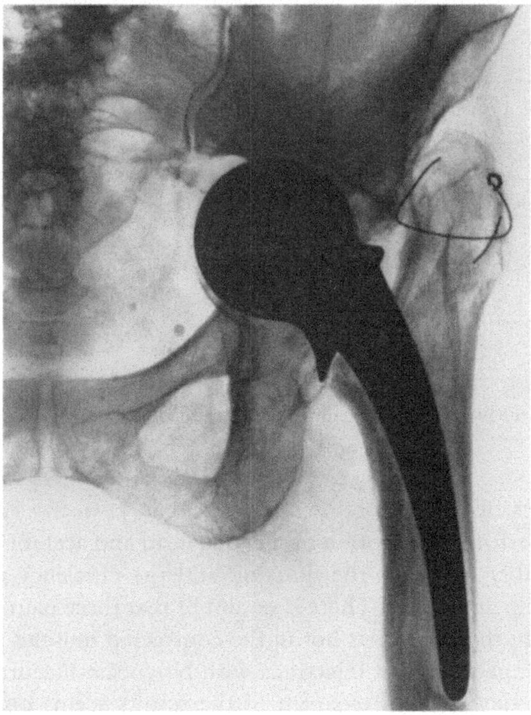

Fig. 2. This prosthesis wandered in the course of 6 years through the socket of the hip bone in a female with congenital dysplasia of the acetabulum

in nearly all other papers and round-table discussions. But this is not quite true as I will demonstrate in a film. No doubt the results differ widely.

In an analysis of our cases in 1960 it was demonstrated that age, weight and physical strength were of less importance compared to the angle and the perfection of the anatomical reconstruction in comparison with the opposite hip.

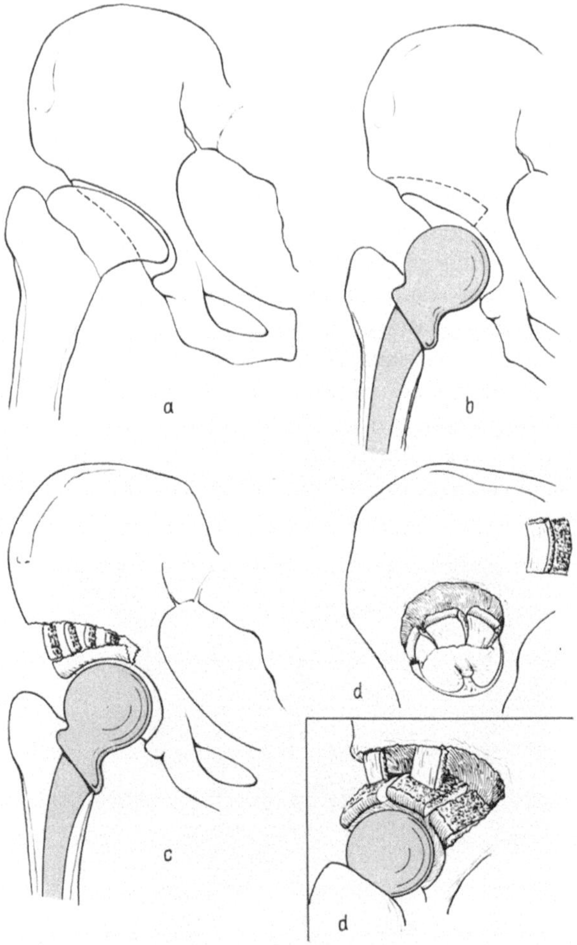

Fig. 3. Scheme of moulding a severely deformed acetabulum with preservation of the cortical lining

A little shortness of the femoral neck, a less than perfectly correct antetorsion angle, a carelessly performed adaption of metallic head and acetabulum will — in the long run — inevitably influence the function and the efficiency of the leg with a painful contracted hip at the end. There is no doubt that these pains have their origin not in the bone or in the prosthesis but in the contracted muscles as can be demonstrated by the prolonged effect of injections with Novocain-Decortin.

In our point of view an improvement of the results seems only possible if this kind of plastic surgery is done with much more care in the restoration of the anatomical dimensions of the individual than was done up to now.

With this in mind we ascertain individually the diameter of the femoral head, angle of neck, anteversion angle and so on by special X-ray examination in order to have the necessary guide lines during the operation. Some things may be mentioned in detail:

The necessity of a careful adaptation of femoral head to the acetabulum.

Physiologically the femoral head is kept in position by the atmospheric-pressure with a power of 17 kg. If this is not taken into consideration it will result in a hip which I tried to characterize as a "muscular wobble prosthesis". Those patients are frightened to take the first step. The reason for this is that under these circumstances a patient at first has to bring his joint under muscular tension through an effort of his will and this is accompanied by an uncomfortable feeling which he never brings under control.

On the other hand the adaptation of head and acetabulum should under no circumstances be forced by molding the acetabulum. If the lining cortex is destroyed, an uncontrolled sliding of the metallic head, sometimes for years, was the inevitable result in our series.

If there is a great discrepancy as shown in Fig. 4a a reconstruction with preservation of the cortical lining illustrated in Fig. 3 may lead to a satisfactory result, as demonstrated in Fig. 4b.

Apart from my own investigations I was unable to find discussions of the fate of the cartilage lining the acetabulum. According to my observations a malnutrition in the border line between metallic head and cartilage of the acetabulum seems to be the rule. In a re-operated case we saw a complete necrosis of the whole cartilage in the acetabulum although no infection was evident.

Therefore in principle we remove or diminish the cartilage in the acetabulum during operation.

In the end the bottom of the acetabulum is covered by a vital connective tissue or a very thin layer of cartilage.

Further investigation of the damage to the cartilage at the level of the metallic head seems necessary. I found only a hint about similar disturbances by LUNCEFIELD JR. in Journal of bone and joint surgery **47**, 842 (1965).

These problems can be dealt with surgically if we are acquainted with important details. It is, however, in many cases impossible to surmount the difficulties in the restoration of the correct length and angle of the femoral neck. Our follow-up made quite clear that an insufficiency of gluteal muscles indicates that the length of femoral neck was not correctly estimated. We found a decrease in walking in 50% of our operated patients. The difficulties arise from the construction of the metallic prosthesis. There we have a great variety in diameter of the head at our disposal but by no means in length of the femoral neck (Fig. 5).

The distance between the highest point of the head and the supporting neck of the protheses is in every device 5 cm.

If there is a sufficient amount of the neck at your disposal you may be able to level the situation by sparing a certain amount of the femoral neck, always comparing with the normal side, if present.

If a strong dwindling of the femoral neck down to the intertrochanteric line is present, an adjustment may sometimes be possible by using a prosthesis of the Gosse-type.

In general such a procedure will lead to an insufficiency of the involved muscles.

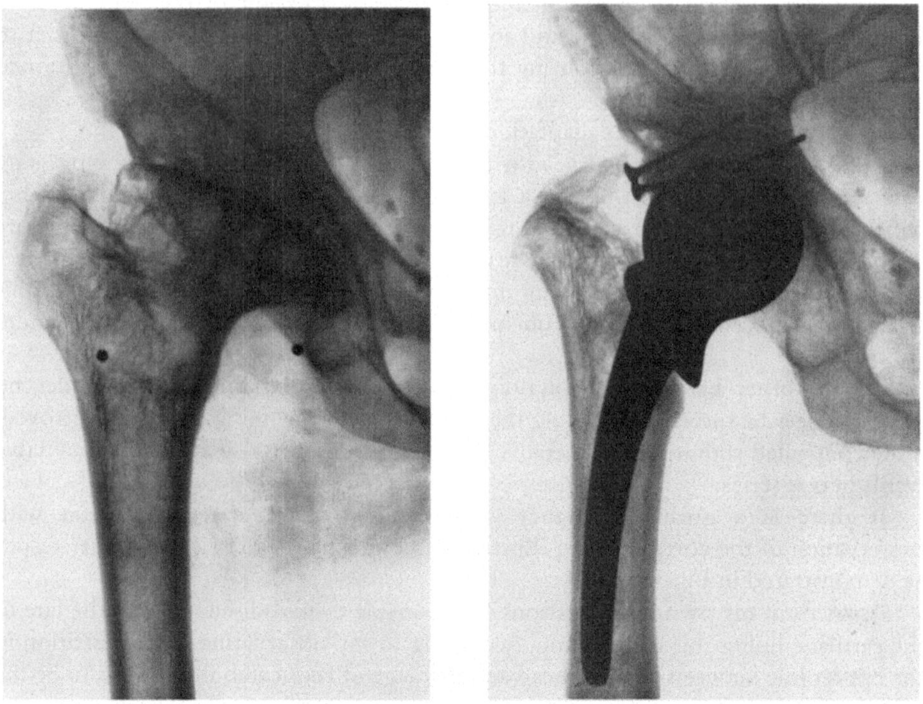

Fig. 4. Procedure as given in Fig. 3. Male, 46 years: a) *Left:* situation before, b) *Right:* 2 years after operation

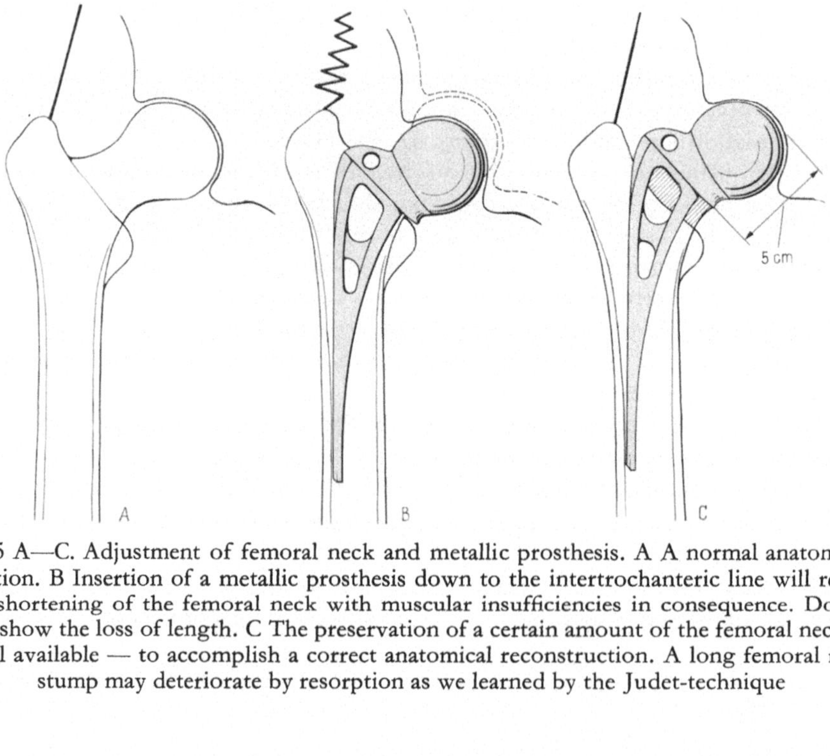

Fig. 5 A—C. Adjustment of femoral neck and metallic prosthesis. A A normal anatomical situation. B Insertion of a metallic prosthesis down to the intertrochanteric line will result in a shortening of the femoral neck with muscular insufficiencies in consequence. Dotted lines show the loss of length. C The preservation of a certain amount of the femoral neck — if still available — to accomplish a correct anatomical reconstruction. A long femoral neck stump may deteriorate by resorption as we learned by the Judet-technique

I want to emphasize here that, in principle, all metallic prostheses at our disposal today do not meet with sufficient accuracy the necessity of an individual reconstruction of the hip.

New investigations regarding these problems seem necessary.

In connection with the problems of the adaptation of the femoral neck and angles the question arises whether, in view of the good experiences with "muscular decompression" of Voss in painful hips, it is wise to shorten the femoral neck more than 0.5 to 1 cm during operation.

We studied this problem in several cases and found that such a procedure seems to be unfavourable. The reconstruction of normal tension in the gluteal muscle is the main difficulty which obviously can not always be met by adaptation of the femoral neck alone.

The under-correction of this muscular tension seems to be the rule and not the over-correction. If a prosthesis was inserted in an incorrect anteversion angle the damage to the muscle will be as fatal as a shortening of the femoral neck.

The patient will not be able to compensate this failure in rotary balance.

It seems to be necessary to control the position of the inserted prosthesis during operation by X-ray, but this is still a doubtful method.

We are operating and controlling with a special X-ray image intensifier. But until now we are not able to control the insertion with sufficient accuracy. On top of this the construction of the prothesis does not meet the physiological conditions in the anteversion angle.

Wittepol — a Dutch author — made an improvement of this kind in construction of a new prosthesis.

To sum up we must emphasize that in our follow-up and analysis of 243 patients with reconstruction of a defective hip joint by endoprosthesis a well-balanced muscular function seems to be the main problem. We have demonstrated that a joint with normal range and function can be obtained even in the long run. But it can only be obtained if all anatomical changes are taken into consideration individually and correlated with the normal hip.

Frequent errors, in our series 50%, are an imperfect adaptation in length and angle of the femoral neck and the angle of anteversion. This muscular imbalance leads nearly inevitably to a contracted painful hip as the final result. According to our experience, however, we must emphasize that adolescents should be given an endoprosthesis, if a balanced anatomical reconstruction seems possible.

Traumatic Injuries of the Groin Including the Genitalia*

Nicholas G. Georgiade, and Richard A. Mladick

Traumatic losses in the groin area may be generalized as in burns (Fig. 1) or localized as in most penetrating wounds and gunshot injuries. Involvement of larger areas of injury usually occur with automotive injuries, farm or industrial accidents. Unprotected rotary mechanical devices may catch a portion of the clothing which then entangles and avulses the loose skin of genitalia. Because the skin is loose in this

* From the Department of Surgery, Division of Plastic Surgery, Duke University Medical Center, Durham, North Carolina 27706.

area it is easily separated superficial to Buck's fascia of the penis, and inferior to the tunica dartos of the scrotum. The classic injury is of the degloving type and usually spares the body of the penis and the testes. Prompt reconstruction of this degloved external covering may give the patient normal functioning genitalia.

Resurfacing of the denuded areas of the penis and scrotal areas is considered to be an emergency procedure. Previous literature has described a number of procedures in the management of this type of problem [*1*, *10*, *16*, *17*, *18*].

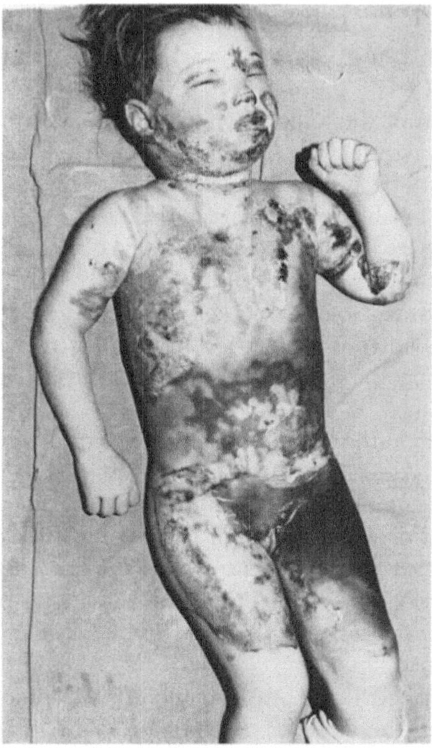

Fig. 1. Generalized extensive third degree burn involving the entire groin, genitalia area as well as abdomen and chest

Penile Repair

Avulsion of the skin of the penis usually extends to the coronal margin of the glans penis. Split thickness skin grafts of moderate thickness are used to resurface the denuded areas. The technical aspect involves the insertion of an indwelling urethral catheter prior to any application of the skin grafts. These grafts are applied circumferentially after the penis is extended to its longest possible length. The grafts are applied in an interdigitating manner to prevent a straight line scar contracture from occurring and allowing greater length of the scar during expansion of the penis (Figs. 2 A, B, C). The grafts are dressed over a bolus of mechanics waste and not dressed for 7 days as replacement dressings are more difficult to obtain satisfactorily. This also allows sufficient time for the graft to "take" to the underlying surface. Replacing of a second dressing over the grafted area is not as satisfactory.

Not infrequently a tragic accident will cause the loss of the shaft of the penis. The reconstruction of the total penis involves a number of reconstructive procedures with the techniques previously described by FRUMKIN [*12*], GILLIES [*13*], and others [*11*, *14*, *15*, *16*] having been found to be the most satisfactory. This usually consists of elevating a tubed abdominal pedicle flap, a tubed urethral flap, and then implantation of an autogenous cartilage or plastic implant at the superior portion of the tube prior to transfer or at a later stage. The composite skin tube should be inserted into the

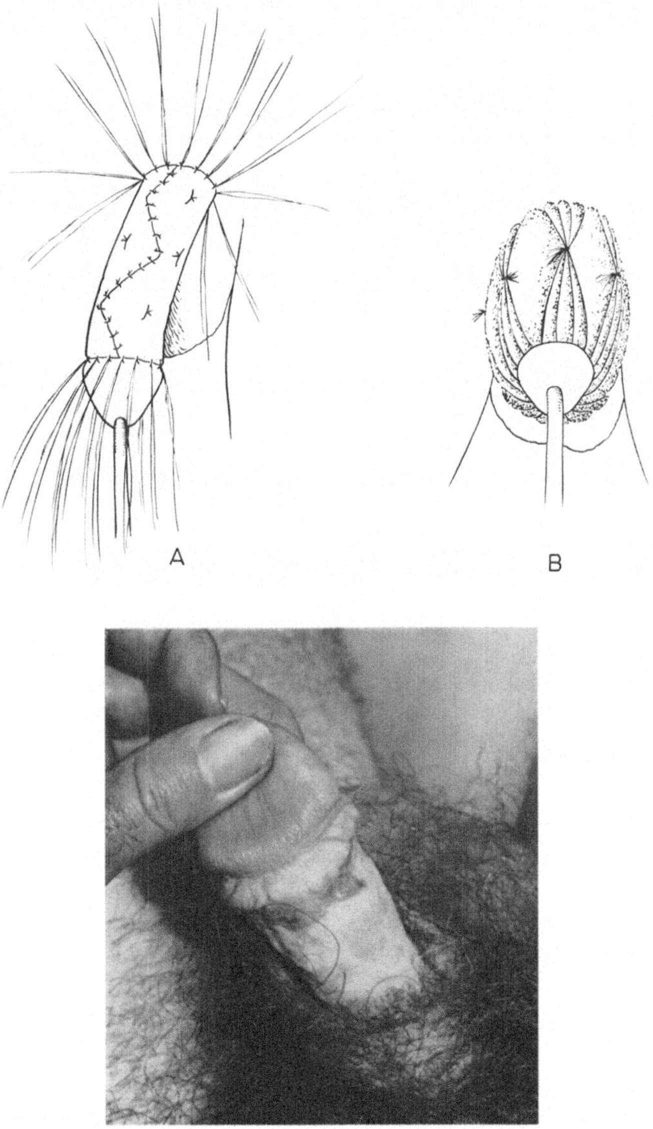

c

Fig. 2. A Technique for applying split thickness skin grafts to penis with interdigitating of grafts. B The type of bolus used to secure the graft applied on the extended penis. C Post-operative appearance of split thickness graft to penis remaining cavernous body area anastomosing the urethral remnant with the new tube (Figs. 3 A, B, C, D). A diverting perineal urethrostomy is carried out prior to this urethral junction. In children it may be possible to spare complicated tube reconstruction by using scrotal flaps when available. In any case it is always important to look for and use any residual portions of corpora that are spared. Exploration of the ischial region and lengthening procedures may increase the available length of these remnants of corpora.

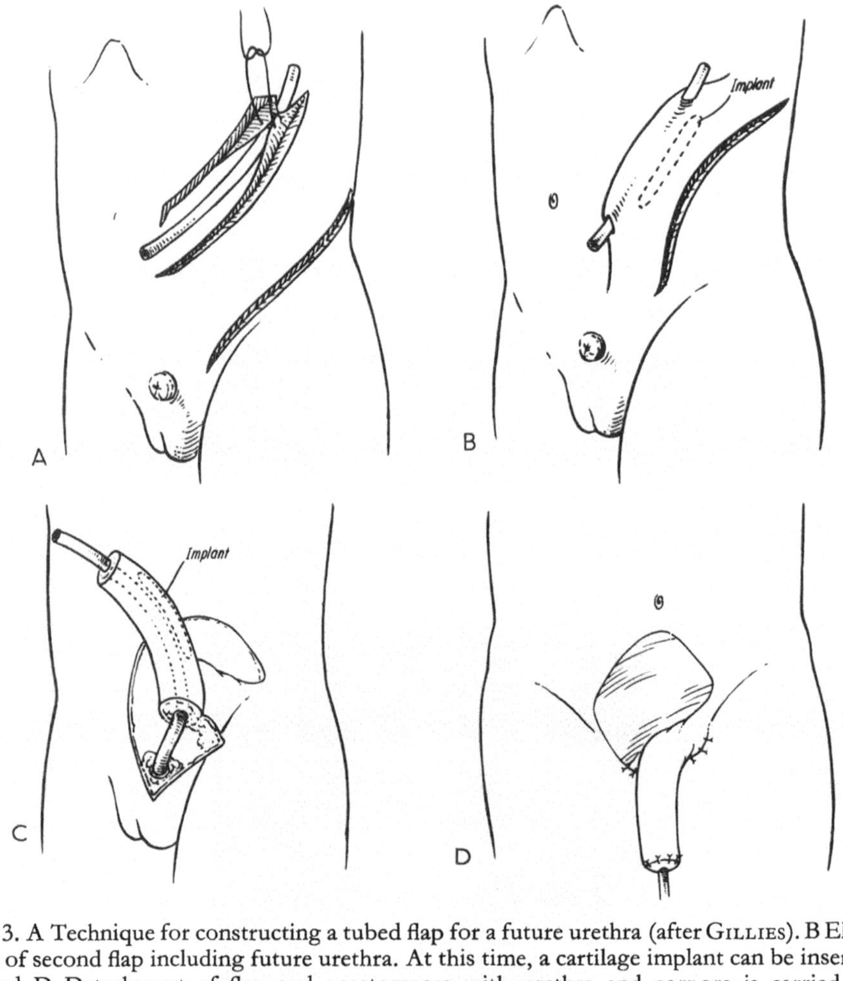

Fig. 3. A Technique for constructing a tubed flap for a future urethra (after GILLIES). B Elevation of second flap including future urethra. At this time, a cartilage implant can be inserted. C and D Detachment of flap and anastomoses with urethra and corpora is carried out

Scrotal Repair

Avulsion of the scrotal skin involves not only coverage of the denuded area but also protection of the exposed testicles and the spermatic cords. Partial avulsion of the skin may allow repair of the scrotum with the remaining skin affording protection to the testes. Initially, there may be considerable tightness as a result of the repair, however, this skin used in the repair will gradually loosen over a period of months. Subtotal skin loss may also be treated with split thickness skin grafts in most cases.

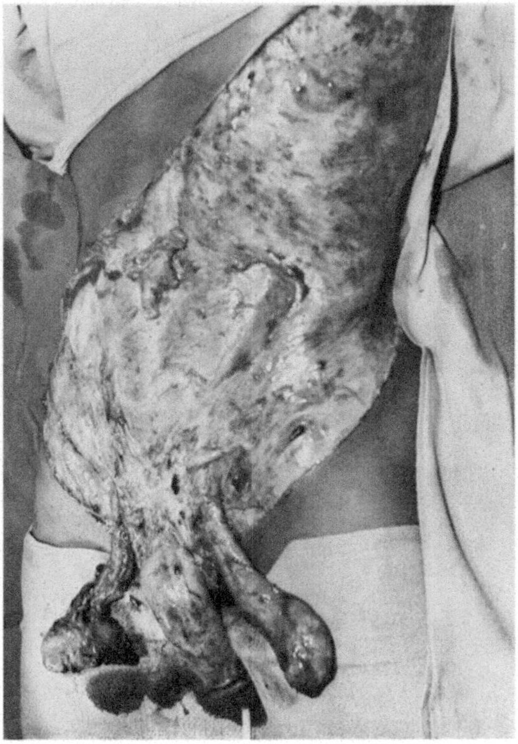

4A

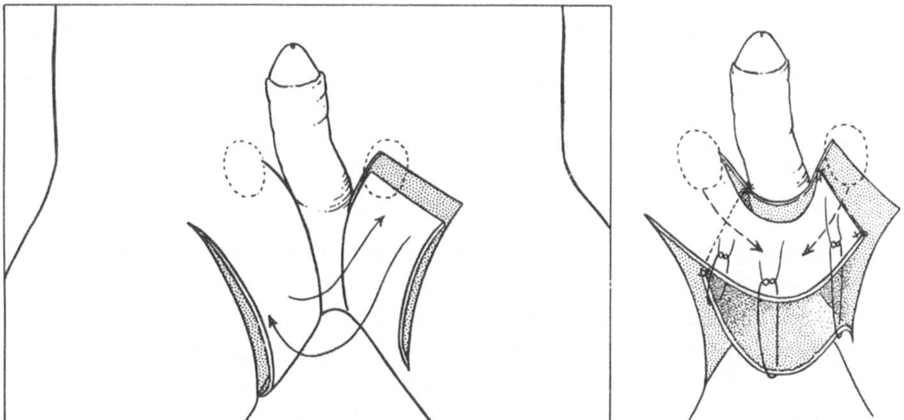

4B

Fig. 4. A Traumatic avulsion of soft tissues of groin, shaft of penis, and testes. A + B Elevation, delay and transposition of thigh flaps as the base of the penis for formation of new scrotum. C Size, location, and position of thigh flaps illustrated with the testes safely positioned just under the skin. D Final position of thigh flaps prior to and after releasing lateral margins one month later. E Position of flaps shown at the time of original transfer. F and G Final appearance of reconstructed groin, penile and scrotal defects with split thickness skin grafts and thigh flaps to reconstruct scrotum

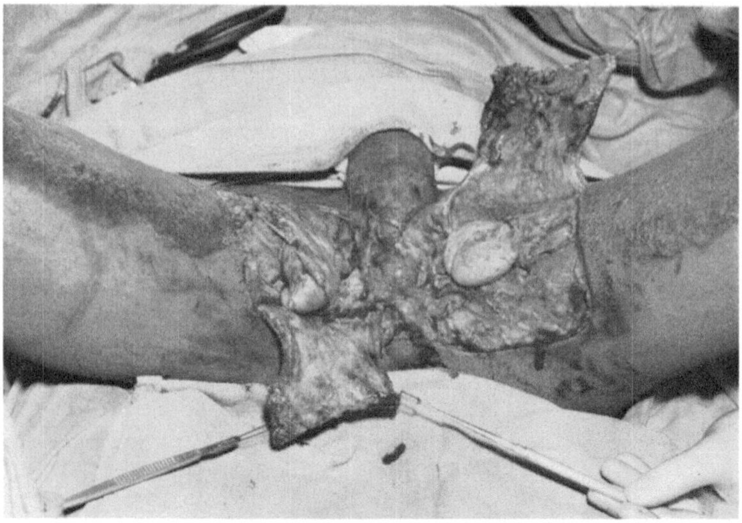

4C

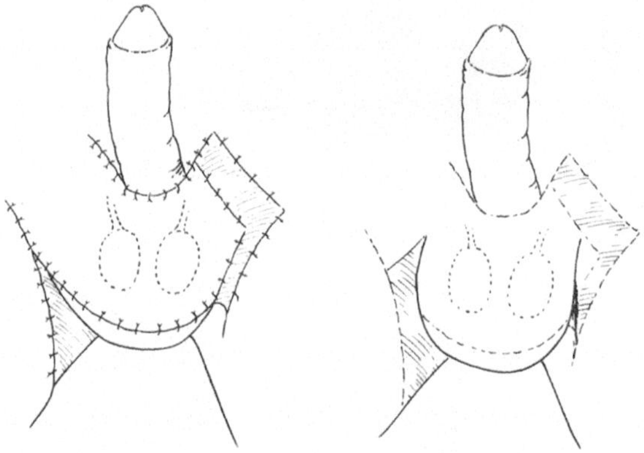

4D

In situations where there is total loss of scrotal skin exposing the vessels and the denuded testes the procedure of choice is the immediate formation of subcutaneous thigh pockets immediately under the skin just lateral and superior to their normal positions. This location between the skin and subcutaneous tissues has been found to be within a suitable temperature range which will not affect spermatogenesis. If buried below the subcutaneous fat the increased temperature may be harmful as to future spermatogenesis.

Completed reconstruction involves the formation of a suitable compartment or pocket. This can be carried out in stages by outlining superiorly based flaps after the method of ROBERTSON [3] and ROBINSON [6] over the buried testes. The flaps containing the testes and vas deferens and vessels are rotated medially. They are then sutured together in the midline constructing a new scrotal sac. A technique found to be satisfactory in our hands involves the use of high medial thigh flaps which are delayed, one based superiorly and one inferiorly. The flaps are elevated and attached

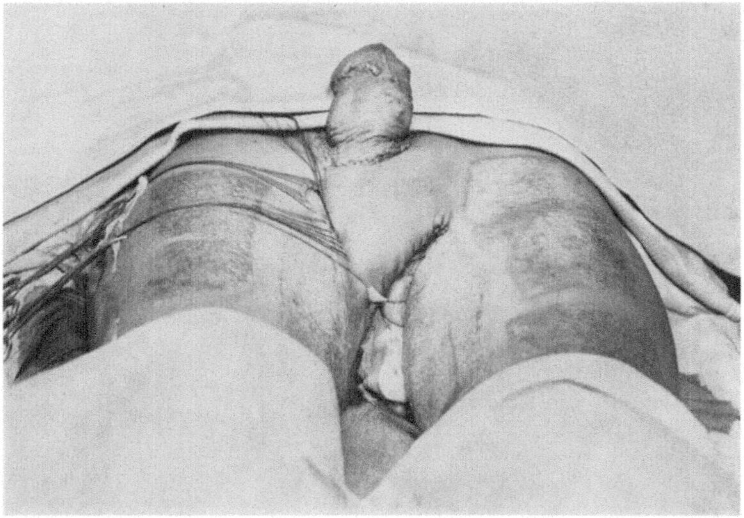

4E

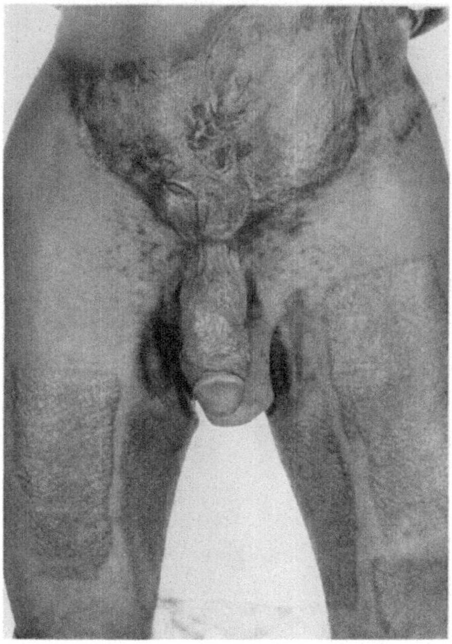

4F

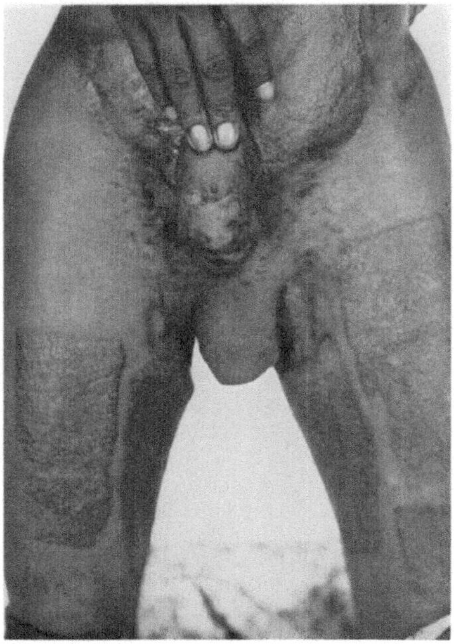

4G

with one flap superimposed on the other and containing the testicles. Partial detachment from the thighs is then carried out at a later date to contour the new scrotum (Figs. 4 A, B, C, D, E, F, G).

Associated Inguinal and Perineal Loss

If these areas have sustained trauma as a result of thermal burns the usual procedure is debridement and resurfacing with split thickness skin grafts. Automotive and mechanical injuries may cause more extensive damage quite often involving the

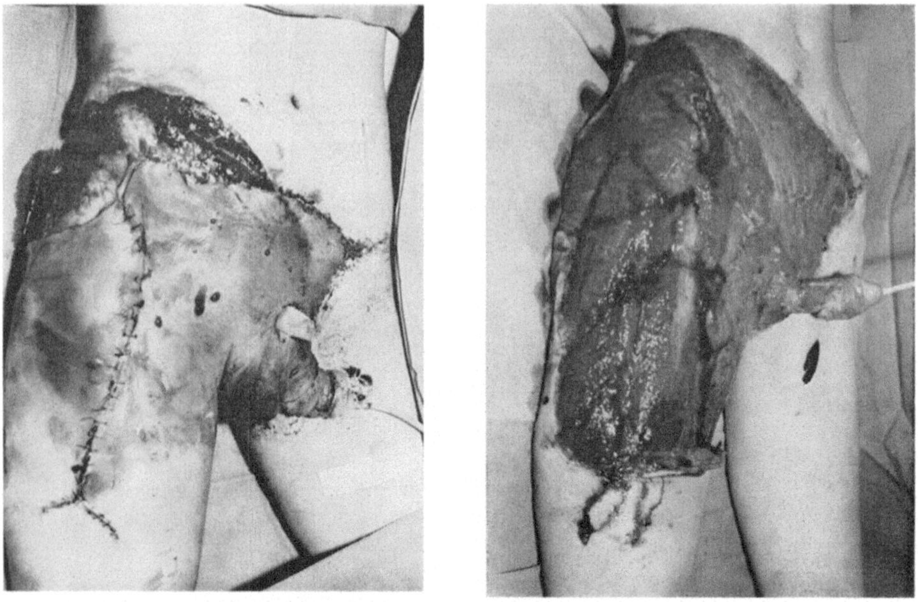

A B

Fig. 5. A and B Automotive injury with resultant necrosis of tissues of groin, scrotum, and shaft of the penis

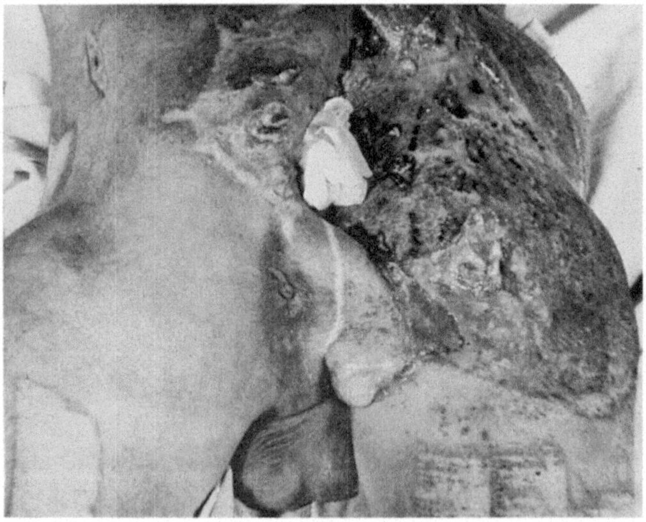

6A

Fig. 6. A and B Extensive avulsing injuries of perineal, buttock, and back complicated by a severe clostridial infection

closely associated genitalia. In these situations selective debridement and early resurfacing usually with skin grafts is indicated (Figs. 5 A, B). In some extensive cases a temporary diverting colostomy is indicated prior to resurfacing procedures. A serious complication of these injuries is gas gangrene which we have treated in the

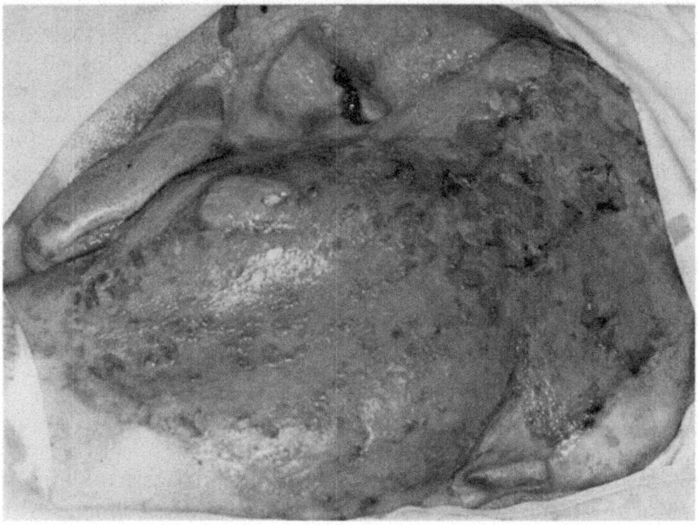

6 B

hyperbaric unit with 2 to 3 atmospheres of oxygen for varying periods of time (usually 2 to 3 h) (Figs. 6 A, B). The hyperbaric oxygen is felt to be an important adjunct in treating clostridial infections and is used prior to and after the debridement. It is felt this treatment may decrease or stop the clostridial population and minimize the necessary debridement.

Technically we have found abduction of the legs and thighs by retraction, skeletal fixation, or splints valuable in obtaining a good "take" of split thickness grafts. This technique decreases the temperature and moisture of the perineal area and facilitates wound care.

In every perineal injury sphincteric damage is a potential problem. When the sphincters are badly involved it is best to perform a diverting colostomy and carry out the simplest repair possible at that time. Later evaluation of the sphincter function will then disclose whether a secondary procedure such as the Stone fascial sling procedure or a gracilis muscle transplant is indicated.

Acknowledgement. To Dr. Kenneth L. Pickrell for the use of one of his patients shown in the illustrations.

References

1. Gibbs, R. W.: Charleston Med. J. Rev. **10**, 154 (1855).
2. Borgoras, N.: Zbl. Chir. **63**, 1271 (1936).
3. Robertson, J. F.: Sth. Med. Surg. **93**, 527 (1931).
4. Roth, R., and K. Warren: J. Urol. (Baltimore) **52**, 162 (1944).
5. Owens, N.: Surgery **12**, 88 (1942).
6. Robinson, D. W., K. L. Stephenson, and E. C. Padgett: Plast. reconstr. Surg. **1**, 58 (1946).
7. Brown, J. B.: Surg. Gynec. Obstet. **65**, 362 (1937).
8. Davis, A., and R. Berner: Plast. reconstr. Surg. **3**, 417 (1948).
9. Sutton, S.: N. Y. St. J. Med. **43**, 2279 (1943).
10. Davis, A., and R. Berner: Plast. reconstr. Surg. **3**, 417 (1948).
11. Robertson, J. F.: Sth. Med. Surg. **93**, 527 (1931).
12. Frumkin, A. P.: Amer. Rev. Sov. Med. **1944**, II, 14.

13. Gillies, H., and R. J. Harrison: Brit. J. plast. Surg. **1**, 8 (1948).
14. Loeffler, R. A., and E. S. Soyegh: J. Urol. (Baltimore) **84**, 559 (1960).
15. Gelb, J., M. Malament, and S. LaVerme: Plast. reconstr. Surg. **24**, 62 (1959).
16. Masters, F., and D. Robinson: J. Trauma **8**, 430 (1968).
17. Huffman, W., D. Culp, and R. Flocks: Injuries to the male genitalia. Reconstructive plastic surgery, pp. 2057—2073. Philadelphia: W. B. Saunders Company 1964.
18. Millard, D. R.: Plast. Reconstr. Surg. **38**, 10 (1966).

Reconstructive Surgery of the Legs Following Trauma*

Kenneth Pickrell, Richard Mladick, Lawrence Thompson, and Morton Kasdan

In our modern-mechanized era, fractures, lacerations and avulsing injuries of the lower extremities are the most frequent; next come burns. While there have been many changes in therapy during the past decade, these consist of innovations and augmentations of the fundamental principles of wound care, which, in themselves, remain essentially unchanged because they are based on sound surgical judgement. The treatment of all injuries, regardless of type, must be individualized. This will encourage the physician to broaden his scope, which will allow flexibility of the general rules. The purpose of this presentation is to outline and re-emphasize some of the general principles in the management in treatment of soft tissue injuries of the legs.

The aim of surgical treatment of soft tissue trauma is to convert the accidental wound into a clean surgical wound, and then to repair it. While the creation of a surgical wound is not always possible, certain rules of therapy will closely approach the ideal if carefully followed.

Cleansing. Proper cleansing of the traumatic wound is essential. While many bacteriostatic and bacteriocidal agents are used widely as "mild" antiseptics, yet any agent powerful enough to kill bacteria may also traumatize the raw surface of a wound. The routine of antiseptics within the wound is to be condemned, although these same antiseptics may be valuable in the cleansing and preparation of the surrounding intact skin. Phisohex is an excellent cleansing agent[1]. The use of Pre-op Surgical Sponges are very good to cleanse the skin. The wounds should then be irrigated copiously with isotonic saline or Ringer's solution.

Debridement. The second step in the general care of soft tissue injuries is widely advocated, but frequently practiced too conservatively. The entire purpose of debriding a traumatic wound is to convert it into a clean surgical wound, yet all too often either the press of time or fear of creating additional deformity leads to the mere trimming of jagged, contused skin edges and the removal of bits of fat, muscle and bone that are obviously no longer viable.

Closure. The principles of closure of a traumatic wound are essentially the same regardless of the part of the body involved. Every attempt should be made to obtain

* From the Division of Plastic and Reconstructive Surgery, Duke University Medical Center, Durham, N. C. 27706.

This study supported in part by National Institute of Dental Research, National Institutes of Health, Bethesda, Maryland (Grant No. DE 01899).

[1] Phisohex. Sterling-Winthrop Co., 90 Park Ave., New York, N. Y. 10016 Pre-op Textured Surgical Sponge. Davis & Geck Co., Danbury, Conn.

a careful layer-by-layer closure. The best results are obtained by meticulous approximation of all wound edges, using small suture materials and small instruments. In general, only absorbable collagen or catgut sutures should be buried in these contaminated wounds.

Hematoma. One of the commoner mechanical inhibitors of wound healing is the subcutaneous collection of serum or blood. The pressure from a large hematoma may cause venous thrombosis and delay or failure of tissue union. A Hematoma may become infected or it can organize and degenerate into a fluid-filled, cystic mass that may require surgical removal. Hemostasis should be absolute to prevent mechanical interference with the healing of a traumatic wound.

Dead Space. In large avulsing wounds, the loss of subcutaneous tissue acts as a deterrent to wound healing. This space fills rapidly with blood or serous exudate, which is an ideal culture medium for bacteria, and also it prevents raw surface-to-raw surface opposition which is necessary for firm primary healing and union. Some large unavoidable dead spaces, e.g., when large amounts of subcutaneous tissue are avulsed, are best treated with suction drainage and light compression dressings.

Tension. Mechanical tension at the suture line is one of the commonest causes of wound separation and is second only to infection as a cause of postoperative keloid or hypertrophic scar formation. If the sutures are too tight, they may act as miniature tourniquets, thus strangulating the tissues and preventing the normal process of repair. If a wound cannot be closed without undue tension, some form of relaxation incisions or grafting procedure is essential.

Dressings. The postoperative dressing of the traumatic wound is almost as important as the original reparative procedure. A good initial result can be preserved or lost by the dressing care it receives. A dressing should not only protect the sutured wound from external contamination, but it should also promote healing by immobilization of the surrounding area. Putting injured tissue at rest increases its rate of healing; this is accomplished best by a careful and adequate postoperative dressing. Immobilization may be accomplished by either a bulky dressing, which mechanically limits motion in the entire area, or localized splinting. Adequate immobilization adds to the patient's comfort, since excessive motion of any injured area is painful. One of the commonest defects in dressing care is probably attributable to the surgeon's natural curiosity. It is, indeed, a temptation to change dressings quite often to "make sure that things are going well." The motion and mechanical irritation associated with frequent dressing changes prolongs healing, adds to the patient's discomfort and may increase postoperative scarring. Unless there is some specific indication such as pain, swelling, unexplained fever or tenderness, there is no reason to change a comfortable dressing oftener than every 2 or 3 days.

The use of Sulfamylon ointment has proven very beneficial, especially in burns; also in the preparation of ulcers and granulating surfaces for grafting[2]. We have been so impressed by its effectiveness in controlling surface infections, predominently due to Pseudomonas, its use has now been extended to donor areas, as an ointment-impregnated dressing following clean elective operations as well as those reparative procedures following trauma.

---

[2] Sulfamylon, Sterling-Winthrop Co., 90 Park Ave., New York, N. Y. 10016.

Grafting the Lower Extremities

The use of split grafts to resurface burns, areas of avulsion and ulcers is a procedure of election. A number of ingenious dermatomes: Padget-Hood, the Brown electro-dermatome and the relatively new Brown Air dermatome have all simplified split grafting procedures[3]. There are a number of meshing devices available which can perforate a skin graft to allow it to be easily stretched to cover one and one-half times its original size.

Pedicle Grafts. Pedicle grafts are always procedures of necessity. A common error is to use local flaps without due consideration of the defect to be covered. When an injured lower extremity must act as both donor and recipient, a good result is often unobtainable. The use of local flaps, although useful in other parts of the body, are fraught with danger on the lower extremities. Local rotation flaps rarely succeed except in the case of small defects on the plantar surface; the lateral advancement flap is effective only for defects of the proximal leg; and the bipedicle sliding flap, is reserved for defects of the mid-leg. Even though a local flap may first appear to flourish following transfer, usually its success is illusory, since it is likely to be too small to provide the resilient coverage needed. Mere rearrangement of the soft tissues on an already damaged leg is unprofitable when larger pieces of tissue with a good blood supply can be brought in from other areas: the contralateral leg or thigh, or the abdominal wall or torso.

Torso Pedicles. Among pedicle flaps raised on the torso are the open or closed jump flap, attached to the forearm as a carrier along most of its length; the tubed abdominal pedicle-with or without a "pancake". All require a vascular carrier, usually the wrist or forearm, which nourishes the flap en route to the desired recipient site.

Cross-leg and Cross-thigh Pedicles. A cross-leg or cross-thigh flap is used only if the opposite member is unscarred and unaffected by varicosities, cellulitis, peripheral vascular disease or if the patient is not older than 50 years. Knees and hip joints must be sufficiently mobile to permit close approximation of the two extremities at the point of pedicle attachment. The danger of venous thrombosis and possible embolism is always a treat in trying to immobilize extremities in patients over 50 years [7].

As outlined previously, a cross-extremity flap is always a procedure of necessity and should only be used when a split graft has ulcerated, when scar lies over the bony tibia or malleoli, or the tendon of Achilles; and when further reconstruction will involve operative orthopedic procedures. Pedicle grafts of skin and a heavy layer of subcutaneous adipose tissue will (1) provide a vascular bed to support additional surgical procedures on bone, tendon or nerve; and (2) withstand the surgical retraction and reparative processes required for these secondary procedures. Methods of planning, elevation, formation and transfer of pedicle flaps of all varieties are well documented in many plastic surgery articles and texts.

Each step of the procedure is vital to the life or death of the flap. Improperly based flaps, infection, kinking, insufficient delays, hurried detachments and improper fixation are all well known pitfalls in lower extremity reconstruction. The sound plastic surgical principles of flap reconstruction that were found valid in the past largely from the experience of two World Wars, still hold true and little new has been

---

[3] Padget-Hood Dermatome. Kansas City Assemblage Co., Kansas City, Mo. Brown Air Dermatome. Zimmer Manufacturing Co., Warsaw, Ind.

added. Today, however, the surgeon now has promising new tests for determining the fate of flap circulation, e.g. the Xenon test, [*1*] and he still has his ingenuity to help him in designing new flaps [*2*, *3*] and new types of fixation.

The following examples show how flexibility and ingenuity can help solve two difficult cases of lower extremity reconstruction. These cases illustrate (1) an

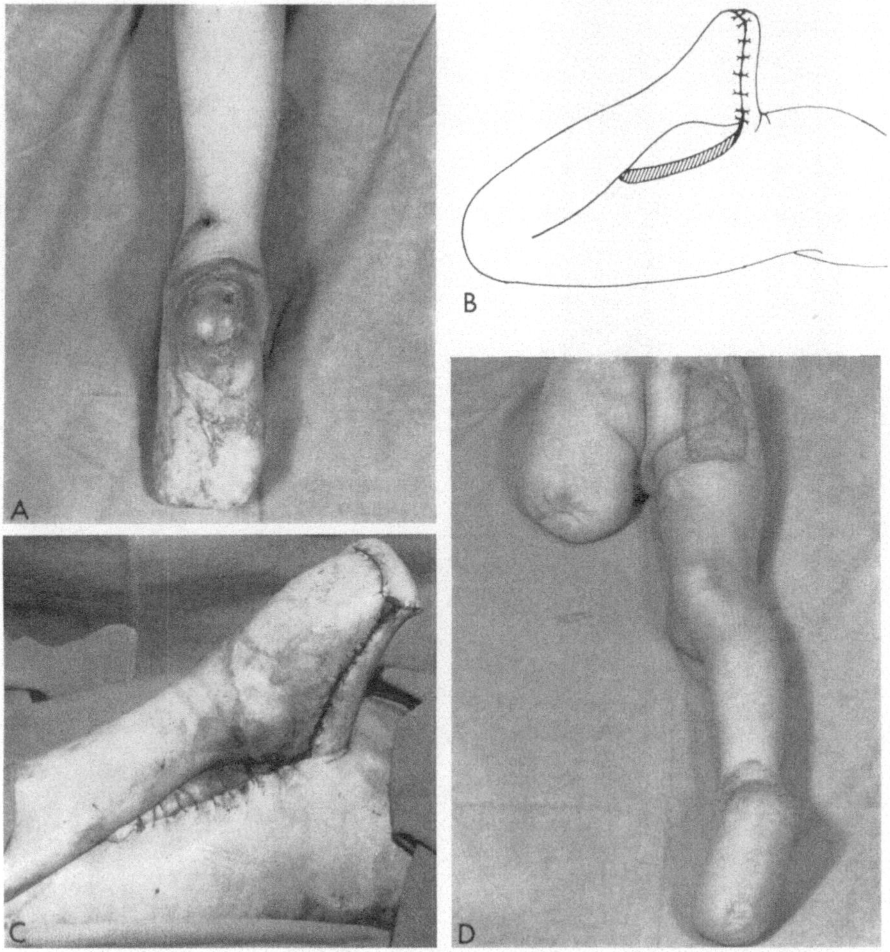

Fig. 1. A The right foot is shown. The left leg has been amputated above the knee. The foot is covered by a tenuous layer of scar tissue and skin grafts that were applied as temporary cover after the necrotic de-gloved skin was debrided. The os calcis partially exposed and the foot is tender and unable to bear weight. Pedicle flap coverage was clearly indicated. B Diagramatic representation of the acute flexion of the right knee enabling the entire plantar surface of the foot to be resurfaced by the ipsilateral posterior thigh flap. The cross hatch area represents the skin grafted donor flap site. C The operative view of the total plantar resurfacing by the posterior ipsilateral thigh flap. D The patient is shown lying prone 3 weeks following the detachment of the flap. The picture demonstrates (1) the healed donor area, (2) the complete range of knee extension and (3) the completely resurfaced sole of the right foot. The patient began weight-bearing approximately 2 weeks later and at approximately 3 months after his surgery, was walking well with the use of a prosthetic leg. Minimal sensation returned to the resurfaced foot which was otherwise painless

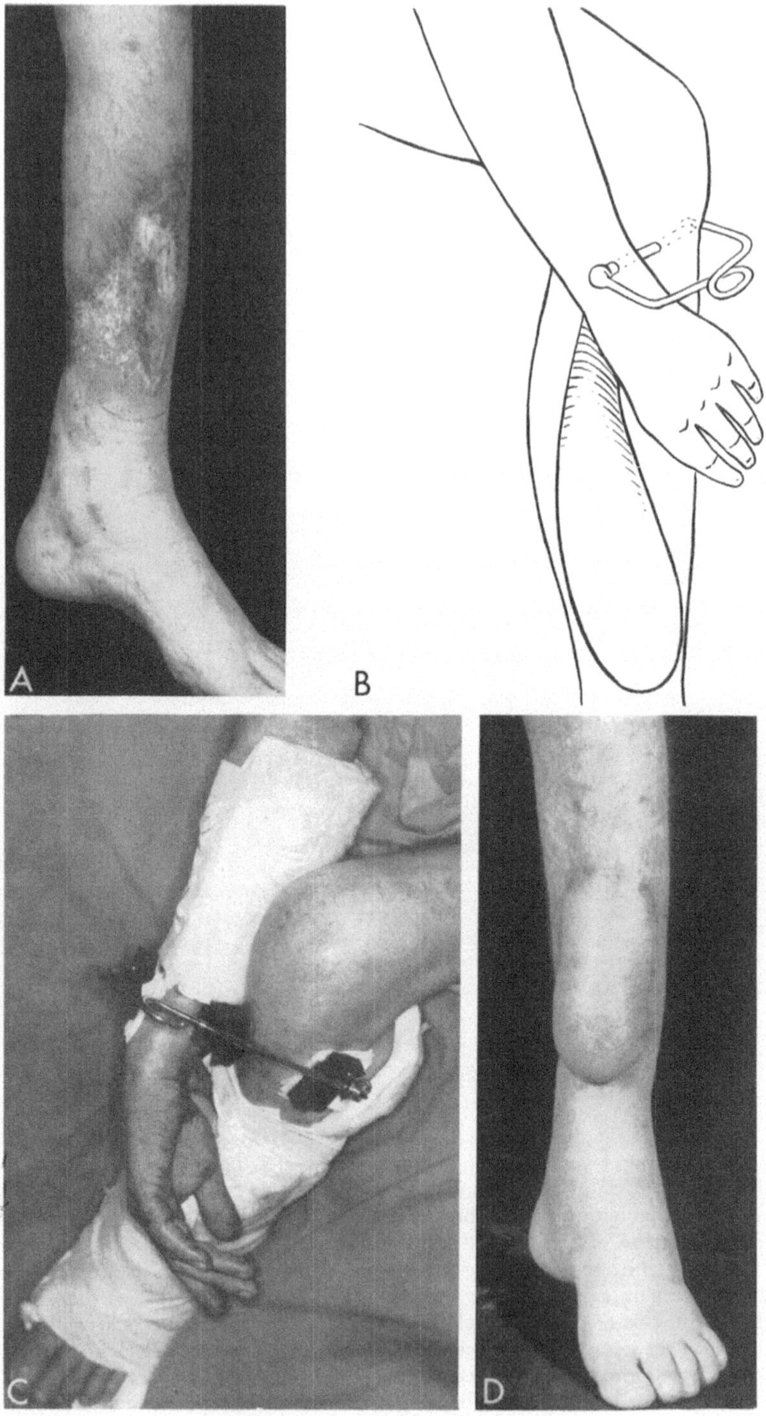
A
B
C
D

interesting new approach in flap planning and (2) a recent innovation in the fixation of extremities undergoing flap reconstruction.

Case I: WRB was an 8-year old boy who was playing on railroad tracks when he slipped and fell under a passing train. The left leg was crushed and had to be surgically amputated above the knee while the right foot was degloved of skin and subcutaneous tissue. The replaced de-gloved skin and subcutaneous tissue became necrotic and required total debridement. As a temporary cover, the foot was skin grafted with split skin grafts (Fig. 1 A). The skin grafted foot had virtually no subcutaneous tissue and never completely healed with the os calcis being exposed. The foot was painful and unable to support weight-bearing. It was considered necessary to apply healthy padding and skin to this foot for weight-bearing and flap coverage was therefore indicated. As the opposite thigh stump would have to bear the weight and trauma of a prosthetic leg, it was felt to be inadvisable to scar this stump further with a cross-thigh flap. With the cross-thigh flap contraindicated, it was felt the next logical solution to covering the entire plantar surface of the right foot was an abdominal tube flap on a wrist carrier. However, a simpler more direct solution was found. The patient had limber joints typical of an 8-year old boy and it was found that he could easily flex the right foot against his buttocks. Therefore, a 3 to 1 pedicle flap was designed — based superiorly on the gluteal vessels. After one delay procedure, the leg was flexed against the buttocks; the plantar surface of the foot was debrided and the flap lifted up covered the entire plantar surface of the right foot (Figs. 1 B, C). The leg was left in position for 3 weeks and the flap then cut loose and set in. The flap healed nicely giving excellent coverage to the entire plantar surface and full range of joint motion returned to the right knee within 2 weeks time (Fig. 1 D). 3 months afterwards, the child was walking well on his newly covered foot and a prosthetic leg.

Case II: RL was a 47-year old white male who suffered a shotgun injury to both lower extremities. The right leg suffered only skin and subcutaneous damage while the left leg suffered skin and subcutaneous loss and a fracture of both tibia and fibula (Fig. 2 A). Skin coverage was inadequate over the exposed fracture site and flap coverage was thoroughly a necessity. Cross-leg flap could not be used to the injured opposite extremity. Therefore, an abdominal tube brought down on a wrist carrier was elected. After a number of delay procedures, the abdominal tube was brought

---

Fig. 2. A The left leg is shown approximately 6 weeks following the shotgun blast which fractured both tibia and fibula and injured the opposite extremity. The tibia is exposed near the fracture site and there is insufficient coverage by scar tissue epithelium to permit bony healing. Cross-leg flap could not be used and the patient was not able to flex his knee sufficiently to permit a cross-thigh flap. Abdominal tube was indicated. B Diagramatic representation of the abdominal tube brought down on the left wrist. After the abdominal tube was set in, the only fixation was one Steinman pin drilled carefully through the ulna to avoid the ulnar nerve and artery and through-and-through the tibia. The Steinman pin ends were then connected by a Steinman pin bow. C The immediate postoperative view of the left wrist fixed in place by the Steinman pins which are connected by the Steinman pin bow. Felt padding has been placed between the forearm and knee. A posterior plaster splint helps hold the foot in the proper position to prevent foot drop. The pedicle of the abdominal tube is just barely visible coming off the radial side of the wrist. D 1 month after the division and set in of the abdominal tube to the injured area. The Steinman pin fixation holds in the wrist and lower leg area healed uneventfully as soon as the pin was removed. Full range of knee and wrist motion returned within a short time down on the left wrist. The flap was placed in the propose position and the left wrist fixed in place by drilling a Steinman pin through-and-through the ulna and through-and-through the tibia (Figs. 2 B, C). This Steinman pin was then connected with a Steinman pin bow. This was the only fixation used on this patient and was extremely comportable and allowed maximum exposure for cleaning and care of the wounds. At 3 weeks time, the flap was divided and set in; the Steinman pin was removed and the wound on the left wrist and the left tibia areas healed uneventfully (Fig. 2 D).

The use of skeletal fixation was reported by ALMS [*4*] when he used Steinman pins, connected with steel rods and univeral clamps for fixing crossleg flaps. ERIKSON [*5*] used the Hoffman transfixation method and CONSTANT and GRABB [*6*] recently described the use of two Steinman pins for cross-leg flap fixation. This would appear to be the first report of the use of a single Steinman pin for an arm-to-leg fixation.

References

1. MLADICK, R., R. CORTEN, and K. PICKRELL: Surg. Forum **17**, 489 (1966).
2. PICKRELL, K., and N. GEORGIADE: Postgrad. Med. **20**, 26 (1956).
3. MASTERS, F., N. GEORGIADE, and K. PICKRELL: J. Amer. med. Ass. **156**, 105 (1954).
4. ALMS, M.: Canad. med. Ass. J. **89**, 419 (1963).
5. ERIKSON, F., G. ERIKSON, and B. NYLEN: Plast. reconstr. Surg. **38**, 410 (1966).
6. CONSTANT, E., and W. GRABB: Plast. reconstr. Surg. **41**, 179 (1968).
7. PICKRELL, K.: Babcock's principles and practice of surgery. K. JONAS, Ed. Plastic, maxillofacial and reconstructive surgery, Chapter II, pp. 169—257. Philadelphia: Lea & Febiger 1954.

Operative Treatment of Fractures

Indications for Conservative and Operative Treatment of Fractures

G. Maurer and Fritz Lechner

The operative treatment of fractures is increasingly gaining ground in accident surgery, where it is replacing conservative treatment since atraumatic operative techniques, corrosion resistant metal implants, improved instruments, and better knowledge of the healing of fractured bones have been attained. Operative treatment has become more acceptable to the surgeon by his better training, to the patient by his greater understanding.

Operative treatment has the advantage of achieving early functional stability. There is no longer any need for long-lasting immobilization with the damage that it may cause, such as atrophy, limitation of movement, and disorders of circulation. The dangers of long confinement to bed, especially in the old, are avoided.

The disadvantages of operative treatment are well known. There is the danger of infection, which even the best technique and an antibiotic protection cannot prevent with certainty, the exclusion of bone fragments from proper nutrition, so that healing is delayed, the creation of additional soft tissue wounds and scars, the possibility of foreign body reaction from the exogenous material of osteosynthesis, and the necessity to remove this later, with the danger of the fracture recurring, e.g. in the vicinity of the matrix canals for screws or bolts.

Obviously, it is necessary to pay careful attention to the fundamental rules of conservative treatment of fractures.

It is not possible to lay down a general rule for the treatment of fractures, so as to obtain the best anatomical and functional results. Treatment plans adapted to each individual case and his peculiarities should stipulate the therapeutic measures, weighing up all advantages and disadvantages, that would achieve optimal curative results.

The following points must be considered: in old age and under favourable general conditions osteosynthesis, that is functionally and stresswise stable, is recommended so that the threatening consequences of immobilization may be prevented.

Conservative procedures are more likely to be decided upon in fractures of young people.

The general state of the patient may limit the indications for operative treatment. Contraindications are: shock, severe additional injuries, other disorders unconnected with the accident, such as diabetes, vascular changes, cardiovascular disorders, liver or kidney diseases, thyrotoxicosis.

The mental attitude and the degree of intelligence of the patient are also of importance and should not be underestimated. The injured person will have to understand that he must not apply stress, even if the fracture is stabilized functionally by means of screws or bolts. If he is not disciplined enough, there is the risk that he will turn up for treatment after a few weeks with bolts or screws that are torn out of position and with an early pseudarthrosis.

The interval between the accident and the start of treatment is also of importance. The usefulness of operative treatment becomes doubtful 2 to 3 weeks after the accident. In the case of multiple fractures operative treatment of all fractures of joints and shafts is indicated, if it is possible, especially as healing may be delayed.

In equilateral fractures of femur and tibia surgeon should decide on *one* procedure for both fractures, as otherwise, on account of instability of the fracture treated conservatively, the disadvantages of immobilization will have to be accepted for the part that has been treated operatively.

In transverse lesions of the cord operative treatment is also preferable. Plaster casts and the inability to change position whilst in extension position favour formation of bed sores.

Furthermore, the local condition in the immediate vicinity of the fracture is of importance. The surgeon should make sure of the state of the soft tissues, the type and the localization of the fracture before he decides to carry out his procedure. In open fractures with large soft tissue defects that require extensive decompression incisions or grafting (free or pedicle grafts etc.), the limb should be stabilized by operation, so that fragments will not shift and pressure on soft tissues, where blood flow is already disturbed, is avoided. Plaster casts that might interfere with plastic surgery should also be avoided. If the damage to tissues is minor, e.g. in stab wounds, treatment will depend upon the site of the injury.

When the joint is damaged, e.g. in fractures of the patella, the olecranon, or in open joint and dislocation fractures, we usually fix the fracture during operation, because late operations usually do not achieve good functional results.

In open fractures, too, functional stability is very useful, as early and painless movement of muscles and joints in the vicinity of the fracture will prevent post-traumatic disorders of blood flow.

Even if the wound is not open, the condition of the skin will have to be considered. Tension bullae with swelling of soft tissues indicate severe tissue damage and necessitate greater care, if operation is intended.

The dystrophic skin of old people also restricts the indication for operation, especially of the lower leg.

So far as fractures are concerned, operative intervention is indicated:

1. if it is impossible to achieve satisfactory positioning conservatively, e.g. if there is some impediment that prevents reduction or in severe displacement,

2. in fractures where experience has shown that reduction is not going to remain stable or will require repeated manoeuvres, and

3. when healing is disturbed.

The treatment of fractures of the shaft depends upon site and type of fracture. Fractures of the upper limb differ fundamentally from those of the lower limb in that statics are not so important, so that minor defective positionings may be accepted without great disadvantage, especially of the clavicle and the humerus. We treat surgically fractures of the clavicle or of the upper arm only, if nerves or blood-vessels are injured by fragments, if there is pressure on the brachial plexus, or if the fracture is greatly displaced and not sufficiently reducible. When there is deformity of the shoulder or torticollis, operation is sometimes unavoidable. We fix fractures of the clavicle with *Kirschner wire* or an AO. *plate*, as the rigid Küntscher nail often does not conform to the physiological curvature (Fig. 1a, b). Hypertrophic pseudarthroses of the clavicle are best treated by means of a *compression plate*; in atrophic pseudarthrosis insertion of a chip of cancellous bone substance is useful.

We also treat fractures of the shaft of the humerus conservatively with Böhler's U splint, or Desault's bandage. We operate only in special cases, e.g. in paresis of the

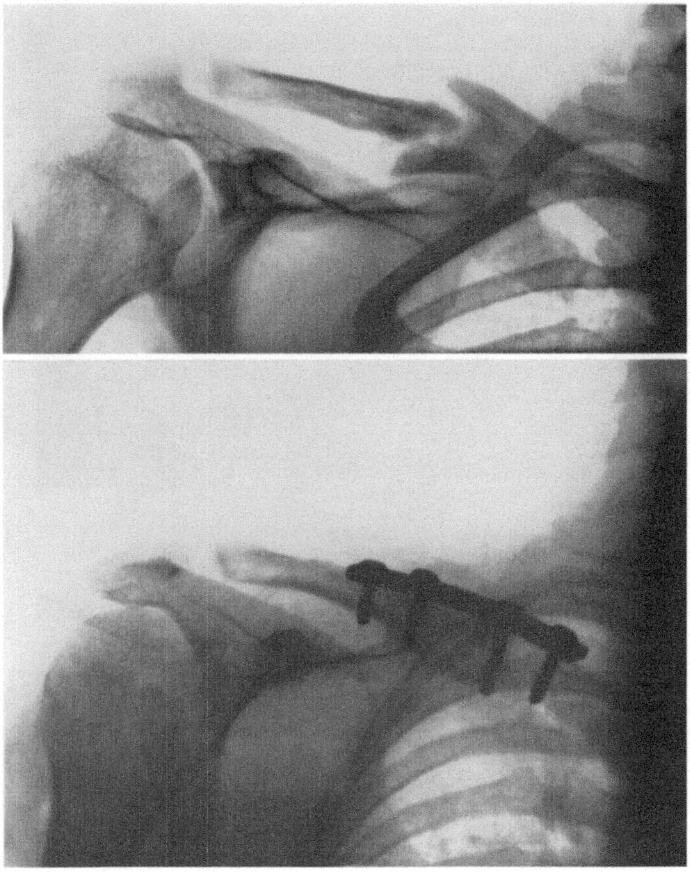

a

b

Fig. 1. a Hypertrophic pseudarthrosis of the clavicle. b Osteosynthesis with AO.-compression-plate

radial nerve, or if the patient needs surgical stabilization of the fracture for occupational reasons. In these cases the AO. plate and multiple nailing according to Hackethal have proved useful.

In contrast to these fractures, fractures of the lower arm, except for subperiosteal fractures of young people, are an absolute indication for operation, because reduction is generally difficult, fixation is commonly unsatisfactory, and repeated efforts at reduction do not benefit healing.

Angulation of the fragments in the plaster cast, which may produce a definitive callus, should be prevented, as it may cause persistent disturbance of function.

Failures of medullary nailing in *fractures of the forearm*, and failures of Rush pinning, where we had 17.5% pseudarthroses, have made us give up medullary

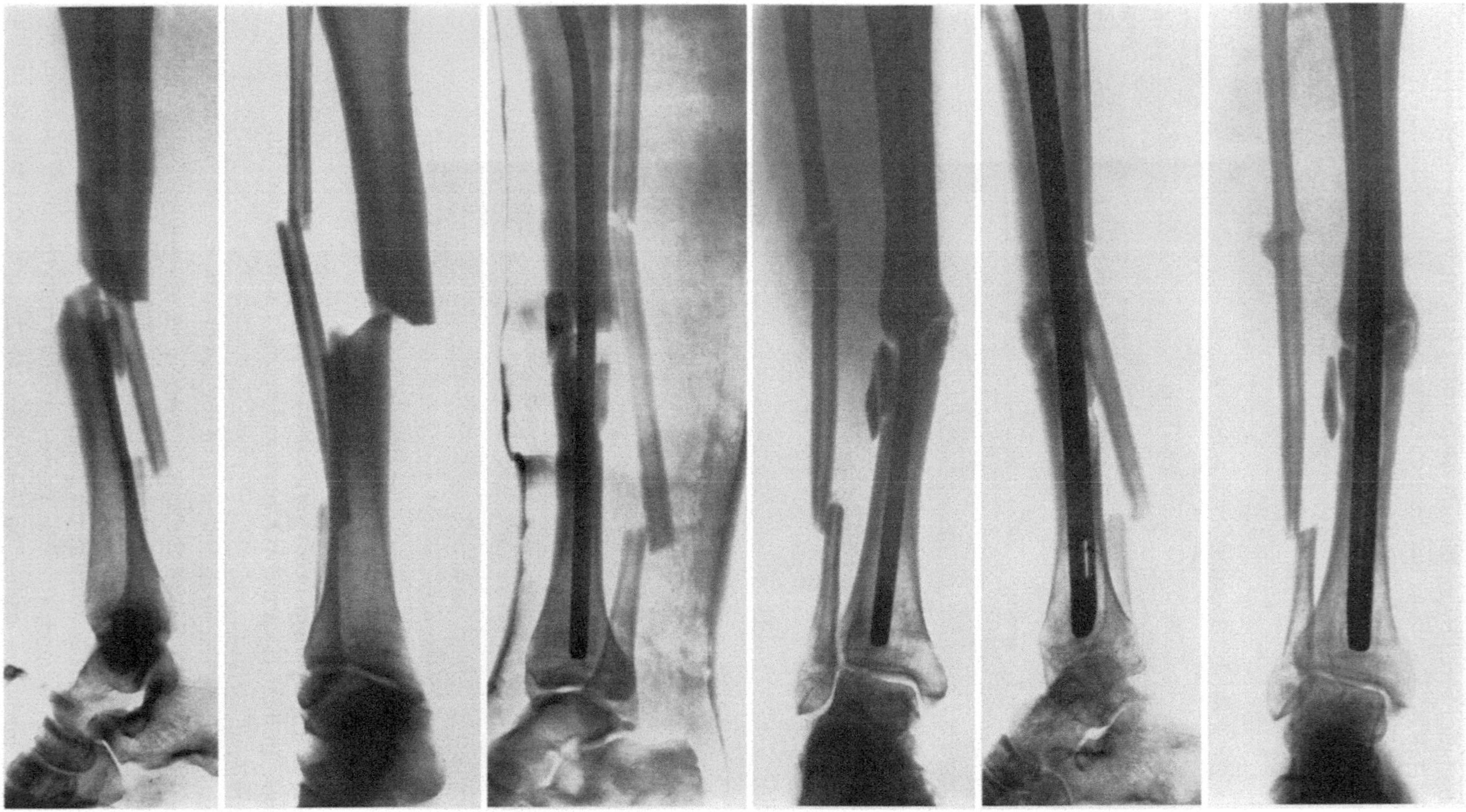

a b c

Fig. 2. a Fracture of tibia and fibula in middle-third. b Osteosynthesis with a Küntscher nail. This is too thin and a pseudarthrosis results. c Renewed nailing with a wider nail and resection-osteotomy of the fibula leads to bony union of the fracture nailing of fractures of the forearm. We are now using *compression plates*, developed from the AO., with which furthermore unobjectionable rotation stability is obtained.

We also use this procedure for isolated fractures of the radius or the ulna, because it prevents dislocation of the distal fragment of the radius, produced by the pull of the pronator quadratus muscle.

We use conservative measures in the typical compression fractures of the radius, when Kirschner wire need to be inserted additionally only if the fracture is intra-

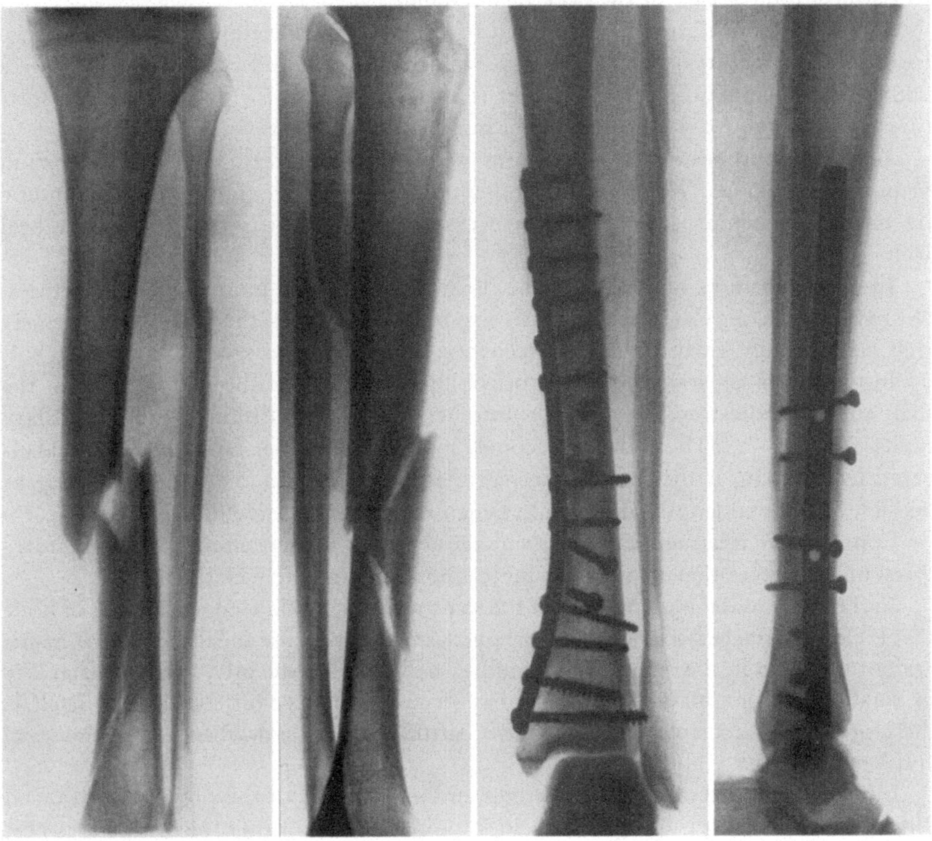

a b

Fig. 3. a Tibial fracture with a long torsion fragment. b Osteosynthesis with AO.-plate and compression screws

articularly comminuted. Operative treatment is then superfluous, if only because the small fragments cannot be fixed by any means at our disposal.

Completely different considerations apply to fractures of the shaft of the leg. It is most important here to prevent malalignment, so that static conditions are created that will prevent the development of secondary arthropathy.

This cannot always be achieved completely by conservative treatment; for this reason operative treatment is appropriate for *fractures of the shaft of the femur*. In our view transverse and oblique fractures of the middle third of the femur are best treated by closed Küntscher nailing. In fractures in which the fracture line is perpendicular to the direction of the trauma and where there are large wedge-shaped fragments open nailing with the proscribed *additional wire sling*, fixed over a Kieler chip, may be necessary.

If there are also fractures of the neck of the femur, we use one of the following three methods:

1. Küntscher's Y-nail,
2. the angular or straight AO. plates, or
3. a Küntscher nail, inserted below the trochanteric mass and a flanged nail so as to stabilize the fracture of the neck of the femur.

In our opinion subtrochanteric fractures are definite indications for operation; we treat oblique fractures with Küntscher nails and torsion and comminuted fractures with the angular AO. plate. The latter is also very useful for peritrochanteric fractures and may be fixed with Palacos in high-grade osteoporosis.

We had good results in these cases with extension treatment when operation seemed inauspicious. We agree with other authors that operation in peritrochanteric fractures of the femur is not absolutely necessary, as this type of fracture tends to heal well.

In distal fractures of the femur, i.e. in supra-, dia-, and monocondylar fractures, we have used condylar plates exclusively, because they fix the fractures extremely well and promise early functional recovery.

In the lower leg transverse or short oblique fractures of the middle-third of the shaft are also indications for closed Küntscher nailing after drilling of the medullary cavity (Fig. 2a—c). The fracture becomes more stable under stress and less endangered by rotation, if the part of the nail that is attached to the bone is as long as possible. The total length of the nail as such is not the decisive factor.

Conservative treatment has no advantages here, as in these short oblique fractures the shearing forces that impede healing cannot be completely eliminated.

In fractures of the middle-third of the shaft with arcuation wedges the part of bone that is closely attached to the medullary pin is smaller, because the detached fragments are not included in the stabilizing medullary splint. Consequently, there is instability of rotation and angulation, and this may occur even later on. Nailing by itself is therefore only defensible when there are small wedges, and when early functional and stress stability is desired.

If in the presence of arcuated wedges and in fractures of the proximal and distal third of the lower leg the surgeon decides to operate, then firm osteosynthesis is best achieved by fixation with compression screws and plates (Fig. 3a and b). It should not be forgotten that there is danger, especially in comminuted fractures — even for experienced surgeons — of exclusion of fragments from nutrition and that the danger of infection does increase with the duration of the operation.

For this reason conservative treatment with extension bandages and plaster casts is less dangerous in simple torsion fractures, in fractures with one or several arcuated wedges, and particularly in comminuted fractures of the shaft of the tibia. Comminuted fractures of the shaft of the tibia may be reduced without difficulty by extension, they heal within a reasonable time when treated conservatively, and they are able to bear stress at a time when osteosynthesis progresses most favourably.

Wire suturing according to GOETZE, which is again under discussion in Germany and Austria, is in our view suitable only in certain circumstances (AHRER has recently reported on 400 cases with 4% of pseudarthroses), because the accepted aims of operative osteosynthesis are not properly achieved, and because the surgeon by using the method commits the old mistake of trying to combine two incompatible procedures.

a

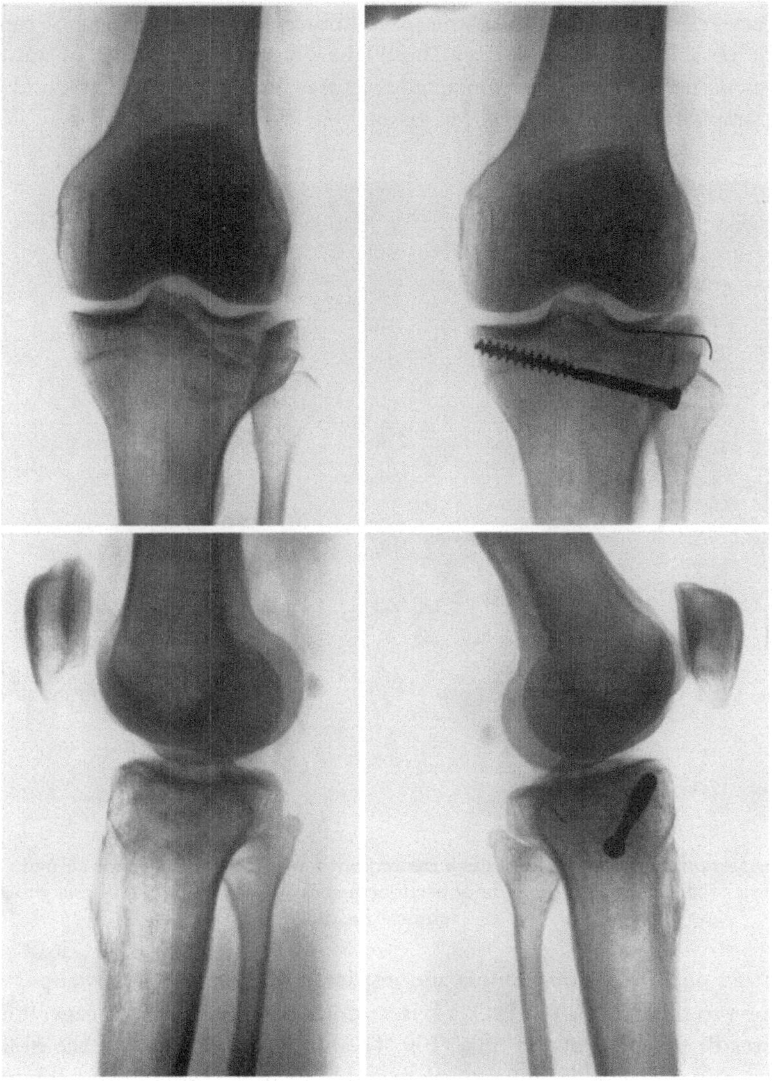

b

Fig. 4. a Repressed fracture of lateral tibial plateau. b The fracture has been reduced with interposition of cancellous bone and fixed by means of a spongiosa screw

In contrast to shaft fractures, when the question of conservative or operative treatment is open to discussion, articular fractures with displacement are a clear-cut indication for operation. In comminuted fractures it seems sensible to attempt reconstruction. If it is unsuccessful, arthrodesis may always be carried out later.

Supra-, dia-, and monocondylar fractures of the humerus and the femur belong to this group. In *supracondylar fractures of the humerus* of children insertion of Kirschner wire after successful reduction, as recommended by Jörg Böhler, is usually sufficient. In adults operative procedures are generally unavoidable, and screws with or without plates have proved to be the best means of achieving stable osteosynthesis. Early movement is of decisive importance for the degree to which movement of the joint will be possible later on.

In fractures with impaction of the joint surface with large defects of cancellous tissue the repositioned joint surface should be given an underlayer of autogenous cancellous tissue, because these impacted fractures usually have not as good a prognosis as simple fractures of cancellous tissue.

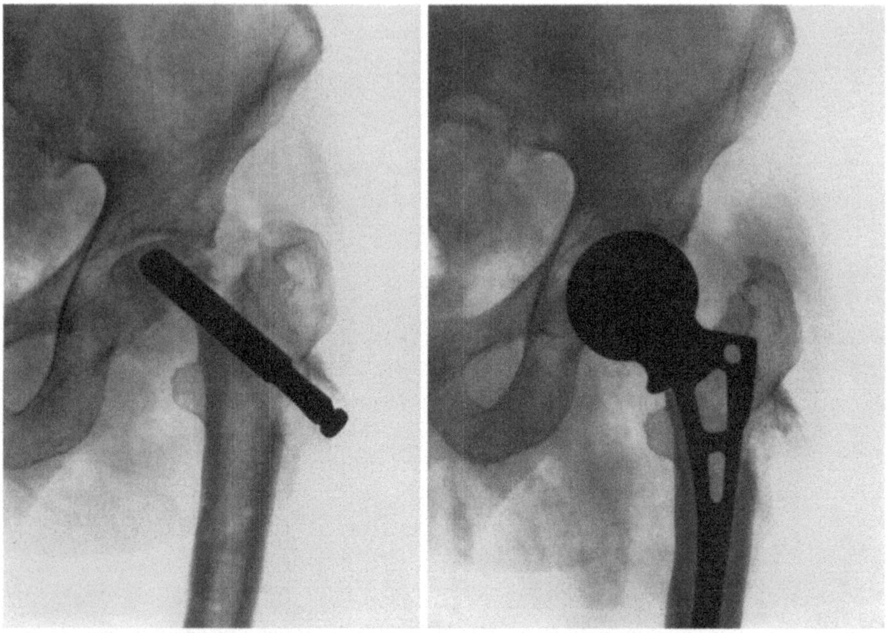

a b

Fig. 5. a Lateral fracture of femoral neck treated with a Smith-Petersen type of nail. The nail has become dislocated and there is a pseudarthrosis. b Vitallium prosthesis replaces the femoral head

Fractures of the head of the tibia and impacted fractures of the distal parts of the tibia belong to this group. The AO. advises additional pinning of the cancellous bone in fractures of the head of the tibia (Fig. 4a and b), stabilization of the fibula with Rush pins, and medial splinting with plate and bolts in the case of distal fractures.

In cases of transverse comminuted fractures of the distal third of the tibia with multiple small fragments, it is better not to carry out operative osteosynthesis, because no manner of osteosynthesis will achieve good stabilization. In these cases conservative treatment is preferable.

The articular fractures, which must be treated operatively, are in contrast to fractures of the head of the humerus, which we treat with conservative procedures only. Early functional treatment after 10 days' rest in Desault's bandage gives excellent results. Operative treatment has no advantages, because the material used for osteosynthesis cannot be fixed properly in the head, as this is often osteoporotic, as blood flow is diminished by the surgical intervention, and as fresh scars will develop in the joint capsule.

In dislocation fractures of the head of the humerus, especially in older patients, resection of the head and subsequent functional exercises are usually better than operative surgery or even substitution of the head by a vitallium endoprosthesis.

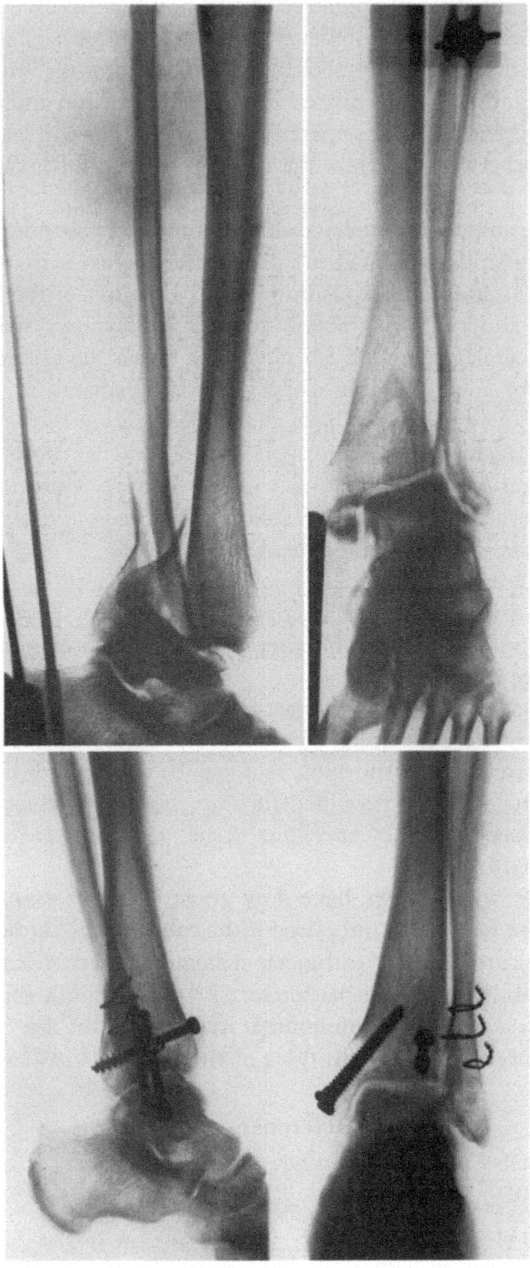

a

b

Fig. 6. a Bimalleolar dislocation fracture of the ankle. b Osteosynthesis with malleolar and spongiosa screws as well as hemicerclages

In medial fractures of the neck of the femur there is no doubt about the indication for operation. We prefer treatment with a flanged nail. Use of the vitallium endoprosthesis for the head of the femur with reduced nutrition and its fixation with Palacos is a measure nowadays fully accepted in all orthopedic departments (Fig. 5a and b).

In fractures of the acetabulum it is often impossible to obtain exact reconstruction of the joint, even operatively, and operative efforts, however involved, are useless and will lead to a poor final result. If, however, there is a prospect of restitution of the acetabulum, from a technical and biomechanical point of view it should be attempted. In fractures of the acetabulum with posterior luxation of the hip and comminution of the posterior part of the acetabulum operative treatment that will lead to reconstruction is promising. Otherwise we treat the majority of central luxations of the hip joint conservatively.

In fractures of the ankle joint we have almost completely abandoned conservative treatment and rely on Müller and Weber's procedure. We use screws for fractures of the medial malleolus after careful reposition; we fix fractures of the lateral malleolus according to height and type by traction strapping, Kirschner wire, semi-circular plates, semi-circular cerclages, and Rush pins. It is nearly always possible to obtain ideal reduction and to achieve stable osteosynthesis, so that it is possible to start early movement (Fig. 6a and b). We have abandoned bolting of the syndesmosis on account of the high incidence of arthroses (35%!), and we now suture the torn ligamental apparatus after careful treatment of the fracture. Unfortunately, it is not possible to avoid the use of a plaster U splint, which fixes the malleolar fork and which permits a certain degree of movement.

In dislocation fractures of the ankle joint we also proceed as described, and in addition we pin the displaced posterior triangle of the tibia. Here, too, immediate movement is usually possible. If forceful attempts during postoperative-treatment are omitted the results are usually good.

In fractures of the talus we prefer conservative treatment, provided the fractures are not displaced and are reducible. Operation should be decided upon early in displaced dislocation fractures of the talus, as it may be anticipated that these will heal with little tendency to necrosis, provided they are carefully reduced surgically and properly fixed with screws in the cancellous tissue, and provided that early movement therapy is carried out.

In fractures of the calcaneus we have now given up all procedures for straightening. Screwing of the fracture is only used if the tuber of the calcaneus is torn. We reduce all other fractures of the calcaneus manually in accordance with Ehalt's directives, and immobilize them in plaster casts. We also think that the most promising procedure in extensive comminuted fractures with the least amount of unpleasant consequences is early arthrodesis of the talo-calcaneo-navicular joint.

References

Allgöwer, M.: Langenbecks Arch. klin. Chir. **308**, 423 (1964).

Axhausen, W.: Chirurg **37**, 400 (1966).

Böhler, J.: Langenbecks Arch. klin. Chir. **304**, 517 (1963).

— Akt. Chir. **1**, 15/365 (1966).

Böhler, L.: Langenbecks Arch. klin. Chir. **304**, 630 (1963).

—, u. J. Böhler: Technik der Knochenbruchbehandlung, 12/13. Aufl. mit Ergänzungsband. Wien: Maudrich 1963.

Bürkle de la Camp, H., u. M. Schwaiger: Handbuch der gesamten Unfallheilkunde. Stuttgart: Enke 1965.
Hackethal, K. H.: Die Bündelnagelung. Berlin-Göttingen-Heidelberg: Springer 1961.
Kemlein, W.: Chirurg **38**, 463 (1967).
Küntscher, G.: Praxis der Marknagelung. Stuttgart: Schattauer 1962.
— Chirurg **37**, 69 (1966).
Lange, M.: Orthopädisch-chirurgische Operationslehre. München: Bergmann 1962.
—, u. E. Hipp: Dtsch. med. J. **17**, 292 (1966).
v. Lanz, T., u. W. Wachsmuth: Praktische Anatomie, Bd. I/3. Berlin-Göttingen-Heidelberg: Springer 1959.
Müller, M. E., M. Allgöwer und H. Willenegger: Technik der operativen Frakturenbehandlung. Berlin-Göttingen-Heidelberg: Springer 1963.
Schenk, R.: Langenbecks Arch. klin. Chir. **308**, 440 (1964).
Tscherne, H., F. Magerl und P. Feischl: Langenbecks Arch. klin. Chir. **317**, 209 (1967).
Viernstein, K., u. W. Keyl: Z. Orthop. **102**, 119 (1966).
Weber, B. G.: Die Verletzungen des oberen Sprunggelenkes. Bern:Huber 1966.
— Chirurg **38**, 441 (1967).
Weller, S.: Mschr. Unfallheilk. **70**, 233 (1967).
— Chirurg **38**, 445 (1967).
Wilhelm, A.: Münch. med. Wschr. **6**, 357 (1968).
Willenegger, H.: Chirurg **38**, 341 (1967).
Witt, A. N., u. M. Jäger: Arch. orthop. Unfall-Chir. **60**, 49 (1966).

Discussion

Carlo Scuderi

In discussing this excellent paper, one is obliged to discuss it on a philosophical basis, because I wholeheartedly agree with the material presented.

The objective in the treatment of any fracture is to obtain an anatomical reduction. This insures proper alignment of the fragments, and as a result, a more rapid return of function.

As a basic principle, the more comminuted a fracture is, less is the indication for internal fixation. Frequently skeletal traction is best used in order to restore length, and alignment.

Many wonderful adjuncts have become available to orthopedic surgeons since World War II. The refinement in metallurgy has given us non-irritating strong screws, plates and rods. Antibiotics have advanced very rapidly so we now have a wide selection of anti-bacterial drugs. The innovation of the hemovac permits us to have an efficient method of keeping large wounds free of hematoma formation.

For the above reasons the natural trend in the management of fractures is more and more to open reduction and fixation.

In well regulated orthopedic services, operative infections at the present time are almost unknown. Careful dissection along anatomical planes, gentle handling of tissues and firm internal fixation are the keynotes to success.

The prophylactic use of broad spectrum antibiotics are added insurance for primary wound healing. The older men of this group have unpleasant memories of what postoperative infection means in orthopedic cases. They also recall the problems of vanadium and similar metals from which screws and plates were made. Not only was their tensile strength poor, and hence frequently broke, but the metals in a high percentage of cases were rejected by the tissues. Fortunate indeed is the present orthopedic surgeon with strong, non-irritating screws, plates and rods.

The hemovac has been another fine tool in the hands of all of us. The ability to keep large operative wounds relatively free of blood clots has increased the speed of wound healing and has lessened the material available for organisms to grow in.

Perhaps no field of surgery has made such phenomenal progress as orthopedic surgery, since or because of World War II. May our future advancements come from the peaceful coexistence of mankind, who may have tranquility and the opportunity to sit quietly and think out the answers to our present existing orthopedic problems.

Immediate Surgical Care of Fractures Involving the Socket of the Hip-joint

J. Rehn

We were able to record in our clinical material an increase of 85.5% in the number of injuries to the hip-joint within the past few years. As in the case of statistics comprising all injuries we found also in this type of injury that traffic accidents involving impact of the knees made up nowadays about 70%.

Table 1. *Injuries of the hip-joint "Bergmannsheil" Bochum. 1945 to 1964*

	Number	Percentage %
Fractures of the socket		
Unilateral	67	34.01
Bilateral	7	3.05
Fracture dislocations		
Group 1 (accord. to Böhler)	51	25.89
Group 2 to 5	36	18.28
Group 6 to 9	20	10.0
Central dislocations		
Group 1 (accord. to Böhler)	6	3.05
Group 2	8	4.06
Group 3	2	1.02

Injuries of the hip-joint: altogether 197 cases.

We found in addition numerous other causes of fracture dislocations of the hip-joint (Table 1). In our area in particular we encountered frequently injuries at work which were the result of direct trauma of the trochanter major. While in the case of a mere dislocation a torsion force predominates, a fracture dislocation will have an impact with lever action as its cause. The direction of the thrust and the position of the femur in relation to the hip-joint will largely determine the type of injury.

The hip-joint is protected by a thick cushion of muscles and is in addition due to its shape an extraordinarily stable and static joint. Great force is required to produce a fracture dislocation. This explains the severe multiple injuries which are usually encountered at the same time. Fractures of the socket are more common than those of the head of the femur. The greater elasticity of the head plays probably a part in this.

Normally a diagnosis should precede any therapy. In the case of the frequently encountered multiple injuries however some immediate results of the trauma which may endanger life have to be attended to before an exact diagnosis of even severe bony injuries can be made. Apart from a clinical examination, orientating straight X-rays of the pelvis may already provide indications for further specialized X-ray investigations which may be required. A lateral view or one accord to LAUENSTEIN should always be taken. In addition where required we carry out oblique views accord to the directions of URIST and WALLER, which permit a more detailed inspection of the hip-joint and above all a better visualization of fracture lines and displaced fragments. In doubtful cases tomograms may make a pelvic fracture visible for the first time. It is first of all however necessary during the course of an investigation to think of the possible effects of such injuries, particularly in the cases where the trauma strikes the knees, and examine accordingly.

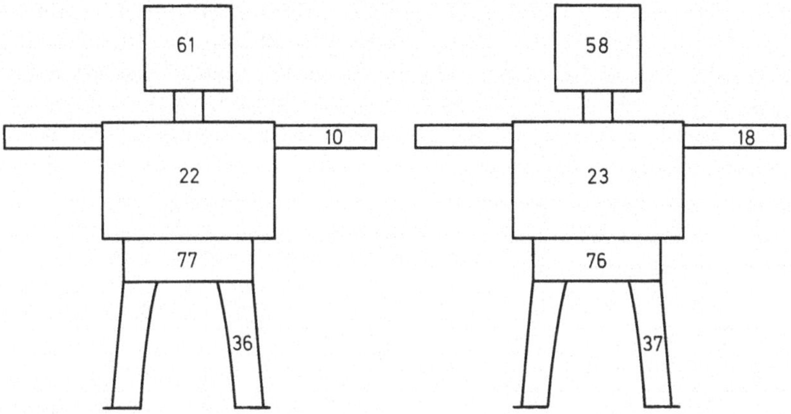

in 197 hip-joint traumas "Bergmannsheil" Bochum

in 128 hip-joint traumas Surgical unit, University Hospital, Heidelberg

Fig. 1. Multiple injuries sustained with hip-joint traumas. Comparison of "Bergmannsheil" Bochum (mainly injuries which occurred at work) with the University Hospital Heidelberg (predominantly traffic accidents) according to JUNGBLUTH and KRATZERT

The numerous simultaneous injuries which have been already mentioned (Fig. 1), they affect on average 50 to 70%, restrict not only diagnostic procedures but also influence our therapeutic measures. Shock, fat embolism or additional severe injuries may for a limited period prevent the immediate surgical treatment of a fracture of the socket. In the case of these injuries too one should not depart from the principle that only life saving operations should be carried out if the patient is in a state of shock. We had therefore sometimes let the time elapse during which the best results can be achieved with an operation resp. osteosynthesis in the region of the hip-joint. In addition, for instance in the case of extensive soft tissue injuries with decollement infections, a considerable time will pass before healing takes place or plastic surgery has covered the area involved.

A large portion of the socket or fracture dislocation of the hip-joint which came under our care also reached us too late to enable us to carry out any primary reconstructive surgery. But it is in fact the hereby gained negative experience which provides the basis for demanding objectively a primary osteosynthesis of fracture dislocations involving the hip-joint.

The multitude of principles according to which these traumas have been divided are mostly related to the localization of the injuries. In the context of this paper it seems important to me that the following two main types should be discussed.

1. Injuries of the socket which do not require any surgical measures.

2. Fractures of the rim or the floor of the acetabulum with or without dislocation of the head of the femur which are urgently in need of osteosynthesis.

When considering the fractures of the acetabulum under this heading, the first group will contain the fractures which either show no significant dislocation or no dislocation at all. We count amongst these simple cracks or fractures for instance are only visible in tomograms. They are mostly the result of a force acting directly on the trochanter. At the time of the examination the built-in elasticity of the acetabulum of the hip-joint has already resulted in a spontaneous reposition.

But also small and also larger fractures in the posterior region of the socket without dislocation do not require osteosynthesis, this also applies to small fragments breaking off the roof of the socket. On the whole the head of the femur retains in these types of fractures its normal and stable relationship to the carrying surface. Amongst 74 simple fractures of the socket we found a significant displacement of the fragments in only 12 of the cases.

Conservative measures which were aimed at repositioning and also relieving pressure on a fracture dislocation of the hip-joint, cannot be expected to lead to a true anatomical restoration.

What can be considered the best time for surgical intervention? An operation as early as possible as long as no danger is involved will give the best results. Numerous authors were able to show that the results of the operations get rapidly worse as time passes — even after 24 h — following the injury. Above all the dislocation of the head of the femur should be eliminated right away, because if the dislocation persists and the tension of the joint capsule and its bloodvessels is not relieved, the incidence of a secondary collapse of the head increases significantly.

Up to which time can restorative surgical operations be carried out? Opinions differ widely on this point. Our own experience shows that the reconstitution of a destroyed acetabulum after repositioning of the head of the femur, undertaken after 3 to 6 weeks or later, will nearly invariably lead to bad late results. For this reason we have now given up carrying out complicated operative surgery in such cases, which were either diagnosed late or where reposition became only feasible at such a time.

The indication for surgical intervention is mainly determined by the type of fracture. Instable fracture dislocations and dislocated fractures of the socket in the region where the body's weight is carried should if possible be stabilized by an operation. One has of course to be aware preoperatively, that even surgical measures will not always lead to an exact reconstitution of the socket. If a really good result cannot be expected from osteosynthesis, then conservative measures should be used. In comminuted fractures a complete restitution may be impossible, so that rarely at once, more often after waiting for a consolidation of the fracture, an arthroplasty or arthrodesis has to be carried out later, according to the age of the patient. In addition extensive damage to the cartilage or bone of the head and acetabulum cannot be expected to recover. On the other hand displaced fragments which get into the way, larger dislocated fragments like in the case of a central dislocation of the hip or transarticular fracture of the pelvis, fractures of the roof of the socket and fractures of the lower portions of the acetabulum, all amount to a definite indication for surgical reconstruction. Smaller displaced fragments can be removed. If the neck of the femur after penetration of the acetabulum by the head of the femur is held in position like in a button hole, reposition can only be carried out through open surgery as the necessary strong pull will nearly certainly result in a fracture of the neck of the femur.

At this stage it should also be pointed out that in the presence of any of the already mentioned contraindications to surgery, it should be at least the attempt made to achieve an adequate reposition by using conservative measures. If satisfactory results can be achieved conservatively, there will be no need for later surgery.

An absolute criterion for surgical intervention is also the partial or complete paralysis of the sciatic nerve. This complication does not only constitute a definite indication for operative surgery, but has also an important diagnostic significance.

Before the operation it is recommended to make blood available for a transfusion and particularly in the case of recently injured give an easily tolerated anaesthetic like e.g. neurolept-analgesia. The loss of blood in the case of multiple injuries must be determined by a volumetric device and made up before the operation. The surgical operation will lead to an additional blood loss. In the case of older patients a preliminary examination by a physician and suitable premedication where it is indicated is obviously necessary.

The surgical approach will be determined by the localization of the injury. The latero-dorsal approach will usually be suitable. A different path will have to be used in the case of posterior displacements than in the case of a fracture of the socket roof. Very rarely it will even be necessary to deal with extensive fractures by using both an anterior and posterior access.

What types of stabilization are nowadays available after operative exposure? It would not do here to try to make detailed suggestions. In the first place we must aim at stabilizing the hip-joint socket as far as possible by the use of wiring and screws. But suitably shaped semicircular tubes and other plates can also be used for the fixation of the carefully aligned fragments. In the case of extensive fracture lines which involve the whole of the os ileum, the pelvic rim is after reposition first fixed in place by a plate. This makes the remaining repair distally much easier. Before plating the fracture of the acetabulum the exact intraarticular reposition of the fragments has to be checked.

The so achieved osteosynthesis should remain stable on exercise and obviate the need for supporting bandages. If this is not possible then a pelvic Plaster of Paris must be applied. With postoperative traction and simultaneous easing of the joint, the results of the reposition will remain more stable. Opinions are divided on the necessary length of bedrest and complete stabilization of the joint by traction. In conservatively treated fractures of the acetabulum without dislocation, full weight carrying will be achieved from between 8 weeks to 3 months after the injury. It is however recommended in cases with severe injuries to the socket of the hip-joint not to permit any weightbearing of the joint for at least 3 months. In the case of severe fracture dislocations with a good reposition result, we try for a whole year with the aid of suitable apparatus to achieve as much as possible a support of the hip-joint. We aim hereby at a regeneration of the damaged head of the femur and in this way try to avoid a later necrosis of the head.

What kind of complications and later effects dominate nowadays the picture in injuries of the hip-joint?

Amongst the early complications, which appear immediately after the accident, we observed on rare occasions impaired circulation in the distal parts of the limbs due to the pressure of the dislocated head on the large blood vessels. Damage to the sciatic nerve occurs in about 10 to 15% of the cases and is three times more common in fracture dislocations than in dislocations only. In posterior fracture dislocations and also in fractures of the roof of the socket a partial paralysis mainly of the peroneal nerves or more often a complete paralysis can occur as a result of the marked displacement of the broken fragments. The peroneal portion of the sciatic nerve runs more ventrally and laterally and lies therefore nearest to the acetabulum and most exposed to the traumatic effects. It is indicated to carry out an operative exposure and freeing of the nerves as soon as possible to avoid any permanent damage.

The special characteristic of the necrosis of the head which is a relatively common later complication consists in not being recognizable at first. It manifests itself only at a later date. According to our present state of knowledge it would appear that already at the time of the trauma severe compression of the head with reversible deformities due to cartilage and spongiosa fractures will occur, which much later give rise to the much feared partial necrosis of the head. In addition the damage to the blood supply, particularly in the case of dislocation through tearing the blood-vessels of the joint capsule constitute an important cause. We cannot base our primary surgical measures on the knowledge of these complications which at that time cannot be recognized. After months or more often after years a necrosis of the head will occur even after the best possible primary care. If the reduction of the fracture dislocation is delayed until about 6 to 7 h after the injury, the incidence of necrosis of the head increases. According to TRUETA osteocytes can exist only up to 6 h without a blood supply. The frequency with which these complications will occur depends largely on the severity of the injury. It ranges from 12 to 70%.

Myositis ossificans within the area of the injury to the hip-joint is a relatively common occurrence. The pathogenesis is not clear. Undoubtedly the heavy haemorrhage and other effects of the trauma play a part. On the other hand large numbers of patients who received identical treatment are not affected, so that an individual disposition to it must be considered an essential factor.

Arthrosis is a complication which depends essentially on the extent of the primary injury and the quality of the initial surgical treatment. Inadequate adaptation of the fragments with remaining projections can lead to grinding-off arthrosis. Partial necrosis of the acetabulum cartilage or the head can lead to arthrosis. The necrosis of the cartilage is usually induced by a severe initial trauma. A partial necrosis of the head will of course also cause arthrosis. The incongruity of the joint surfaces is here an essential factor.

The treatment of the so-called old fracture dislocation where secondary changes in the joint have already occurred remains problematical, that is surgical restorative measures nearly invariably produce poor results. In the young patient where the injury affected only one side, an arthrodesis will be carried out, in the older patient, that is over the age of 65 to 70, an endo or total prosthesis will be used. Cup and "Lexer" plastic operations have also their place here. These examples are only intended to be representative of the multitude of restorative and corrective measures which have been used in this field.

In conclusion a few words about the late results (Table 2). Our own list is made up of injuries of varying severity. The late results refer mainly to conservatively treated injuries.

The difficulty one faces in all statistics of this nature is due to the different interpretation of the late effects, the varying indications for surgical measures according to the length of time which passes between the injury and the time of examination (Table 3). Usually there is a clinical material that has been treated both surgically and

Table 2. *Late effects occurring in 105 patients with injuries of the hip-joint, who were reviewed between 3 and 15 years after the original trauma*

Type of late effect	Number	Percentage %
Coxarthrosis	23	21.9
Necroses of the head	8	7.6
Arthrosis with simultaneous necrosis	4	3.8
Myositis ossificans	6	5.7
Ossification of the capsule	4	3.8

Table 3. *Incidence of late effects following injuries to the hip-joint according to various authors*

Author	Type of injury	Arthrosis %	Necrosis of head of the femur %	Ossification of soft tissues %
Urist (1946)	H D	63.2	—	4.4
Armstrong (1948)	H FD*	25.0	—	1.9
	H FD*	60.0		
Trojan and Persch (1956)	H FD	22.7	12.1	9.2
Fineschi (1957)	H D + H FD	35.5	9.7	16.1
Germann (1961)	H FD	61.6	7.7	23.1
Brav (1962)	H FD*	50.5	25.3	12.6
	H FD*	72.4	65.5	27.6

H D Dislocation of hip.
H FD Fracture dislocation of hip.
* Of different severity.

conservatively. Severe injuries are certainly followed by a higher percentage of arthroses and necroses of the head. It is probable that with the increase of open reduction and osteosynthesis better results can be expected in a portion of the socket fractures. On the other hand we have to be aware that dislocation of the hip and fracture dislocation can only be the result of the most severe trauma, so that destruction in the region of the head and acetabulum and specially in the area of the cartilage is caused at the time of the injury and will partly cause late effects. A most exact and subtile X-ray diagnosis should enable us to reduce the number of injuries to the hip-joint which have been overlooked to an absolute minimum. The after care has to be considered also as an essential part of the whole therapeutic concept. Only a relatively early mobilization with weight bearing later can help to reduce the incidence of necroses of the head.

Amongst our clinical material of 197 hip-joint injuries 17 patients died as a result of additional severe injuries (Table 4).

I sum up as follows:

1. The saving of life is the prime task. The immediate surgical intervention can only be justified if no danger is attached to it.

2. Whenever an instable fracture of the acetabulum or fracture dislocation with cracks, steplike projections or displaced fragments in the acetabulum are present or paralysis of the sciatic nerve occurs, surgery has to be undertaken and osteosynthesis should be carried out as far as possible without any step formation, to achieve stabilization.

Table 4. *197 hip-joint injuries treated at "Bergmannsheil" Bochum from 1945 to 1964. Type of trauma and number of deaths*

Type of injury	Number	Percentage %	Death due to other injuries
Dislocations	51	25.89	3
Acetabulum fractures	74	37.56	—
Unilateral: 67			
Bilateral: 7			
Fracture dislocations	43	21.83	4
Central fracture disl.	16	8.12	4
Combined fractures of acetabulum, Femur and injury to other hip	13	6.60	1
Altogether	197	100.0	12

3. Late operative surgery, weeks after the accident, in an attempt to restore normal use of the limbs, can only be justified if an exact reconstruction of the socket of the joint can be achieved.

References

Böhler, J.: Wiederherstellungschir. u. Traum. **4**, 75—108 (1957).
— Verh. dtsch. orthop. Ges. **50**, 243—253, 260—261 (1962).
Brav, E.A.: J. Bone Jt Surg. **44 A**, 1115—1134 (1962).
Brinkmann, W. H.: Mschr. Unfallheilk. **70**, 273—289 (1967).
Chapchal, G.: Orthopädische Chirurgie und Traumatologie der Hüfte. Stuttgart: Enke 1965.
Derian, P. S., and Th. Purser III: J. Bone Jt Surg. **48 A**, 1614—1618 (1966).
Ehalt, W., u. G. Gelehrter: Arch. orthop. Unfall-Chir. **48**, 561—581 (1956).
Fineschi, G.: Wiederherstellungschir. u. Traum. **4**, 44—74 (1957).
Fries, G.: Arch. orthop. Unfall-Chir. **59**, 229—239 (1966).
Germann, W.: Helv. chir. Acta **28**, 672—738 (1961).
Jungbluth, K. H., u. R. Kratzert: Hefte Unfallheilk. **91**, 38—41 (1967).
Kollmann, K.: Arch. orthop. Unfall-Chir. **59**, 312—315 (1966).
Merle-D'Aubigné, R.: Wiederherstellungschir. u. Traum. **5**, 61—73 (1960).
— Verh. dtsch. orthop. Ges. **50**, 265—270 (1962).
Motta, C.: Z. Orthop. **100**, 133—153 (1965).
Müller, H. J.: Hefte Unfallheilk. **91**, 14—24 (1967).

Müller, M. E.: Hefte Unfallheilk. **91**, 25—28 (1967).
Neff, G.: Helv. chir. Acta **29**, 165—175 (1962).
Nigst, H.: Spezielle Frakturen- und Luxationslehre. Bd. III: Hüftgelenk und proximaler Oberschenkel. Stuttgart: Thieme 1964.
Rehn, J.: Hefte Unfallheilk. **91**, 35—38 (1967).
Reimers, C.: Unfallschäden des Beckens und des Hüftgelenkes. In: Handbuch der gesamten Unfallheilkunde, Bd. III, 3. Aufl., S. 232—367. Stuttgart: Enke 1965.
— Hefte Unfallheilk. **91**, 32—35 (1967).
Sommelet, J., M. Bessot et G. Streit: J. Chir. (Paris) **92**, 473—480 (1966).
Stewart, M., and L. Milford: J. Bone Jt Surg. **36 A**, 315—342 (1954).
Trueta, J.: Verh. dtsch. orthop. Ges. **50**, 263—265 (1962).
Urist, M. R.: Amer. J. Surg. **74**, 586—597 (1947).
— Ann. Surg. **127**, 1150—1164 (1948).
Viernstein, K., u. P. M. Jantzen: Wiederherstellungschir. u. Traum. **5**, 117—137 (1960).
Waller, A.: Acta chir. scand. Suppl. **205**, 1—94 (1955).
Weller, S.: Hefte Unfallheilk. **91**, 30—32 (1967).

Discussion

Edwin F. Cave

Acetabular fractures can be classified as follows:

1. Undisplaced.
2. Posterior.
3. Inner wall.
4. Superior.
5. Central with intrapelvic displacement of femoral head.

The prognosis is different for each type of fracture. For instance, the undisplaced fractures of the central portion of the acetabulum usually carry a good prognosis, no matter what form of treatment is applied; whereas those which involve the superior and posterior weightbearing surfaces of the acetabular cup, with or without associated dislocation of the hip, carry a guarded prognosis unless prompt and accurate repositioning of the femoral head and of the acetabular cup is carried out. Even if there is prompt reduction of the dislocation, there often follows aseptic necrosis of the femoral head, which ultimately leads to traumatic arthritis involving the hip-joint. Therefore, the fracture of the posterior and superior acetabular cup, with or without dislocation of the femoral head, is the type of fracture with which we are chiefly concerned and which, in my opinion, offers the most frequent indication for operative treatment. A fracture of the superior-posterior rim of the acetabulum with dislocation of the femoral head is often associated with sciatic nerve injury and if the sensory and motor functions of the nerve do not return after replacement of the femoral head, exploration of the posterior rim of the acetabulum and replacement of the fragment are indicated.

Probably the only other indication for immediate operative treatment of acetabular fractures is for those which involve extensive fracture of the pelvis and are associated with intrapelvic hemorrhage. Operative repair of lacerated blood vessels may be indicated, but this in our experience has not often been necessary. The severely comminuted fracture of the acetabulum with or without fracture of the femoral head may on occasion be best treated by primary arthroplasty if in the opinion of the surgeon instability and traumatic arthritis are more than likely to follow. Such a procedure is probably best delayed until the primary state of shock from injury has passed.

We believe that fractures involving the inner wall, although markedly displaced, are best treated by skeletal traction, longitudinal and lateral, which must be initiated early. This requires general or spinal anesthesia, the application of a Kirschner wire through the distal end of the femur and possibly through the greater trochanteric area. Heavy traction may be necessary and it is maintained for a period of 6 weeks until the acetabulum has consolidated in its restored position. We believe that the operative treatment of this type of fracture is rarely if ever indicated, realizing at the same time that in a small number of cases eventual arthroplasty of the joint may have to be done if pain and deformity follow the socalled conservative, or traction, form of treatment.

In a series of 91 patients with 93 acetabular fractures reported recently from the Massachusetts General Hospital by Rowe and Lowell, the following complications were recorded:

Traumatic arthritis and femoral head necrosis: 24 or 26%.

Myositis ossificans: In 3 of 61 cases treated conservatively (5%); in 11 of 32 cases (34%) treated by operation.

Femoral head damage: In 13, 10 of which eventually had a poor end result.

Sciatic nerve damage: In 16 or 17%. In 10 of these the paralysis was temporary. 7 were explored.

Massive hemorrhage was very rare.

Thrombophlebitis developed in 9 cases.

The real problem, therefore, in fractures of the acetabulum results from severe trauma to the posterior-superior acetabular support and through the neglected, prolonged displacement of the femoral head, the blood supply to which has been interrupted. Immediate operative treatment is indicated if after reduction of the femoral head there remains displaced a major fragment of the posterior and superior rim of the acetabulum.

Is Prosthesis Treatment of Fresh Femoral Neck Fractures Justified?

R. Merle D'Aubigné

Good results obtained with prostheses in old femoral neck fractures have lately given rise to the idea of applying this method as primary treatment of femoral neck fractures, thus avoiding the unfortunately frequent complication of necrosis or pseudarthrosis. In France this view has been held by Leger and Sicard since 1949 and has found many supporters among general surgeons.

Up to 1960 I myself disagreed with this approach. I always used osteosynthesis in fresh fractures, and a prosthesis only as secondary treatment in failures.

It must be admitted, however, that the failures of osteosynthesis, i.e. early displacement, pseudarthrosis or necrosis, are in the long run hardly tolerable for old patients. Repeated surgical intervention is not without danger for such patients. They have to be kept under observation for 2 or 3 years after the operation. The patient and his family are bitterly disappointed when a seemingly good result gradually deteriorates owing to the development of necrosis.

All these considerations prompt the surgeon to find a quick and sure solution even if it is only moderately satisfactory.

For these reasons we decided in 1960 to treat with prostheses patients over 70 yea s of age, suffering from fresh femoral neck fractures.

We use the Moore vitallium prosthesis. Patients with femoral neck fractures are immediately operated on, by postero-lateral incision without dividing the glutei. The indications for the operation were very extensive. The average age was 78,5 patients were over 90 years old. Only moribund patients were not treated.

The results of the method in 104 cases were examined in 1965.

We tried to compare this series of 104 cases treated with prosthesis with a series of 108 cases treated with osteosynthesis before 1964. In order to get a real comparison we included only femoral neck fractures with displacement, and over 65 years.

Two points were considered for this comparison:

1. Mortality
2. Functional results.

1. Mortality

Mortality figures given by various authors differ considerably: Reynolds 8.3%, Hinchey 10%, Poilleux 22%.

These differences are not explained by technical reasons. They must be due to the indications for the operation. Some surgeons observe their patients for several days and decide to operate only after mature consideration. Their material is therefore carefully selected and thus shows a smaller mortality.

Table 1. *275 cases of medial displaced fractures of the femoral neck in patients 65 to 98 years of age. Mortality according to treatment*

	Conservative		Fixation		Prosthesis	
Death rate in the first 3 months	15 cases	46%	108 cases	15%	167 cases	19%
Average age of the dead	81		79.5		79.7	

Clinique Chirurgicale Orthopédique et Réparatrice, Professeur Merle d'Aubigné, Hôpital Cochin.

One must also remember to correlate the mortality with the average age of the patients. Statistically at 80 years of age mortality is 2.8% during the first 3 months.

The mortality in our series is stated in Table 1. This includes all non-operated cases as well as those with osteosynthesis and prosthesis in patients aged 65 or more. Mortality for osteosynthesis is 15%, for prosthesis 19%. This difference in favour of osteosynthesis cannot be described as significant. The difference in severity of the two operations is too slight compared with the part played by the patient's general condition. It is therefore necessary to base one's findings on the functional results if the actual merits of osteosynthesis and prosthesis are to be assessed.

The average duration of hospitalisation was 26 days for prosthesis against 62 for osteosynthesis. This can be regarded as an advantage of the method.

2. Functional Results

a) Prosthesis

Out of a total of 167 patients only 104 could be used for the evaluation of functional results. 29 patients died before the control examination. 34 others were lost.

Table 2. *Compared functional results*

	Nr. of cases	Excellent	Good	Fair	Poor
Primary fixation	68	46%	26%	22%	5 %
Secondary prosthesis	22				
Primary prosthesis	104	9%	72%	12%	5,4%

Clinique Chirurgicale Orthopédique et Réparatrice, Professeur Merle d'Aubigné, Hôpital Cochin.

The period of observation of the 104 patients whose functional results could be evaluated varied between 26 months and 6 years.

The distribution of results is seen in Table 2. The percentage of 5.4% failures is due mainly to complications: 4 infections, 7 dislocations. 80% of results can be described as satisfactory, with 72% showing only slight disturbances, i.e. mild pain, the need for a stick when walking outside. Only 9 cases with a perfectly normal hip were found.

b) Osteosynthesis

From the functional point of view the series of patients treated with prosthesis can be compared with 68 femoral neck fractures treated by the osteosynthesis method. The number is very limited as only those cases could be considered which remained under observation for at least 2 years, and only fractures with displacement of fragments in old patients. With this kind of selection the results are, of course, not very brilliant although one must differentiate between anatomical and functional results.

The anatomical results, to judge from radiographs, show complete bony union with restitutio ad integrum in only 50%. In 16% of cases there developed a limited and often well tolerated necrosis of the femoral head during the 2 years following fracture consolidation. In 34% of cases, however, a pseudarthrosis or extensive necrosis of the femoral head developed.

Functional results were very good in 26 cases, good in 10, fair in 9 and poor in 23. Of these 23 cases 22 required a second operation. This consisted of head and neck resection in 1 case because of infection, renewed osteosynthesis in 6 cases and prosthesis insertion in 15 cases because of necrosis or pseudarthrosis.

In 68 patients, 22 of whom required a second operation, an excellent result was achieved in 46%, i.e. restitution of a normal hip. There were good results in 26%, fair results in 22% and poor results in 5%.

Conclusion

The mortality is comparable in the two methods and depends in no way on the type of operation but on the age and general condition of the patient.

The functional results with prosthesis are worse than those with osteosynthesis inasmuch as excellent results are much rarer and early complications more frequent. But, fair results are regulary obtained with only one operation and a short hospitalisation. With osteosynthesis, while excellent results are obtained in one case out of two, late complications make reoperation necessary in one case out of three.

From this we may draw the following personal conclusion. In an old patient in good general condition, still very active and living in reasonably comfortable circumstances, who can face a second operation without detriment to his health or his material situation, we prefer osteosynthesis as it produces excellent functional results, sometimes after a second operation. On the other hand, in old patients with only moderate resistance for whom a second operation would be dangerous and whose living conditions would make prolonged postoperative surveillance difficult, we believe we are justified in using primary prosthesis.

Discussion

George Hammond

Dr. D'Aubigné has attempted to answer the important question of whether acute displaced fractures of the femoral neck are best treated by reduction and internal fixation or by replacement of the head and neck using an Austin Moore prosthesis. To find the solution, he compared the mortality and functional results in two groups of patients of comparable ages treated by these two methods.

I. Mortality

There was not much difference in the mortality within 3 months of injury, since the mortality after prosthetic replacement was 19% and after osteosynthesis was 15%.

II. Functional Results

A. Prosthetic replacement. There were 104 fractures of the hip treated by prosthetic replacement available for followup study. The table of results indicated that the followup of prosthetic replacements was 6 months to 6 years, with an average follow-up of 26 months. I believe the minimal followup period should have been 2 years because there are many complications with a prosthesis that appear after the first 6 postoperative months.

A considerable number of complications of prosthetic replacements occurred in the series. It would have been of great interest to know more about the seven dislocations, since with the posterior approach used in these patients dislocation is relatively rare. Was the method or length of postoperative splinting at fault? How were these dislocations treated, and what was the explanation for the high mortality and poor results in this group? The two fractures of the femur at operation are not too unusual, but I am sure everyone would be interested in a more detailed explanation and analysis of the five fractures of the femur that occurred on resumption of weight bearing and which are most unusual. It would be important to know the cause and the outcome of paralysis of the sciatic nerve in three patients. No mention is made of other common complications, and I wonder if this group of patients was so fortunate as to have had no errors of selection and insertion of the prosthesis and no problems caused by bone absorption, such as loosening, settling, and intrapelvic protrusion of the prosthesis.

The functional results in 104 patients with prosthetic replacement with good or excellent results in 64% are average. Some might question if a prosthetic replacement ever results in a normal hip, which is the author's definition of an excellent result (9 cases).

B. Osteosynthesis. 67 patients with displaced fractures of the femoral neck treated by closed reduction and internal fixation were available for end-result study with a followup period of 2 years or more. 50% of these patients obtained healed fractures without avascular necrosis, and 15% had healed fractures with limited necrosis. In 34% (23 patients) nonunion or major avascular necrosis resulted. No other complications were reported. The functional results in these 67 patients were good or excellent in 53%, fair in 13%, and poor in 34%.

It should be noted that the number of excellent results with internal fixation is much higher than in patients with prosthetic replacement (38% versus 8.6%) and that good and excellent results constituted 53% of the total. These statistics are ample arguments against the routine use of prosthetic replacement in all fractures of the femoral neck.

I wholeheartedly agree with the author when he concludes that there should be a definite indication for a prosthetic replacement and that many patients are best treated by closed reduction and internal fixation.

In the United States it is recognized that prosthetic replacement for displaced fractures of the femoral neck has a definite place, but it is also agreed that the best result is a healed fracture without avascular necrosis. To use a prosthesis as a routine procedure for all such fractures is to deny about 55% (our own statistics) of the patients the advantage of the best possible result.

There *are* varying degrees of avascular necrosis, and a patient with such a complication may have a satisfactory result and not need a second operation. It is also true that nonunion of the femoral neck does not always demand a second operation. Thus, in the series of 387 displaced fractures treated by internal fixation reported by Boyd and Salvatore*, only 18% (and not 45%) of the patients required a second operative procedure for these complications. It must be emphasized that the results of *prompt* prosthetic replacement in patients with poor results of osteosynthesis caused by nonunion and avascular necrosis are comparable to the results with the use of a prosthesis as the primary procedure. Thus, many poor results from osteosynthesis can be salvaged satisfactorily, whereas if prosthetic replacement fails, a major problem is created, a second operation may be necessary, and it is difficult to obtain a good result by the various salvage operations. Certainly, prosthetic replacement is far from a panacea. The best results after prosthetic replacement are not comparable with the best results after osteosynthesis, nor are we as yet certain how long a good result from a prosthesis will last.

We recognize that there are certain indications for the use of prosthetic replacement as the primary procedure in displaced fractures of the neck of the femur. A word of caution — since this operation is so easy and the postoperative care less arduous than after internal fixation, it is easy to expand the true indications unjustifiably to include patients who should be treated by internal fixation. Some of the more important indications for prosthetic replacement in acute, displaced fractures of femoral neck are:

1. Major comminution of femoral neck making stable reduction and internal fixation impossible.

2. Inability to obtain excellent reduction or rigid internal fixation.

3. An untreated displaced fracture that is 3 or more weeks old.

4. Traumatic dislocation of the hip with fracture of the superior, weightbearing portion of the femoral head.

---

* Boyd, H. B., and J. E. Salvatore: J. Bone Joint Surg. **46A**, 1066—1068 (1964).

5. Dislocation of the hip with fracture of the femoral neck.

6. Old age in itself is not an indication, but there are certain senile patients who will not be able to use crutches after internal fixation and who will benefit by a primary prosthetic replacement. Many of these patients had very little capacity to ambulate before fracture and have a short life expectancy.

7. Poor general health that demands early mobilization and early return to near normal activities.

Conclusions

In conclusion, I agree with Dr. D'Aubigné that the best treatment for acute displaced fracture of the neck of the femur is reduction and internal fixation. Although there are certain indications for prosthetic replacement as the primary treatment, the sacrifice of the head and neck of the femur is not the proper solution for the majority of patients.

References

Anderson, L. D., W. R. Hamsa Jr., and T. L. Waring: J. Bone Joint Surg. **46 A**, 1049—1065 (1964).

Campbell, W. C.: Operative orthopaedics. Ed. 4, 1778 pp. St. Louis: C. V. Mosby Co. 1963.

Eaton, G. O.: J. Bone Joint Surg. **47 A**, 218—219 (1965).

Hinchey, J. J., and P. L. Day: J. Bone Joint Surg. **46 A**, 223—240 (1964).

Lunceford, E. M., Jr.: J. Bone Joint Surg. **47 A**, 832—841 (1965).

Moore, A. T.: The Moore self-locking vitallium prosthesis in fresh femoral neck fractures. Instructional Course Lectures, American Academy of Orthopedic Surgeons, Vol. 16, pp. 309—321. St. Louis: C. V. Mosby Co. 1959.

Rowe, C. R.: J. Bone Joint Surg. **47 A**, 1043—1059 (1965).

Long Term Experience with Internal Nail Fixation of Fractures of the Femur and Tibia

Richard Maatz

This report on my experience with medullary nailing of the lower limb is based on 491 nailings of the femur and 1081 of the tibia.

The clinical material was derived from the hospital in Kiel, and some establishments in the neighbourhood of Kiel with whom we closely collaborated during the years which immediately followed the war, and from my own hospital in Berlin. My records of cases treated by me during the war in hospital ships, military hospitals and in my capacity as assistant to the consulting surgeon to the German Navy, Prof. A. W. Fischer, have unfortunately all been lost with the exception of the records of 30 suppurating gunshot wounds involving fractures which had been treated by nailing.

Let me first make the following statement: "A fracture that can be nailed cannot be better treated than with a medullary nail". Only this will produce a weight bearing osteosynthesis, while with all other methods at best only a functionally stable osteosynthesis can be achieved. This distinction is most important. To avoid any misunderstanding it should be however stressed that we are all in favour of a functionally stable osteosynthesis if the fracture is not suitable for nailing. There exists also an indeterminate field where medullary nailing is indicated even though a weight bearing osteosynthesis cannot be at once achieved. But I shall return to that later.

The nailing of the femur achieved a rapid success and became accepted within a few years all over the world. In the case of the tibia this was more difficult. Important opinions counselled against it. During the Congress of Northwest German surgeons at Lübeck in 1961 however Küntscher rightly stated that in a kind of "underground movement" this form of nailing had begun to be accepted by the younger surgeons, and today after the introduction of the rigid pin with clover leaf profile and the opening up of the marrow cavity with the use of flexible drills, nobody really has any doubts about the value of the method even in that part of the skeletal system.

Let us first consider the indications:

In the femur the range has been increased during the past few years. No doubt exists in the case of transverse and oblique fractures in the area covered by the nail. Hereby I should like to stress that not the smooth transverse fracture but the short oblique fracture constitutes the "ideal case". The latter can never cause failure of rotation while the first unfortunately sometimes does. A large flexure triangle has only the disadvantage that *the nail alone* guarantees stability. This is important when deciding on the date for weight bearing. Fractures with displacement can produce technical problems, the indication for nailing will however nearly invariably be absolute. Comminuted fractures show marked local reaction with good healing tendencies. I therefore do not nail them.

Supracondylar fractures I used to stabilize with two Rush pins for a number of years. I have now reverted to using a Küntscher pin. We know that the osteosynthesis achieved in this way is initially only stable at rest and after 2 weeks only functionally stable, but nothing more can be achieved with the Rush pins either. The use of a Küntscher pin has however the great advantage that the field of operation is far removed from the area of reduction. This is a decisive advantage from the asepsis point of view.

Cranially situated fractures of the femur have only recently and in my opinion successfully made suitable for nailing by Küntscher. I refer here to the long, bent pin which is introduced at the level of the medial femoral condylus in a medial-ventral direction.

This method has again the advantage that the field of operation and area of reduction are separate. In addition the soft tissue injury is small when compared with the subtrochanteric wound. It is in fact just a small puncturelike incision.

Having convinced myself of the effectiveness of this method in the treatment of pertrochanteric fractures, I have used this long pin also successfully for per- or subtrochanteric oblique osteotomies of varus or valgus inclination. The nail seems to me also indicated in the case of a torsion fracture if the medullar space is wide enough. Such a torsion fracture shows an unwelcome tendency towards rotation failure. With this technique however the rotation component is reliably eliminated, because the pin is lodged sideways in the femoral neck and the femoral condylus. The inadequate fit of the pin in the bony shaft has to be accepted.

In the tibia the area of the nailable fractures begins cranially at the level of the border between 1st and 2nd third, if we do not choose a temporary transarticular method, which in some special cases both with supracondylar fractures of the femur or fractures of the tibia near the knee-joint can be fully justified. We must be aware of carrying the use of the thick and rigid pin to excess in cranially situated fractures, as it can result in the bursting of the bony shaft ventral-cranially or dorsal-caudally. We prefer the use of a wedge pin, that is we use 2 of the old type of tibial pins and then drive 1 or 2 shorter pins of the same shape in between the first 2. In this way we achieve the necessary wedge shape, which assures the good fit and resistance to bending of the total pin.

The rigid Küntscher pin with clover leaf profile can be used for the rest of the tibia with the exception of fractures near the ankle-joint, that is below the border between 3rd and 4th quarter of the tibia. These we treat by using a spreading nail with inclined planes. It enables us to achieve a functionally stable osteosynthesis within the first few weeks. The position of the level of the pin is governed by the position and shape of the fracture.

Now just a few words about the question whether fractures in children should be nailed. The indications can be given in the same way both for the femur and the tibia.

We nail invariably if a nailable fracture cannot be reduced and stabilized by purely conservative measures. In our experience wire extension using the calcaneus is more likely to cause osteomyelitis than the nailing of the tibia.

In my opinion there is no better treatment for a nailable open fracture than nailing. This also applies to the tibia. This is shown by the data given in table.

Table. *Compound fractures of the tibia*

	Maatz, Kemmerisch, Trischkat	Böhler	
Number	335		500
Sec. amp.	2.4%		8.9%
Infections: soft tissue	23.0%	mild	21.8%
osteomyelitis	3.0%	severe	15.6%
Duration of illness	125.4 days		234 days

In compound fractures the wound secretions are drained during the first few days via a Redon drainage which can be within the pin pushed up right to the fracture level. Above all however one has to, even more carefully than in the case of a closed fracture, try to achieve a stable osteosynthesis. If it comes to suppuration of the wound or even to suppuration of the bone this will mean then a much prolonged period of invalidity, the osseous union of the fracture however will still usually take place. This is in marked contrast to the results with all other operative methods and shows most clearly the strong case for medullary nailing. Evidently it would be quite wrong to remove on account of suppuration a pin before osseous union has taken place.

On the right time for nailing:

Compound fractures must be immediately treated. If a contraindication is present then nailing should be carried out 2 to 3 weeks later after the wound has healed. During the war we nailed suppurating fractures caused by gunshot wounds. In the preantibiotic era this endangered life if carried out on the femur and endangered the leg when the tibia was involved. On the humerus and the forearm the same technique was however unexpectedly successful without exception in 40 cases. This is probably explained by the fact that in suppurating gunshot wounds of the upper limb diseased fragments are removed and the resulting shortening of the limb is accepted. Under the conditions which prevail nowadays I cannot agree to the nailing of a compound fracture which is suppurating in the area of the fracture, as it could lead to a spread of the infection.

A closed fracture of the tibia is treated immediately after admission. If the injury is bilateral first only one leg is nailed, the other after a few days. In 1943 we had one death due to fat embolism after the immediate nailing of both tibiae.

Closed fractures of the femur we do not nail primarily on account of the danger of fat embolism. The patients are first treated with wire extension and then nailing is carried out on the 4th to 5th day.

Now a few words on the technique of the nailing:

The nailing is carried out as a closed procedure in principle. This offers no problem in the case of the tibia and is possible in the case of the femur with suitable preliminary treatment consisting of extension under a good anaesthetic and using muscle relaxants. This is usually most successful with very few exceptions.

The ability to reduce the fracture should be tested before the operation starts. An exception is the cranially situated oblique fracture of the femur where the pin which is introduced into the proximal fragment provides the means for achieving the reduction. Cranially situated oblique fractures I like to expose first and then use a conical trochanter pin.

The maintenance of asepsis is made easier by the use of of the magnifyer but still not adequately assured. Whenever possible I separate the field of operation from the field of reduction into an aseptic and septic part. The more distal the fracture is situated the easier this is to achieve. There should be preferred therefore only one surgeon too because this makes it easier to keep to the discipline of keeping the two regions separate.

The determination of the length and thickness of the pin is possible by sample drilling of the medullar space. The mandrin is pushed in, up to the required length and the required measurements can then be worked out. We do not use excessive thicknesses of the pins if they can only be made possible by extensive drilling. Extremely large medullar spaces require however extremely thick pins. If in the presence of an adequately wide medullar space there remains any doubt about the caliber of pin that should be used, we rather go in once more with the drill. In any case nowadays it should not any more become necessary to have to saw off the pin because it got too firmly wedged into the bone. I was called in to advise in two cases where indeed the nail would neither move forward or background. In both cases I split the shaft of the bone over the point of the pin with an oscillating saw lengthwise and relieved the pressure in this way.

Additional traction may be indicated very occasionally in fractures of the femur with a tendency to shortening.

An additional Plaster of Paris we use in compound fractures of the tibia even after achieving a stable reduction, in every case, because the complete avoidance of all movements for the first 2 to 3 weeks is indicated in view of the infection of the soft tissues. Closed fractures of the tibia required in our clinical material an additional Plaster of Paris in 15% of the cases due to the inadequate stability resulting from a widening of the medullar space. Previously the percentage was 31%.

We permit walking after fractures of the femur as soon as the wound has healed, that is after about 2 weeks, in the case of the tibia after 3 weeks.

I shall now discuss possible complications.

The at the beginning most feared complication is fat embolism. It was in fact observed with a lethal outcome in fractures of the femur, in one case in a military hospital even in the severe form of an air and fat embolism. Every one of us who has ever withdrawn a medullary nail quickly, knows the sound of the air rushing in. In this way repeated insertion and withdrawal of the nail can lead to a kind of pumping effect.

We have not had any death from fat embolism during the past 20 years since we

1. decided to nail closed fractures of the femur only after a few days,
2. open up the bone of the trochanter over the trocar with a rasp,
3. give the bone marrow time to drain and
4. use driving purposeful blows of the hammer instead of many small blows.

Infection after nailing constitutes a severe but not catastrophic complication. It is a remarkable fact that the tendency towards infection varies with the different bones of the extremity. So it is greater in the femur and humerus than in the radius, ulna, and tibia. It would serve no purpose to give all the figures derived from our quite large clinical material, because this would include all the mistakes which were made during the period while this method was perfected and therefore not give a correct picture of the situation as it is today. Amongst the past 200 closed medullary nailed fractures of the tibia we encountered two superficial wound infections at the place where the pin had been introduced and one bland abscess 3 months after the operation.

In favourably positioned and suitably placed fractures the nailing will force the fragments into the only correct position. Wrong positions are of course more likely to arise where the fracture lies beyond the narrowest part of the marrow cavity.

The greatest care must be taken to achieve a good primary result. Unfortunately the viewer with its close circuit television link up produces a rather distorted picture which can simulate a correct axis when actually a bent one is present. But even the rigid nail which lies in the bone of the tibia can be correctively bent if a great force is carefully applied (set of pulleys) over a wide area.

To what extent a rotation fault must be corrected by operation we do not yet know. A 40° external rotation of the femur forced us to take action on account of increasing manifestations of stress in the knee joint. In the case of the tibia we were never forced to carry out any correction if the rotation was under 30°.

Discussion

MOORE MOORE JR.

Today Professor Dr. MAATZ has shared with us his very considerable experience, technical knowledge and wisdom in the field of long bone fixation. He is to be complimented on his presentation and especially in pointing out how to avoid some of the pitfalls of intramedullary nailing as well as how to get out of trouble in this field.

My own preference for intramedullary femoral fixation has been the Hansen-Street diamond-shaped nail which was developed in Memphis by STREET while at the Veteran's Administration hospital there. His technique was also largely the so-called blind or stab wound method but most private practitioners in the area preferred the open procedure with retrograde insertion of the nail but only after reaming the canal first to avoid wedging the nail in the isthmus of the femur. Fractures involving the lower third of the femur have usually been fixed by the Veseley modification of the diamond-shaped nail, namely splitting the distal nail so that the two parts tend to hold the lower fragment by lateral spread. This is in effect the two pin Rush technique but approaches the fracture from above rather than below.

We have been hesitant to allow weight bearing of an early fracture, usually waiting about 6 weeks and requiring crutches until adequate callus is seen.

The diamond profile nail has the ability to prevent rotation of fragments if fitted properly.

It is interesting to note that intramedullary nailing of femoral fractures (even bilateral ones) has been carried out successfully by STEVENSON et al. on a large orthopaedic service (U.S. Naval Hospital, Portsmouth) as a reliable means of controlling position in patients who had concomitant severe intracranial injuries and were therefore uncontrollable by other means.

Most sub- and practically all intertrochanteric fractures have, in our experience, been treated successfully by the Jewett nail (MOORE) for the past 15 years or more.

In the tibia the Lottes (St. Louis) or trifin profile nail has enjoyed greatest use in our area. His technique is also largely the blind or stab wound type nailing. This manner of fixation is especially helpful in segmented tibial fractures and of course its corollary in the femur with similar fractures.

As regards fat embolism, our experience parallels that noted and we do not find it as frequent complication.

I must enter a plea for closed conservative treatment of long bone shaft fractures in children. Only in very rare instances (as when one is convinced of massive persistent muscle interposition) do I open children's fractures in long bones and then we do not use an intramedullary nail.

Osteomyelitis has not been noted as a complication of skeletal traction though one may see an occasional and relatively innocuous wire or pin tract infection which clears promptly.

References

LOTTES, J. O.: J. Amer. med. Ass. **155**, 1039 (1954).

— Intramedullary nailing of the tibia. American Academy of Orthopaedic Surgeons Instructional Course Lectures, vol. XV, p. 65. Ann Arbor: J. W. Edwards 1958.

MOORE, M., JR.: Amer. J. Surg. **84**, 449—452 (1952).

STEVENSON, C. A.: Personal communication. Also symposium on intramedullary nailing at 1962 meeting of Society of Military Orthopaedic Surgeons.

VESELEY, D., G.: Sth. med. J. (Bgham. Ala.) **59**, 394—399 (1966).

Prevention and Management of Infection in Osteosynthesis*

H. WILLENEGGER

"The most effective prophylaxis against wound infection after internal fixation is the conservative treatment of fractures." This is a rather pointed oversimplification popular among many advocates of conservative treatment in opposition to the internal fixation of fractures in general, and of closed fractures in particular.

---

* From the Surgical Department of the Kantonsspital Liestal/Basle, Switzerland (Head: Prof. H. WILLENEGGER).

It is quite obvious and has indeed never been disputed that wound infection is a danger to be taken seriously and that it is one of the causes of a great number of failures after internal fixation. But it is not the only cause; incorrectly performed internal fixations are no less frequently to blame.

On the other hand, there are a great many fractures in which optimal functional results can only be achieved by internal fixation. We therefore have no choice but to come to terms with internal fixation and its disadvantages and risks, not only in the field of traumatology, but in all areas of orthopaedic surgery.

The general principles of asepsis, sterility and non-infection that apply to all forms of surgery must be studiously observed in connection with internal fixation. Once infection has set in, the situation is very close to disaster. The prevention of infection is therefore of vital importance in the surgery of bones and joints and no effort to this end is too small to be worth making.

The chief danger lies in hospital infections. For this reason, complete separation of septic and aseptic areas of the hospital can already bring about a significant reduction of the risk of infection. In one of our series of patients, the incidence of infections was reduced from about 4% to less than 1% solely as a result of the aseptic and septic areas being located on different floors. Wherever internal fixations are performed it is essential that the accommodation, equipment and measures taken to ensure asepsis should be carefully planned and constantly reviewed.

Rigorous and uncompromising demands must be made on the personal discipline of each and every member of the staff involved, to the extent that the principle of non-infection and all it implies become second nature to all concerned. Precise instructions must be given in this respect. Nose and throat swabs must be examined periodically. The wearing of face masks is mandatory, even in the preparation rooms.

Proper preparation of the patient is no less important. In emergency admissions, any contact whatsoever with the general emergency ward should be avoided. It is preferable to have the patient, clothes and all, brought straight into the aseptic department, regardless of whether the fracture concerned is a closed or compound one. With compound fractures especially, the danger of infection by hospital germs is far greater than that of bacterial contamination following the accident. In our experience, in only one quarter of all compound fractures (from the simple perforation to gaping wounds) was contamination demonstrable on culture. Prior to elective surgery, we recommend the following procedures: the skin should be prepared on the day before the operation with a depilatory ointment, then sprayed down, painted with a potent (penetrant and bactericidal) disinfectant and covered with a sterile dressing. We use the razor, which must be sterilized, only in emergency cases.

During the actual operation, we regard the following procedures as mandatory: the skin must be covered with a sterile adhesive draping and suction drainage must be instituted after surgery; for this purpose Jost-Redon's automatic suction drainage (Fig. 1b) has proved by far the most effective method. In preventing infection of the wound, another extremely important factor is that soft tissues have to be treated with the utmost care, above all where they are in direct contact with the bone; denudation of the bone must be restricted to the minimum. Vital soft-tissue, vital bone and thorough drainage of haematoma and secretory spaces contribute very significantly towards preventing the multiplication of any germs present and facilitating their destruction by the natural tissue defences. In the treatment of compound fractures, the importance of complete, meticulous debridement cannot be emphasized enough.

Postoperative elevation of the extremity in question not only promotes wound-healing as such, but is also of prophylactic value. Superinfection via the drain exit is not to be feared if the channel is long enough and the point of exit adequately attended to, e.g. by regular treatment with bactericidal spray. In the event of late haematomata forming after the removal of the suction drain, appropriate punctures should be made until they have been completely eliminated, especially in the case of subcutaneously situated bones, such as the medial surface of the tibia. The safety of the punctures can be enhanced if a stab incision is made first under local anaesthesia.

The prophylactic value of systematically administered antibiotics is, to say the least, dubious; they can certainly never replace the measures for preventing infection

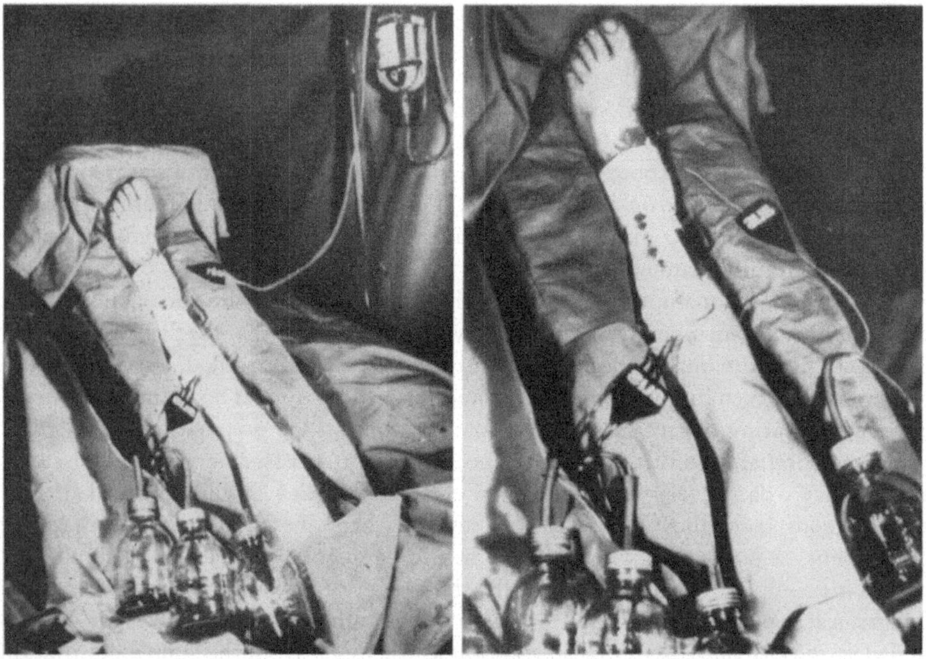

a b

Fig. 1 (see text)

already mentioned. The question that remains to be discussed is the topical application of antibiotics. During the operation we recommend the irrigation of the surgical wound with a 0.25‰ to 1.0‰ solution of nebacetin or a combination of bacitracin, polymyxin and neomycin. After long-lasting operations, after extensive surgical wounds and after primary internal fixation of compound fractures we tend to use the same solution for a temporary, postoperative instillation drainage. The procedure is simple: the most central drain is used as an instillation drain for a short time (Fig 1 a). As a rule, rapid drip infusion of 1 to 2 bottles of 1,000 ml is sufficient. Thereafter, the instillation drain is connected to a vacuum bottle. If the bottles are properly changed — this must be carefully taught — superinfections can certainly be prevented.

Treatment: Should infection nevertheless set in, there are still effective means of averting disaster and achieving good functional results, at least in the great majority of cases.

A distinction must be made between suspected and manifest infections.

Treatment of suspected infections: Inadequate regression of inflammatory reactions (which occur after all fractures, not only after internal fixations), rising temperature and increasing number of leucocytes (daily determinations should be made) after internal fixation are the events that arouse suspicion of slowly progressive wound infections. In such cases systemic antibiotic therapy is clearly indicated. The causative organisms are most frequently hospital germs. Their sensitivity to antibiotics should be known in most hospitals, so that the most suitable antibiotic can be selected in suspect cases. In our hospital we are using the following antibiotics:

a) Penicillin	20 to 60 million units	daily i.v.
Streptomycin	1 G.	
Sulphonamide	1 G.	
b) Chloromycetin	2 G. daily i.v.	
c) Synthetic penicillins.		

Treatment of Manifest Infections

If wound infection is confirmed, we adopt the following measures as a standard procedure: 1) implants are left in place to ensure immobilization of the infected areas, which is extremely important; 2) antibiotic instillation drainage of the infected area is instituted; 3) systemic antibiotics.

The mode of action of antibiotic instillation drainage consists in bacteriostatic or bactericidal treatment of the infected surfaces on the one hand and mechanical cleansing on the other; both are important.

In setting up the instillation drains, the following principles should be observed: 1) all infected spaces must be irrigated, including all layers and fissures down to the microscopic level; 2) drainage must take place from the centre of the infection site towards the periphery. — A distinction must be made between open and closed drainage, the open technique being much more commonly used (Fig. 2).

The effectiveness of instillation drainage is basically that the virulently infected surface is converted into a blandly infected surface (Table). Even with bactericidal antibiotics, complete sterility is seldom achieved. On the other hand it is not absolutely necessary. Effective instillation drainage stops the proliferation of the pathogens in the surrounding tissue. Soft-tissue cellulitis and osteitis subside. Even severely affected osteitic bones can be revitalized and integrated, provided contact with vital soft tissue is rapidly established. In this respect, however, the method has definite limitations. Necrotic bone splinters and fragments must be removed, together with the usual treatment for osteitis. Remaining defects call for plastic reconstruction; for this purpose, autologous cancellous-bone grafts have proved to be the most effective and reliable method.

In principle, the choice of the antibiotic solution depends on the results of sensitivity tests. For a number of years we have chiefly used a $0.25^0/_{00}$ solution of chloromycetin, since bacteriological tests invariably showed this to be the most effective drug. We are now testing a combination of bacitracin, polymyxin and neomycin, in particular with the Danish preparation Citomyxin and the English Polybactrin. To what extent these preparations inhibit the mesenchymal elements responsible for regeneration cannot be assessed definitively at present. From the clinical point of view, their use entails no significant disadvantages.

Antibiotic instillation drainage over a period of 6 to 7 days is enough to produce a bacteriostatic effect. The antibiotic should then be replaced by physiological saline. If antibiotics are given for longer periods, resistant strains tend to emerge, amongst which Proteus and Pyocyaneus are particularly undesirable.

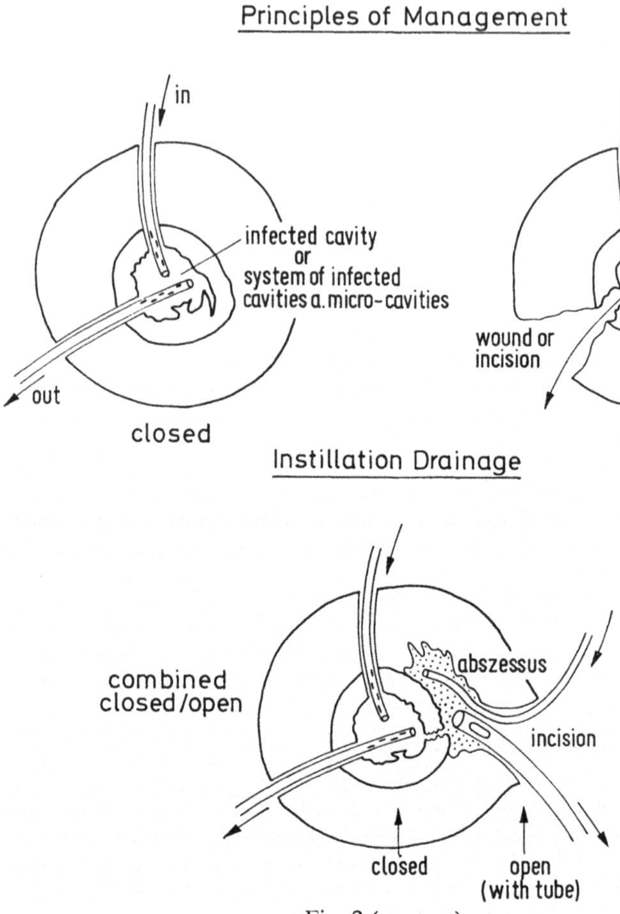

Fig. 2 (see text)

Table. *Effectiveness of Instillation Drainage*

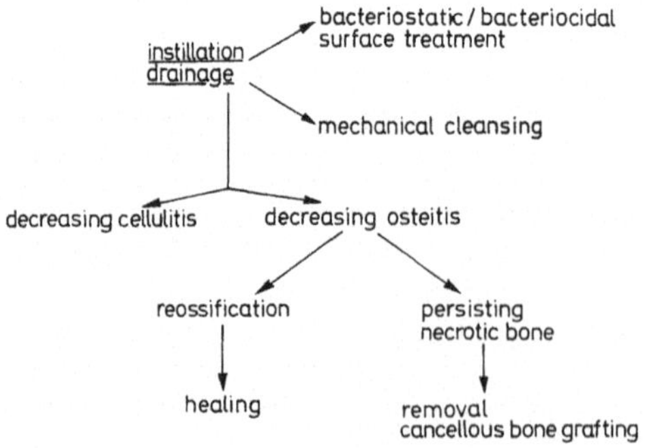

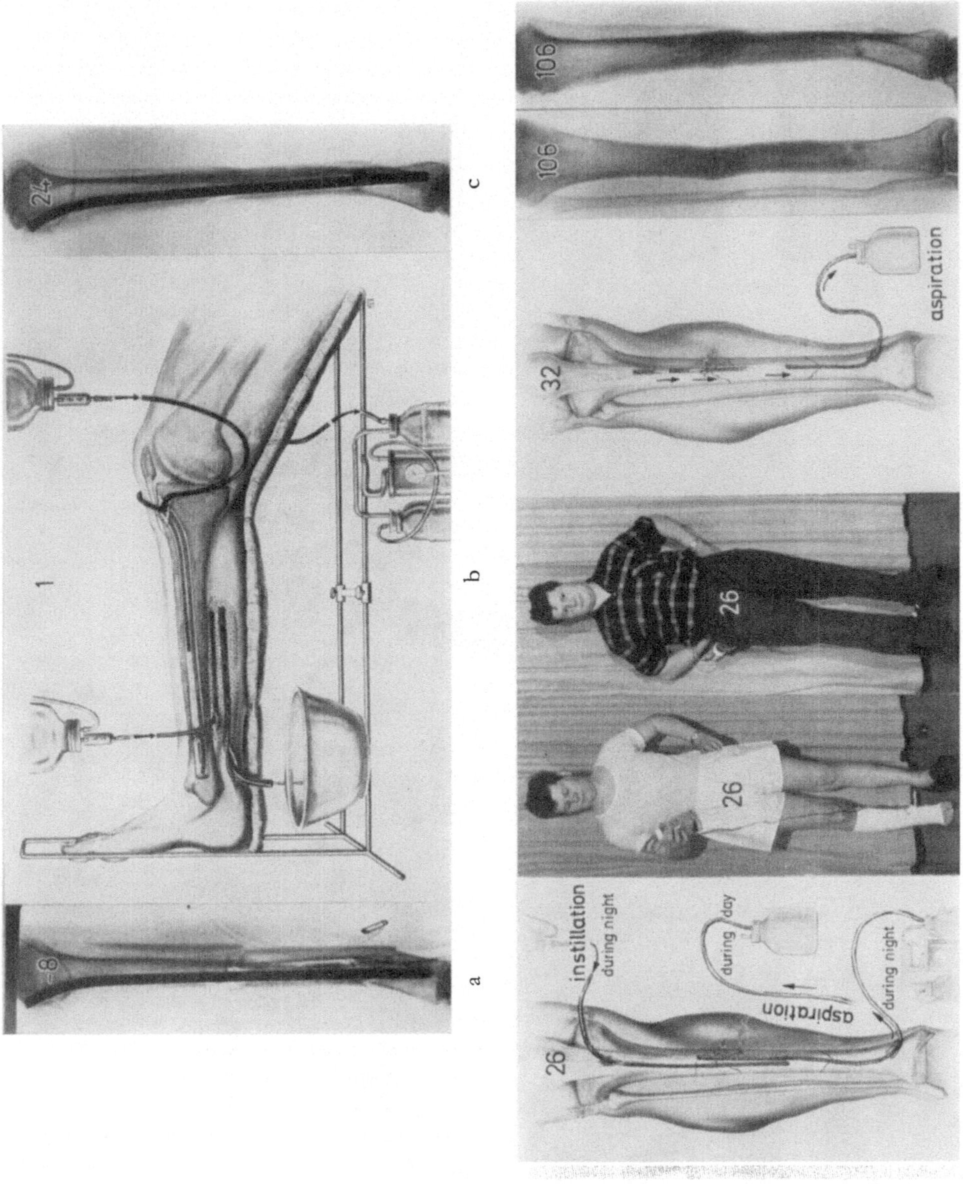

Fig. 3a—g. Severe infection after intramedullary nailing. a Infected and necrotic bone 8 weeks after nailing: instillation drainage begun. b 1 week after institution of instillation drainage: closed system through the nail-bore, open system in a periosteal abscess. c Bone-healing 24 weeks after beginning of instillation drainage; nail removed. d 26 weeks after instillation drainage or 2 weeks after removal of the nail. It is essential that the medullary space should be drained from the lowest point. For this purpose an opening is bored on the medial side of the tibia. Instillation drainage during night; during day aspiration only; e The patient is up and about, carrying the aspiration bottle with him. f Successive retraction of drain. g Perfect bone-healing and full restoration of function

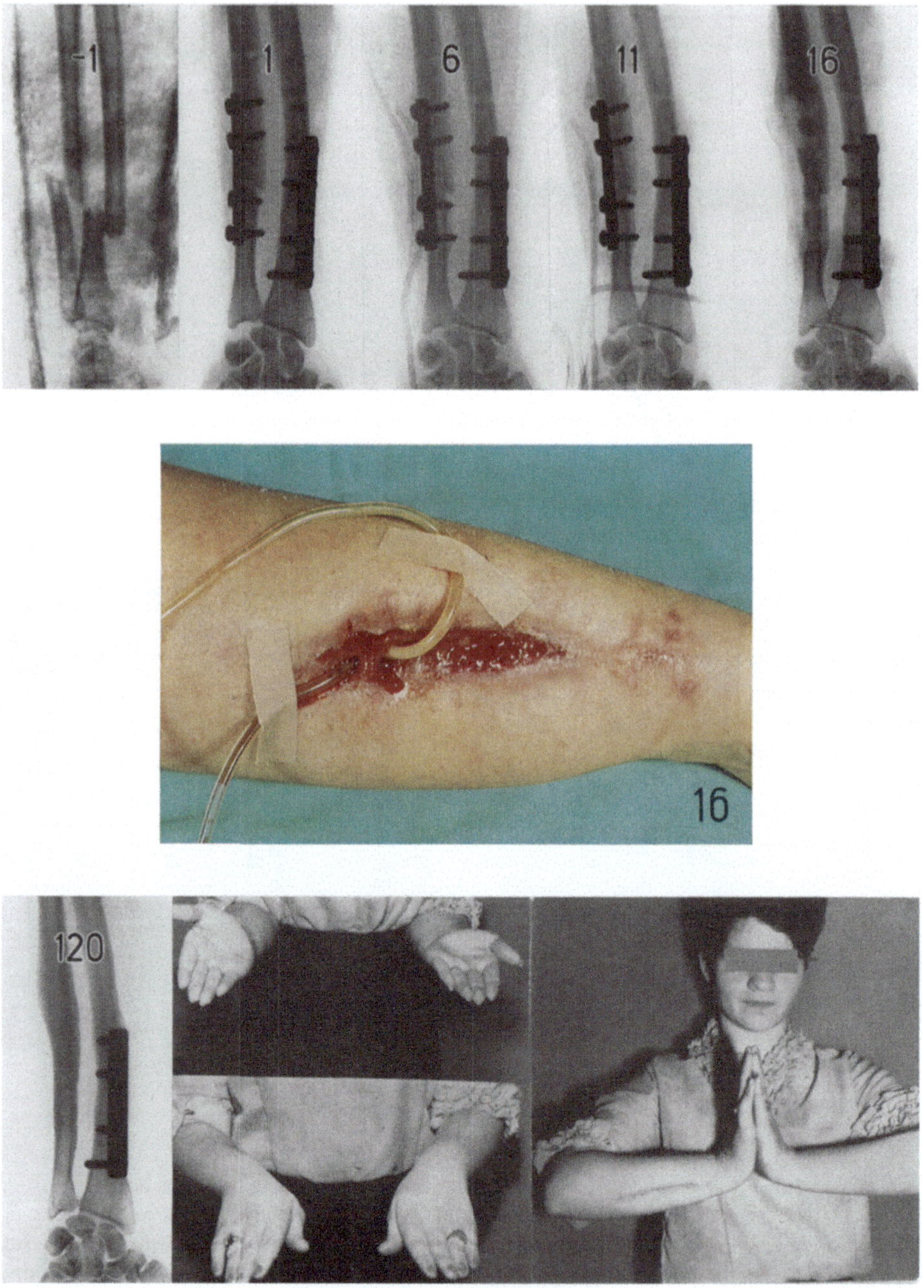

Fig. 4. Internal fixation after unsuccessful conservative treatment (figures denote weeks before and after internal fixation). Infection only at the ulna, becoming manifest 10 days after internal fixation; instillation drainage set up immediately. 16 weeks after internal fixation ossification sufficient to allow removal of the plate. Colour photo shows instillation drainage after removal of the plate. End result 120 weeks after internal fixation; some functional impairement of supination only

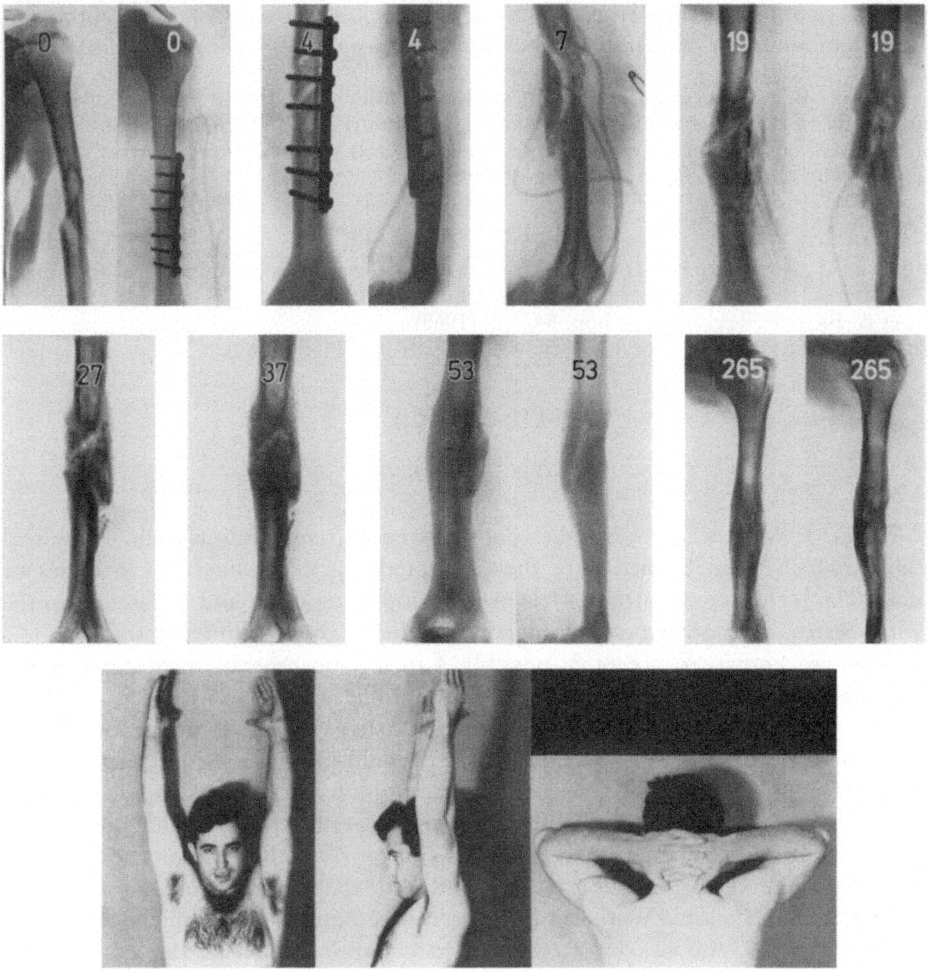

Fig. 5. Severe wound infection after poorly indicated internal fixation of oblique fracture of humerus. See text

The overall duration of instillation drainage varies to a great extent and depends above all on the progress of bone healing.

As soon as there is evidence of consolidation of the bone, the implants are removed. Antibiotic instillation drainage is then reinstituted to ensure that the fresh surgical wound remains bland.

The management and the prospects of successful treatment can be illustrated briefly by reference to a few particular cases:

Case 1: J. W., male, age 23. The situation is easiest to deal with in fresh infections after intramedullary nailing (Fig. 3). The nail itself serves as a cannula. A periosteal infection must be treated separately. Early weight-bearing is usually possible and this promotes healing of the bone. After removal of the intramedullary nail, antibiotic irrigation is renewed. Successive retraction of the drain is effected through a distal opening, bored at the time of removing the nail.

This basic technique also yields successful results in other fresh infections:

Case 2: Z. U., female, age 17. Failure in conservative treatment of a forearm fracture. Then internal fixation (Fig. 4). Wound infection confined only to the ulna. Rapid healing and ossification under open instillation drainage. No sequestra. Minimal functional impairment.

Case 3: B. A., male, age 21. In this case we consider that the advisability of primary internal fixation was debatable. Severe wound infection (Fig. 5). Open instillation drainage. Striking reossification of the severely infected bone. Only two small, unimportant sequestra needed to be removed. Full restoration of function.

References

Müller, M. E., M. Allgöwer, and H. Willenegger: Technique of internal fixation of fractures. Berlin, Heidelberg, New York: Springer 1965.

—, et A. Britzy: Rev. Chir. orthop. **54**, 139 (1968).

Willenegger, H., u. W. Roth: Dtsch. med. Wschr. **87**, 1485 (1962).

Discussion

Moore Moore Jr.

Professor Willenegger is to be congratulated on reminding us again of the real tragedy which is established once there is noted a genuine infection in bones or joints. The incidence of infection has been variously reported and apparently in the United States it is reported as a bit higher than the 1% quoted in this instance. Some hospitals are known to accept 3, possibly 3 to 6% postoperative infection as the irreducible minimum. In orthopaedics we should not accept this at all.

Of course the best treatment for infection in osteosynthesis is prevention. At the risk of over simplication and seeming naive I would like to point out that the first and best line of resistance to infection is intact, good skin. Therefore, when one is confronted with a fracture he should examine it carefully to determine whether or not open surgery is actually the method of choice or whether an alternative closed method would give as satisfactory a result with little differential in loss of time or loss of function. If the closed method can be used it certainly is preferable. Secondly, if one is confronted with an open wound it is essential that adequate skin coverage be present prior to any later surgery, for it is certainly agreed that all bone injuries and infections heal better with good skin overlying them. In this instance I would like to cite the recent work of Parkes at U.S. Naval Hospital, St. Albans, New York in covering large skin defects by open grafting with the involved extremity suspended by means of 2 or more Kirschner wires or Steinman pins, as the case may be. Skin graft is placed on without suturing and very meticulous attention is paid to gently pushing out the collections of serum and/or blood which may develop underneath the skin in 3 or 4 days. These grafts have been seen by me and take very readily. Then one has a good skin surface which promotes better viability of the bone underneath it no matter what its condition. It is also interesting to note that according to Parkes that wards on either side of his, which are not using this technique have difficulties with a fair number of bone infections, whereas he has not experienced such tragedies. As a final comment it is quite interesting to note that independently Professor Willenegger and Bingham have reported essentially the same idea in prevention of bone and joint infections, although Bingham (Amer. J. Orthop., June 1967) relates his technique as a prevention and prophylactic method rather than a treating method. However, I am sure it can and has been adapted to this. He reports on some 3,000 cases of traumatic and surgical wounds with favorable results by use of a dilute solution of penicillin to irrigate the wound at the time of surgery. It is his opinion that most of the penicillin, which is in dilute saline or lactate Ringer's solution, is washed out at the time by the actual irrigation process and by serum, etc., but that there remains a thin film or coating in the wound with the antibiotic being fixed to proteins in this region. Virtually no reactions to penicillin have been noted. There is immediate protection. He feels that this adds only 4 or 5 min to the surgical procedure. However, other potent antibiotics can be used locally if there is a strong history of penicillin sensitivity. These would be Aureomycin, Terramycin, Lincococin and Erythromycin. Possibly Terramycin or Oxytetracycline would be the best. The lack of allergic reaction to penicillin is attributed to the entrapment of the solution locally and its relative lack of absorption into the system generally.

In conclusion let me say that this has been a most interesting and stimulating paper. I feel that all of us will profit by adherence to the principles expressed by Professor WILLENEGGER.

References

BINGHAM, R.: Amer. J. Orthop. (1967).
PARKES, J.: Pers. communication.

Surgery for Rheumatoid Arthritis of the Lower Extremities

PHILIP D. WILSON JR.

We are now again in an era when surgeons must play important roles in the planning of treatment for patients with Rheumatoid Arthritis. The two past decades have witnessed first, the astounding development of cortico-steroids; second, a stage of optimism occasioned by the dramatic effect of these hormones on the synovitis of rheumatoid arthritis; and finally, a phase of disillusionment because of the nonspecific suppressive nature of their action and the many serious complications attendant to their use. All too often the progression of illness to a crippling stage has not been prevented. But since no other effective drugs have been developed to take the place of cortico-steroids, responsible rheumatologists have turned back to the surgeon for help.

We have, therefore, been challenged to find suitable indications for operative intervention and new and better answer to the many various problems that this unpredictable disease may present. As a consequence, the whole field of synovectomy of joints has been redeveloped in the past several years. The suitability of this type of procedure to the eradication of the early stages of joint inflammation — thereby to prevent articular damage — has added another whole surgical dimension to what was formerly a reconstructive field only. Certain rheumatoid syndromes, on the other hand, do not lend themselves well to synovectomy. Experience has shown that such joints tend to stiffen and deform despite the best of medical and surgical treatment. For these we must continue to turn to the more classical principle of treatment by arthroplasty. But not necessarily by the same old types of arthroplasty, since here again the situation is in a state of change and the exciting new techniques of whole joint replacement give great promise for the future.

These then are the two main categories of operations useful in the surgical treatment of rheumatoid arthritis; one, the "prophylactic" i.e. synovectomy; and two, the "reconstructive" i.e. arthroplasty. However, the joints of many patients for which operation is indicated are neither good enough to be ideal for synovectomy, nor bad enough for joint replacement. It is this type of joint which we see the most frequently and which will therefore occupy most of my ensuing attention in the discussion of the surgical treatment of the weight bearing joints.

The general condition of the patient as a whole must be considered first. Treatment must obviously be individualized to the sex, age and stature of a patient, and to the particular nature and stage of the disease. Socio-economic factors also play an important part in the planning of surgical programs involving multiple operations and long periods of hospitalization and disability.

An accurate evaluation of the suitability of the upper extremities for the use of walking aids is of primary importance before undertaking operations on the lower extremities. Shoulder stiffness without pain does not impair this significantly. Weakness of elbow extension, and of wrist stabilization and grasp, however, do. When the wrist is too painful for use of conventional crutches or canes, the power of elbow extension may be sufficient to permit the use of forearm support crutches. Stabilization of the wrist and operations designed to improve grip not only may be carried out while such crutches are in use, but may be helpful in giving the patient better control of them.

The next step of importance is the preoperative estimation of the degree of interdependence of multiple joint deformities or malfunctions, and what effect the correction of one will have on another. For instance, there is little purpose in correcting a hip flexion contracture without planning to correct companion flexion contractures of an ipsilateral knee or a contralateral hip. Severe pain in one hip may prevent the recovery of a very satisfactory arthroplasty of the other or a painful knee may prevent the proper use of a nicely reconstructed hip on the same side. These factors must all be considered in preoperative planning and the purpose of treatment clearly defined so as to derive maximum benefit from a series of operations. There is equally as much danger of not doing enough as of doing too much. Generally speaking knee flexion contractures should be corrected before those of the hips, and the excision of bony prominences in the soles of the feet is not indicated unless the preoperative plan includes the functional restoration of the knees and hips. Where deformity is not a significant factor in disability, the most symptomatic joint should be operated upon first.

Complications may prove disastrous and so disarrange a soundly planned program of surgical reconstruction as to render it completely ineffective. Every precaution must be taken to prevent their occurrence — a task of no small dimensions, when one considers the debilitated physical condition of many arthritics, who frequently suffer from chronic hyperadrenocorticoidism and other systemic conditions affecting wound healing or susceptability to infection. The prophylactic use of massive doses of antibiotics would seem a justifiable practice when metallic prostheses are left in situ in such patients.

It is beyond the scope of this presentation to go into great detail about the surgical correction of each joint, but I should like to touch on the major indications for specific procedures, and on certain points of operative technique which my colleagues at the Hospital for Special Surgery and I have found useful.

The excision of bony prominences in the feet is a particularly effective and reliable procedure for the relief of pain from calluses. When the problem is confined to 1 or 2 rays the approach through a single linear dorsal incision placed between the metatarsal rays sufficies, but when all metatarsophalangeal joints must be excised a plantar incision gives excellent exposure, heals rapidly, and avoids the dorsal contractures which often follow linear incisions on the tops of the toes, HOFFMAN (1911). The line of incision crosses the sole from side to side just anterior to the metatarsal heads and just posterior to the web spaces. The scar does not sustain pressure in weight bearing. The joints are approached singly between the digital bundles which, with rare exception, are displaced well upward between the rays so that their retraction is simplified. It is possible to level off the metatarsal stumps under direct vision, and arrive at a very even distribution of pressure over all of them when walking is resumed. Although HOFFMAN recommended the removal of bone from the metatarsal head and neck only, we have followed the practice of excising the whole metatarsophalangeal joint including the metatarsal head, the base of the phalanx and the joint capsule. One should err on the side of removing too much rather than too little bone.

The lack of attention in the literature to treatment of the ankle in rheumatoid arthritis reflects the fact that it is seldom the site of sole or predominant complaint. We have done only a few synovectomies early in the course of disease, but if pain and swelling are sufficiently bothersome it has proven a worthwhile procedure. For adequate exposure we have used two incisions, anteromedial and posterolateral. If the articular surfaces are already eroded, ankle fusion is preferable to synovectomy, and fixation by means of two criss-crossing threaded pins should be used to shorten the duration of plaster fixation. The preferred position for arthrodesis is one of sufficient plantar flexion (10 to 25 degrees) to permit use of shoes with usual heel height when the foot is in normal weight bearing position.

As a preface to my remarks on the surgery of the arthritic hip or knee, I must say that I find myself in complete agreement with the conclusions drawn from the 2nd International Symposium on "Synovectomy and Arthroplasty in Rheumatoid Arthritis" held in Basle, last year, CHAPCHAL (1967). The current indications for, and the limitations of these procedures are clearly presented. Essentially synovectomy is most effective early in the course of disease and particularly useful in treatment of disease of the knee joint. Alone, it is of relatively little, if any, value in disease of the hip.

Just how early should a synovectomy of the knee be carried out? This is a question that must be answered individually for each patient and the answer must depend on the extent and variability of joint involvement; the failure of the synovitis of the knee to respond to suitable medical management; the dose of steroids required and the ability of the patient to tolerate it; and the severity of pain and incapacity that the synovial swelling is presently causing or likely to cause in the future by destruction of the joint. The last point is the one on which it is sometimes difficult to draw a reliable conclusion.

Although most effective in the treatment of early stages of joint involvement before secondary capsular and osteochondral changes have taken place, the usefulness of synovectomy in more advanced forms of the disease should not be ignored. In combination with posterior capsulotomy to correct flexion contractures of under 30 degrees, useful function can be restored and pain relieved. If there is gross instability, the synovectomy may be combined with medial, lateral, or "bilateral" tibial plateau prosthetic replacement and a nice result obtained, McIntosh (1967). The only prerequisite is an adequate preoperative range of flexion (90° plus). Postoperative manipulation of the knee is especially helpful in the recovery of motion in these late and more difficult cases.

For ease of exposure of the entire knee we prefer medial and lateral incisions placed 3 to 4 cm away from the margins of the patella. This provides access to the posterior knee compartments through separate capsular incisions posterior to the collateral ligaments as well as affording adequate exposure of the anterior knee joint structures. It permits as complete a synovectomy as possible and also gives adequate exposure for posterior capsulotomies and the insertion of McIntosh prostheses.

Whereas synovectomy finds its primary usefulness in the treatment of disease of the knee joint, arthroplasty is the procedure of choice for treatment of arthritis of the hip. Here again, as in the knee, the problems presented to the surgeon and the results of operative intervention depend on the local pathological situation, which appears in three distinctive patterns. One, the painful, mobile, cracking osteoporotic hip with loss of joint cartilage, which in the advanced stage develops a protrusio deformity; two, the ankylosing and deforming disease with or without bone bridging of the articular space; and three, the arrested hip of juvenile arthritis in which there are secondary degenerative changes and distorted anatomic features such as valgus and anteversion of the femoral neck. Treatment of the three types must be discussed separately.

In the first situation vitallium mold arthroplasty in our hands has given adequate results comparable to those of other reported series, Schwartzmann (1959), Solomon and Aufranc (1962), Bickel and Bryan (1966). Relief of pain is usually excellent and the restoration of active mobility, stance and walking function relatively satisfactory. The procedure should be combined with a complete capsulectomy and for adequate exposure I prefer a lateral approach with osteotomy of the greater trochanter and reflection of all the muscles closely clinging to the capsule from the iliopsoas anteromedially to the obturator externus posteromedially. Central reposition of the hip is important and the acetabulum must be reconstructed against the inner table of the ilium. A large cup is usually needed. If the subchondral bone of the head is intact, nicely fitting joint surfaces can be made. However, in certain cases with advanced destruction of the femoral head it becomes rather small, and fits loosely unless a Stinchfield differential mold is used. Whether the use of the latter affords much advantage in the long run is still uncertain in my mind, but it seems to restore better joint mechanics at the time of operation and accelerates postoperative functional recovery. Its heavy weight, however, offers a potential disadvantage which may not become apparent until we have a longer follow up.

In the severe grades of protrusio deformity, a very similar procedure has given us surprisingly good results. The acetabulum must be enlarged so that pressure is distributed outward to the iliac part of the acetabulum, and of course central displacement is not necessary. However, it is in this situation that total hip replacement combined with self-curing plastic fixation in bone offers us exciting new prospects for the future, McKee and Watson-Farrar (1966), Charnley (1960, 1966). My own experience with this procedure is too small to give anything but superficial endorsement to these reports. Although we should continue to be apprehensive about the long term durability of such devices, their use in these seriously disabled patients seems not only justified but indicated.

The average age of rheumatoid patients who need hip reconstruction is relatively young it is true, but their general disablement is usually extensive enough so that they need every advantage, while at the same time arduous overuse of replacement parts is unlikely. Current and future bioengineering research should gradually diminish the importance of the problem of wear, and permit the freer use of total joint replacement.

In the second pathological situation associated with adhesive capsulitis and ankylosis, treatment by mold arthroplasty is not nearly as satisfactory as in the first. The indication for intervention is usually as much the lack of mobility as it is pain, and the tendency to postoperative reankylosis is, with occasional dramatic exceptions, quite disappointing and reoperation is often necessary. Resection-osteotomy is too destructive a procedure to have anything but a rare application, Batchelor (1945), Milch (1955). We have reserved it for desperate situations only. It will be interesting to see if total hip replacement can help us out of this dilemma.

In the third type of hip disease, the problem is essentially analogous to that of the treatment of a degenerated hip joint, and the results from mold arthroplasty are very similar — that is satisfactory in the majority of cases. From the point of view of postoperative treatment, the program must be simplified from that which is ideal to that which suits the condition of these frequently very disabled patients. Often both hips have been operated upon within a short space of each other, and other joints have also been involved in the surgical program. Therefore, early weight bearing is mandatory. It seems to be tolerated very well — I think because of the fact that patients are usually capable of only such restricted activity. Walking aids are usually required for a long long time, sometimes indefinitely, but this reflects the incapacity due to generalized joint involvement and weak musculature rather than that due to impairment of hip function alone.

The position of arthroplasty in the treatment of the arthritic knee is not as well established as that of the hip. The major deterrent to advance in this field of surgery has been the relatively subcutaneous position of the joint which increases the risk of infection, the lack of innate stability of the bony parts which places great demands on the design of the mechanical apparatus, and the pronounced bone atrophy which inhibits adequate prosthetic fixation. We have had no experience with hinged prostheses, Walldius (1960), Shiers (1960), Young (1963), Girzadas et al. (1968). Our very limited trial of femoral condylar prostheses has not been encouraging. The need for continued research in this field is self evident. The prospect of using selfcuring plastic to facilitate the seating of a metallic prosthetic knee hinge seems to offer some hope, Editorial (1967), but for the present we have restricted ourselves to the use of the McIntosh tibial plateau prostheses, despite the fact that they obviously do not suit all situations.

The procedure of osteotomy plays a very small part in the treatment of patients with rheumatoid arthritis. Bones are osteoporotic and therefore internal fixation is difficult. The diseased joints stiffen rapidly with immobilization. These are the problems. The chief indications for this type of procedure in my experience have been: one, to correct knee flexion contractures of over 30 degrees in patients with arrested disease and where the knees have at least 80 degrees of motion; two, to correct severe knee valgus with tibial collateral ligament weakness, after a previous synovectomy has arrested the local inflammation and restored good extension and flexion; and three, to adjust the ankylosed position of the ankles and feet when equinus or varus prevent adequate weight bearing function. One point of technique deserves emphasis. If the osteotomies are performed in the juxta articular regions (i.e. above the patellar tendon attachment to the knee, and through the condylar ridges in the femur) large apposable cancellous surfaces can be impacted and the need for elaborate internal fixation avoided. Immobilization in plaster may be discountinued after 2 to 4 weeks and functional restoration started relatively quickly.

In conclusion, good surgical care plays a more important role than ever before in the treatment of the patient with rheumatoid arthritis. As long as the cause remains obscure and medical treatment essentially suppressive, this state of affairs is bound to continue. The indications for different types of operations are continually being better defined. The results of each type of operation depend almost directly on the suitability of its indication. In the early phases of disease, synovectomy is the procedure of choice; in the later stages, arthroplasty; and in — between there are varying indications for techniques modified from these two extremes. Each weight bearing joint carries its special problems and indications which must be continually borne in mind to derive the best results from operative intervention.

References

BATCHELOR, J. S.: Proc. roy. Soc. Med. **38**, 689—690 (1945).

BICKEL, W. H., and R. S. BRYAN: Surg. Gynec. Obstet. **123**, 243—250 (1966).

CHAPCHAL, G.: Synovectomy and arthroplasty in rheumatoid arthritis. 2nd International Symposium. Stuttgart: Thieme. New York: Intercontinental Medical Book Corp. 1967.

CHARNLEY, J.: J. Bone Jt Surg. **42B**, 28—30 (1960).

— Total prosthetic replacement for advanced coxarthrosis, p. 311. In: Proceedings of the X Congress of SICOT — Brussels, Les Publications Acta Medica Belgica 1966

Editorial: Brit. Med. J. **2**, 525 (1967).

GIRZADAS, D. V., S. GREENS, M. CLAYTON, and J. D. LEIDHOLT: J. Bone Jt Surg. **50A**, 355—364 (1968).

HOFFMAN, P.: Amer. J. orthop. Surg. **9**, 441—449 (1911).

MCINTOSH: In: CHAPCHAL, G., Synovectomy and arthroplasty in rheumatoid arthritis (see above).

MCKEE, G. K., and J. WATSON-FARRAR: J. Bone Jt Surg. **48B**, 245—259 (1966).

MILCH, H.: J. Bone Jt Surg. **37A**, 699—717 (1955).

SCHIERS, L. C. P.: J. Bone Jt Surg. **42B**, 31—39 (1960).

SCHWARTZMANN, J. R.: J. Bone Jt Surg. **41A**, 705—721 (1959).

— J. Bone Jt Surg. **49A**, 398—410 (1967).

SOLOMON, L., and O. E. AUFRANC: Arthr. and Rheum. **5**, 37—54 (1962).

WALLDIUS, B.: Acta orthop. scand. **30**, 137—148 (1960).

YOUNG, H. H.: J. Bone Jt Surg. **45A**, 1627—1642 (1963).

Synovial Tumors: Diagnosis, Treatment, and Prognosis

EDGAR G. HARRISON, JR., and MARK B. COVENTRY*

A variety of rare tumors and tumorlike conditions of the synovium may occur in the region of articulations, in bursae or tendon sheaths, or in their anlage in pluripotential mesenchymal tissues. When located within a joint, these lesions may imitate some other condition, such as monoarticular arthritis, and remain undiagnosed or

* Mayo Clinic and Mayo Foundation: Section of Surgical Pathology (Dr. HARRISON), and of Orthopedic Surgery (Dr. COVENTRY).

inappropriately treated. Differential features of some tumors in this category, which were encountered at the Mayo Clinic, are the subject of this discussion.

Histogenesis

The normal synovium (Fig. 1) is a complex, specialized lining which forms from the interzonal cavities of the future joint from the 5. to the 7. weeks of fetal life. The synovial cell layer is closely related to underlying fibroblasts or "stromal cells" which may produce xanthic tumors or osteochondromatosis. The subsynovial layer is composed of fibroareolar tissue with collagen, fat, nerves, and blood and lymphatic vessels which may give rise to some of the benign tumors listed in the diagram (Fig. 1). Malignant synovial tumors — for example, synovial sarcoma — are not

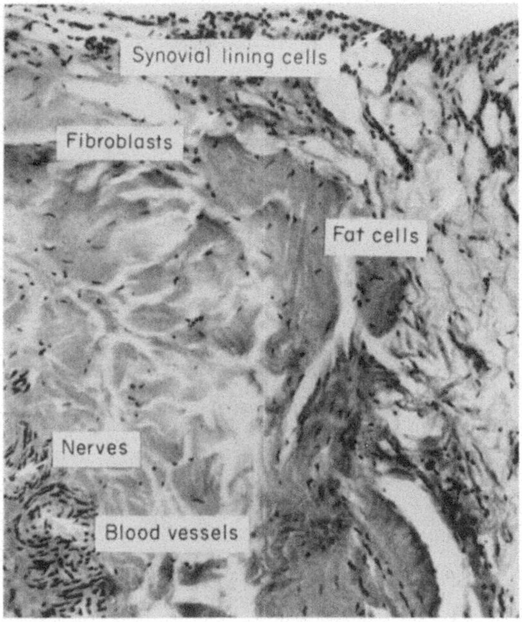

Fig. 1. Classification of synovial tumors and tumorlike conditions related to synovial histology

commonly encountered in relationship to a joint. Direct invasion of a joint from an adjacent malignant tumor may at times occur, but metastases from distant tumors — for example, from bronchogenic carcinoma or hypernephroma — are extremely rare.

Benign Tumors and Tumorlike Conditions

The most frequent site of intraarticular benign tumors is the knee, and these should be considered a diagnostic possibility for any patient with articular pain, swelling, or dysfunction evidenced by limitation of motion or "catching". A normal roentgenographic appearance and the absence of a specific history of trauma, with certain exceptions, should enhance suspicion (Coventry et al.).

For the years 1945 through 1964, there were 95 benign synovial tumors recorded in the files of the Mayo Clinic (table). Overall, there was an almost equal sex distribution and the ages of patients ranged from 3 through 70 years. Xanthic tumors,

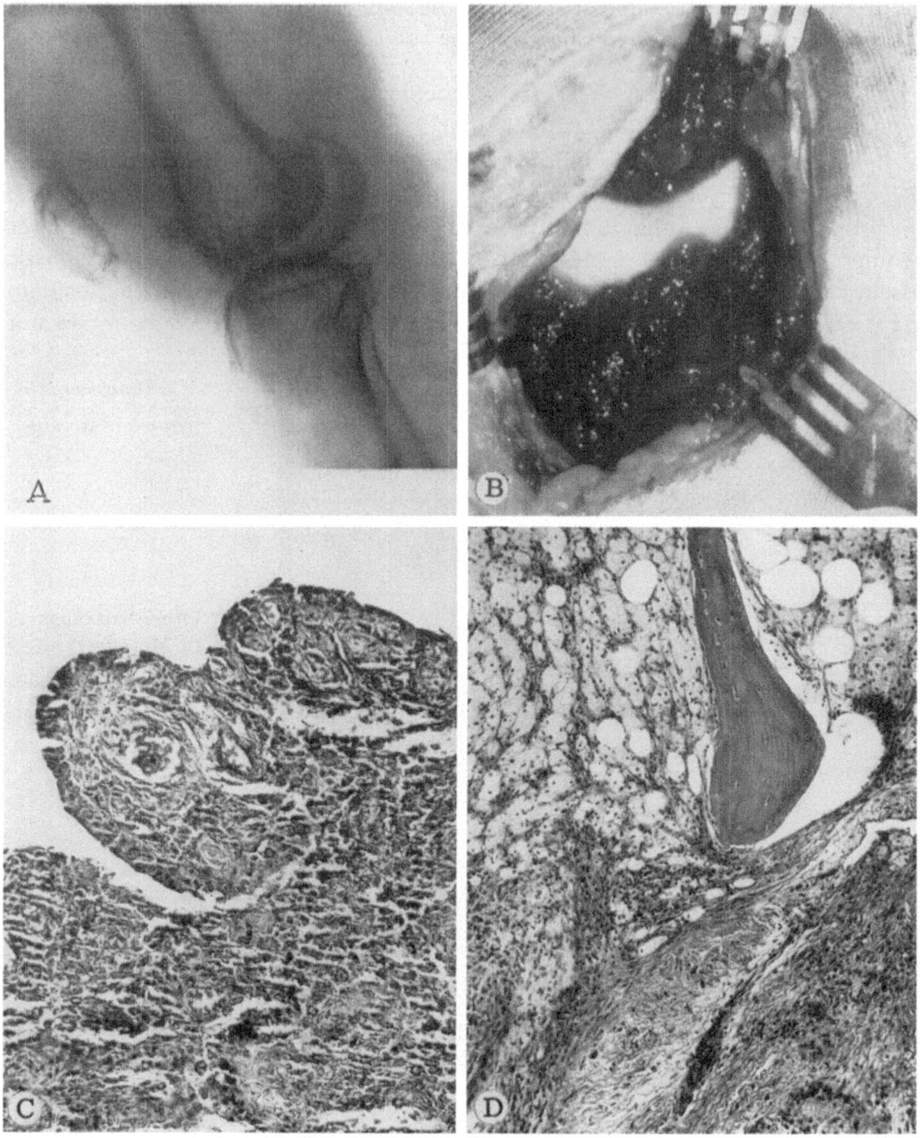

Fig. 2. (Legends see page 423)

including pigmented villonodular synovitis and xanthoma (localized nodular synovitis), were the most frequent and comprised almost half of the lesions. Osteochondromatosis accounted for 28%, hemangioma for almost 12%, and lipomas for 8%. Other rare types included plexiform neuroma, vascular myoma, and myxoma. An instance of a rare synovial glomus tumor was previously reported by HOFFMANN and GHORMLEY.

Pigmented villonodular synovitis. A pigmented xanthic inflammatory tumorlike proliferation of stromal cells (JAFFE et al.), this lesion is almost invariably unilateral and in the lower extremity, the knee being the most commonly involved joint (72%). Rarely it may be encountered in other joints such as the hip, ankle, or shoulder. In-

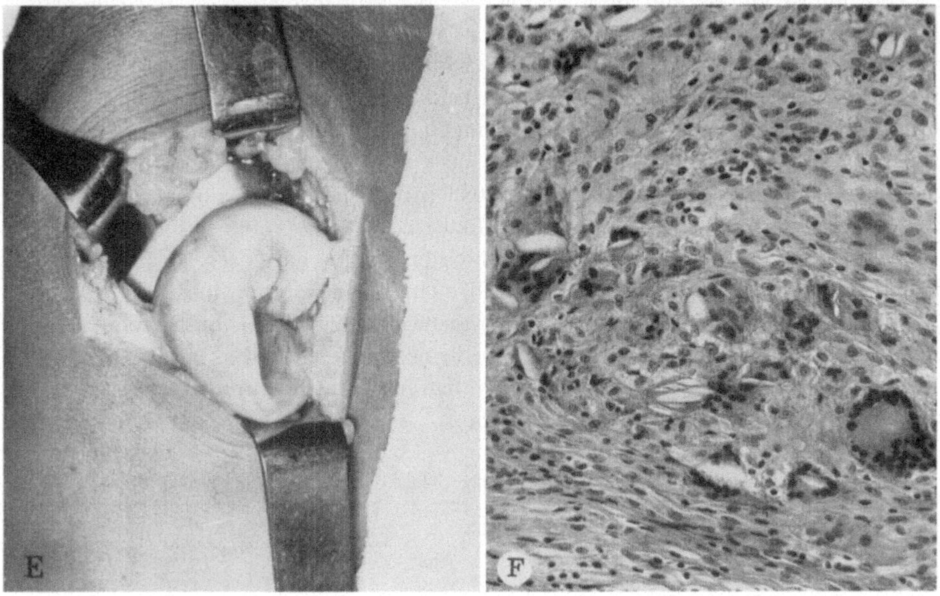

Fig. 2 A—F. Synovial xanthic tumors. A Erosion of articular surface and juxtaarticular cystic changes in case of pigmented villonodular synovitis. B Shaggy reddish-brown mass characteristic of pigmented villonodular synovitis. (Patient was 28-year-old man with pain and swelling of left knee for 2.5 years. Total synovectomy included removal of involved popliteal cyst. Patient was doing well 2 years after operation.) C Proliferation of stromal cells, hemosiderin deposition, and giant cells in pigmented villonodular synovitis. (Hematoxylin and eosin; reduced from × 150.) D Involvement of bone in case illustrated in A. (Hematoxylin and eosin; reduced from × 100.) E Xanthoma, pedunculated mass arising near anterior attachment of medial meniscus, of 30-year-old women. (Patient had intermittent swelling of right knee for 4 years and palpable tender mass at knee. She has been asymptomatic for 4 years since local excision of three xanthomas.) F Stromal cells of fibroblastic and histiocytic types with foam cells and giant cells in section of xanthoma. Note cholesterol clefts and scattered lymphocytes. (Hematoxylin and eosin; reduced from × 200.) [Parts B, C, E, and F from COVENTRY, M. B., E. G. HARRISON, JR., and J. F. MARTIN: J. Bone Jt Surg. **48 A**, 1350—1358 (1966). By permission of the publisher, The Journal of Bone and Joint Surgery, Inc.]

frequent bursal or extraarticular origin also may occur (ATMORE et al.; CHUNG and JANES; PETERSON et al.).

The condition may affect persons of either sex at almost any age exclusive of childhood — from 16 to more than 80 years. Chronic swelling and pain may be present from a few months to 25 years or more. Aspiration may reveal a dark-brown serosanguinous fluid, and the roentgenogram may be normal or show bone erosion and juxtaarticular cystic changes (Fig. 2 A).

At arthrotomy the synovium usually presents an abundant diffuse reddish-brown, shaggy-bearded or grapelike appearance (Fig. 2 B) which may vary with fusion of the tumorous masses. At times a more localized form may be seen. Brown discoloration of the synovium due to intraarticular hemorrhage from a variety of causes — for example, hemophilia, previous acute synovitis, or trauma — must be excluded in the differential diagnosis.

The diffuse villous and nodular microscopic transformation of the synovialis (Fig. 2 C and D) results from proliferation of synovial lining and stromal cells which fill the interstices and infiltrate the subsynovial fat. These fibroxanthic components are histiocytic, form multinucleated giant cells, and contain abundant lipoids and hemosiderin. There is also an accompanying inflammatory component of lymphocytes and some plasma cells.

Xanthoma. Localized nodular synovitis, comprising tenosynovial and intra-articular synovial xanthomas, is a benign localized usually circumscribed tumorlike proliferation of synovial stromal cells, which is considered closely related to pigmented villonodular synovitis (JAFFE et al.). The most common locations of tenosynovial xanthomas are the fingers, at the metacarpophalangeal joints, followed in frequency by the palms, wrists, toes, ankles, arms, and legs (CHARACHE; GALLOWAY et al.). Somewhat more common in women than in men, this tumor may be encountered at any age, although rarely in childhood.

Table. *Benign synovial tumors of the knee: Mayo Clinic 1945 through 1964*

Tumor	Patients		Sex		Knee	
	No.	Age, yr	M	F	R	L
Osteochondromatosis	27	14 to 65 Av. 40.0	20	7	14	13
Pigmented villonodular synovitis	27	22 to 63 Av. 42.1	12	15	14	13
Xanthoma	19	20 to 70 Av. 41.6	7	12	8	11
Hemangioma	11	3 to 48 Av. 27.6	4	7	6	5
Lipoma	8	9 to 49 Av. 27.3	5	3	6	2
Plexiform neuroma	1	37	0	1	0	1
Vascular myoma	1	37	0	1	1	0
Myxoma	1	42	1	0	0	1
Total	95	3 to 70	49	46	49	46

Tenosynovial xanthomas are usually painless masses, while intraarticular synovali xanthomas are almost exclusively of the knee and produce obscure swelling, pain, and occasional locking of the joint. Often a movable mass may be palpable medial to the patellar tendon. Duration of symptoms varies from a few weeks up to many years.

The tenosynovial and synovial articular xanthomas (Fig. 2 E) are similar and at operation usually consist of ovoid or rounded yellowish-white to brown moderately firm masses, 1 to 2 cm in diameter. They may be multiple and either encapsulated or polypoid in their synovial attachment. Microscopically their stromal components show transitions from fibroblasts through histiocytes, foam cells containing lipoid, and multinucleated giant cells (Fig. 2 F). There are cholesterol clefts, hemosiderin deposits, and scattered lymphocytes.

Synovial osteochondromatosis. This benign tumorous multifocal chondro-osseous metaplastic proliferation involves the subsynovial connective tissue of joints, tendon sheaths, or bursae. The knee is involved in almost 70% of cases and the hip in 16% (MURPHY et al.). Less frequent sites are the ankle, shoulder, and wrist. Differential

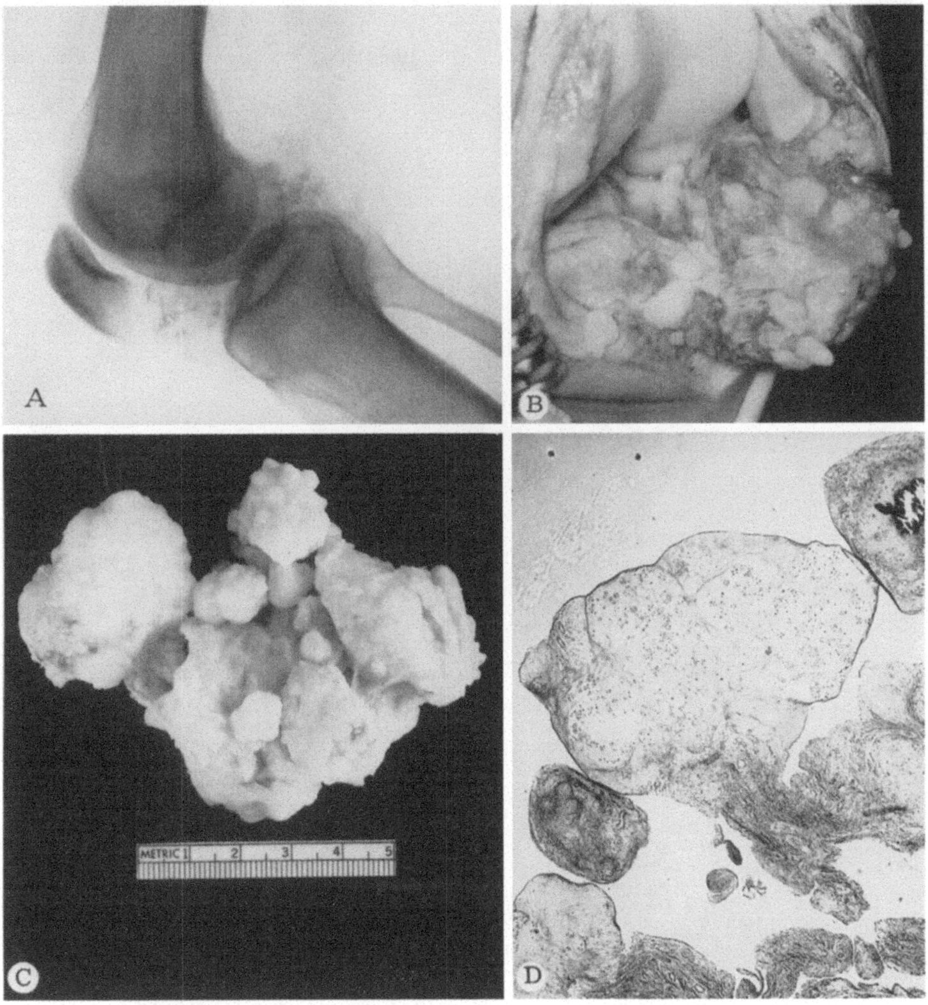

Fig. 3 A—D. Synovial osteochondromatosis. A Multiple calcified bodies in joint. B Multiple osteochondromatosis nodules extending over synovial surfaces of knee at arthrotomy. (Patient, a 54-year-old man, had increasing pain of knee and intermittent swelling and limitation of motion for 2 years before synovectomy.) C Surgically excised conglomerate lesion shown in B. D Nodules of hyaline cartilage in subsynovial layer. (Hematoxylin and eosin; reduced from × 25.) [Parts A and C from Coventry, M. B., E. G. Harrison, Jr. and J. F. Martin: J. Bone Jt Surg. **48 A**, 1350—1358 (1966). By permission of the publisher, The Journal of Bone add Joint Surgery, Inc.)

diagnosis includes loose bodies from degenerative joint disease, osteochondritis dissecans, arthritis, and fracture. Occasionally, the process may extend through a joint capsule and suggest some other tumor, such as in a case of synovial osteochondromatosis of the hip which we encountered that presented clinically as a pelvic tumor.

The ages of our patients ranged from 14 to 65 years, average 40 years, and men were affected more often than women. The major symptoms, pain, swelling, and

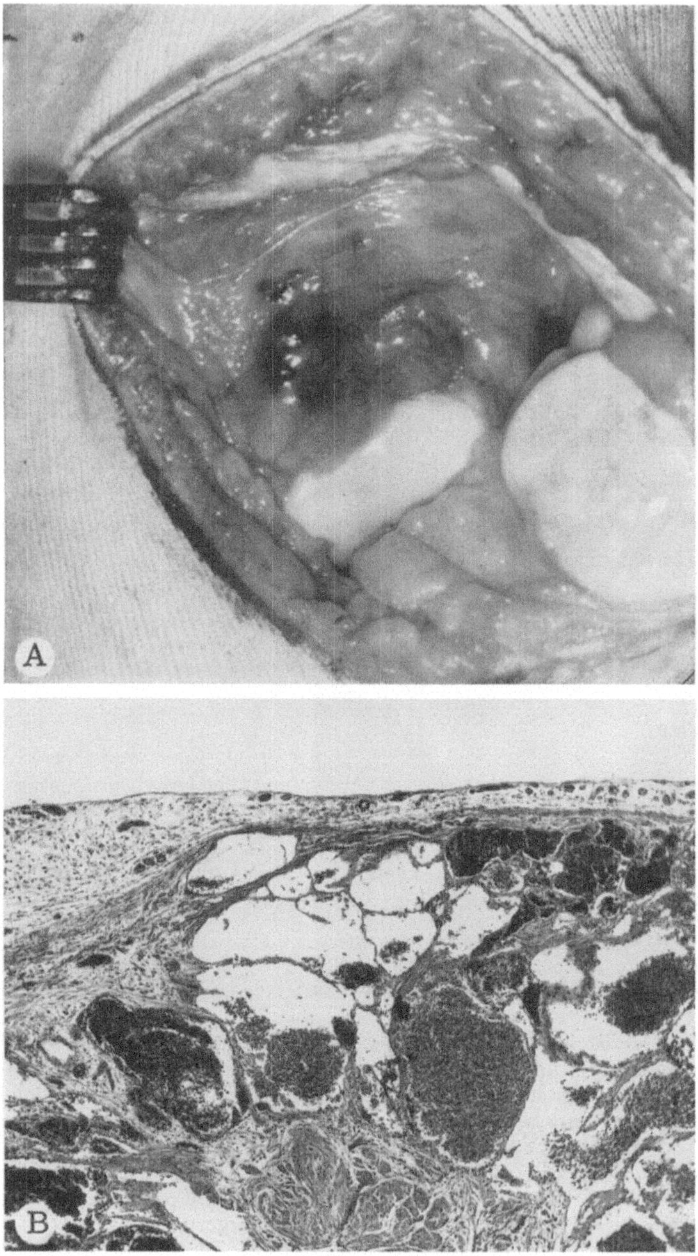

Fig. 4 A—B. Hemangioma. A Blood-filled hemangioma at arthrotomy. (Patient, 26-year-old women, had had episodic pain in knee and slight swelling since age 10 years. Extremity had become increasingly weak, and patient received X-ray therapy elsewhere for "arthritis". Suprapatellar pouch was tender and thickened. Synovectomy for hemangioma and patellectomy for chondromalacia were curative — 13-year follow-up.) B Microscopic appearance of cavernous hemangioma in subsynovial layer. (Hematoxylin and eosin; × 50.) [Parts A and B from Coventry, M. B., E. G. Harrison, Jr. and J. F. Martin: J. Bone Jt Surg. **48 A**, 1350—1358 (1966). By permission of the publisher, The Journal of Bone and Joint Surgery, Inc.]

limitation of motion, were present for 1 month to 47 years. Two thirds of the roentgenograms evidenced radiopaque masses (Fig. 3 A).

Arthrotomy reveals multiple to myriad nodular osteocartilaginous bodies (Fig. 3 B and C), either projecting from the synovial surface or detached from it. These bodies range in size from a few millimeters to more than 5 cm and are pearly-white firm nodules. Microscopically, the cartilaginous bosselation is found within the

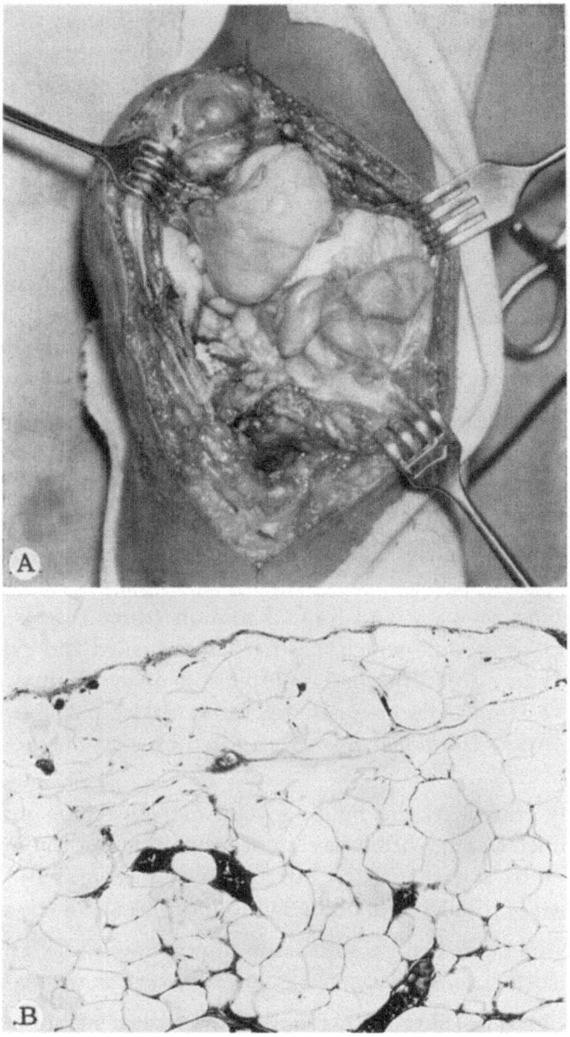

Fig. 5 A—B. Lipoma. A Appearance of arborescent lipoma at arthrotomy. (Patient, 9-year-old girl, probably had familial lipomatosis. Painless enlargement of left knee had been evident for 6 years. Patient had had previous excision of recurrent lipoma of thigh. At time of operation, she had multiple soft subcutaneous masses in thigh, groin, and trunk. Synovectomy removed lipoma; extension through capsule into thigh also was excised. Mass gradually recurred and was reexcised elsewhere 7 years later.) B Mature fat cells of lipoma. (Hematoxylin and eosin; reduced from × 100.) [Part A from Coventry, M. B., E. G. Harrison Jr., and J. F. Martin: J. Bone Jt Surg. **48 A**, 1350—1358 (1966). By permission of the publisher, The Journal of Bone and Joint Surgery, Inc.]

subsynovial layer (Fig. 3 D). Chondrocytes often appear plump and at times binuclear in regions of active growth; these findings can be mistaken for malignant changes. Foci of ossification and calcification may be seen in larger nodules.

Hemangioma. A benign overgrowth of blood vessels, which has more features of a hamartoma or vascular malformation than of a true neoplasm, synovial hemangioma is rare, usually affecting the knee. It may involve the elbow, the ankle (LEWIS et al.), or even the shoulder (COVENTRY et al.).

Patients with synovial hemangiomata usually have a history of joint dysfunction dating from early childhood, although the cause is not recognized until adolescence or young adulthood. Pain and swelling are present and may be intermittent. One third of patients have locking of the knee and 80% have limited motion. Tenderness on palpation over a poorly defined articular mass is a helpful sign. Quadriceps muscle atrophy is often present, and in more than one fourth of the cases hemangiomata may be noted elsewhere on the body.

At arthrotomy (Fig. 4 A) multiple dark-red blood-filled spaces are seen which have an intact synovial covering. The mass is often doughy in consistency, poorly outlined, and up to 6 cm in diameter. Microscopically (Fig. 4 B) there are usually abundant mixed capillary and cavernous, rarely venous, vascular spaces irregularly distributed in the subsynovial layer and commonly containing organizing thrombi.

Lipoma. Benign and often lobulated or arborescent, this neoplasm is composed of well-differentiated lipocytes. Although this is the most common benign tumor of the soft tissues of the extremities (SOULE), it rarely occurs in synovial tissue, except for infrequent involvement in the knee.

Our 8 patients with synovial lipoma, 5 male and 3 female, ranged in age from 9 to 49 years. Symptoms, present from 6 months to as long as 12 years, included pain (four cases), swelling or mass, and limited motion (three cases). 1 patient had an asymptomatic palpable nodule which was partially calcified and evident on a roentgenogram of the knee. 2 patients had multiple soft-tissue lipomas, 1 of which was considered to have familial lipomatosis. Of three masses palpable near the patella, two were tender. An intraarticular mass was noted on a roentgenogram of the knee in three cases.

At arthrotomy (Fig. 5 A) the bulging yellowish glistening masses range from 2 to 15 cm in diameter. They often have more than one bud or segment extending throughout the subsynovial tissue. Microscopically (Fig. 5 B) the subsynovial lipoma is composed of lobules containing adult lipocytes and a few capillaries.

Other. Any of the other benign soft-tissue tumors rarely may arise from elements of the synovialis, such as *plexiform neuroma*, *myxoma*, *vascular myoma*, and *glomus tumor*.

Treatment and prognosis. Surgical excision is the treatment of choice for localized benign tumors, whether xanthoma, hemangioma, lipoma, or other. A complete synovectomy is usually needed for diffuse lesions, such as pigmented villonodular synovitis and osteochondromatosis, since incomplete excision, especially of the diffuse lesions just named, may result in recurrence and necessitate a second operation. X-ray therapy was used rarely in our cases, except in a few instances of residual pigmented villonodular synovitis where it may have had some beneficial effect.

The prognosis is excellent after adequate surgical therapy for benign synovial tumor.

Malignant Neoplasms

Diagnosis. Primary malignant disease of intraarticular synovium is extremely rare and should be, therefore, a reluctant diagnosis when made by the pathologist.

Confusion of a benign tumor with sarcoma is a real problem which may arise particularly in the case of synovial chondromatosis, for a small biopsy specimen of this lesion may histologically mimic well-differentiated chondrosarcoma of bone. Also in cases of pigmented villonodular synovitis, the cellularity, giant cells, and scattered mitoses may cause one to mistake the lesion for a malignant process. In its early descriptions in the literature it gained such terms as "fibrohemosideric sarcoma" and "giant cell sarcoma". Confusing terms such as "benign synovioma" which has at times been applied to xanthoma should be relegated to the limbo of the past in order to avoid conveying the impression of a relationship to synovial sarcoma.

Also, benign cystic lesions, such as a myxoid cyst of the meniscus (GHORMLEY and DOCKERTY) should be recognized and not mistaken for a mucinous neoplasm.

Synovial chondrosarcoma. Rarely if ever does an initially benign synovial tumor become malignant. GOLDMAN and LICHTENSTEIN in 1964 reported on three adult men with primary synovial chondrosarcoma of the knee treated by amputation or wide local excision. Although these tumors simulated synovial osteochondromas, they apparently arose sui generis, rather than from preexistent benign tumors. Cytologic anaplasia and invasion of muscle or bone are features of the malignant growth.

Synovial sarcoma. This lesion (CADMAN et al.) usually arises in the extremities and limb girdles but may occur rarely in the trunk and neck. About 70% of the tumors involve the lower extremity, usually the thigh, followed in decreasing frequency by the knee, foot, hand, and leg. In only 11.9% of the 134 Mayo Clinic cases reported by CADMAN et al. was there suggestive evidence of origin from anatomic synovium: 7 tumors involved tendon sheaths, 6 the knee joints, and 3 bursae. It is generally agreed that this malignant tumor usually develops de novo from the ubiquitous mesenchyme of the somatic soft tissues rather than from preexistent synovial tissue.

Ages of 134 patients with synovial sarcoma (CADMAN et al.) ranged from 8 months to 72 years; 5.2% were less than 10 years of age and most were young or middle-aged adults. The male:female ratio was 1.5:1. Predominant symptoms were the presence of a mass or swelling (97%) and pain or tenderness (59%). The average duration of symptoms before operation was 2.5 years, ranging from less than 1 year to 20 years. Roentgenograms demonstrated evidence of calcification in 31.6% of 57 cases (Fig. 6 A).

The typical synovial sarcoma (Fig. 6 B) is a lobular, circumscribed grayish tumor, measuring 1.5 to 18 cm in diameter. It may show zones of hemorrhage, necrosis, calcification, or cyst formation. Microscopically (Fig. 6 C and D) it is characteristically bimorphic, the cells ranging from plump spindle cells to epithelial-like elements lining glandlike spaces or clefts.

Metastases to the lungs occur in 81.1% of cases, to regional lymph nodes in 23%, and to bone in 20%.

Treatment and prognosis. Synovial sarcoma typically has a prolonged course with multiple recurrences particularly after local excision. In fatal cases in the series reported by CADMAN et al., mean duration from onset of symptoms to death was 6.5 years. One fourth of the patients lived 5 years and 11.2% 10 years or more.

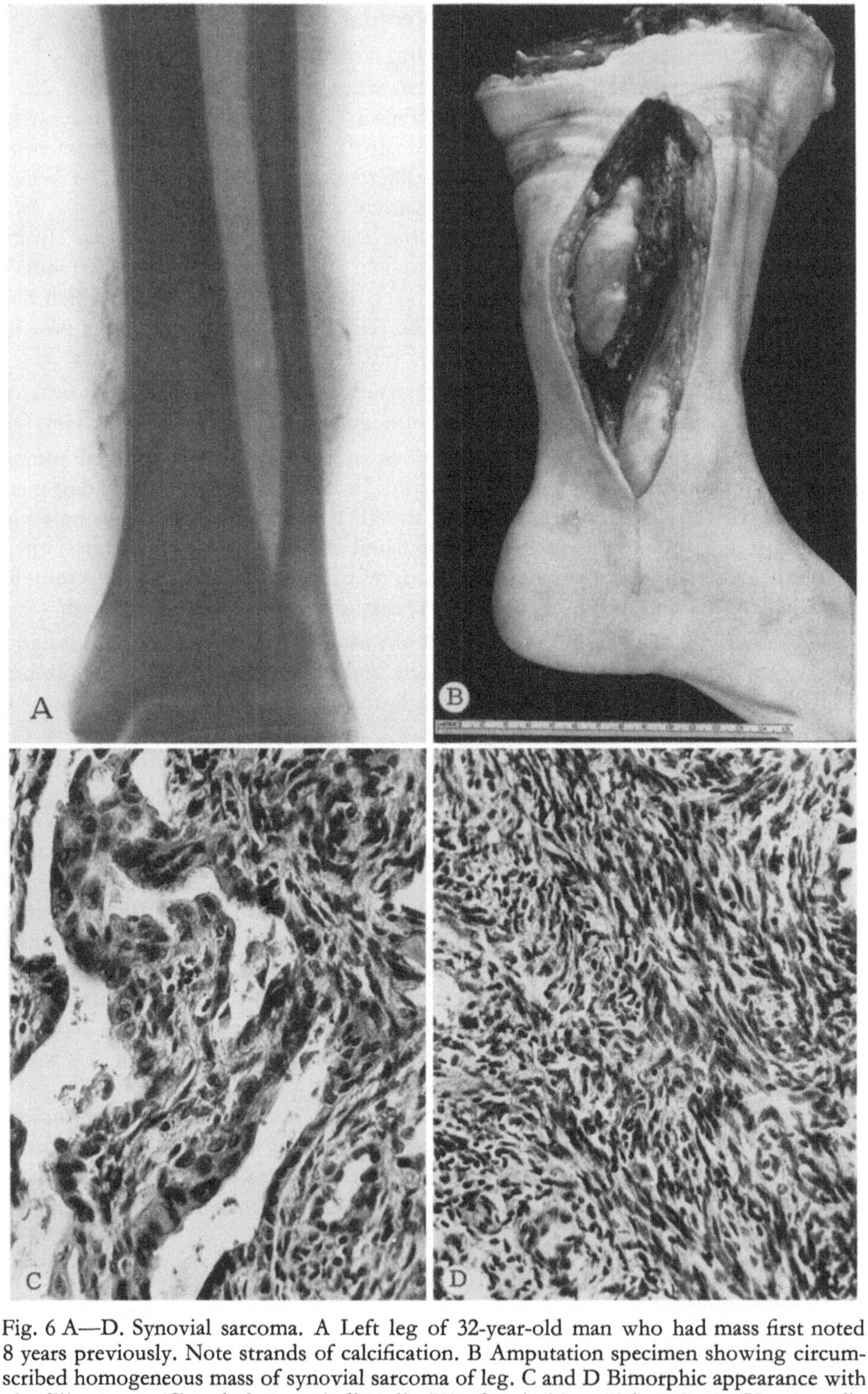

Fig. 6 A—D. Synovial sarcoma. A Left leg of 32-year-old man who had mass first noted 8 years previously. Note strands of calcification. B Amputation specimen showing circumscribed homogeneous mass of synovial sarcoma of leg. C and D Bimorphic appearance with glandlike spaces (C) and plump spindle cells (D) of typical synovial sarcoma. (Hematoxylin and eosin; reduced from × 350)

Early amputation achieved somewhat better results than did amputation after recurrence. Regional lymph node dissection should be included. Postoperative irradiation decreased the frequency of local recurrence but did not improve survival rates.

References

ATMORE, W. G., D. C. DAHLIN, and R. K. GHORMLEY: Minn. Med. **39**, 196—202 (1956).

CADMAN, N. L., E. H. SOULE, and P. J. KELLY: Cancer (Philad.) **18**, 613—627 (1965).

CHARACHE, H.: Arch. Surg. **44**, 1038—1052 (1942).

CHUNG, S. M. K., and J. M. JANES: J. Bone Jt Surg. **47 A**, 293—303 (1965).

COVENTRY, M. B., E. G. HARRISON, JR., and J. F. MARTIN: J. Bone Jt Surg. **48 A**, 1350—1358 (1966).

GALLOWAY, J. D. B., A. C. BRODERS, and R. K. GHORMLEY: Arch. Surg. **40**, 485—538 (1940).

GHORMLEY, R. K., and M. B. DOCKERTY: J. Bone Jt Surg. n.s. **25**, 306—318 (1943).

GOLDMAN, R. L., and L. LICHTENSTEIN: Cancer (Philad.) **17**, 1233—1240 (1964).

HOFFMANN, H. O. E., and R. K. GHORMLEY: Proc. Mayo Clin. **16**, 13—16 (1941).

JAFFE, H. L., L. LICHTENSTEIN, and C. J. SUTRO: Arch. Path. **31**, 731—765 (1941).

LEWIS, R. C., JR., M. B. COVENTRY, and E. H. SOULE: J. Bone Jt Surg. **41 A**, 264—271 (1959).

MURPHY, F. P., D. C. DAHLIN, and C. R. SULLIVAN: J. Bone Jt Surg. **44 A**, 77—86 (1962).

PETERSON, L. F. A., E. W. JOHNSON, JR., and L. B. WOOLNER: Amer. J. clin. Path. **30**, 158—162 (1958).

SOULE, E. H.: Primary soft-tissue tumors of the extremities: Classification, histogenesis and indicence. In: American Academy of Orthopaedic Surgeons: Instructional Course Lectures, vol. 11, pp. 3—11. Ann Arbor, Michigan: J. W. Edwards 1954.

Injuries of Growth Cartilage

JOHN C. WILSON JR.

The growing end of a long bone is made up of an epiphysis, a growth plate, and a metaphysis. The plate is weaker than bone. Yet, injuries to the growing end of bone account for no more than 15% of all fractures of childhood. This paradox is explained by the nature of epiphysial injuries which occur largely following shearing or avulsion stresses, or from a crushing force. 10% of epiphysial injuries leave permanent residuals in the nature of angular deformity or shortening, or both. The type and extent of growth abnormality can often be anticipated and prevented. A crushed growth plate from forceful injury is irreversible. A crushed growth plate from a forceful surgeon is preventable.

The growth plate is weaker than capsule, ligament and tendon. Therefore, dislocations of joints and tears of major ligaments are uncommon in children. Dislocations of the elbow, and rarely of the hip and knee, are recognized; but dislocation of the shoulder is practically non-existent. A force sufficiently strong to tear the medial collateral ligament of the knee in an adult separates the distal femoral epiphysis in the child. Stress which would cause anterior dislocation of the shoulder in an adult avulses the proximal humeral epiphysis in the child.

Two types of epiphyses contribute to bone growth. Articular epiphyses comprise the end of long bones. They are within joints and contribute to longitudinal bone growth. Extra-articular epiphyses, or apophyses as they are sometimes called, serve as attachments for tendons. The ischial epiphysis, the apophysis of the os calcis, and the medial epicondyle of the humerus are example of this type.

Injuries to growth cartilage can be divided into four major categories: *1*, those involving the epiphysis only. Examples of this injury are fractures involving the eminence of the proximal tibial epiphysis and osteochondral fracture of the distal femoral epiphysis, which sometimes complicates forceful lateral dislocation of the patella; *2*, separations of the growth plate without fracture; *3*, fractures that cross the growth plate and involve the epiphysis or metaphysis, or both; *4*, crushing injuries to the growth plate.

Knowledge of the histology of the normal growth plate is helpful, for shearing forces separate the plate uniformly in the third layer of cells. The four layers are: (1) Cells at rest; (2) Cells in proliferation; (3) Cells in hypertrophy, and (4) Endochondral ossification. The cells are bound in a matrix of longitudinally arranged collagen fibrils and a cement containing chondroitin sulfuric acid. The matrix, and not the cells, give strength to the plate. However, in the layer of hypertrophy, the matrix is scant and the plate is fragile. On the metaphysial side of this layer, calcification has occurred, making this portion of the layer firmer than that portion toward the epiphysis. Shearing stresses, therefore, separate this third layer at the junction of the fragile and firm portions.

With this separation, the growing cells remain attached to the epiphysis. Unless the epiphysial blood supply is impaired by the force of injury, normal growth usually continues. Furthermore, the periosteum tears on the side of displacement but remains intact on the opposite side, providing a firm membrane against which reduction can be accomplished and over-reduction prevented.

TRUETA and MORGAN [*9*] have accurately described the blood supply to the growth plate. It comes from two sources. The epiphysial vessels arise within the epiphysis and penetrate the plate to end in capillary tufts in the first layer of cells at rest. Metaphysial vessels arise in the marrow to end in the layer of endochondral ossification. The blood supply to the majority of articular epiphyses enter through the soft tissues at some distance from the plate. However, the proximal femur and proximal radius are covered totally by cartilage, and have no soft tissue coverings. Therefore, these two epiphyses are particularly susceptible to avascular necrosis following injury. The blood vessels which supply these intra-articular epiphyses enter by traversing the rim of the plate, and are frequently torn at the time of injury.

The history of injury in the child is often totally lacking, inaccurate, or purposely deceptive. The physical examination and X-ray interpretation are of first importance in making an accurate diagnosis. If there is swelling at the end of a long bone, or within a joint, epiphysial injury must be included in the differential diagnosis.

The location of an epiphysis determines, to a great extent, its susceptibility to injury. The size and shape, the position of the epiphysis, the amount of potential growth, and whether the epiphysis is weight bearing or non-weight bearing are all important factors in determining the diagnosis, treatment and prognosis.

The epiphyses of the upper extremity are more prone to injury. In order of frequency, the injuries are: the distal radius; distal ulna; distal humerus; proximal radius; phalangeal epiphyses of the fingers, and proximal humerus. In the lower extremity, the order of frequency of injury is: Distal tibia, distal fibula, and proximal femur.

The distal radius is the commonest site of epiphysial injury, and occurs with greater frequency than all other epiphysial injuries together. Growth plate injuries occur more frequently during difficult delivery, in the first year of life, in infants subjected to inflicted trauma, and during periods of rapid skeletal growth, including the pre-pubertal growth spurt.

The epiphysis can separate and reduce spontaneously, leaving little evidence for diagnosis except swelling, local tenderness, and sometimes a chip of metaphysial bone on the side of displacement, a hallmark of trauma known as *The Sign of Thurston Holland* (Fig. 1).

The roentgenographic appearance of growing bone is confusing to the physician unfamiliar with children. The epiphysis, growth plate, apophysis, nutrient arteries, cast confusing shadoes which require thoughtful interpretation. X-rays in two

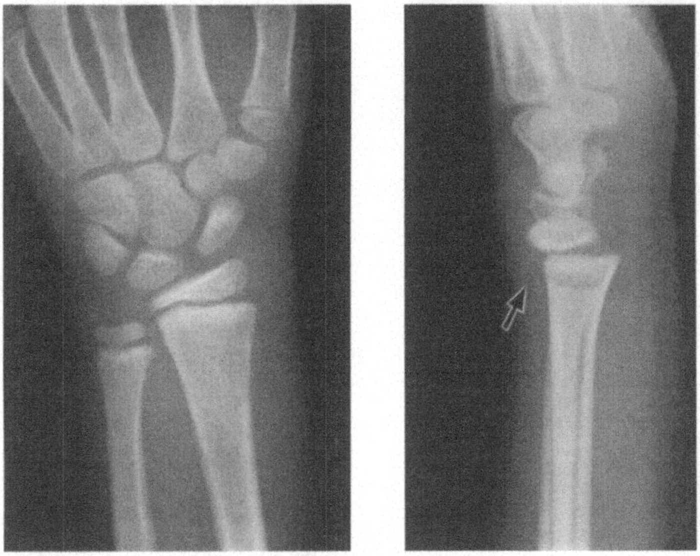

Fig. 1. Anteroposterior and lateral views showing separation of the distal radial epiphysis with a chip of metaphysis on the side of displacement. The sign of Thurston Holland

planes and comparative views of the uninjured extremity are helpful in making an accurate diagnosis. In the neonate and young infant whose bone ends are entirely cartilaginous, the diagnosis of epiphysial separation, or fracture, can be difficult. In these injuries, the location and degree of swelling, plus deformity of the adjacent joint help to make a diagnosis.

In differentiating the various types of growth plate injuries, Salter's classification is clear and helpful [*8*]. *Type 1* is a complete separation of the epiphysis through the third layer of the plate, without fracture. This injury occurs during difficult breach delivery and in the first 2 years of childhood, when the growth plate is particularly thick. Furthermore, type 1 injuries often occur from inflicted trauma, or from any major shearing stress to an epiphysial plate throughout early childhood (Fig. 2).

The displacement of the epiphysis is usually not great, in the young infant, because the periosteum is intact. The periosteum, however, is often torn in the infant subjected to inflicted trauma or in children struck down by automobiles.

The distal humerus, distal femur, proximal humerus, and proximal femur most often demonstrate Type 1 injuries. Gentle reduction is imperative. Healing occurs quickly, within 3 to 4 weeks, and accurate anatomic reduction is not required as the bone rapidly remodels.

A sub-type, 1 (a), relates to injuries of the epiphysis only. True epiphysial fractures are relatively rare. An avulsion of the proximal tibial epiphysis at the cruciate ligament insertions is an example of this type, or an osteochondral fracture of the distal femoral epiphysis complicating forceful dislocation of the patella. These injuries occasionally require surgical intervention, either to replace a large epiphysial fragment or to remove a smaller fragment from the joint. The prognosis if most injuries of type 1 and 1 (a) is good, unless circulation to the plate has been disturbed by the force of trauma.

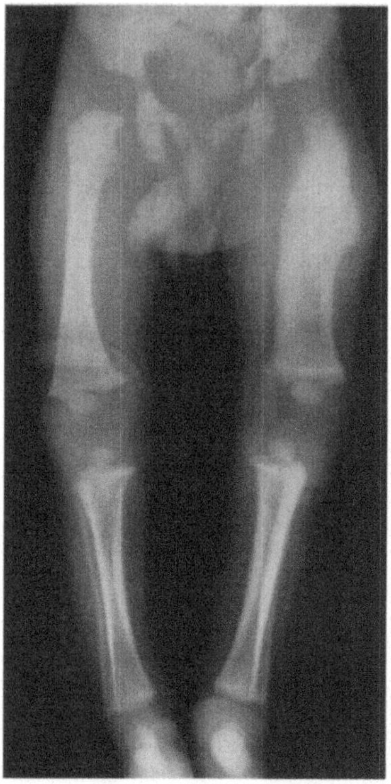

Fig. 2. Extensive epiphyseal injury in a young infant subjected to inflicted trauma. Note the deformity of the proximal femur on the left due to forceful separation of the upper femora epiphysis. There is irregularity of the plate at the distal femur on the left with metaphyseal fractures associated with trauma of this type. The proximal tibial epiphysis on the left also shows evidence of injury

(Fig. 3). *Type 2 injuries* are characterized by separation of the growth plate with fracture of a relatively small fragment of metaphysis. The distal radius and distal femur are examples of this type, and these injuries occur usually toward the end of the first and during the early years of the second decade of life. In the non-weight bearing epiphyses, accurate reduction is unimportant and rapid remodeling and healing occur. In a Type 2 injury of the distal femur, careful reduction with intralen fixation using fine metallic wires is sometimes necessary. Growth arrest can follow Type 2 injuries, as is demonstrated in Fig. 3.

Type 3 injuries are rare. The fracture is entirely intraarticular, usually involving the knee or ankle. The injury occurs from major trauma and is seen in the older child. The epiphysis is split and displaced, the plate separates in the fragile layer, the metaphysis is not fractured. The joint is disrupted and open reduction is often required. The prognosis is usually quite good, as the injury is seen toward the end of the growing period (Figs. 4 and 5).

Type 4 injuries involve the epiphysis, the growth plate, and the metaphysis. A fracture of the capitellum of the humerus is an example of this type of injury. It requires accurate reduction with internal fixation and, if properly treated, carries usually a favorable prognosis. However, if Type 4 injuries are unreduced, the longitudinal displacement of one fragment causes healing of the epiphysis of the distal fragment to the metaphysis of the proximal fragment. This leads to premature closure of the growth plate, with resultant angular deformity and shortening. It is important, in Type 4 injuries, that the epiphysis be approached and handled with great care and that the soft tissues not be stripped from the epiphysial fragments during the operation. Internal fixation with fine Kirchner wires through the metaphysis, or actually

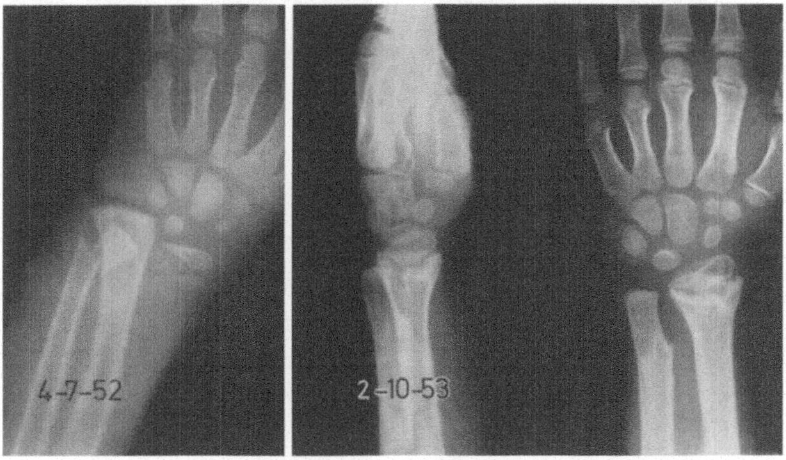

Fig. 3. A type 2 injury, with separation of the distal radial epiphysis and with it, a metaphyseal fragment. The distal ulan is fractured 1 cm proximal to the epiphyseal plate. X-rays 10 month later reveal growth arrest of the distal radial epiphysis

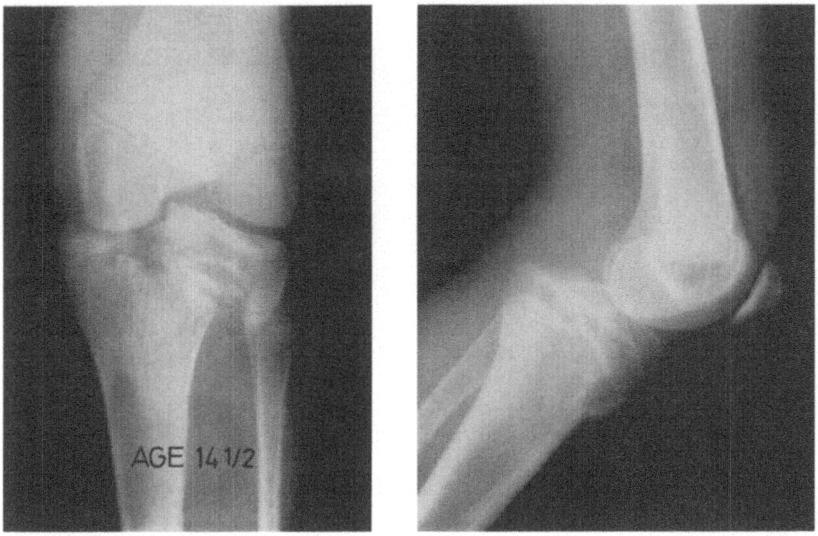

Fig. 4. A type 3 injury with fracture and displacement of the proximal tibial epiphysis. This is the type of injury which requires open reduction with internal fixation. (Patient of Doctor Robert Nippell)

through the plate, do not cause growth disturbance. The wires can be removed at the end of the third week (see Fig. 6).

Type 5 injuries occur very infrequently. Occasionally, one plane joints, such as the knee and ankle, are subjected to severe valgus or varus stresses which damage the growth plate without displacing the epiphysis and without causing metaphysial fracture. These injuries are treacherous, for they are frequently interpreted as sprains. A favorable prognosis is given and the child discharged from care only to return

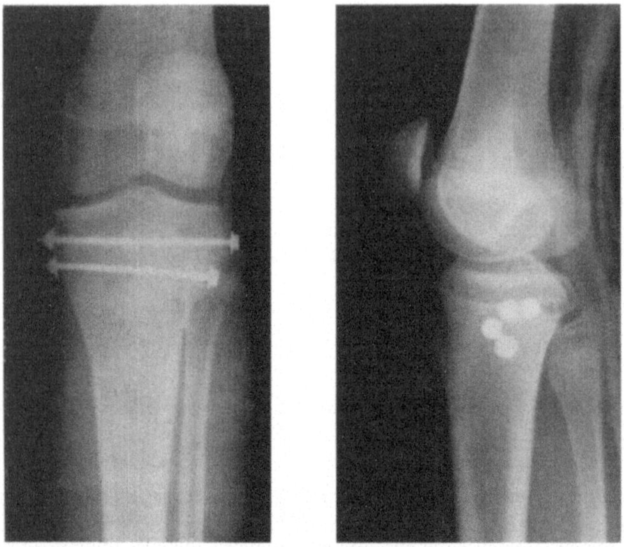

Fig. 5. The same fracture, showing the type of internal fixation utilized

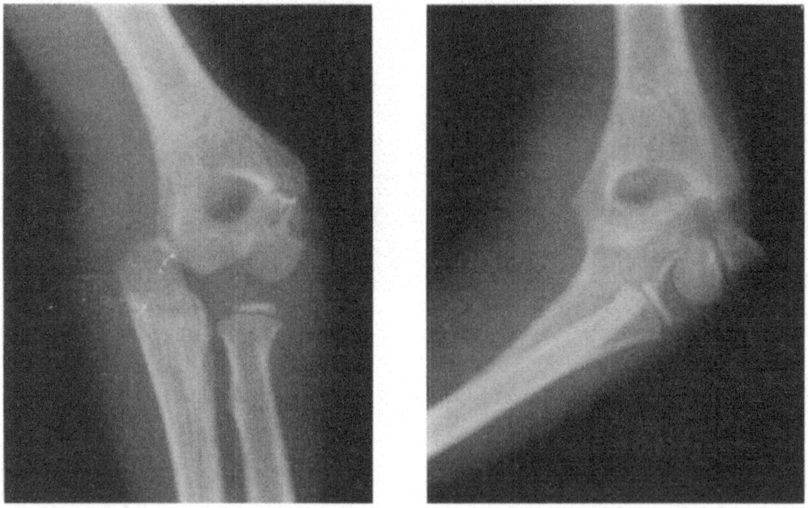

Fig. 6. A dislocation of the elbow complicated by a type 4 injury: a fracture through the capitellar epiphysis, the plate, and the metaphysis. This type of injury requires open reduction with internal fixation utilizing fine metallic wires

history is often obtainable in these injuries, for they occur in the young athlete who can give some description of what type of injury he suffered. Moderate or severe within a few months, manifesting a deformity of increasing severity. An accurate swelling about the knee or ankle with pain and inability to walk, in the absence of significant X-ray findings of fracture should cause the physician to be highly suspicious of a crushing injury to the growth plate. Possibly bone scanning techniques may eventually be sufficiently refined to provide helpful information in this type of growth plate injury.

Some mention must also be made of a poorly understood entity which is referred to as the "over-exercised elbow". This injury, usually the result of excessive forceful exercise, such as the use of the arm surfing or throwing a baseball, causes injury to all of the epiphyses of the elbow. The child manifests a chondrolysis with gradual narrowing of the joint space, chronic synovitis, and permanent limitation of motion within the joint. The only treatment which seems helpful is protection of the elbow

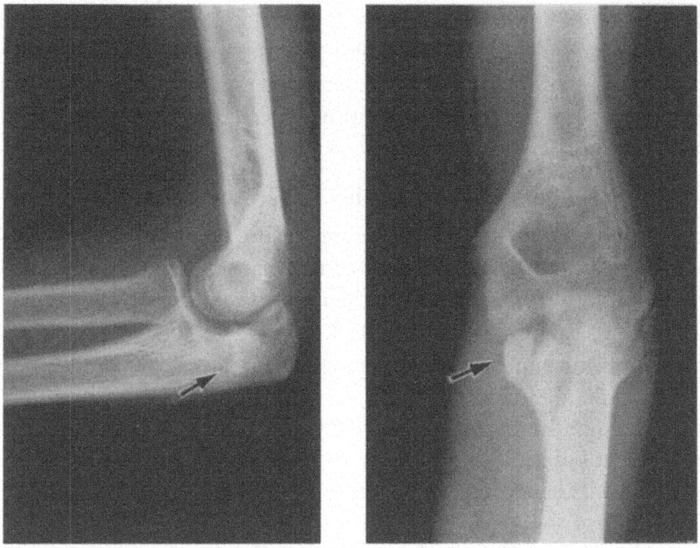

Fig. 7. A displaced medial epicondyle in the elbow joint 6 month following injury. The seriousness of the injury was not appreciated by the physician who first saw the patient. The boy, age 12, was subjected to arthrotomy with removal of the fragment and transplantation of the ulnar nerve

in a removable plaster splint for several months, and the avoidance of repetitious forceful exercise to the joint.

Injuries to traction epiphyses, or extra-articular epiphyses, occur with frequency. The medial epicondyle of the humerus is avulsed commonly following a valgus stress on a flexed elbow. This injury can occur before or after ossification of the epiphysial center. The diagnosis is difficult before the appearance of the ossification center on X-ray. The injury may be mild, without significant displacement, or it may complication dislocation of the elbow, in which the fragment remains trapped within the joint. Such injuries require open operation, with either replacement of the fragment and fixation, or excision of the fragment. Excision of the fragment leads to no significant cosmetic or functional deformity of the elbow. In old, unrecognized avulsion injuries of the medial epicondyle, the fragment should be carefully removed from the elbow joint and the ulnar nerve transplanted anteriorly (Fig. 7).

The lesser trochanteri epiphysis of the femur, the major insertion of the iliopsoas tendon, can be avulsed by sudden, forceful contraction of the muscle. This injury frequently occurs in the young athlete engaged in the high jump or in running hurdles. The treatment simply consists of rest with the hip in flexion for 3 weeks and with the avoidance of athletic acitivities for an additional 6 weeks.

Principles of Treatment

Prompt, early, gentle reduction is imperative. Epiphysial fractures are difficult to reduce after the 5th day, and impossible by the 10th day following injury. In Types 1 and 2, perfect reduction is not always possible but remodeling takes place promptly and healing occurs within 3 to 4 weeks. Type 3 and 4 injuries require accurate open reduction with internal fixation. The epiphysial fragments are to be handled with great care to avoid injury to the plate and to avoid the stripping of the soft tissues which would lead to an avascular necrosis. Type 1, 2, and 3 injuries heal in approximately half the time required for union of a fracture through the metaphysis of the same bone. In Type 4 injury, involving a large metaphysial fragment, healing takes the same amount of time as would a metaphysial fracture or a diaphysial fracture of the same bone.

Complications of Injuries to Growth Cartilage

Growth may cease completely in the injured plate, or it may continue for a time at a diminished rate and then cease, or a part of the plate may continue to grow and the remainder close. Obviously, the younger the child, the more growth remains and the greater the deformity that can be anticipated.

Angulation, or shortening of the bone, or both, can occur, and are progressive throughout the child's growing period.

Progressive angulation is best managed by an opening wedge osteotomy to gain as much length as possible. It is advisable to overcorrect the deformity, particularly in the younger child. Furthermore, corrective osteotomies may have to be performed more than once before the growth period is over.

Progressive shortening of a single weight-bearing bone can be managed best by an epiphysial arrest on the normal limb at the appropriate time. Femoral and tibial lengthening on the shortened side are not recommended as the risk of complication is far too high.

In paired bones, such as the radius and ulna, the tibia and fibula, osteotomy with closure of the distal fibular or distal ulnar epiphysis, or resection of the distal ulna after growth has been complete, serve to correct the appropriate deformities.

References

1. Aitken, A. P.: J. Bone Jt Surg. **17**, 302—308 (1935).
2. — J. Bone Jt Surg. **18**, 685—691 (1936).
3. — J. Bone Jt Surg. **18**, 1036—1041 (1936).
4. Blount, W. P.: Fractures in children. Baltimore: The Williams and Wilkins Co. 1955.
5. Eliason, E. L., and L. K. Ferguson: Surg. Gynec. Obstet. **58**, 85—90 (1934).
6. Larson, R. L., and others: J. Amer. med. Ass. **196**, 607 (1966).
7. MacAuslffnd, W. R.: Surg. Gynec. Obstet. **23**, 147—1/5 (1916).
8. Salter, R. B., and W. R. Harris: J. Bone Jt Surg. **45 A,** 587—622 (1963).
9. Trueta, J., and J. D. Morgan: J. Bone Jt Surg. **42 B,** 97—109 (1960).
10. Wilson, J. C., and D. P. McDonnell: J. Bone Jt Surg. **30 A,** 347 (1948).
11. Wilson, J. C., Jr.: Pediat. Clin. N. Amer. **14**, 659—682 (1967).
12. —, and Krueger, J. C.: Amer. J. Surg. **112**, 326—332 (1966).

The Pathogenesis of Adolescent Scoliosis

I. V. Ponseti

Idiopathic scoliosis may be subdivided into infantile scoliosis when the deformity starts in infancy or early childhood, and adolescent scoliosis when it starts after the age of 7 or 8 years. Adolescent scoliosis is by far the most prevalent type of spinal deformity seen in the United States. A mild deformity may be detected shortly before 10 years of age, but the scoliosis develops during the adolescent growth spurt.

Any scoliosis, irrespective of its primary cause, increases considerably during the adolescent growth spurt. Increased rate of spinal and pelvic growth accounts for the adolescent growth spurt. The increase at about puberty in the growth rate of the trunk, but not of the long bones, may be related to the differences in structure of the growth plates of the vertrebrae and ilium, and the long bones.

The iliac crest is histologically similar to the vertebral rim and in both a secondary ossification center develops during adolescence. Interstitial cartilage growth increase in the iliac crest and vertebral plates during both periods of rapid growth, infancy and adolescence. Bone forms in the iliac crest cartilage as in the vertebral rims. Both the iliac crest and the vertebral rim may be considered special forms of traction epiphysis. Enchondral ossification, as seen in the long bones, occurs in the iliac crest growth plate in between areas where calcification and ossification take place, resembling that at the insertions of certain ligaments. Most of the growth of the ilium occurs in this growth plate and in a group of children studied by Anderson et al., increase in height of the pelvis accounted for 21.5% of the total growth of the trunk in girls between 8 and 18 years of age.

The galactosamine concentration[1] in the iliac crest cartilage of normal children decreases sharply during the first 2 years of life. It then declines gradually until to 12 years of age, and again increases until 16 years of age. This curve corresponds closely to the rate of trunk growth. It corresponds also to the rate of deterioration of most scoliosis deformities.

All the iliac crest specimens obtained from patients with adolescent scoliosis had a content of galactosamine higher than the normal controls. The average increase of the samples studied was 20% over the normals. The glucosamine content did not change significantly. The hydroxyproline values were found to be within normal limits[1].

The dominant features of scoliosis are excessive vertebral rotation with torsion of the intervertebral discs, and a relative lengthening of the anterior components of the spine (vertebral bodies and discs) compared with the posterior elements (neural arches and interspinous ligaments). Roaf explained convincingly that both features are inter-related. Previously the same explanation had been given by Heuer, Erlacher, and Somerville. In a normal spine the length of the anterior longitudinal ligament and that of the supraspinous ligaments are nearly equal, while Roaf has found that the anterior longitudinal ligament was 10.2 cm longer on the average than that of the supraspinous ligaments in five scoliotic spines of adults. The excessive vertebral rotation seen in scoliosis implies severe laxity of the intervertebral discs.

[1] In cartilage, galactosamine and glucosamine can be taken as indexes of the content of chondroitinsulfates and keratosulfate respectively. Hydroxyproline is the index of the total collagen content.

Based on the similarities observed between the iliac crest cartilage and the vertebral plate, and since in both an increase of interstitial cartilage growth occurs during adolescence, we may speculate that the galactosamine content of the vertebral plate increases as it does in the iliac crest to sustain the trunk growth spurt. The hypothesis is presented, therefore, that the mucopolysaccharide content of the vertebral plates and possibly also of the annulus, since both structures are joined together, increases during adolescence in normal children, and more so in children with adolescent scoliosis. The increased mucopolysaccharide content implies a change in the mucopolysaccharide-collagen ratio which may alter the physical properties of the annulus and may cause the disc to expand, owing to increased hydration. Increase in length of the anterior elements of the spine could result first from increased hydration of the intervertebral discs and later on from an excessive growth in the plates and even in the vertebrae, owing to the increased content of chondroitin sulfates. Since the posterior elements of the spine do not expand and grow normally, the vertebrae are forced to rotate, as explained by ROAF. Vertebral rotation could be facilitated by the laxity of the annulus. In adolescent scoliosis these changes might be severe enough to disrupt the normal alignment of the spine.

References

ANDERSON, M., SHIH-CHEN HWANG, and W. T. GREEN: J. Bone Jt Surg. **47 A,** 1555—1564 (1965).

ERLACHER, P.: Verh. dtsch. orthop. Ges. **25**, 282—306 (1931).

HEUER, F.: Z. orthop. Chir. **52**, 513—533 (1930).

ROAF, R.: J. Bone Jt Surg. **48** B, 786—792 (1966).

SOMERVILLE, E.: J. Bone Jt Surg. **34** B, 421—427 (1952).

Intertrochanteric Osteotomy in Arthrosis of the Hip-Joint

M. E. MÜLLER

Total prosthesis will probably, if not certainly, guarantee a firm, mobile and painless hip for a few years at least; but inspite of the great success achieved by this treatment, intertrochanteric osteotomy still remains the best and most reliable hip surgery for certain forms of arthrosis of the hip joint. Only by this technique can we fundamentally alter the mechanics of the hip joint and influence the disease. It remains the method of choice for quite some time, particularly in most dysplastic hip joints, or after epiphyseolysis and Perthes' diseases have run their course. In young people after fractures of the neck of femur and partial necroses of the femoral head, and after certain acetabular fractures it is often possible to normalize the situation to a large extent by intertrochanteric osteotomy.

There are *three types of intertrochanteric osteotomy:*

Varisation osteotomy, the *McMurray osteotomy* and *valgisation osteotomy*

The osteotomies have different purposes, effects and indications.

Varisation osteotomy is designed to improve the congruence between the acetabulum and the femoral head, to increase the amount of joint under pressure, to extend the length of the muscle lever arm and to relax the adjoining muscles. At the same time, changing the effective forces of pulling and pushing induces a change in the internal structure of the head and neck of the femur.

Intertrochanteric varisation osteotomy was developed by PAUWELS and is always the method of choice when the aims described above can be achieved in this way. In the coxa valga luxans, the roof of the acetabulum must not be too short, otherwise the varisation osteotomy should be combined with plastic surgery of the roof of the acetabulum. Particularly where there is incipient hip joint arthrosis with medial narrowing of the articular space, where a fracture has healed in valgus with incipient hip joint arthrosis but no necrosis of the head of femur, and in polyarthritis which is

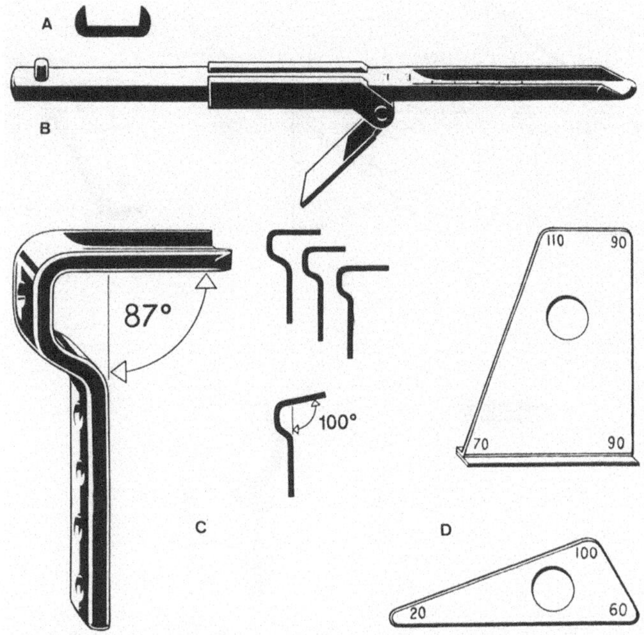

Fig. 1. a U-profile of the blade of the rectangular plate. b Standard rectangular plate suitable for all intertrochanteric osteotomies in hip joint arthrosis and variants with different arch depths. c Plate site instrument for preparing the site of the plate blade in the neck of the femur and its aligning apparatus for determining the sagittal plane. d Metal triangle and quadrilateral for determining the angle

not too advanced, we try to stop the progression and if possible introduce a regression of the arthrotic process, by means of varisation osteotomy. From the technical point of view, it is important to know that in every intertrochanteric osteotomy there are six possibilities for correction: valgus/varus, adduction/abduction, external/internal rotation, lengthening/shortening, displacement medially/laterally, displacement ventrally/dorsally. These possible corrections must be accurately computed and established before and during the operation. Also, the blade of the plate must be exactly in the middle of the neck of the femur.

The *McMurray — or displacement osteotomy* is characterized by 4 factors:

1. Fracture separation in the intertrochanteric region.
2. Flexion of the proximal fragment.
3. Correction of all malpositions so that the bone lies axially after the operation.

Valgisation osteotomy allows us to set the medial portion of the head of the femur under pressure. This operation is indicated primarily in adduction contractures and it must then be combined with a muscle-relaxing operation at the level of the iliopsoas and the adductors, sometimes even at the level of the hip abductors.

All three types of osteotomy mentioned are carried out in the intertrochanteric region by means of a rectangular plate with a U-shaped blade profile. The site of the

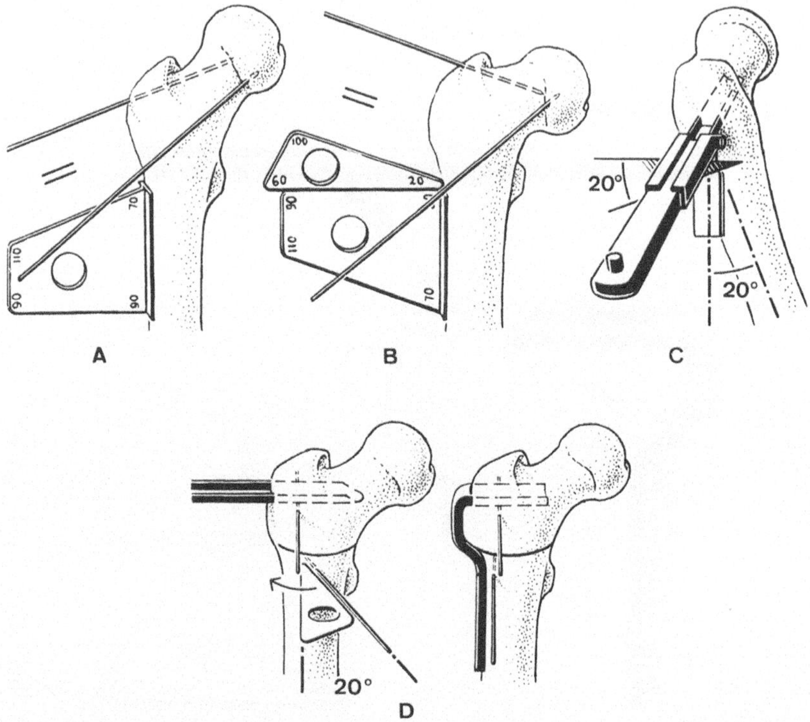

Fig. 2a—d. Establishing the four standard planes in intertrochanteric osteotomies. a In a varisation osteotomy of 20°: the Kirschner wire, placed over the neck of the femur, indicates its direction (horizontal plane). b With the aid of a metal quadrilateral, a 70° angle can be determined between shaft and plate blade. The second Kirschner wire is then driven into the greater trochanter (massive) parallel to the upper edge of the metal quadrilateral *(frontal plane)* and parallel to the first wire. c The flap of the small aligning apparatus is mounted on the plate site instrument, forming an open angle of 20° with the femur shaft to the rear (sagittal plane). In this way, the proximal or the distal fragment is extended by 20°. d To determine the rotation plane, one Kirschner wire is introduced on either side of the proposed osteotomy line. These form an angle with one another which corresponds to the required correction (here 20° outwards rotation)

plate must be prepared before the osteotomy with a '*plate site instrument*' (Fig. 1). This must be introduced in the three calculated planes (horizontal, frontal and sagittal plane) (Fig. 2).

We use the rectangular AO plate for all three types of osteotomy. According to the medial displacement necessary, there is a choice of three models.

Results: in a group of 1000 osteotomies we found that, having achieved good mobility of the joint and the purpose of the osteotomy, extensive freedom from symptoms and regression of the pathological process can be expected in 75% of the cases.

The results were the same after more than 5 years and it is not possible to predict whether there will be recurrence of the hip joint arthrosis later on. But whenever the mobility is severely limited before the operation we are able to achieve substantial relief of symptoms, although after a preliminary recovery of the arthrosis, perhaps

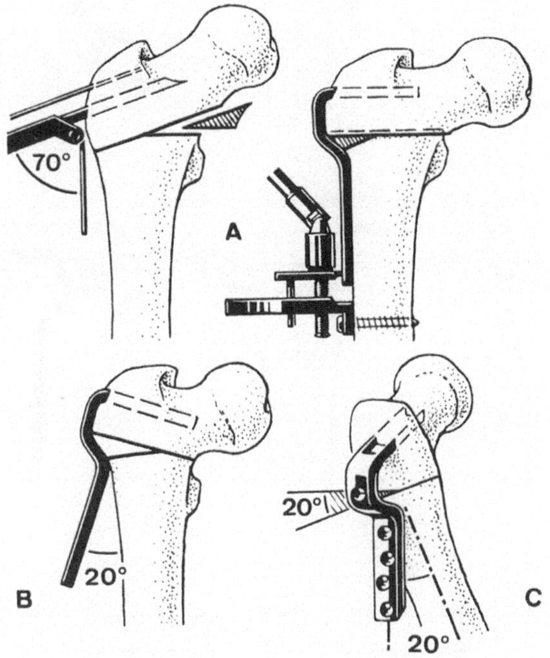

Fig. 3 a—c. The three intertrochanteric standard osteotomies. a Varisation osteotomy with removal of a wedge with medial base. Axial compression by means of plate stretchers. b Valgisation osteotomy; the plate is driven in cranially into the neck of the femur. c Extending osteotomy with resection of a dorsal wedge of bone by 20°

lasting for years and demonstrated radiologically, we found that there was deterioration later in life.

Today we are cautious in our use of osteotomy after the 6th decade, since it will only produce regression of the pathological process in elderly patients under the most favourable conditions, i.e. in incipient hip joint arthrosis or where the head is massive. Thus, elderly patients with hip joint arthrosis are usually treated by total prosthesis. Before the patient is 60 years old we do not feel justified in offering him a prosthesis unless there is a case for 'head and neck of femur resection' according to Girdlestone. However, in younger patients, particularly where the mechanical situation can be completely restored, there is no operation to match osteotomy in long term results.

References

Müller, M. E.: Hüftnahe Femurosteotomien. Stuttgart: Thieme 1957.
— Manual der Osteosynthese. AO-Technik. Berlin-Heidelberg-New York: Springer 1969.

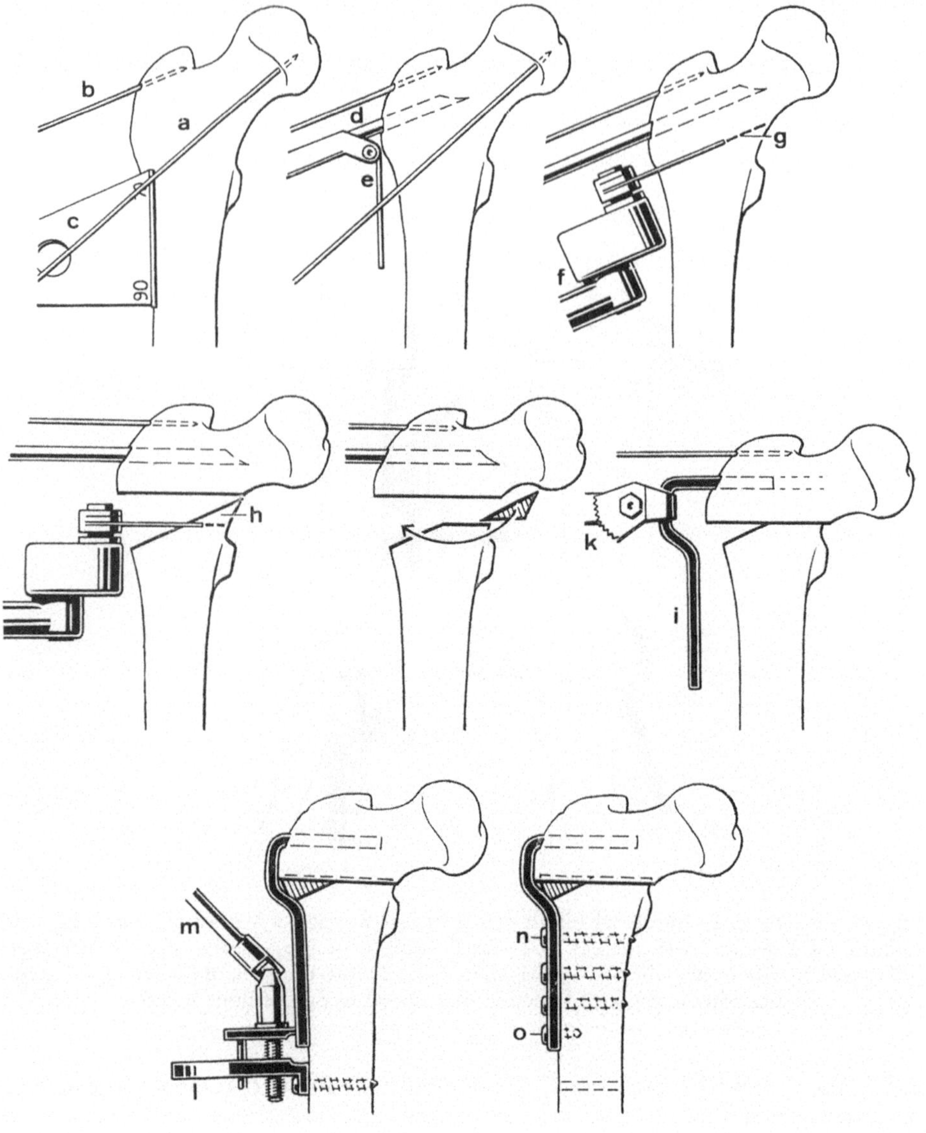

Fig. 4. Technique of varisation osteotomy. The Kirschner wire (a) shows the direction of the neck of the femur, Kirschner wire (b) lies parallel to (a) and to the upper edge of the metal quadrilateral (c). The plate site instrument (d) is driven into the femur neck parallel to (b) when the flap of the aligning apparatus (e) is parallel to the upper femur shaft. With the oscillating saw (f), the intertrochanteric osteotomy (g) is set parallel to the plate site instrument, as proximal as possible. After tilting the femur head fragment, the bone triangle (h) with medial base can be sawn off. This wedge is inserted laterally later. After knocking out the plate site instrument with the slit hammer, the plate held with the fastener, follows (i). By means of the threaded tension apparatus (l) and the cardan key (m), the osteotomy surfaces are set under pressure. At the end of the operation the screws (n) are screwed in, the tension apparatus removed and the short screw (o) fixes the distal end of the plate

Neurological Complications of Cervical Spine Injuries: Diagnosis and Treatment

Robert W. Bailey*

Neurological complications following cervical spine injuries may be divided into acute or chronic. This presentation will be developed in this manner.

The most important structures whose functions might be compromised in cervical fracture or dislocation are the spinal cord and nerve roots. Frequently two surgical disciplines are concerned, Neurosurgery and Orthopaedic Surgery, and this is true at The University of Michigan. As a result of the close co-operation between members of these services, improved treatment can be effected and further valuable new information can be gained about the pathomechanics of certain injuries.

A precise neurological examination is an absolute essential, and then frequent repeat evaluations in order to note any changes. Recognition of the level of the lesion in which there has been complete transection of the cord is not difficult, but, unfortunately, too often on cursory neurological examination, errors in evaluation are committed when the examiner fails to note that certain functions of the spinal cord have remained intact. A major objective of this presentation is to emphasize the need for thoroughness in clinical evaluation. As a further aid to correctly identify levels of complete paralysis, certain characteristic postures of the extremities are observed. In a fracture dislocation of the sixth on the seventh cervical vertebrae, the fifth and sixth cord segments which innervate the biceps are usually spared. The position of the patient in such instances is usually with the arms held in a flexed position lying across the chest and with the hands lying motionless and half closed. When the fracture dislocation is between the fifth and sixth cervical vertebrae, the arms may be held at right angles to the long axis of the body and the forearms moderately flexed with the hands lying at the level of the head. With fracture dislocation between the fourth and fifth cervical vertebrae and there is paralysis, the arms lie motionless at the side. Fracture dislocation at the level of the third and fourth cervical vertebrae with paralysis is usually fatal, but here, too, the arms are flail and at the side.

There is no universal opinion among neurosurgeons or orthopaedic surgeons with respect to the indications for carrying out laminectomy. Most would agree that prompt reduction of the fracture dislocation accomplishes a most important step in decompression of the cord and nerve roots by restoration of the neural canal. Immediately upon establishing the correct diagnosis, the patient is placed in Vinke tongs traction, and by using weights of increasing increments, the fracture dislocation is reduced under radiographic control.

In the acute fracture or dislocation with neurological damage, the question of laminectomy is always raised. As already stated, the neurological examination must be accurate and the patient's condition watched carefully for any changes which may occur with the passage of time. The author agrees that when the cervical cord damage is immediate and complete and lasts for a period of 24 h, there is virtually no hope for recovery and laminectomy therefore has really nothing to offer. The most important factor in effecting cord decompression is restoration of the normal diameter of the neural canal.

---

* Prof. of Surgery, Department of Surgery, Section of Orthopaedic Surgery, The University of Michigan Medical School.

Perhaps the most important factor in arriving at a decision involving carrying out a laminectomy in the total complete and immediate paralysis type of case relates to the impact of the injury on the psyche of the patient and his relatives. These extrinsic pressures at the time of injury or even later on may warrant laminectomy after vertebral realignment has been achieved if only to answer any gnawing doubts of the

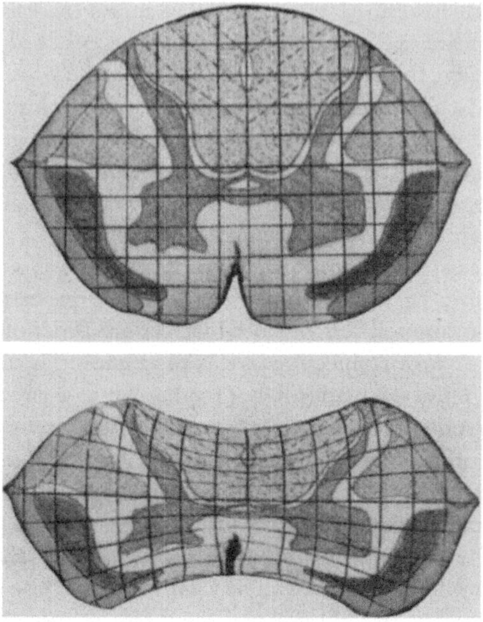

a

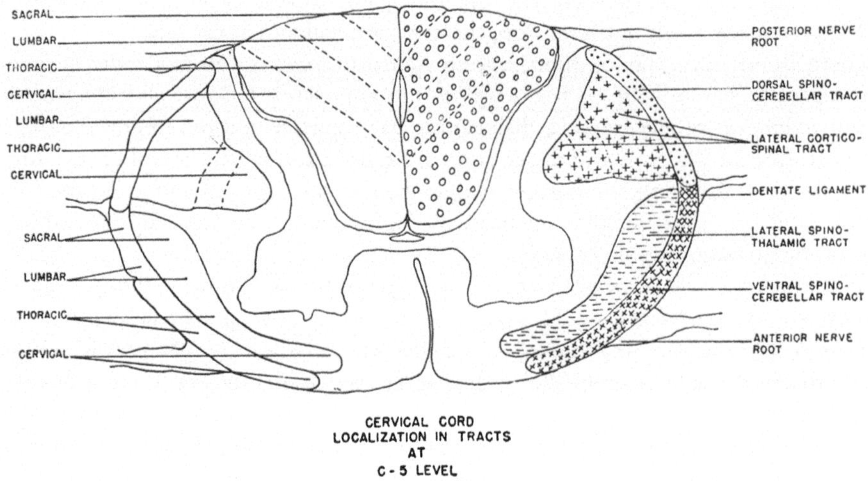

b

Fig. 1. Cervical spinal cord section and model of cross section of cord demonstrating compression by both anterior and posterior force (Reproduced from Schneider, R. C., G. Cherry, and H. Pantek: J. Neurosurg. **11**, 546, 1954) patient and/or his relatives as to whether he might have been better if the surgeon had visibly inspected the spinal cord to see if whatever was wrong could have been righted.

In acute trauma to the cervical spine with neurological findings, other syndromes which must be recognized are: (A) The Acute Central Cord Compression Syndrome as described by R. C. SCHNEIDER; and (B) Acute Anterior Cervical Cord Compression Syndrome described by E. A. KAHN. The pathology of acute central cervical cord compression make recognition of this important since laminectomy can only serve to hurt rather than to improve the patient. The neurological picture is essentially one of paralysis in the arms being greater than in the legs and of an ascending order of neurological improvement with return of bowel and bladder function followed by improvement in the lower extremities and finally in the arms. SCHNEIDER demonstrated by mechanical means and with post mortom specimens that the effect on the spinal cord with the central portion of the cord suffering the greatest change, as described by TAYLOR, the more peripheral portion is relatively spared since it is peripherally where the nerve fibers to the legs lie most superficially in the pyramidal tracts (Fig. 1). The central portion of the cord, which includes the anterior horn cells and the medial portion of the pyramidal tracts, is most severely involved and accounts for the profound weakness in the arms and a lesser involvement in the legs.

In 1947, E. A. KAHN described the role of the dentate ligaments in producing chronic cervical compression. An acute form of anterior cervical cord injury on a similar basis has since been described by KAHN and SCHNEIDER. The syndrome of acute anterior cord injury consists of immediate complete paralysis with hypalgesia and hypesthesia to the level of the lesion with preservation of motion, position and vibratory sense. There is no block on jugular compression and the symtoms are immediate and do not progress. If reduction of the fracture dislocation has been achieved, laminectomy is advisable if the paralysis does not improve, but this is done only after the patient's general condition has stabilized.

The bursting fracture of the vertebral body or the tear-drop fracture, also described by SCHNEIDER, may produce acute compression of the anterior portion of the spinal cord by postero displacement of a portion of the vertebral body. The cord may be crushed against the lamina, but if the dentate ligaments hold attaching cord to dura, the trauma may be dissipated into the anterior part of the cord, sparing the posterior columns. Below the lesion there is paralysis with loss of pain and temperature but preservation of posterior column function with position touch and position senses preserved. Immediate application of cervical traction and reduction of the fracture dislocation is important. Early fusion should be performed when the patient's condition has stabilized. The technique of a thrust type of bone graft using an anterior approach as described by BADGLEY and BAILEY is advised (Fig. 2). Then, later, if neurological improvement does not occur or late neurological sequela develops, laminectomy can be done and the stability of the spine is not altered.

Since 1939, under the influence of BADGLEY at The University of Michigan, many cervical fractures have been treated by cervical fusion in order to protect the cord or roots from any later damage. BADGLEY; CONE and TURNER; GALLIE, ROGERS; and others, in the 1930's, pointed out that many cervical fractures and dislocations heal poorly and are prone to early or late recurrence and sometimes with disastrous neurological consequences. The key factor to such re-displacement is the injury to the intervertebral disc whose healing potential is poor, much like the semilunar cartilage of the knee (Fig. 3). The role of the disc acting as a bond between the

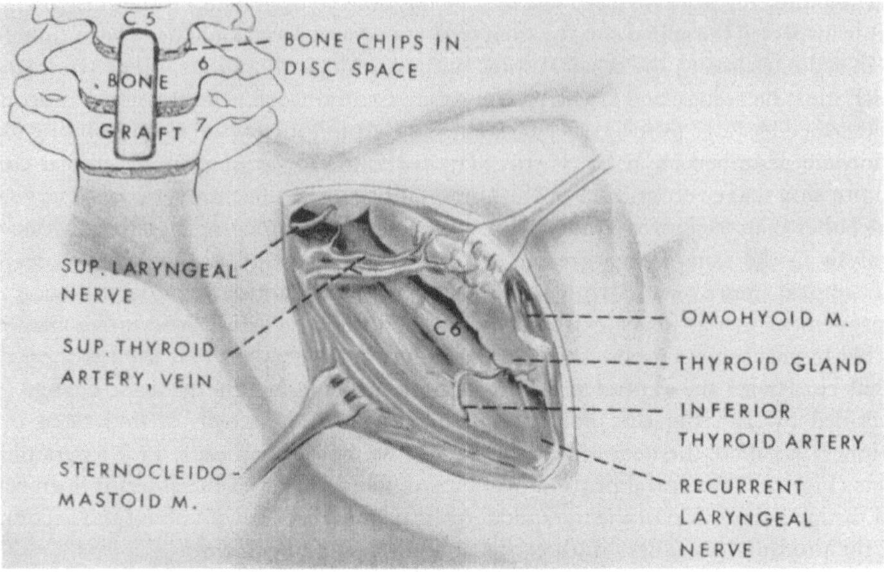

Fig. 2. Anterolateral approach to the cervical spine. The inset indicates the method of fusion with an iliac bone graft mortised into a carefully prepared bed and cancellous chips gently packed into the disc spaces

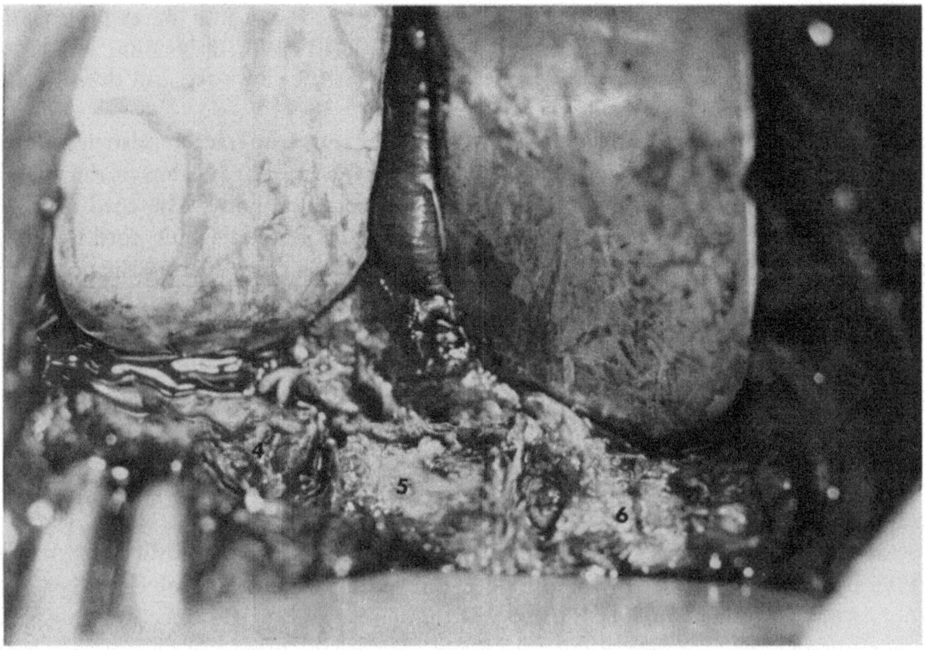

Fig. 3. With cervical traction applied, the intervertebral disc space opens to a greater extent between the fifth and sixth cervical than between the fourth and fifth cervical vertebrae. As traction was alternately increased and decreased, the nucleus pulposus would pop forward like a "pea from a pod", indicating inadequate repair of injury to the intervertebral disc (From Bailey, R. W.; J. Bone and Joint Surg. **42-A**, 565-594, 1960)

vertebral bodies, aiding in maintaining vertebral integrity, and the significance of disruption in this bond, I have previously reported. Posterior and anterior cervical fusions have commonly been performed when the injury has resulted in disruption of the disc. Anterior cervical fusion has certain advantages: (1) following previous laminectomy, especially when the dura has been left open; (2) the surgeon has been allowed to go wider laterally in bone removal in the course of laminectomy, well recognizing that anterior fusion could later be performed; and (3) in the tear-drop fracture, anterior fusion can be done with the realization that later, should neurological findings develop, laminectomy could be carried out without loss of stability.

TAYLOR, in 1951, reported a case of severe spinal cord damage without any evidence of cervical fracture or dislocation. He hypothesized that the neurological damage was secondary to the cord being compressed between a bone spur anteriorly and the ligamentum flavum behind. His myelographic studies showed this very

Table 1. *Indications for laminectomy in the cervical area*

1. Open fracture in a fracture dislocation due to a penetrating wound.
2. Presence of bone fragments in the spinal canal.
3. In the uncommon instances where the neurological lesion is progressive, e.g., acute anterior spinal cord injury syndrome, immediate laminectomy should be performed.
4. Psychological factors.

Table 2. *Contraindications for laminectomy in the cervical area*

1. With total immediate and complete paralysis lasting for 24 h. No hope of improvement unless at C5-6 level, where foraminotomy may effect root decompression which is important in rehabilitation.
2. Acute central cervical spinal cord injury.
3. Fracture dislocation at or above the fourth cervical vertebra, or with evidence of a cervico-medullary syndrome.
4. When the patient's general condition will not permit surgery.
5. If the hospital facilities and/or personnel are not equipped to handle this type of case.

adequately. SCHNEIDER has also reported on a number of similar cases which he has termed "chronic anterior cervical-cord injury or compression syndrome", with improvement following laminectomy and removal of the spurs anteriorly (Fig. 4).

The syndrome has a history of previous injury. The cord was compressed anteriorly between the spur and the ligamentum flavum from behind, producing destruction in the central portion of the cord with surrounding edema. "Since the nerve fibers to the fingers, hand, and arm lie more medially in each lateral corticospinal tract than do those to the trunk and lower extremities, recovery follows the characteristic pattern of this syndrome with movement in the lower extremities returning first, followed next by return of bladder function, and then by motor power in the arms and hands". An interval follows, then symptoms develop consisting of increasing spasticity with weakness of the extremities with bilateral hyper-reflexia and extensor plantar reflexes. An area of chronic localized compression of the anterior cervical cord in the midline by the spur with secondary zones of stress in the lateral corticospinals tracts occur due to the pull of the dentate ligaments at their insertions. Laminectomy with section of the dentate ligaments and removal of the anterior spurs has been helpful.

The experimental work of TARLOV producing compression lesions of the cord by means of inflation of a balloon within the spinal canal of dogs deserves consideration in relation to cervical laminectomy. He showed that when large compressive forces were used, recovery could take place if the compression was released within 30 min. When spinal cord compression was of a lesser magnitude, recovery occurred after periods of compression for as long as 2 h. This work should be given thought and, if possible, a correlation between the experimental animal and investigative procedures, and of fracture dislocation in man then be made. I agree with KAHN's comment — "how would it be feasible to decompress a spinal cord even 2 h after injury, and what would the mortality be?"

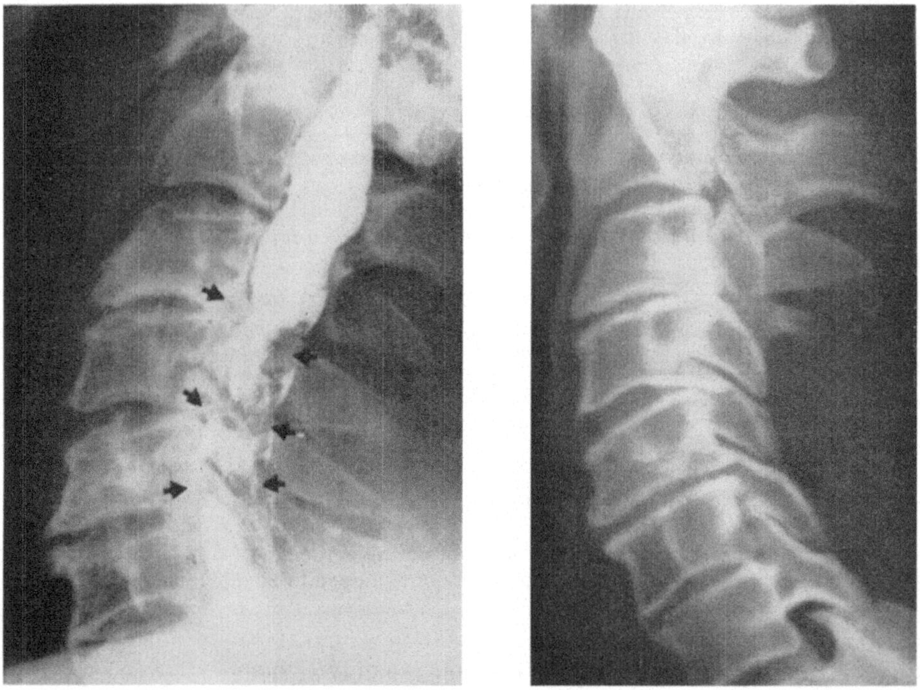

Fig. 4. Cervical myelogram showing simultaneous encroachments on the spinal canal anteriorly and posteriorly

STOVER, METTEN and I, in 1962, reviewed all cervical fractures and fracture dislocations seen between 1939 and 1963, and this work was reported at the annual meeting of the American Academy of Orthopaedic Surgeons in January 1963. There were 335 cases in this study and all were studied from various aspects including neurological abnormalities. Objective neurological findings were present in 147 cases, 70 of which had quadriparesis. In the majority of those without severe neurological damage, the findings were frequently those of diminished reflexive biceps or triceps; hypesthesia in an area of the arm; or weakness usually in the distribution of a specific nerve root which corresponded to the area of dislocation. In fractures or fracture dislocations of the atlantoaxial articulation, the only complaint may have been of severe headache along the course of the greater occipital nerve unilaterally or bilaterally. Of the 335 cases, there were 14 deaths attributed directly or indirectly to the cervical spine injury: 9 occurred in patients with serious neurological damage, of which 6 had not had surgical treatment other than tongs traction. There were 3 deaths in patients with neurological injury who had been treated by laminectomy. Death in 2 others was due to pulmonary embolus, and in the third, attributed to renal failure. 1 patient died following cervical fusion of a pulmonary embolus. In 10 of those who expired, the level of dislocation was between the fourth and fifth cervical vertebrae. The over-all death rate was 4.17%, which may seem surprisingly low, but no doubt reflects the referral nature of the hospitals and the fact that many of these patients did not come under treatment within the first 24 h following injury.

Since 1962, a great many more fusions (a total of 60) have been done anteriorly for acute fractures and dislocations.

References

BADGLEY, C. E.: Personal Cummunication.
BAILEY, R. W., and C. E. BADGLEY: J. Bone Jt Surg. **42 A,** 565—594 (1960).
—, C. N. STOVER, and C. F. METTEN: J. Bone Jt Surg. **45 A,** 1550 (1963).
CONE, W., and W. G. TURNER: J. Bone Jt Surg. **19,** 584—602 (1937).
GALLIE, W. E.: Amer. J. Surg. **46,** 495—499 (1939).
KAHN, E. A.: J. Neurosurg. **4,** 191—199 (1947).
ROGERS, W. A.: J. Bone Jt Surg. **24,** 245—258 (1942).
SCHNEIDER, R. C.: J. Neurosurg. **12,** 95—122 (1955).
—, and E. A. KAHN: J. Bone Jt Surg. **38 A,** 985—997 (1956).
—, G. CHERRY, and H. PANTEK, M.S.E.: J. Neurosurg. **11,** 546—577 (1954).
TARLOV, I. M.: Spinal cord compression. Springfield, Illinois: Charles C. Thomas 1957.
TAYLOR, A. R.: Ann. Surg. **90,** 321—340 (1929).
— J. Bone Jt Surg. **33 B,** 543—547 (1951).

Urologic Injuries

Diagnosis of Injuries to the Kidney: a Review of 125 Cases*

A. T. K. Cockett, S. A. Brosman, and W. E. Goodwin

The increased speed of the automobile today is associated with an era of rapid transportation. Our highly mobile population has created new problems. Modern super-highways are now commonplace. Late model high-powered automobiles are often devastating following collision with the average pedestrian. Auto versus auto collisions occur with increasing frequency and provide ample opportunity to evaluate and treat multiple body system injuries.

Harbor General Hospital, a 750-bed facility, is located adjacent to a busy expressway. 1 mile north is a second superhighway which cuts diagonally away from the hospital. 3 miles eastward are two expressways which are heavily used during rush hours.

During the past 7 years approximately 125 cases of renal trauma have presented themselves in the emergency room. 60% of these patients had injury in at least a second organ system; most often the injury was orthopedic in nature.

The purpose of our study is to outline a diagnostic approach to the evaluation of renal injuries. This plan has evolved over the past 7 years.

The X-ray scout film or KUB obtained on admission is invaluable. Presence of rib fractures (T-11 and T-12), or fractures of the transverse lumbar processes (L-1 and L-2), when coupled with gross hematuria, are highly suggestive of renal injury on the ipsilateral side. Scoliosis may be present and is a valuable sign denoting psoas major muscle spasm and injury to the kidney on that side. A ground-glass appearing soft tissue mass obscuring the lateral margin of the psoas muscle is also helpful in focusing attention on an injured and bleeding kidney.

Approximately 15 years ago one of us (WEG) performed translumbar aortography as a diagnostic procedure in selected renal trauma patients. In several instances the injected contrast media revealed no evidence of significant renal injury. However, the procedure was diagnostic from a second standpoint. The X-ray films revealed evidence for a splenic rupture. Recently, liver lacerations coexisting with injury in the upper right kidney were documented in a patient.

In the early years when urographic contrast media were less than ideal, emphasis was placed on the performance of retrograde pyelograms [*1*]. The presence of retrograde extravasation of contrast media into the renal parenchyma was indicative of a severe laceration justifying surgical exploration. This view is still adhered to by many.

Recently we have been impressed with the diagnostic value of the renal scan [*2*]. An experimental renal trauma study by our group compared the scan and the renal

* From the Department of Surgery/Urology, Harbor General Hospital, Torrance and the UCLA School of Medicine, Los Angeles, California.

arteriogram. We especially noted the sensitivity of this technique; minor lacerations and contusions could be localized by the scan. A major laceration through the capsule had to occur before the renal arteriogram was helpful; in this latter instance the cold area was also clearly demarcated by the renal scan.

Observations and Results

The distribution of 125 renal trauma cases is shown in Fig. 1. 78 patients were over 17 years of age. Renal exploration was performed in 50 instances. The majority (43) had sustained a laceration.

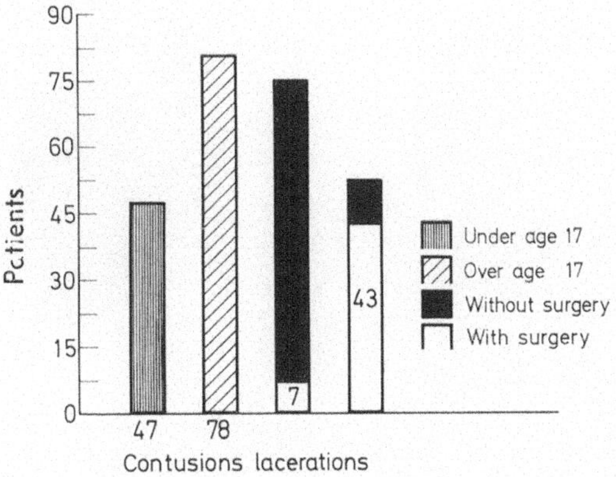

Fig. 1. Bar graph — Distribution of 125 renal trauma cases. Cases divided into contusions and lacerations. Number of cases explored in each group are shown

Table 1. *Value of diagnostic tests in renal injuries*

	Significant	Not significant	Accuracy %
Renal scan	25	0	100
Aortogram	15 (+ 3)	3	83 (86)
Retrograde pyelogram	27	5	84
Conventional IVP	32	24	57
Infusion pyelogram	48	7	87

Table 2. *Urologic procedures performed in 50 patients*

Surgical procedures		Mortality	
Nephrectomy	10	Secondary to renal injury	0
Partial Nephrectomy	17	Associated injury	4
Hemostasis and drainage	23		

Table 1 lists the diagnostic tests performed in our study. Renal scans were significant in 25 out of 25 instances. The aortogram was helpful in 15 of 18 cases. In an additional two patients the aortogram demonstrated puddling of contrast media in the spleen. Lacerated spleens were removed in both patients. In a third instance aortography was suggestive for the presence of liver lacerations and a right upper renal laceration. The lacerations diagnosed preoperatively were found at surgery, and surgical hemostasis was obtained.

Table 2 lists the urological procedures performed in 50 patients. Hemostasis and simple drainage were performed in 23 instances.

Several typical case reports demonstrate the usefulness of aortography and renal scanning.

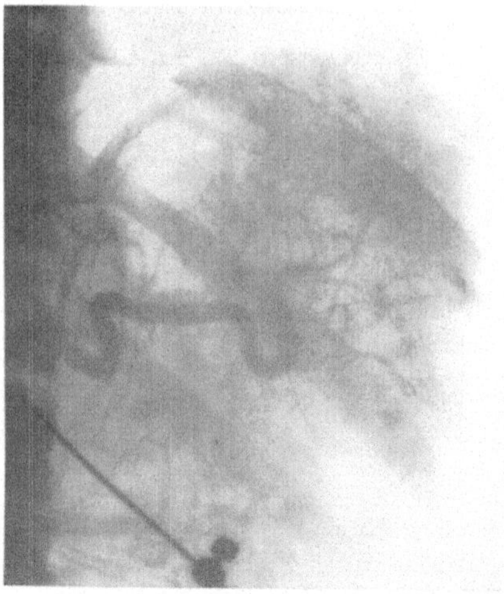

Fig. 2

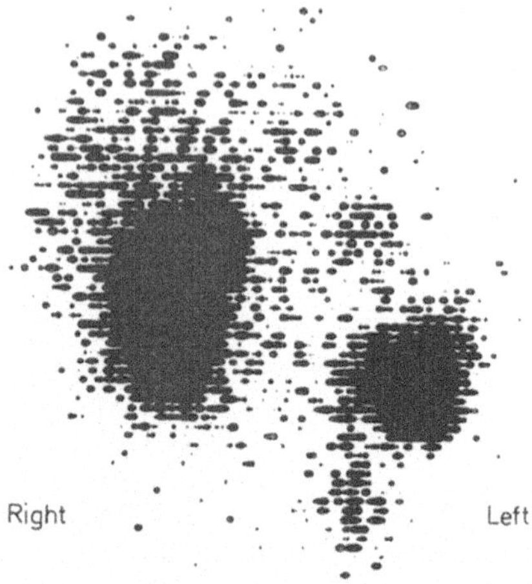

Fig. 3

Fig. 2. Splenic arteriogram demonstrating puddling in periphery

Fig. 3. Kidney scan demonstrating cold area in upper left kidney region

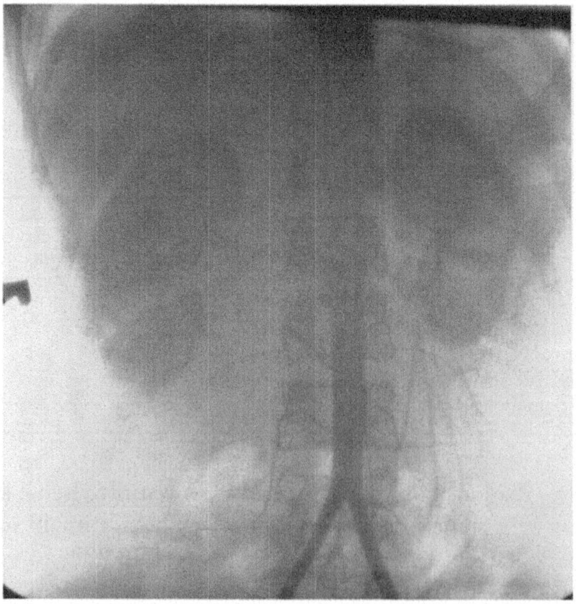

Fig. 4. Aortogram demonstrating transverse laceration of right kidney

J. C., a 19 year-old male, was noted to have gross hematuria several hours after an auto accident. Intravenous urography revealed normal visualization of contrast media in both kidneys. Translumbar aortography demonstrated a normal renal arterial vasculature bilaterally. Pooling however, in several areas of the spleen was observed (Fig. 2). Surgical exploration was performed because of increasing tachycardia and a reduction in blood pressure. A torn spleen was removed. Blood (1500 ml) was evacuated from the peritoneal cavity.

B. H., a 9 year-old girl, was struck by an automobile. She sustained a fracture of the left femur. Gross hematuria was also observed on admission. Increasing tachycardia associated with a reduction of blood pressure soon ensued. A cystogram was normal. Intravenous urography revealed non-visualization of the left renal area. The left psoas muscle border was obliterated. A renal scan was obtained the next day (Fig. 3). No radioactivity was seen in the left upper renal area. Aortography was also

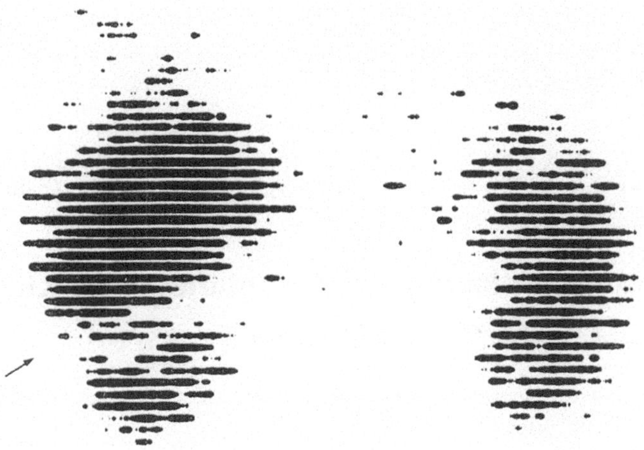

Fig. 5. Renal scan delineating transverse laceration in right lower kidney

performed. Urinary extravasation in the left renal pelvic area was demonstrated. At surgery an upper renal heminephrectomy was completed, and the exposed calyx was carefully closed.

H. M., a 38 year-old male, was involved in an auto versus auto collision. Right flank pain was a major complaint. Gross hematuria was associated with a reduced blood pressure (88/60). Non-visualization of the right kidney was evident following intravenous urography. The aortogram was suggestive for the presence of a large transverse laceration (Fig. 4). A second renal artery was observed to the lower pole. The renal scan clearly delineated the area of laceration (Fig. 5). At surgery the partially separated ends of the kidney were sutured together in circumferential fashion.

Discussion

Comment has been made in the literature regarding the increased susceptibility of a diseased or congenitally deformed kidney to injury. We have been impressed by this fact. Malformed or diseased kidneys injure more easily.

The scout film (KUB) obtained at the time of intravenous urography is valuable in patients who sustain renal trauma. Fractured ribs (T-11 and T-12) overlying the posterior upper kidney probably impale and injure the kidney during impact.

Our experience with conventional intravenous urography has been disappointing. Constant infusion of larger volumes of contrast media however, has improved our ability to assess the extent of renal injury (Table 1).

In our experience the renal scan and the abdominal aortogram are the two best diagnostic tests in patients harboring an injured kidney. The scan is probably more sensitive than the aortogram. However, selective renal arteriography improves the surgeon's ability to assess the extent of injury. The aortogram is also useful in providing selective visualization of the liver or splenic vasculature. Delayed films obtained during aortography are the equivalent of an intravenous urogram. 60% of our patients had injury in a second organ or system. The aortogram can be beneficial in selected instances when intra-abdominal visceral injury is suspected.

We believe that the best urological approach to a patient with renal injury will be based on accurately assessing the extent of renal injury. If the boundaries of injury can be accurately determined, then the type of surgery to be performed is fairly obvious. The renal scan and the aortogram appear to be the best diagnostic procedures presently available in providing such information. In our series the infusion pyelogram is the third procedure of choice.

References

1. Hodges, C. V., D. R. Gilbert, and W. W. Scott: J. Urol. (Baltimore) **66**, 627 (1951).
2. Kazmin, M. H., L. E. Swanson, and A. T. K. Cockett: J. Urol. (Baltimore) **97**, 189 (1967).

Conservative Management of Injuries to the Kidney

W. Lutzeyer

The indication for *primary conservative treatment* of renal trauma results from the following *three* basic rules:

1. Conservative treatment will not be considered for *penetrating* renal injuries (approximately 10%).

2. Immediate surgical treatment is advised in patients with combined injuries, i.e., renal trauma combined with trauma to the skull, the bony skeleton or to intra-abdominal organs (64%).

3. Conservative treatment is only indicated in patients who suffered *blunt renal trauma* and who, on the basis of the local and clinical findings, do *not require immediate treatment.*

However, in these cases exact observation of the patient's condition *must determine* the change from primary conservative to secondary surgical treatment!

This outline once again shows a summary of my personal classification of the various forms of renal injuries, which range from contusion to internal or external rupture, to laceration of the kidney and to total renal or ureteral avulsion.

Thus, in patients with closed renal trauma the *strict indication* usually includes only the first two types:

1. *Contusion*, the mild form of which is frequently not recognized clinically if it occurs by itself and which accounts for approximately 65% of the cases with mild renal trauma.

Urologische Klinik der Medizinischen Fakultät der Rheinisch-Westfälischen Technischen Hochschule Aachen. (Vorstand: Prof. Dr. med. W. Lutzeyer).

Smaller radial subcapsular tears or subcapsular hematomas are the pathological-anatomical basis of this process.

2. Mild or severe renal rupture may be treated conservatively if the rupture presents as a closed injury, i.e., it drains itself into the kidney pelvis and does not produce extrarenal urine and blood paravasation. It can also be treated conservatively

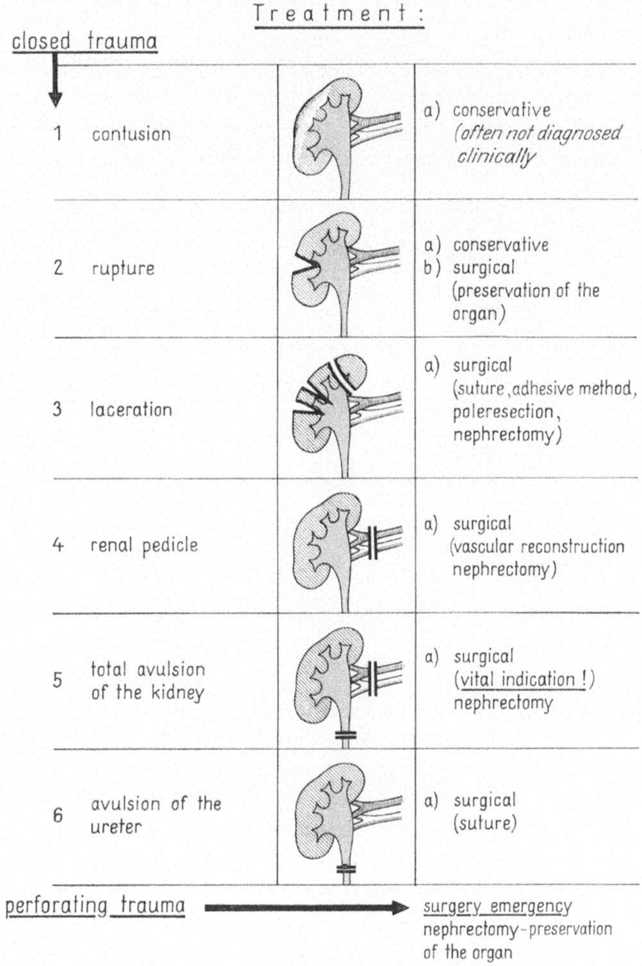

Fig. 1. The relation between the pathological-anatomical injury type and the indication for treatment in patients with renal trauma. After W. LUTZEYER: Act. Chir. **3**, 19 (1968)

if, in cases with a through and through rupture, the wound closes spontaneously on account of compression by the hematoma.

Whereas the *former criteria* for the indication of "conservative treatment — surgical exposure" were usually determined by intravenous pyelogram, nephrotomography and possibly retrograde pyelography. There emphasis was placed on the extravasation of the dye at the present time *transfemoral renal serial angiography* (OLSSON, BERGMANN, RODECK) is the decisive *diagnostic factor* for a decision about the respective indication.

Without knowledge of the important main aspects of the symptomatology, *critical observation of the course of the patient* is impossible. On account of this we would like to present the groups in such a manner in this paper that they show from the left upper corner (predominantly local symptoms) to the right lower corner the severity or the change of the disease and thus permit, in every case, the assessment of the respective indication.

In patients with isolated blunt renal trauma *hematuria, pain and tumour* are a group of symptoms forming a triad.

If the clinical appearance remains mainly limited to these symptoms, conservative treatment can be continued. However, if the patient develop signs of shock or collapse (second group), and finally signs of peritoneal irritation or disorders of renal function with changes of the general condition appear, observation of the patient

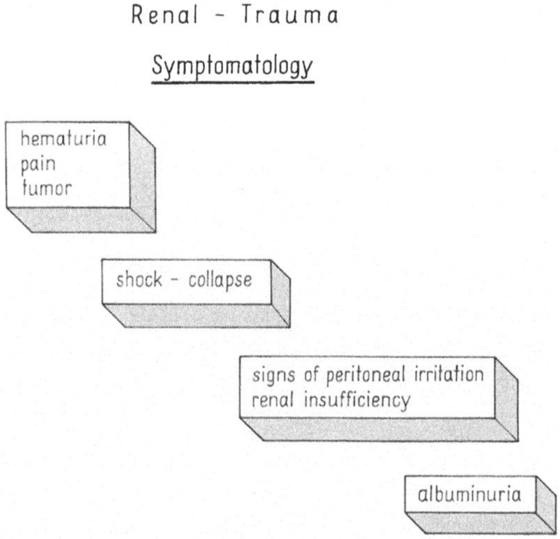

Fig. 2. The symptoms of blunt renal trauma with regard to the control of the course. After W. LUTZEYER: Act. Chir. **3**, 19 (1968)

may force us to a change of indication: i.e., we abandon the conservative approach and have to undertake suitable surgical treatment.

According to an outline which was modified by MCANICH, a brief summary of the indication for surgery would be stated as follows: If, as far as the local symptoms are concerned, the tumour in the loin is decreasing and at the same time the patient also complains of increased pain; if widely spread extravasation of the contrast medium is seen in the radiogram, which practically indicated increasing urinary extravasation and progression of the hematoma, and if hematuria lasts more than 96 h, it is important to make the *clinical findings* one of the main aspects of the indication: If the general condition of the patient deteriorates despite continuous administration of blood and plasma, if *pulse-rate and* bloodpressure reache critical values, if the hematocrit and hemoglobin as well as the erythrocyte count show a constant decrease, and if the urine output begins to cease, *conservative treatment which had hitherto been undertaken* must be abandoned in favour of *surgical* intervention.

This table shows in what manner we define *control of the clinical course* in patients with blunt renal trauma. However, the order of sequence in which the various points are listed is not intended to indicate their importance:

1. Urinary output and fluid balance, i.e., measuring the fluid intake and output is just as important as

2. the severity of hematuria and, most of all,

3. the continuous charting of pulse, bloodpressure and temperature.

At the present time when complicated laboratory examinations are predominant, it is frequently no longer considered important that, in the final analysis, pulse and bloodpressure determinations as well as temperature determinations are the centre of observing the clinical course.

4. The blood status usually includes hemoglobin, erythrocyte count and hematocrit.

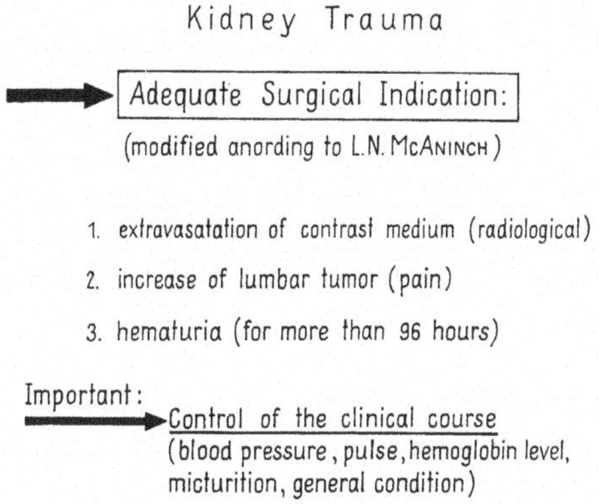

Fig. 3. Change of indication from hitherto conservative to emergency surgical treatment

Table 1. *Renal trauma: control of the clinical course*

1. *Urine output* (fluid balance).
2. *Severity of hematuria.*
3. *Pulse — blood pressure — temperature* (continuous registration).
4. *Hemoglobin,*
   erythrocyte count,
   hematocrit.
5. *Urea,*
   serum creatinine,
   serum electrolytes.
6. *Abdominal symptoms.*
7. *Circumference of the abdominal and loin region* (loin tumour).
8. *General condition!!*

5. For the determination of renal function we feel that at least urea controls, controls of the serum creatinine values and, most of all, the serum-electrolytes are important.

6. The severity and duration of abdominal symptoms, i.e., symptoms of peritoneal irritation or of ileus, are just as important criteria as

7. the abdominal circumference, including the loin.

8. Even though all these points may provide an evaluation of the *general condition* of the patient, one should, however, never forget, despite the existence of the controls, to observe the patient with regard to the general situation, i.e., cold perspiration, facial pallor, general restlessness, etc.

However, if one decides on conservative treatment of renal trauma — naturally always with the possibility of surgical intervention — the following guidelines are valid for us:

1. Absolute bedrest with the old and somewhat outmoded ice-bag.

2. Treatment of shock according to the general principles, e.g., volume replacement, adrenal corticosteroids.

Table 2. *Renal trauma: conservative treatment*

1. *Absolute bedrest* (ice-bag).
2. *Treatment of shock* e.g., volume replacement adrenal corticosteroids.
3. *Blood replacement* (selective).
4. *Stimulation of diuresis* e.g., 10 to 20% mannitol intravenous drips, sodium lactate intravenous drips.
5. *Antibiotics* (broad spectrum — high doses).
6. *Bowel function.*
7. *Food supply* parenteral,
   mild diet.
8. In patients with anuria — extracorporal dialysis.
9. Coagulating agents are contraindicated — occlusion anuria.

3. Selective blood replacement and

4. stimulation of diuresis with a 20% mannitol intravenous drip or with an alkalizing sodium lactate intravenous drip.

5. Prophylactic antibiotics should be administered, preferably in the form of high doses of broad spectrum antibiotics.

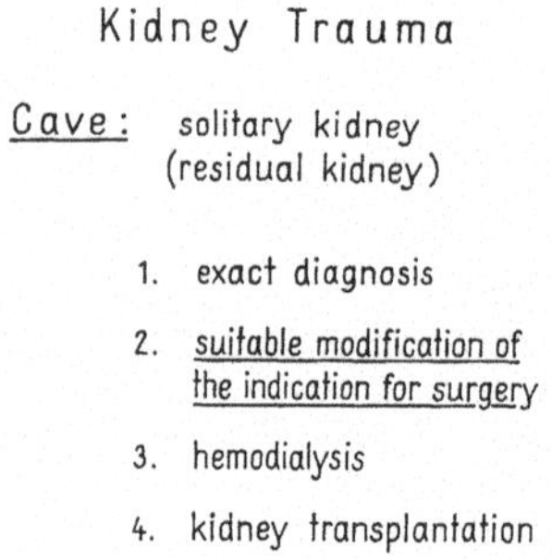

Fig. 4. Therapeutic approach to patients who have suffered blunt renal trauma and who have one residual (solitary) kidney. After W. Lutzeyer: Act. Chir. **3**, 19 (1968)

That, 6th and 7th, the control of bowel function and of the food supply, either parenteral or by a mild diet, may be decisive factors, is natural to the expert.

8. If the patient develops *anuria* one has to determine whether one is dealing with occlusion anuria due to blood clots, possibly due to reflex involvement of the contralateral side.

If this is not the case, extracorporeal dialysis is indicated.

In this context we would like to warn against the use of highly effective coagulants as e.g., ε-amino-capronic acid or their derivatives which in patients with *intrapelvic* hemorrhages may produce immediate coagulation and thus may result in tamponade of the renal pelvis and occlusion anuria.

If one is dealing with a solitary or single remaining kidney the *exact diagnosis* determines the subsequent approach.

If one is merely dealing with a contusion, and observation of the patient's course does not show deterioration of the condition, I would treat the patient conservatively according to the previously shown principle. The question whether one should use *aortography* as a diagnostic measure must be decided individually in view of the potential complications of aortography and the severity of the injury to the remaining kidney. It is up to the individual physician to make a decision on that.

However, if one is dealing with a *more severe, progressive hemorrhage* with avulsion of a renal pole with sequestration, I feel that *surgical intervention*, possibly under hypothermia and with temporary dialysis, is indicated.

Thus, the possibilities of hemodialysis may prolong the time before a renal transplant is required.

The following should be valid as additional rules of treatment. Bedrest should be continued for at least 8 days since one does not know whether one may be dealing with secondary rupture. The patient should stay in hospital for 2 weeks in order to diagnose possible *early complications*, which are subsequently listed, in due time: Infiltration of urine, perirenal hematoma or abscess are those complications which, according to BRINKMANN, are *secondary indications* for surgical intervention and thus render *further conservative treatment useless*.

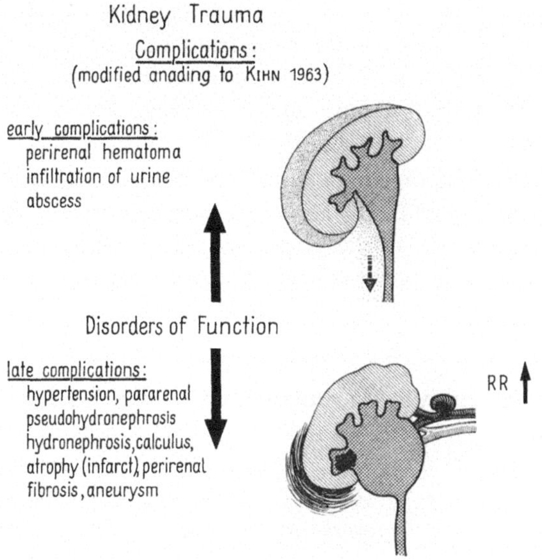

Fig. 5. Potential early and late complications after blunt renal trauma. After W. LUTZEYER: Act. Chir. **3**, 19 (1968)

With reference to possible *late complications* which range from hypertension to pararenal pseudohydronephrosis, hydronephrosis, calculi, atrophy to aneurism of the renal artery and which naturally imply a *functional disorder*, I suggest that in patients who were *treated conservatively* the following examinations be carried out before the patient is discharged from hospital:

a) Urinalysis,

b) intravenous excretion-urogram with nephrotomogram and late radiogram,

c) complete blood chemistry.

If these examinations give rise to suspicion of a serious parenchymal or vascular lesion, I feel that aortography is not only indicated for possible immediate treatment but also for a later evaluation.

The objection that late complications in patients with blunt renal trauma can be avoided by a relatively wide indication for surgical treatment is not always valid since a number of authors, such as RUMMELHARDT and DEVENS, have shown that the examined patient groups, surgical on one hand, conservative on the other hand, are not always exactly comparable.

I come to the following conclusions:

1. By the use of serial renal angiography and its importance, the indication for conservative treatment after blunt renal trauma is, at the present time, increasingly replaced by the tendency for primary surgical treatment.

There is a tendency to early exposure of the kidney and organ-preserving revision.

2. Even though 65% of the cases with *blunt renal injuries* usually are contusions, exact observation of the clinical course with all criteria is the decisive factor which either carries responsible conservative treatment to its conclusion or, on the basis of essential vital indications by necessity results in surgical intervention.

3. Conservative treatment is a responsible task that cannot be separated from observation of the clinical course and can only be placed in the hands of a well-trained physician and perhaps should be carried out on intensive care wards or monitoring wards. It requires the whole scale of modern shock treatment as well as treatment of threatened renal failure and knowledge about general surgical and traumatological aspects.

4. Only the comparison of larger groups of *patients with renal injuries who were treated surgically and who were treated conservatively*, with reference to the severity and the time of examination as well as the respective treatment type, can *provide critical indications for new concepts of conservative and surgical treatment* for the future.

The Operative Management of Renal Injuries

PAUL C. PETERS, M. O. PERRY, and H. M. SPENCE*

Parkland Memorial Hospital serves as the major teaching hospital for the University of Texas Southwestern Medical School at Dallas and is the major trauma center for the Southwestern United States. There are approximately 500 emergency room visits to this hospital each day. There have been for the past 8 years an average of 2,500 cases of trauma each year requiring major surgery. 1,400 of these cases have required exploratory laparotomy each year. Four times as many patient bed days are

Table 1. *PMH major general surgical and urological procedures 1967*

Total general surgical operations		9,831
Elective	5,106	
Emergency	4,725	
Total urological operations		593
Elective	518	
Emergency	75	

* Divisions of Urology and Surgery (Vascular), Southwestern Medical School, University of Texas at Dallas, Dallas, Texas 75235.

required for the trauma patients as for new born children and patients with heart disease. A typical year's experience is illustrated, including general surgical and urological operations for 1967.

During the period of 1955—67 182 cases of trauma were seen in which the renal injury was the predominant one. These were classified into two main groups: 1) Penetrating renal injuries — those due to a missle or stab wound, and 2) Non-penetrating renal injuries — those due to a blunt external force [*6*].

Etiologies in the two groups were as follows:

Penetrating injury 98 cases		*Non-penetrating injury 84 cases*	
Gunshot wound	80	Auto accident	55
Stabwound	16	Fall	15
Needle biopsy	2	Fighting	4
		Boating accident	2
		Football injury	7
		Struck by plank	1

When a patient presents to Parkland Memorial Hospital with a history or physical evidence of blunt or penetrating trauma he is immediately triaged to the surgical emergency area. There a history and physical examination is done by a member of the trauma team. The presence of blood in the urine results in prompt urologic consultation. Those patients with blunt renal trauma are initially managed conservatively following a voiding cystogram and excretory urogram which are done in that order; 96% of these patients have done well on non-operative management with bedrest and proper fluid and electrolyte replacement as needed until gross hematuria clears. Necessity for operative intervention is dictated by subsequent chemical clinical deterioration and evidence of massive hemorrhage, urinary extravasation, sepsis or shock. The retrograde femoral arteriogram used occasionally as a diagnostic study in this group has been of greatest help in detecting a polar rupture or a major arterial injury. The philosophy of management of a patient with a penetrating renal injury is simple. The patient is explored. This patient is frequently taken to the operating room under emergent conditions. Pre-operative supportive measures include rapid replacement of calculated losses of blood and balanced salt solution, the insertion of a small (18F) retention catheter in the bladder, and the establishment of an adequate airway (by tracheostomy if necessary). A small plastic catheter is placed into the superior vena cava to monitor central venous pressure. This monitoring of central venous pressure in combination with careful monitoring of the urine output allows more intelligent calculation of the adequacy of blood and electrolyte replacement. An adequate urine output is 30 cc per hour with a central venous pressure in the range of 7 to 12 cm of water. Once the patient is in the operating theater, the abdomen is usually prepared for a trans-abdominal approach (Fig. 1). A mid-line upper abdominal incision is made and extended as far inferiorly towards the symphysis pubis as is necessary for thorough abdominal exploration, which is always a part of the surgical management of penetrating genitourinary injuries. Associated visceral organ injury is common in penetrating renal injury; it was present in 35% of the patients in our series. The liver and spleen were most commonly injured. Pre-operatively the patients with associated liver or spleen injury have a positive four quadrant tap showing blood in the peritoneal cavity and have higher total white counts (usually greater than 20,000) than do the patients with an isolated renal injury and no associated visceral organ injury. The latter group have white blood cell counts of 7 to 11,000. The excretory urogram is a reliable guide as to the site of the injury when it is used. It often consists of a single film of the abdomen made on the operating table after contrast material has been injected in the emergency room. When after careful examination of the aorta, vena cava, spleen, and liver, the renal lesion is seen to be the dominant one, attention is quickly directed to obtaining control of the renal artery. This may be done by going through the root of the mesentery for either the right or left renal artery or the colon may be reflected medially by an incision on its antimesenteric border and the artery located just superior and posterior to the renal vein.

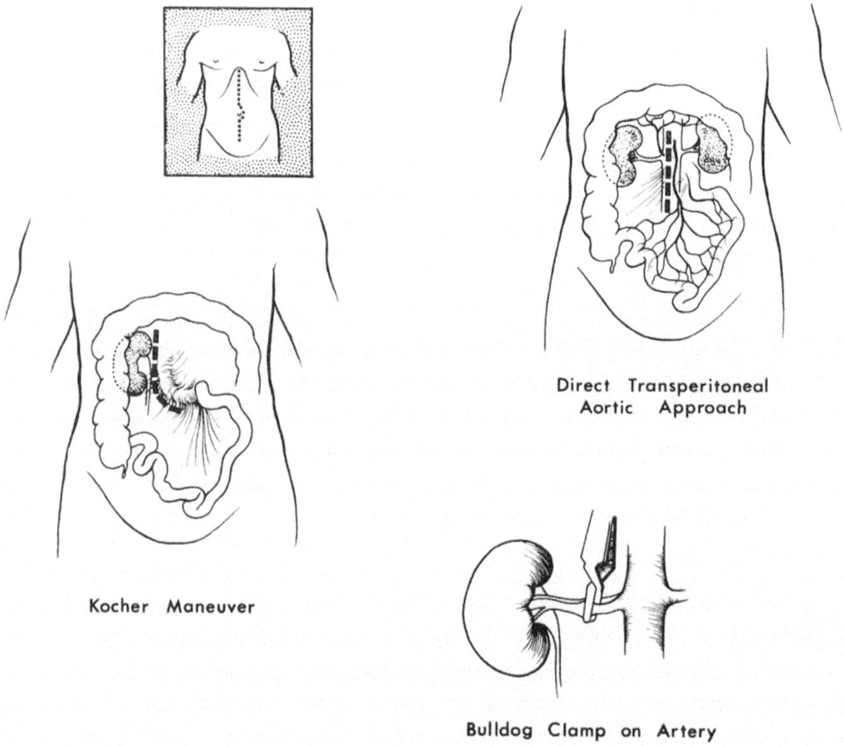

Fig. 1. Diagram illustrating the incision for transabdominal approach (upper left insert) with either transperitoneal aortic approach (upper right) or mobilization of duodenum (lower left) to allow clamping of the renal artery (lower right)

Mobilization of the descending duodenum on the right side aids in exposure of the right renal artery. Once the renal artery is controlled, assessment of the type of renal damage present is then performed. When hemorrhage remains massive after securing the renal artery, an isolation of the renal vein, vena cava and when on the left side isolation of the lumbo azygous vein draining into the left renal vein is immediately necessary. When the pedicle is controlled one may then elect to cool the kidney if inspection suggests a time consuming repair and debridement is necessary. This is simply accomplished by pouring Ringers Lactate cooled to 4 °C into the renal fossa to immerse the kidney. Others have advocated the use of external cooling appliances perfused with various refrigerants [*1*, *2*, *4*, *10*].

A temperature of 17 °C or less is desired and cannot be accomplished unless the artery is temporarily occluded. Function studies by SEMB [*7*, *8*] and HANLEY [*2*] suggest that a previously normal kidney may tolerate an occlusion of the renal artery for 25 min at surgery without permanent damage. The kidney with pre-existing disease however, is much more susceptible to ischemia. We have observed extensive tubular necrosis in a kidney containing stones in which it was necessary to occlude the renal artery for 23 min only. HANLEY [*2*] has suggested that a kidney cooled to 20 °C will tolerate 84 min of surgery without apparent loss of function.

When one completes the necessary mobilization of the kidney, the following types of injuries are found (Fig. 2): 1) parenchymal lacerations, these may be single

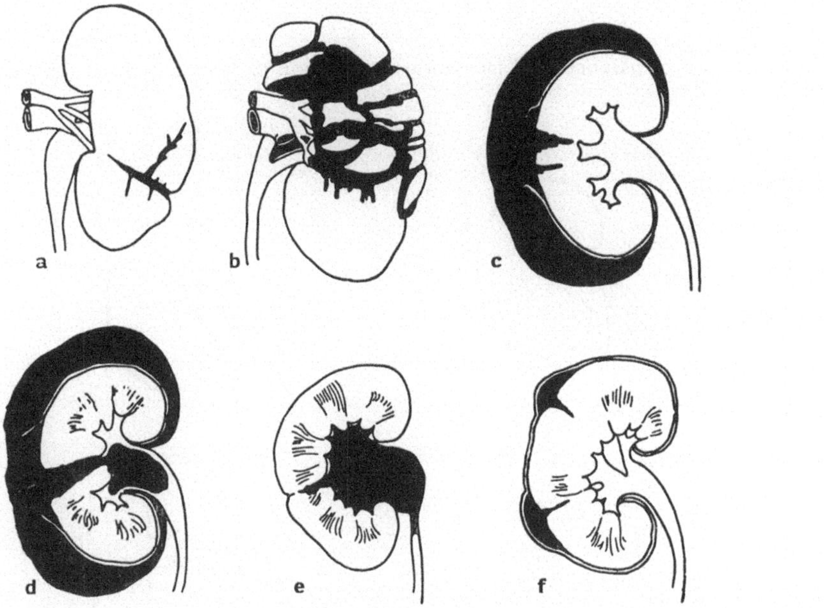

Fig. 2 a—f. Types of renal injury. (a) Simple parenchymal laceration, (b) Shattered kidney often accompanied by arterial or venous injury, (c) Perirenal hematoma with parenchymal laceration, (d) Perirenal hematoma with rupture through parenchyma into collecting system, (e) Rupture of parenchyma into collecting system, (f) Simple subcapsular hematoma

or multiple lacerations involving parenchyma only or may extend through the collecting system. 2) sub-capsular or perirenal hematoma may be found, which may or may not involve adjacent parenchyma. 3) laceration and/or transection of the collecting system at the ureteral pelvic junction is occasionally found. 4) vascular injury may be found, including complete avulsion of the renal artery and/or the vein or laceration of the artery and/or the vein. The following management is employed; parenchymal lacerations are sutured with 4-0 or 3-0 chromic gut suture. The suture may be a simple one tied down over a piece of fat to prevent tearing of the suture through the kidney capsule. The wound is closed with a penrose drain brought out retroperitoneally through a stab wound (Fig. 3). In patients with a sub-capsular hematoma, the hematoma is drained and the capsule is closed, hemostasis is achieved and a drain is placed retroperitoneally through a stab wound in the flank. With rupture into the collecting system a nephrostomy is performed in addition to retroperitoneal

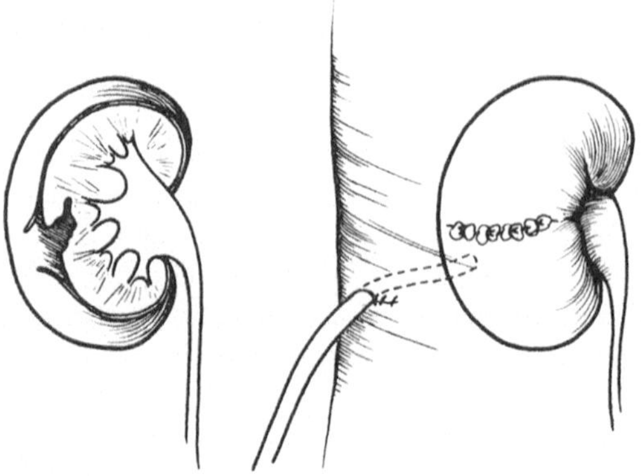

Fig. 3. Closure of parenchymal laceration; evacuation of hematoma and drainage of renal fossa

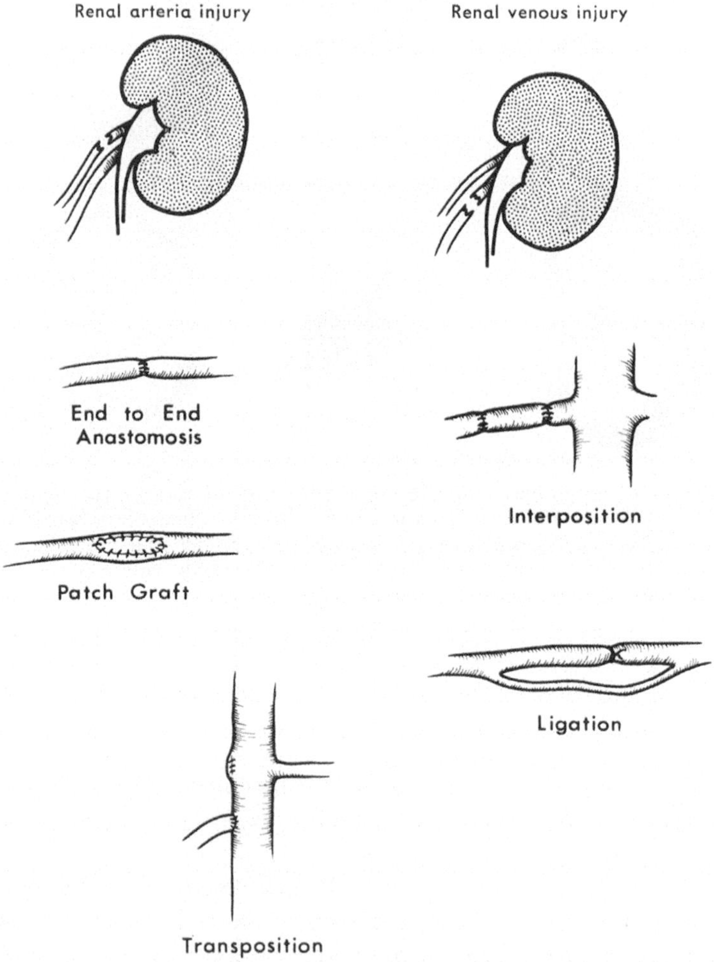

Fig. 4. Techniques of vascular repair in cases of renal arterial or renal venous injury. An everting suture closure of the vascular anastomotic site is performed

drainage. When there is transection of the ureteral pelvic junction one is faced with a difficult problem of management. Because of the possibility of the blast effect, limiting the operator's ability to determine the margin of viability of the tissue at the time of surgery, we prefer to excise obviously injured tissue and perform a dismembered pyeloplasty with splinting and nephrostomy drainage postoperatively. We follow the general principle of using absorbable suture in the kidney and particularly in the repair of the collecting system, because of the fear of stone formation on any suture material which comes in contact with the urine during the post-operative period. We use 4-0 or 5-0 chromic gut suture for plastic repair of the collecting system and 3-0 chromic gut suture for closure of parenchymal lacerations. Nephrectomy is performed only as an absolute necessity. Partial nephrectomy and heminephrectomy is preferred. A shattered kidney or one with an arterial transection of some duration does not lend itself to reconstruction. Nephrectomy has been necessary in 20 of our latest 182 cases of renal trauma. Arterial or venous lesions are usually

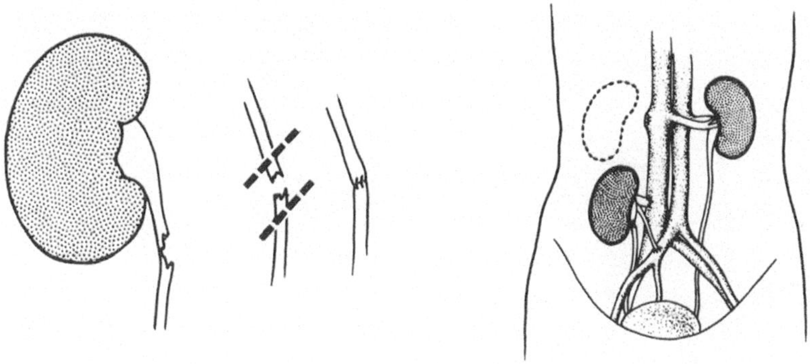

Fig. 5. Autotransplantation; a method of handling vascular or high ureteral injury

lacerations; occasionally complete transection is encountered. Debridement and end-to-end anastomosis is preferred when feasible for complete transections. If the arterial laceration extends for more than 1 cm, a patch graft is advantageous to prevent constriction and stenosis of the repaired vessel. Vena cava or saphenous vein may be used for patching (Fig. 4). If inter-position of a graft is necessary, hypogastric artery or saphenous vein can be used alternately. When using saphenous vein, one must make certain that the valves contained within the vessel are oriented in the proper direction of blood flow. Ovarian vein is too weak and post-operative rupture of this vessel has occurred when it was used for a patch graft [*9*]. Reimplantation into the aorta or autotransplantation may also be considered with extensive arterial injuries or high ureteral injuries (Fig. 5). Successful auto-transplantation of the kidney has been reported in a single case in the recent literature by Hardy [*3*]. For the arterial repair we prefer 5-0 or 6-0 silk or occasionally 5-0 or 6-0 dacron. When using polyester suture, one must be careful to tie four knots as the usual square knot may simply loosen and come untied when this type of synthetic material is used. When faced with the problem of a laceration of a renal vein one may simply tie off the vein if multiple veins are present as intra-renal venous anastomoses are known to be profuse. Arterial collateral anastomoses are rare within the kidney and ligation of a secondary renal artery and branch is apt to be followed by hypertension, particularly if more than 5% of the renal parenchyma is supplied by the vessel ligated. Partial nephrectomy should be combined with the arterial ligation. If a solitary renal vein is found to be injured one must apply the appropriate vascular technique. Main renal artery lesions can be repaired but, injuries to the secondary arterial branches are difficult to reconstruct and are best handled by the use of ligation and partial nephrectomy. It is during the repair of such lesions that cooling of the kidney is especially important to prevent or to minimize the degree of tubular necrosis from ischemia. Complications at surgery due to pre-existing disease in the kidney detected by the pre-operative IVP or angiogram, such as stone or ureteral pelvic junction obstruction are dealt with as they would be in the uninjured kidney providing the condition of the patient permits. At times simple drainage of the kidney in the deteriorating patient is all that can be accomplished and definitive surgery must be postponed. Necrotic polar fragments, either partially or completely avulsed are commonly found in the blunt trauma patients who require exploration.

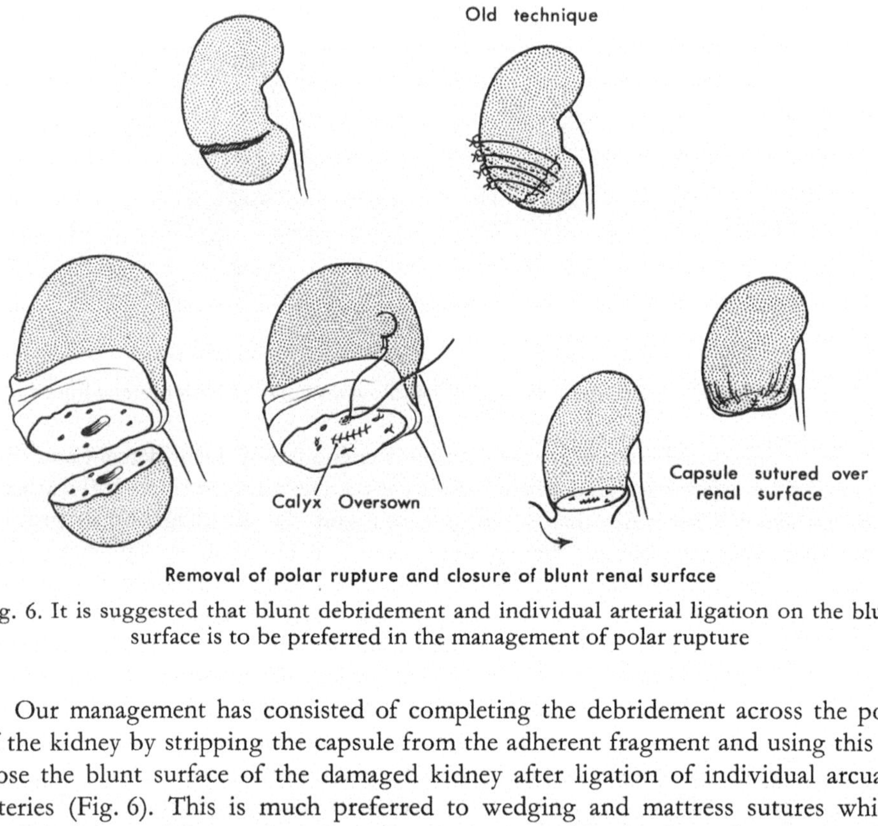

Fig. 6. It is suggested that blunt debridement and individual arterial ligation on the blunt surface is to be preferred in the management of polar rupture

Our management has consisted of completing the debridement across the pole of the kidney by stripping the capsule from the adherent fragment and using this to close the blunt surface of the damaged kidney after ligation of individual arcuate arteries (Fig. 6). This is much preferred to wedging and mattress sutures which result in increased destruction of renal parenchyma and further loss of nephron units. This compares strikingly with the usual complete healing seen to the margin of the wound in the kidney closed by individual arterial ligation and capsule covering as suggested by Murphy and Best in 1957 [5]. It has been suggested in the pre-pubertal child the kidney is particularly susceptible to trauma because of the scant amount of peri-renal fat. Ruptures of the collecting system with extravasation of the urine through the posterior peritoneum into the peritoneal cavity have been described in children and we have encountered two such cases in the past 2 years in our trauma experience. As a potential for growth exists in the child's kidney, every effort should be made to conserve even small portions of remaining parenchyma. One is quite satisfied to perform a partial nephrectomy in the child with the anticipation of further growth of the remaining kidney as the child matures. 18 to 25% of the total functioning renal mass, representing a glomerular filtration rate of 10 to 25 cc a minute, is necessaryf or preservation of satisfactory life in the human.

At closure then, one should have accomplished the following things: 1) hemostasis and evacuation of recently formed hematoma, 2) the necessary plastic reconstruction of the collecting system and vascular system, 3) closure of the source of the extravasation and provision for drainage from post-operative leakage from the collecting system, 4) provision for elimination of post-operative ureteral obstruction by nephropexy and placement of the ureter to avoid its contact with the lower pole of the kidney at the time of closure. This may be accomplished by nephropexy or interposition of fat between the ureter and the lower pole of the kidney. No effort is made to close the peritoneum lateral to the colon. It is simply allowed to fall back in place and the peritoneum will usually be well sealed off during the post-operative course of the patient. The wound is closed with absorbable suture except for the skin. A summary of our operative experience 1955 to 1967 follows:

Table 2. *Operative management of renal injuries*

Nephrectomy	20
Partial nephrectomy	8
Nephrostomy	10
Suture of laceration of parenchyma	31
Exploration of renal fossa	22
Repair of collecting system (pelvis)	2
Repair of vasculature	
Artery	1
Vein	2
Total procedures	96

Post-operative complications peculiar to the renal injury patient which should be borne in mind are: acute tubular necrosis, infarction with secondary renal vascular hypertension, continued extravasation of urine with post-operative sepsis and a complication common to all post-operative surgical patients that of severe post-operative hemorrhage. Only two patients in our series who did not have nephrectomy at the time of the original operation subsequently required a secondary nephrectomy because of hemorrhage.

Again, central venous pressure determination with monitoring of urine output remains a reliable guide to post-operative blood and fluid replacement. Of particular importance is periodic assessment of the blood pressure after the patient leaves the hospital. There were five cases of severe hypertension. One patient whose death was attributed to his renal injury appeared with malignant hypertension and irreversible damage to the opposite kidney 4 years following a traumatic injury to the vascular system of the right kidney. He had returned for only two follow-up visits. The second patient whose death was attributable to his renal injury had a needle biopsy of the kidney, then post-operative hemorrhage followed by a fibrin clot of the collecting system when given Amicar to stop the bleeding. This was followed by onset of uremia because the other kidney was too poor to sustain him and subsequently he died from uremia and gram negative septicemia. The low incidence of uremia is attributable to the prevention of post-operative renal failure and the good status of the opposite kidney in these young individuals.

Table 3. *Complications in operated patients*

Death:	
Related primarily to renal injury	2
Other (multiple injury, stroke, coronary occlusion post-operative)	9
Hypertension	5
Arteriovenous fistula	1
Hemorrhage requiring secondary nephrectomy	2
Uremia	2
Total	21

Summary

182 patients with major renal injury were seen from 1955 to 67 at Parkland Memorial Hospital. 98 of these patients suffered from penetrating renal injury and 84 of these patients suffered from non-penetrating injury. 80 patients had gunshot wounds of the kidney and 55 suffered renal injury in auto accidents. 96 operative procedures on the kidney were performed on traumatized patients during this period. 20 nephrectomies were done on patients in this group and 21 major complications were documented as the result of injuries received to the kidney. The ratio of nephrectomies to other operative procedures was unusually high because of the high incidence of gunshot wounds in this series. Surgical exploration is mandatory in patients with penetrating wounds. 96% of the patients in our series with blunt trauma did well without surgery. A 5 year follow-up is needed to monitor blood pressure changes following renal injury to prevent irreversible damage from secondarily developing renal vascular hypertension.

References

1. Cockett, A. T. K.: Surgery **50**, 905 (1961).
2. Hanley, H. G., A. M. Joekes, and J. E. A. Wickham: J. Urol. (Baltimore) **99**, 517—520 (1968).
3. Hardy, J. D., and S. Eraslan: J. Urol. (Baltimore) **90**, 563—572 (1963).
4. Kerr, W. K., V. N. Kyle, A. G. Keresteci, and C. A. Smythe: J. Urol. (Baltimore) **84**, 236—242 (1960).
5. Murphy, J. J., and R. Best: J. Urol. (Baltimore) **78**, 504—510 (1957).
6. Scott, R. Jr., C. E. Carlton, A. J. Ashmore, and H. H. Duke: J. Urol. (Baltimore) **90**, 535—540 (1963).
7. Semb, C.: Ann. roy. Coll. Surg. Engl. **19**, 137 (1956).
8. —, J. Krog, and K. Johansen: Acta chir. scand. Suppl. **253**, 196 (1960).
9. Straffon, R. L.: Personal verbal communication from the author. February, 1968.
10. Wickham, J. E. A.: J. Urol. (Baltimore) **99**, 246—267 (1968).

Results Following Conservative Surgery of Injuries to the Kidney

Lars Röhl

In case of transverse laceration of the kidney, with a large perirenal haematoma and possible tears of the renal pelvis, the choice of the method of treatment is extremely important. Because of the haemorrhage and the urinary extravasation, conservative therapy in these situations very often leads to early and late complications such as perinephritic abscess hydronephrosis, hypertension, kidney-stone formation, etc. In a large number of these cases further surgery — including nephrectomy — becomes necessary.

Radical surgery, in the form of an early nephrectomy, certainly is an alternative method of treatment to avoid complications and a prolonged hospital stay.

But this has the definite disadvantage of leaving the patient with a solitary kidney. This is especially of importance because, as our experience shows, children and young individuals frequently are subject to this type of kidney-injury.

Table 1. *Clinical material*
Kidney injuries
1. 11. 1962—1. 11. 1967

Total	93
Complete ruptures	19
Nephrectomy	4
1 Hydronephrosis	
1 Renal carcinoma	
1 Profuse bleeding	
1 Multiple ruptures	
Conservative surgery	15

In my opinion, conservative surgery should always be tried in large transverse lacerations of the kidney. We have therefore, in the Heidelberg urological department during the last 5 years, aimed at diagnosing these ruptures as early and as completely as possible and to operate on them without delay. Immediate renal angiography has been of invaluable help in giving us early information on the extent of the laceration. In cases where severe clinical symptoms are present, we give angiography priority over the excretory pyelogram, using the later exposures to show the contralateral kidney. We thank our radiologist, Dr. Wenz, for the skilled cooperation in this matter.

In the following, I would like to summarize the material and the results, as well as giving some comments on typical cases.

The total number of kidney-injuries that we saw during the 5-year period between November 1962 and November 1967 was 93. From these, 19 were diagnosed as complete ruptures and operated upon (Table 1).

Four patients had a nephrectomy: the first had a rupture into a large hydronephrotic kidney; the second had a ruptured renal carcinoma; the third patient had profuse bleeding 14 days after the injury. A large haematoma with urinary extravasation was found at operation. The fourth nephrectomy came to us 2 days after the injury. The upper half of the kidney was completely ruptured and the exposed kidney showed a large haematoma, urinary extravasation and a rupture extending in the main renal vein.

The last two cases illustrate the importance of immediate diagnosis and operation, if conservative surgery is to be of any use in these situations. We believe that a hemi-nephrectomy would have been possible in these cases, if the extensive urinary extravasation could have been avoided through immediate diagnosis.

In 15 of these 19 cases a conservative surgical treatment was possible.

Table 2 shows the different operative measures taken in these 15 cases. In 10 a reconstruction of the lacerated renal pelvis, combined with parenchymal suture was performed. Five patients had partial nephrectomy.

Table 2. *Operative measures*
Conservative surgery

15	
10	5
Reconstruction of the renal pelvis and parenchymal suture	Partial resection

Table 3. *Results*
(Observation time $4^{10}/_{12}$—$^{1}/_{2}$ *years)*

1. Hospital care	(16—21 days)
2. Mortality	0
3. Good kidney function	15
4. Hydronephrosis	0
5. Stone	0
6. Hypertension	0
7. Infection	0

The results are demonstrated in Table 3. The follow-up extends over a period of 4 years and 10 months to half a year. None of the patients were lost. The necessary hospital stay was limited to between 16 and 21 days.

All the "conservatively" treated kidneys showed good function at the time of follow-up.

We saw no post-operative complications, such as hydronephrosis, kidney-stone formation, infection or hypertension.

In the following some illustrative cases, grouped according to severity, were demonstrated including pre- and post-operative excretory pyelograms; pre-operative angiograms and slides of typical operative situations.

Case No. 1: A young man who had an injury to his left kidney while playing soccer. He had macrohaematuria and a tender left groin. Actually, he had a rupture through a renal cyst.

The selective renal angiogram confirmed this finding.

At the operation we saw bleeding into a cyst, the size of a hens egg. The cyst had a small peripheral rupture into a lateral calyx. After closure of the calyx the superficial wall was excised.

Case No. 2 (Fig. 1) illustrates the typical transverse laceration with a tear in the renal pelvis. This case was a 14-year old boy who received his kidney-laceration in a traffic accident. The angiogram showed the typical separation of the kidney margin because of the haematoma in the rupture.

Some technical details have to be underlined. First the perirenal haematoma is removed, leaving the coagulum in the rupture until the main renal artery is prepared and controlled by a sling. The coagulum in the rupture, acting as a plug, reduces the bleeding. Now the rest of the haematoma is removed, the bleeding being controled by traction on the sling. The laceration is then cleaned and inspected. Bleeding points are carefully sutured with stitches. The pelvic tear is closed with atraumatic 4-0 catgut, and the parenchymal edges are adapted with superficial single sutures.

Case No. 3 (Fig. 2) demonstrates a transverse rupture through the elongated connection between the renal pelvis and the upper calyces. Because of the good vascularisation of the upper pole, the renal pelvis was reconstructed and the kidney closed as in the previous case.

The pre-operative excretory pyelogram revealed extravasation of contrast by the right kidney. The X-ray control 6 months after the operation shows a good function in the reconstructed right kidney.

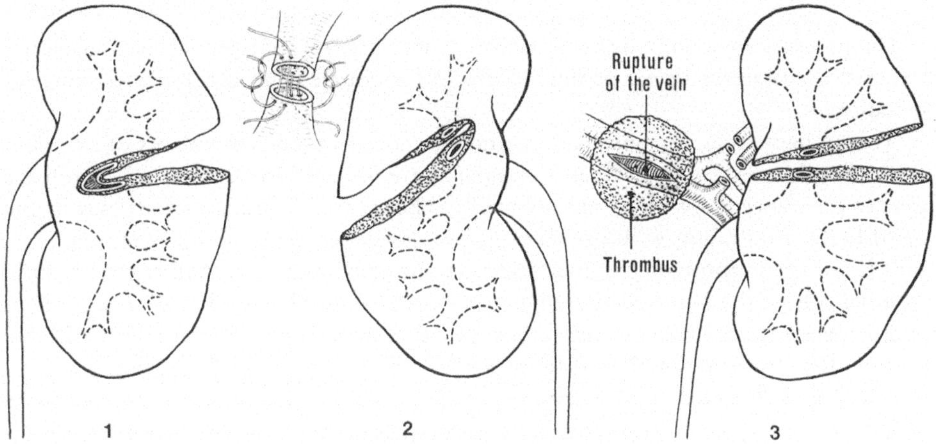

Fig. 1. Typical transverse laceration with a partial tear in the renal pelvis. (Case No. 2)

Fig. 2. Transverse laceration with a total tear of the upper calices. The repair of the renal pelvis schematically drawn. (Case No. 3)

Fig. 3. Complete transverse laceration including the vessels to the upper part of the kidney and a rupture of the main renal vein. (Case No. 4)

Among the five partial resections whe had two heminephrectomies.

The first patient had a complete transverse laceration with a complete tear of the vessels to the upper part of the kidney.

The second heminephrectomy was performed on a 9-year old boy, with the same type of laceration as the previous case but combined with a rupture of the main renal vein (Fig. 3). In the rupture of the vein we found a coagulating thrombus which blocked the vein completly as can be seen in the schematic drawing.

In the angiogram the upper part of the left kidney was not vascularised and the venous flow was actually retarded compared with the right kidney, which already preoperatively gave us a hint of a main renal vein lesion.

At operation the upper half of the kidney was removed. Under the coagulum the renal vein was ruptured. After the removal of the thrombus, the vein was flushed with heparin-saline and sutured.

Summarizing our results of 15 large transverse lacerations of the kidney, treated with conservative surgery, we are convinced that a conservative operation — and not nephrectomy — should always be tried in these situations. We have seen no complications and the hospital care has been short. In all our patients it was possible to conserve a good functioning kidney — or part of the kidney — which to us is especially important as children and young people are frequent victims of this type of kidney laceration.

Immediate diagnosis as to the extent of the laceration by renal vasography and operation without delay, are the most important prerequisites for successful conservative surgery in these cases.

The good old urological rule: A primary consideration should always be to conserve renal tissue, applies especially to large kidney ruptures.

Surgical Injuries to the Ureter

Russell B. Roth

Happiness is an uncomplicated recovery from Surgery. Unhappiness is discovering that one has injured a ureter or the bladder in the course of an otherwise satisfactory operation.

This unhappiness, for both patient and surgeon, has been the subject of excellent comprehensive textbooks such as "Trauma to the Ureter" by Orkin and "Urologic Injuries in Gynecology" by Falk as well as thousands of individual articles in the world literature dealing with prevention, causation, recognition and treatment.

It is not the purpose of this presentation to be encylopedic, but rather to stress the potential role of the Urologist in helping to avoid injuries to the genito-urinary tract, together with some observations on a type of ureteral injury which seems to have been omitted from the published reports which have been available for review.

Injury to the ureter is not a rare event as a complication of surgical procedures carried out on adjacent structures. The gynecologist works in the greatest peril on this score, but the abdominal surgeon, the vascular surgeon and the urologist also share the risk. Reliable incidence figures are lacking for obvious reasons. It is not really unusual for a urologist, in the course of studies for some unrelated problem, to find a functionless kidney with a totally occluded ureter, usually somewhere in its lower third, together with a history of prior pelvic surgery. In evaluating such evidence it is often most reasonable to conclude that the ureter had been inadvertently ligated, and the event had gone unrecognized.

Quite aside from the unrecognized cases it must be evident that such complications are more commonplace in the experience of less competent surgeons and those who only occasionally do this type of work. This is not to say that anyone is immune, regardless of skill or competence. It has been estimated by Orkin that even in well organized hospitals with reliable recording of such matters, ureteral injuries pursuant to gynecological surgery alone run from 1.5 to 3% of all cases, and that in radical pelvic surgery this may approximate 33%. Some of the very best studies of the problem come from the personal experiences of leading surgeons in the gynecological field. It is inevitable that incidence figures derived from such sources tend to understate the overall rate for the surgical world at large. Estimates of ureteral injuries pursuant to general abdominal surgery vary so widely as to be meaningless except to annotate the fact that they happen.

Very brief case reports to illustrate common variants of the problem are included, each for a specific purpose.

Case 1. A 33 year old women was referred to St. Vincent Hospital because of pain in the right costo-vertebral angle region. Urological study showed a right hydronephrosis due to ureteropelvic junction narrowing, and there was no discernible function of the left kidney by intravenous pyelography. Endoscopic study showed a normal left ureteral orifice and ureter for a distance of 7 cm. There was abrupt complete occlusion at this point. The patient gave a history of undergoing hysterectomy and bilateral salpingo-oophorectomy 3 years previously, with a most uncomfortable convalescence attributed to "gas pains".

Our treatment consisted of a right pyeloplasty in November 1953. She was last seen in March of 1968 because of troublesome hypertension which, in the past 5 years, has become refractory to medical management, and the question arises as to the desirability of removing the functionless kidney.

This case is included to stress that ureters may indeed be ligated and that the fact may not be recognized. He who would congratulate himself that he has never had such a case may be on insecure ground. This, of course, has been adequately documented many times before. NEWELL, for example, has reported six unsuspected examples discovered only at autopsy.

Case 2. This 48 year old women was first seen at St. Vincent Hospital in January 1955, 1.5 months after her return from a leading medical center in the eastern United States where she had undergone radical pelvic surgery for carcinoma of the uterus. Her convalescence had been very uncomfortable. Shortly after returning to her home she began to leak all of her urine vaginally.

Our studies showed ureterovaginal fistulae secondary to bilateral ureteral ligation. By great good fortune it was found possible to manipulate ureteral catheters past the area of disruption and to introduce them into the renal pelves. Prolonged drainage by this method permitted adequate healing. It is worthy of comment that at one point when the ureteral catheters were being replaced to advance to a larger size, a left bulb ureterogram was made which produced what may be a wholly unique X-ray, since the dye instilled into the left ureteral orifice not only produced a left ureteropyelogram, but went out the still patent fistula, crossed the pelvis and went up the right ureter to make a right ureteropyelogram as well.

This patient recovered and in 1960 developed a left renal calculus which became impacted in the ureter at the level of the prior damage and had to be removed by ureterolithotomy. At current writing she is alive and well, with no evidence of difficulty to be related either to her original carcinoma or her subsequent urological complications.

This case is included to illustrate the point that accomplished surgeons, professors of their specialty, and authorities in their field, are beset by the same complications as are others.

Case 3. This 66 year old woman had undergone a resection of a malignant lesion in the left colon at one of the great medical centers of the midwestern United States. After her return to her home she suddenly developed severe abdominal pain and distension. Studies at St. Vincent Hospital showed that there had been an unrecognized ligation of the left ureter leading to hydronephrosis and hydroureter with a sudden rupture of the ureter at the site of ligation, permitting all the urine to discharge into the peritoneal cavity. Left nephrectomy and drainage was carried out, with immediate good results, although the patient died 18 months later as a result of metastases from her original neoplasm.

This case is included to emphasize the point that abdominal surgeons as well as gynecologists need to be fully aware that they too may create problems pursuant to ureteral damage.

Case 4. This 59 year old male was studied at St. Vincent Hospital in 1965 because of right flank pain. He had had a left nephrectomy in 1942 and in 1958 had undergone extensive vascular surgery with the insertion of a prosthesis for the bifurcation of the aorta. Examination showed a huge right hydronephrosis with extreme narrowing of the ureter at a level 12 cm above the ureteral orifice and extending for approximately 5 cm above this. At surgical exploration the upper ureter was immensely dilated down to the point of involvement in a dense, almost cartilaginous scar embracing the whole area of prior vascular surgery. A cutaneous ureterostomy was established, which it has been necessary to maintain until the present time with a Silastic ureteral drainage tube because of total atony on the part of the renal pelvis and ureter.

This case illustrates a form of ureteral injury which has escaped general attention. We have previously seen one other patient who would seem to fall in this category because of the delayed development of right hydronephrosis as a result of periureteral fibrosis and constriction in the area of prior surgery for treatment of an abdominal aortic aneurysm.

Personal communications with vascular surgeons and urologists at two major centers for vascular surgery in the United States have dispelled the thought that this might be a common, although delayed complication. HUMPHRIES, despite his extensive experience in Cleveland, reports that he is unaware of such a complication and knows of no attention to this matter in the literature. SCOTT, who has been associated with the vast experience of DEBAKEY and his colleagues in Houston, reports only one comparable case which has come to his attention. He notes, however, that it is not uncommon to find hydronephrosis existing in conjunction with abdominal aortic aneurysm due to associated periureteral involvement in the inflammatory reaction. It has been his experience that this generally subsides without specific attention if the underlying aneurysmal problem is corrected.

It seems obvious that the prevention of ureteral injury is of greater practical significance than diagnosis or treatment, if, indeed, the incidence of such injuries may be effectively reduced. It is the major thesis of this presentation that the urologist may make a significant contribution on this score. There is nothing new in the idea that, prior to surgery in which there is any risk of ureteral injury, it is generally easy to carry out cystoscopy and ureteral catheterization of one or both sides as circumstances may dictate. The ureteral catheter may be left indwelling to facilitate for the surgeon the indentification of the ureter. It is equally well recognized that in patients with pelvic or lower abdominal disease it may be helpful to have preliminary excretory urography to show any possible ureteral involvement, obstruction or displacement. The least helpful attitude is that expressed by the surgeon who regards such precautionary assistance as somehow implying that he lacks the knowledge and ability to locate and handle a ureter properly. Once again no valid statistics are available, but it seems evident that prophylactic ureteral catheterization is not widely employed. This may be, in part, due to a sharing of the attitude expressed in summary fashion by ORKIN as follows: — "Pre-operative ureteral catheterization has been advised by some as a safeguard against ureteral injury but this procedure may have just the opposite effect. The decision as to preoperative ureteral catheterization is an individual one and should be determined by the skill of the surgeon, his experience, and the existing pelvic or abdominal pathology." FALK quotes many who have objected to the procedure, including the judgment of WHARTON that the use of catheters in the ureter has been relegated to the past and is useless and obsolete. The unfortunate fact, however, is that ureteral injuries are not obsolete, and a careful analysis of the objections to ureteral catheterization would seem to permit avoidance of the disadvantages.

Allegation 1. A ureteral catheter may not be palpable, and failure to feel the catheter may lead the surgeon to think that he can cut with safety. Here the comment is that a ureteral catheter for this purpose should be at least six French in caliber, and this is distinctly palpable in a normal thin walled ureter, or in any ureter save the grossly hypertrophied thick walled ureter of disease which should have been fully studied preoperatively.

Allegation 2. A catheter may bow or buckle causing displacement of the ureter, rendering it more susceptible to injury. Here we would comment that ureteral injuries of the type under consideration are virtually always in the lower third of the ureter in gynecological cases, and rarely above the middle third in other surgery. There is no need to advance the catheter all the way to the renal pelvis where it may come to a dead end and bend if it is introduced further. A catheter should generally not be passed more than 15 to 17 cm up the adult ureter.

Allegation 3. The insertion of a ureteral catheter may be the initiating factor in urinary tract infection. To counter this it is clear that no competent urologist would pass a catheter through an infected bladder into a non-infected ureter. Given evidence of existing urinary tract infection the procedure would be regarded as inapplicable and advice would be offered in respect to treating the infection. In addition it is our practice to irrigate the catheter which has been inserted by flushing it with a 2.5% solution of Neomycin Sulfate, to ensure patency as well as to add a modicum of protection against contamination.

Allegation 4. The truly competent surgeon has the knowledge and skill to identify the ureter properly and treat it with kindness. This, unhappily, is self delusion. Pathological processes, especially neoplasia and infection, may so alter normal landmarks and tissue consistencies as to make identification of the ureter a time consuming matter, if not downright impossible. Here the presence of a catheter may not insure identification but it will facilitate recognition of injury if damage is done. It should be noted that an indwelling ureteral catheter makes it very easy for the surgeon to check on any possible incision into, or transection of the ureter. Quite aside from the physical presence of the catheter in the ureter one may inject a highly colored solution in the catheter, such as Indigo Carmine or Methylene Blue. In the event of any break in the integrity of the ureter the dye will promptly appear in the operative field, clearly indicating the site of damage.

It must be admitted that there are occasions on which it is found to be technically impossible to insert indwelling ureteral catheters pre-operatively. The procedure is no more universally applicable, than it is a universal protection against inexperience, incompetence, or quirks of fate. Where it has been used within reasonable limitations and with proper techniques it has been generally good. SISK has reported that during a period in which preoperative ureteral catheterization was routinely employed at Wisconsin General Hospital in "difficult" pelvic surgical cases only one ureteral injury occurred, and in this single instance catheters had not been inserted. Because one cannot always identify the difficult case in advance he advocated routine use of catheters in all cases. To this we subscribe. In no case in which we have preoperatively inserted catheters for our surgical and gynecological colleagues has there been a ureteral injury. In no case has there been a known complication arising from the catheterization.

It is beyond the scope of this paper to consider the medicolegal implications of ureteral injury, but they cannot be ignored, especially in the United States. We would simply comment that the surgeon who has arranged for prophylactic pre-operative ureteral catheterization, but who still has the misfortune to inflict injury to a ureter, has a strong case in his favor for having anticipated the hazards, and for taking all prudent precautionary steps. Technical skill and painstaking procedure are not guarantees against the possibility of ureteral injury. The presence of an indwelling ureteral catheter during surgery is likewise no guarantee of safety. Taken together, the competent surgeon aided by the presence of a ureteral catheter, would seem to have increased opportunity to avoid injury or to recognize it if it occurs.

References

Falk, H. C.: Urologic injuries in gynecology. Philadelphia: F. A. Davis 1964.
Humphries, A. V.: Personal communication.
Newell, Q. U.: Ann. Surg. **109**, 981 (1939).
Orkin, L. A.: Trauma to the ureter. Philadelphia: F. A. Davis 1964.
Scott, R., Jr.: Personal communication.
Sisk, I.: Surg. Gynec. Obstet. **60**, 857 (1935).
Wharton, L. R.: Gynecology. Philadelphia: Saunders 1943.

Renal Stones

Etiology of Renal Calculi

W. J. Brosig

Although urolithiasis has been recognized since antiquity, the etiology of renal calculi is still unexplained in most cases. Patients with certain specific causes, such as hyperparathyroidism, uric acid calculi, cystinuria represent only a small percentage of the total number of "stone formers" (Table 1).

In idiopathic stone disease, the immediate pathophysiological and pathochemical process of urinary stone formation takes place in the kidney and is called "formal genesis" (primary mechanism of stone formation). At present there are two chief hypotheses which are advanced to explain "formal genesis":

1. the hypothesis of primary crystallization;
2. the hypothesis of matrix.

Table 1. *Diseases with hypercalciuria and stone formation*

1. Hyperparathyreoidism.
2. Osteoporosis due to old age, castration, immobilization, Cushing's disease, cortisone therapy, weightlessness.
3. Osteolytic bone diseases.
4. Paget's disease.
5. Sarcoidosis.
6. Vitamin D intoxication.
7. Increased calcium input.
8. Nephropathies
   a) glomerulo-tubular type with secondary hyperparathyroidism,
   b) tubular type (renal acidosis).

Most urinary calculi contain crystalline elements which are "glued" together by a fibrillar organic matrix (2 to 5% of the whole amount of the stone) (Table 2).

According to the hypothesis of crystallization, the formation of a stone is initiated by precipitation of urinary salts, which are fixed together by the protein colloids in the urine. In this case, as also in the matrix hypothesis the concept of urine as a "supersaturated" salt solution is important.

The calciumexcretion in stone formers is often increased (above 300 mg/day). 24% of patients with recurrent stones have a hypercalciuria. With the exception of patients who have oxalosis (600 mg/day) the excretion of oxalate in patients with oxalate calculi is almost normal (10 to 50 mg/day). Phosphate excretion is not increased in patients with phosphate stones (0.5 to 3.0 g/day). The excretion of magnesium is normal (100 mg/day) in patients who have triple phosphate stones. Patients who have gout, lymphoma, leukemia and similar diseases may have an increased uric acid excretion, but most patients who form uric acid stones excrete a normal amount of uric acid in the urine (700 mg/day). By contrast patients with cystin stones do have remarkably elevated cystinuria (300 mg/day and more, 50 mg is normal) [*9*].

Normal urine contains concentrations of calcium phosphate and oxalate which are much higher than their solubility in water. It is not possible to compare solubilitis of salts in water with those in urine by the normal rules of physical chemistry. The following special factors must be taken into account:

1. Ionic concentration.
2. Presence of chelating agents.
3. Solubilizers and inhibitors.
4. pH.

MEYER (1929) showed that urine is a stable solution of salts which cannot be compared with water. This stability is due to reciprocal action of the different salts. The total *concentration of all ions* is important; for when the concentration is increased, the activity of a single ion is less than its specific activity in water [1]. *Chelating agents* fix ions strongly.

Table 2. *The most frequent urinary stones*

I. *Inorganic stones*		
Ca — oxalate (40%)	Whewellit	$Ca(COO)_2\ H_2O$
	Weddellit	$Ca(COO)_2\ 2H_2O$
Ca — phosphate (30%)	Hydroxylapatit	$Ca_{10}(PO_4)_6(OH)_2$
	Brushit	$CaH\ PO_4\ 2H_2O$
	Whitlockit	$Ca_3(PO_4)_2$
Triplephosphate (20%)	Struvit	$MgNH\text{-}PO_4\ 6H_2O$
II. *Organic stones*		
Uric acid (5 to 10%)		
Ammoniumurate		
Cystine		

The citrate ion is a good example of a *solubilizers*. It forms soluble compounds with calcium and thus binds the calcium so that the concentration of "free" calcium ions is decreased. Only the "free" ions are important in stone formation.

Not all stone forming patients are hypercalciuric [2, 3]. Following poliomyelitis some patients produce stones *after* the urinary calcium excretion has reached its peak [4].

Patients with advanced renal stone disease may actually show a decreased calcium excretion because of renal damage due to obstruction and infection [5].

Besides citrate, which can dissolve hydroxylapatit [6], other good *solubilizers* (mediators for dissolution) are magnesium, sodiumchlorid, urea etc.

Hydrogen ion concentration (pH) plays an important role in the solubility of the different salts. For example uric acid calculi, which form in acid urine, can be prevented by alkalization of the urine. Calcium phosphate and triple phosphate are more soluble in an acid than in an alkaline medium [1, 7].

If urine is strongly alkaline, calcium and magnesium phosphate precipitate earlier. Alkalization occurs in paralyzed and immobilized patients and is strongest in urinary infections due to urea splitting bacilli.

The solubility of calcium oxalate is only slightly dependent on pH [7].

The above mentioned factors help to explain the solubility of stone forming salts; however it is questionable whether urine is really supersaturated with calcium oxalate [8]. The saturation of calcium phosphate depends on the pH. FLEISCH believes that not all urine is supersaturated, but he thinks that there is a possibility of calcium oxalate and phosphate supersaturation, because of the connection between urolithiasis and hypercalciuria [*9*].

Urinary oxalate excretion is only slightly increased in the urine of stone formers. However the increased urinary oxalate in normal persons after oxalate ingestion does not cause large oxalate stones even though numerous microcalculi are found [*11*]. The same is true of phosphatic calculi and for calcium and uric calculi [*12, 13*].

Urinary calcium in patients with oxalate and oxalatephosphate calculi is not elevated in comparison to those who form pure phosphate stones [*14*].

Since calcium is bound in the urine by chelating agents, some investigators agree that the urine is undersaturated [*15*]. Boyce et al. manufactured a synthetic ultrafiltrate of urine, which was able to maintain 300 mg of calcium in solution per liter [*16*].

Despite that, Fleisch assumes that there is more calcium phosphate, oxalate and uric acid in the urine than their individual solubilities in pure water. By adding a single crystall of a solid salt to a supersaturated solution one can induce crystallization (nucleation). Fleisch believes that nucleation can only be induced by substances of a certain structure, mostly salts of the corresponding solution. He does not believe that bacteria or epithelial cells can act as a nucleus.

This could also explain formation of stones caused by Randall's plaques. These tiny calcifications on the tips of the papillae could act as a nucleus and thus induce the crystallization of the salts in the urine [*18*]. One should also mention Carr's hypothesis [*19*]. He believes (on the basis of roentgenographic studies of many specimens of kidney tissue) that microcalculi are to be found in the lymphatics of almost every kidney. He thinks that if the renal lymphatics are normal, most of these small calculi are removed by the continues flow of lymph. However, if there is any obstruction (for instance, due to inflammation) the microcalculi in the lymphatics of the renal fornix are able to cause nucleation.

There are also ultrafilterable substances in the urine which may act as inhibitors for the crystallization of calcium phosphate [*14*]. These are not found in normal amounts in the urine of stone patients [*20*]. Fleisch isolated such a substance, a pyrophosphate normally excreted in the urine in the amount of 2 mg/day. In the urine of stone formers, the excretion of pyrophosphate is only half or normal [*17*].

In the *matrix hypothesis* crystallization is secondary. After demineralization, the matrix is found in all urinary stones and usually retains the form and size of the original stone after demineralization [*21*]. Morphologically it consists of concentric fibers and of an amorphic interfibrillary material. The structure is similar to bone and other mineralized tissues. Chemically, the matrix of most renal calculi consists mainly of mucoproteins (uromucoids), which are formed of proteins and polysaccharides. The composition of amino acids and sugars appears to be similar to all inorganic stones. Only the matrix of uric acid calculi has a different composition [*22, 23*]. This suggests a different mechanism of stone formation in these calculi (crystallization).

After feeding rats with oxamide, sulphathiazol, calcium carbonate and calcium oxalate Koch et al. observed the appearance of "colloid bodies" in the urine [*24*]. These clotted in a radial manner, probably a sign of crystallization (spheroliths). By growing in concentric layers, they enlarged to microliths. Because the rapid increase in excretion of these colloid bodies in the urine approached crisis proportions, this situation is called "a stone forming crisis".

Colloid bodies, spheroliths and microliths are also found in human urine. However colloid bodies occur in human urine in several different disturbances and are not limited to calculous formation alone. It is believed that colloid bodies are a compound of proteins and mucopolysaccharides which may be of great importance in connection with the work of

BOYCE, DULCE etc. on the matrix [*21*, *22*]. The hypothesis can only be proved by verification that the colloid bodies are chemically identical with the matrix. In the past 15 years no one has attacked this problem, and the hypothesis remains neither proved nor disproved [*25*].

The excretion of mucoproteins is increased in the urine of patients who have stone disease [*26*]. BOYCE discovered crystallization on the fibrillar matrix of stones, which is similar to mineralization of the bone. He believes that the matrix acts as a nucleus. The mucoprotein matrix in a stone consists only partially of urinary colloids, it does not contain uro acid polysaccharide, however neutral mucopolysaccharides and proteins are found (DULCE, BOYCE). Some believe that the laying down of calcium and phosphorus during stone formation is similar to the mineralization which takes place during bone formation. The similarity between apatit crystals and collagen of the bone [*27*, *28*] leads one to think of a nucleus forming action of the collagen in precipitation of apatit. In order to work as a crystallization center, the collagen has to have a special structure. It is very probable, that the mechanism of mineralization in stone disease is similar to that which occurs in other calcified tissues elsewhere in the body (FLEISCH).

Damage to renal tubules may be the initial cause in stone formation. This observation is most convincing in the condition of hyperparathyreoidism. Hypercalcemia is noxious to the epithelial cells of the renal tubules. By contrast hypercalciuria alone is harmless, as it can be tolerated for a lifetime without ill effects [*29*]. Stone formation is found in patients with renal tubular damage, whereas patients with glomerulonephritis never form calculi. Kidney stones develop in 3 out of 4 patients who have renal tubular acidosis.

After a synthesis of all known experiments and experiences one could imagine that the formation of kidney stones probably occurs somewhat as follow (BOSHAMER, BOYCE, DULCE, FLEISCH, KOCH et al.):

A fibrillar, mucoproteid matrix appears in the urine. It is somehow able to trigger the beginning of crystallization in an unstable solution. This instability of the urine may be caused by an increased excretion of calcium phosphate, oxalate, cystine etc. or by changes of the pH or a decreased excretion of crystalloid solubilizers. The fibrillar matrix, which in the beginning is transparent, is a product of the tubules. It is regarded as a pathological crystallization center, which can induce stone formation only in conjunction with supersaturation and instability of urine. Probably not only one but several factors work together to initiate the process. It also seems clear that some primary stones are formed in the kidney parenchyma rather than in the kidney pelvis (SHIGEMATSU [*30*], KOCH, RANDALL, CARR).

References

1. ELLIOT, J. S., R. F. SHARP, and L. LEWIS: J. Urol. (Baltimore) **81**, 366 (1959).
2. LATHEM, J. E., and J. S. KING JR.: J. Urol. (Baltimore) **89**, 541 (1963).
3. VERMEULEN, C. W., G. H. MILLER, and W. H. CHAPMAN: J. Urol. (Baltimore) **75**, 592 (1956).
4. ELLIOT, J. S., and H. E. TODD: J. Urol. (Baltimore) **86**, 484 (1961).
5. CONWAY, N. S., A. I. L. MAITLAND, and J. B. RENNIE: Brit. J. Urol. **21**, 30 (1949).
6. NEUMAN, W. F., and M. W. NEUMAN: The chemical dynamics of bone mineral. The University of Chicago-Press (Ill.) 1958.
7. PRIEN, E. L.: J. Urol. (Baltimore) **73**, 627 (1955).
8. MILLER, G. H., C. W. VERMEULEN, and J. D. MOORE: J. Urol. (Baltimore) **79**, 667 (1958).
9. FLEISCH, H., u. S. BISAZ: Z. Urol. **59**, 785 (1966).
10. MUGLER, A.: Rein Foie **4**, II/179 (1962).
11. SENGBUSCH, R. v., u. A. TIMMERMANN: Urol. int. (Basel) **5**, 218 (1957).

12. Boyce, W. H., and J. S. King Jr.: Fed. Proc. **18**, 1102 (1929).
13. Atsmon, A., A. De Vries, and M. Frank: Uric acid lithiasis. New York: American Elsevier Publishing Comp. 1963.
14. Pyrah, L. N.: Proc. roy. Soc. Med. **51**, 183 (1958).
15. Raaflaub, J.: Helv. med. Acta **30**, 724 (1963).
16. Boyce, W. H., F. K. Garvey, and C. M. Norfleet: Exp. Med. Surg. **12**, 450 (1954).
17. Fleisch, H.: Schweiz. med. Wschr. **92**, 1197 (1962).
18. Randall, A.: New Engl. J. Med. **214**, 234 (1936).
19. Carr, J. R.: Brit. J. Urol. **26**, 105 (1954).
20. Thomas, W. C., and J. E. Howard: Zit. nach Fleisch [*17*].
21. Boyce, W. H., and J. S. King Jr.: J. Urol. (Baltimore) **81**, 351 (1959).
— — Ann. N. Y. Acad. Sci. **104**, 563 (1963).
22. Dulce, H. J.: Urol. int. (Basel) **7**, 137 (1958).
23. King, J. S., and W. H. Boyce: Proc. Soc. exp. Biol. (N.Y.) **95**, 183 (1957).
24. Koch, F. E.: Z. Urol. Sonderheft **1**, 110 (1950).
—, u. H. Haase: Die Genese der Harnsteinbildung in den Harnwegen nach den neuesten Forschungsergebnissen. Wildunger-Hefte, H. 2, 1953. Weitere Literatur bei K. Boshamer, Handbuch der Urologie X, S. 1ff. Berlin-Göttingen-Heidelberg: Springer 1961.
25. Uebel, H.: Pers. Mittlg.
26. Boyce, W. H., and M. Swanson: J. clin. Invest. **34**, 1581 (1955).
27. Glimcher, M. J.: Calcification in biological systems. The American Ass. for the advancement for Science 1960.
28. Howard, J. E.: J. Urol. (Baltimore) **72**, 999 (1954).
29. King, J. S., Jr.: J. Urol. (Baltimore) **97**, 583 (1967).
30. Shigematsu, S. H.: Elektronenmikroskopische Betrachtungen über die Entstehung der Nierensteine. Z. Urol., Sonderbd., Verh. dtsch. Ges. Urol. S. 269, Wien 1957. Leipzig: Georg Thieme 1958.

Diagnosis of Renal Calculus

Peter L. Scardino

The diagnosis of renal lithiasis depends on a correct interpretation of the results of several inter-related disciplines including urology, roentgenology and biochemistry. If medical orthodoxy and routine laboratory procedures are coupled with the sophisticated interpretation, a correct diagnosis is promptly achieved.

The elicitation of relative factual data, a search for physical clues, and urine studies should be coupled with a meaningful interpretation of accumulated laboratory data, roentgenography, and special studies.

Gout, hyperuricemia and hyperuricuria, excessive use of vitamin D, osteolytic bone disease, leukemia and the immobolized patient require investigations for the presence of possible calculus disease. 20% of stone-formers have a positive genetic reference. Cystine stone disease is not necessarily familial. Cortisone, antihypertensive drugs and carbonic an hydrase inhibiting diuretics may influence the development of renal calculus disease. A florid complexion with moon-face, Buffalo hump and abdominal striae may indicate the presence of Cushing's syndrome in which renal calculi are frequently found. The arthritic who takes steroids may have a Cushinoid appearance and renal calculi. Intrinsic renal disease of the hypertensive, whether vascular or infectious should move the examiner to the need for diagnostic efforts beamed at renal calculus disease. Band keratopathy is an occular lesion that can be seen in 4 of 5 hypercalcemics by an astute physical examiner (Walsh and Howard).

A superficial, hazy, granular, crescent-shaped opacity limited to the paralimbal region on the nasal and temporal sides of the cornea is visible to the untrained eye as is the clear area between the arc of calcification and the corneal-scleral juncture. Not as typical but often seen with band keratopathy is the chalky, dullwhite discrete, grossly visible calcium deposits on the everted eyelid of the hypercalcemic.

Gastrointestinal symptoms are commonplace complaints of the patient with renal calculi. Nausea, vomiting, abdominal distention are second only to urinary symptoms in their frequency of association. The differential diagnosis may be difficult. The flank pain of herpes zoster prior to the development of the herpetic rash is especially trying in the presence of hematuria. More than one intervertebral disc has been removed to cure the pain of relatively silent renal calculi.

Urinalysis is performed by the physician. A urine of pH 5.5 or less may permit the formation of the double-wedged crystals of uric acid clumped in a brick-red rosette battleship formation. The Maltese Cross oxalate crystals as well as the large hexagonal thick plates of cystine are also found in acid urines. In a urine of pH 6.8 to 7.4 following severe vomiting, systemic alkalosis may cause minute calculi to form in the collecting and distal convoluted tubules and may be seen on the roentgenographic study. These concretions however are not to be confused with those seen in the congenitally dilated tubules of the sponge kidney (PYRAH) or the nephrocalcinosis of systemic acidosis. The tubular defect of renal tubular acidosis precludes acidification in one-third of patients with nephrocalcinosis. Concretions that form have a pyramidal distribution in the collecting tubules. Parenchymal nephrocalcinosis is usually bilateral. By etiology and crystalline composition the disease is classified with calcium-phosphate, calcium-oxalate calculi. The crystalline components are usually basic calcium phosphate as hydroxy apatite which after entering the larger drainage ducts acquire additional layers of calcium oxalate. One-fifth of the patients who have nephrocalcinosis have primary hyperparathyroidism and an equal number renal tubular dilatation. The remainder have various disorders which predispose to calcigerous renal calculi (BOYCE).

Excessive urinary excretion of calcium is reflected in the Sulkowitch test using as reagents oxalic acid and ammonium oxalate. In hypercalciuria a precipitate of proportionate density appears. Hypercalciuria is particularly meaningful in a patient with hypercalcemia and hypophosphatemia since the triad is diagnostically significant for hyperparathyroidism.

Hypercalciuria associated with sterile oxalate stone formation commonly appears in the presence of normal urinary volumes. Approximately one-half of these patients respond promptly to oral restriction of calcium. Hypercalciuria in excess of 225 mg per 24 h on an oral intake of 1000 mg of calcium per day requires metabolic ward evaluation. Hypercalciuria in volumes of urine as great as 3000 ml per 24 h is characteristic of hyperparathyroidism. Thirst results from restriction of calcium and fluid intake but little change occurs in urinary calcium excretion. A delay of 24 to 72 h is seen before significant reduction in urinary volume appears.

Less than 100 mg urinary calcium excretion per day is seen in serious renal diseases before there is a significant elevation of blood urea concentration. The reduction in calcium excretion accompanies failing glomerular filtration. Poorly crystalized matrix calculi commonly occur in the presence of urinary calcium excretion of less than 50 mg per 24 h. Urinary tract infection associated with diabetes mellitus in a patient with a non-functioning kidney demonstrated by intravenous pyelography without evidence of opaque calculus can mean the presence of a matrix calculus as the cause of obstruction (Fig. 1). The concretions are composed largely of muco-protein matrix and crystals of hydroxy apatite and magnesium ammonium phosphate. Removal of this non-opaque structure usually permits prompt renal recovery.

All calculi except pure uric acid and matrix concretions are radiopaque including of course those tiny minute calcium stones which do not visualize. An X-ray which

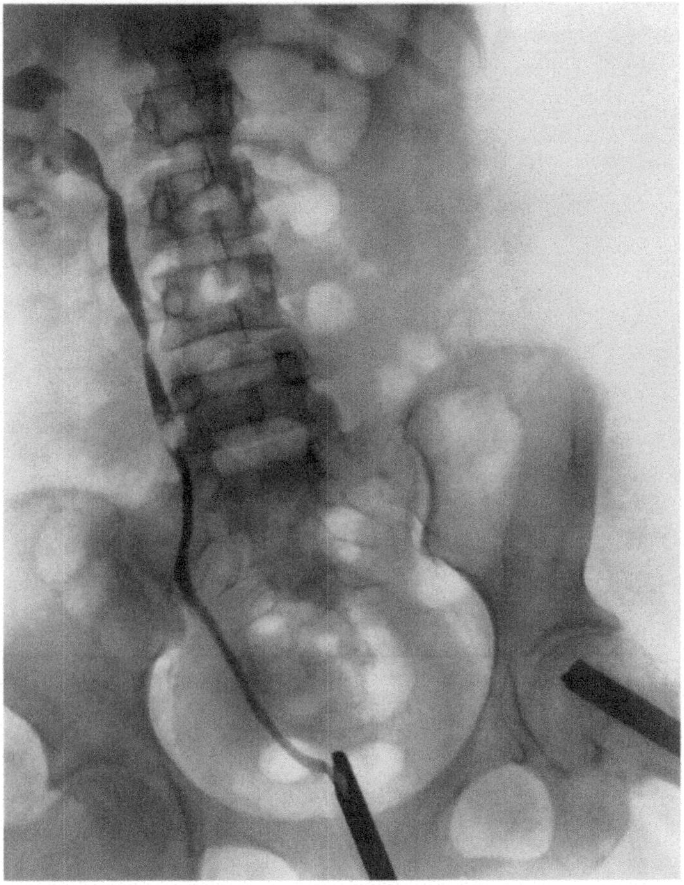

Fig. 1. Matrix calculus. Right retrograde pyelogram of a patient with diabetes mellitus, a non-functioning kidney whose obstruction was secondary to a non-opaque matrix calculus of the renal pelvis

includes the kidney, ureter and bladder followed by excretory urography as soon as the presence of a renal calculus has been suspected will often lead to a prompt diagnosis if the X-rays are obtained under the supervision of a physician. Spot films of the kidneys or points of suspected obstruction, films obtained in various positions such as oblique and lateral or the use of delayed or post-voiding films, cystograms or retrograde pyelograms with contrast media or air contrast are the various techniques that may be required to fill diagnostic demands. The non-opaque and the uric acid calculus with partial or total obstruction can be demonstrated by retrograde air pyelography.

Confusion of roentgenographic interpretation may result from the presence of opacities such as mercury that has escaped a nasogastric bag, retained barium of a gastrointestinal X-ray series or barium enema, gall stones, calcified lymph nodes or foreign bodies.

The staghorn or branched calculus is commonly found among white multiparous lower middle-class residents of the Southeastern United States (Fig. 2). Secondary

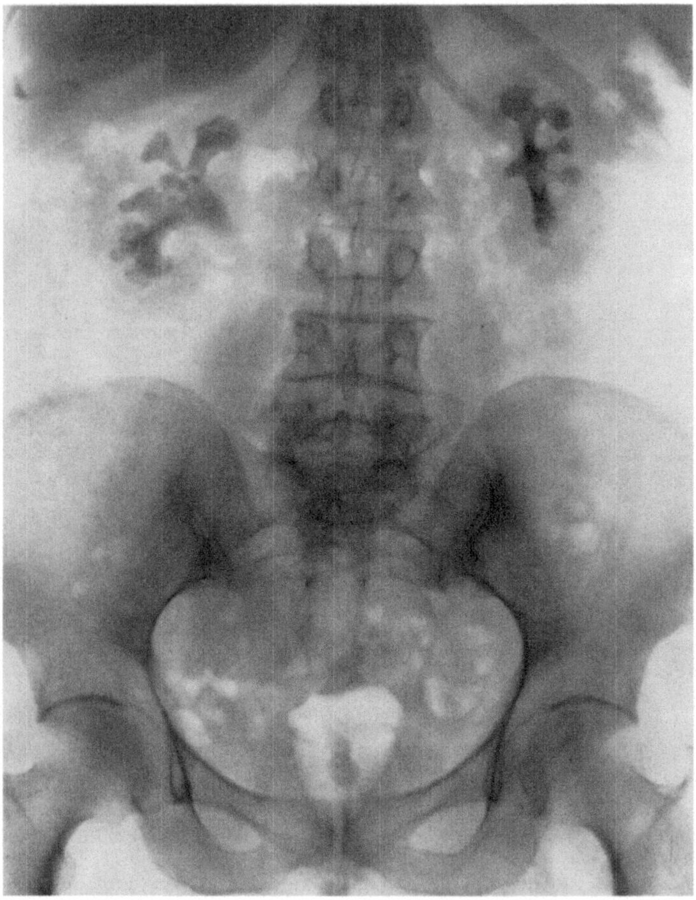

Fig. 2. Staghorn renal calculi, bilateral. Plain X-ray of the kidney, ureter and bladder of a 26-year-old multipara with bilateral branched (staghorn) calculi of magnesium, ammonium phosphate group associated with proteus urinary tract infection

to non-tuberculous pyelonephritis the disease occurs less often in the Negro female, but in a ratio to her male companion paralleling that of the white male and female, a ratio of 5 to 1 (Scardino, et al.). In pregnancy bacteriuria may be present many months before symptoms of pyelonephritis occurs. The incidence of clinical pyelonephritis in asymptomatic bacteriuric women is about 40% (Kass). Almost all patients are infected with proteus sp. Proteus urease (Enzyme) is one of the important agents responsible for the pathogenicity of proteus organisms in the kidney. The enzyme is nephrotoxic and participates in the pathogenesis of pyelonephritis in 2 ways: (1) Proteus becomes intracellular and protected against certain antimicrobial agents and, (2) by creating alkalinity (pH 8.2) in the kidney that leads to necrosis of renal tubular epithelium and to precipitation of magnesium ammonium phosphate with formation of stones on the 'microburns' of the papillae (BRAUDE et al.).

Most female patients with unilateral or bilateral branched staghorn calculi of the magnesium ammonium phosphate group should have nephrolithotomy following complete diagnostic studies. Urine culture, colony counts, sensitivity test, renal scan (Fig. 3), infusion intravenous pyelogram and radio isotope renograms are particularly useful in determining without instrumentation which of two kidneys is a candidate

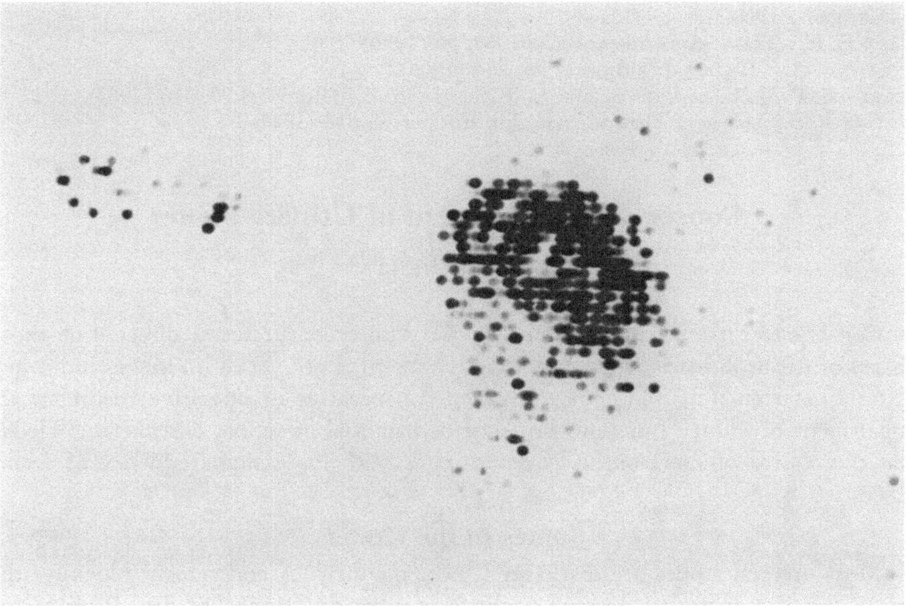

Fig. 3. Renal scan. The same patient seen in Fig. 2. Right renal function reasonably satisfactory. Value of scan: Left nephrectomy necessary

for initial surgery. The solitary kidney with branched or staghorn calculus demands exhaustive diagnostic studies as well as available dialysis techniques for use if necessary in the immediate postoperative period. Diagnosis extends to studies at the operative table and should include organography so that no renal calculi remain following surgery.

Cystine stones are usually seen on preliminary X-rays when more than 300 mg of cystine are excreted in the daily urine. The cystine stone is radiopaque due to its high concentration of sulfur. Milk of calcium stone in a calyceal diverticulum is an X-ray curiosity but one which reflects the presence of innumerable spherules of hydroxy apatite with laminated matrix in a calyceal sac. The apparent fluid-nature of the stones prompts the term "milk of calcium". Correct diagnosis can only be achieved by performing appropriate X-rays in the supine, upright and lateral positions.

Conclusion

The diagnosis of renal calculi is primarily dependent on the examining physician's awareness of the possible presence of stones when presented with certain historical data and physical findings. If the suspected calculus patient is X-rayed, more than an 80% correct diagnosis will be achieved. The presence of crystalluria, bacteriuria, hematuria or pyuria justify urological studies in depth. Specialized roentgenographic and sophisticated biochemical and isotope studies are suggested.

References

Boyce, W. H.: Diagnosis of renal calculi. J. F. Glenn, Ed., Hoeber medical division. New York: Harper and Row 1964.

Braude, A. I., J. Siemienski, and A. B. Shapiro: The role of bacterial urease in the pathogenesis of pyelonephritis, Quinn, E. L., and E. H. Kass, Ed. Boston: Little Brown and Company 1960.

Kass, E. H.: Trans. Ass. Amer. Phycns. **69**, 56 (1956).

Pyrah, L. M.: J. Urol. (Baltimore) **95**, 284 (1966).

Scardino, P. L., C. L. Prince, and C. T. Su: J. Urol. (Baltimore) **90**, 516 (1963).

Walsh, F. B., and J. E. Howard: J. clin. Endocr. **7**, 644 (1947).

Conservative Treatment of Urinary Stones

H. Klosterhalfen

Conservative treatment of calculi in the kidney or ureter is directed at those phases of nephrolithiasis when operative treatment is not yet or no longer indicated. Criteria determinating the choice between conservative or operative treatment are impairment of kidney function, presence of bacterial infection, and the knowledge that the course of nephrolithiasis deteriorates with increasing frequency of recurrences.

Stones in the Ureter

Most ureteral stones are discharged spontaneously. A concrement blocking the ureter completely during passage produces a colic due to abrupt distension of the proximal urinary tract. The colic is best treated by intravenous injection of a spasmolytic or analgetic drug. Morphine should be avoided. Though analgetic, it has no spasmolytic action. It aggravates nausea and vomiting and intensifies impairment of peristalsis. Spasmolytic drugs have the added advantage of inducing the second phase of treatment, i.e. discharge of the stone. Passage of a concrement depends on spasmolysis and in addition on stimulation of peristalsis of the urinary tract. The latter is best achieved by liberal fluid intake, the type of liquid being relatively unimportant. The patient should move about, bed rest is contraindicated.

Treatment with glycerin, still widely used in Europe, is absolutely ineffective. It relies on the hypothesis that orally administered glycerin is secreted with the urine in considerable quantity and has a lubricating effect. We were able to show that a dosage of 150 to 200 gm produces a urinary concentration of 5% only. This amount includes the danger of liver and kidney damage and has no lithagogue effect whatsoever.

In the absence of urinary tract obstruction or infection a conservative attitude is not wrong at least. The urologist finds himself in the role of an obstetrician whose golden rule should be patience. In most cases stones will eventually be discharged spontaneously.

Treatment by Instruments

A trial to induce discharge of an obstructing concrement should, if in vain, be immediately followed by instrumental treatment. Slitting of the ureteric ostium, formerly widely used, is no longer favored. Its use is restricted to stones impacted intramurally and visible in the ostium causing permanent colics.

The remainder of low ureteral calculi are amenable to loop extraction. So-called high extractions, i.e. of stones in the upper or middle third of the ureter, cannot be recommended to the unexperienced. Stones in the lower third of the ureter that offer themselves to loop treatment should no longer be extracted immediately following application of the loop. We prefer to close the loop around the stone and ambulate the patient. In most cases the loop descends quickly and is discharged with the stone. If the loop remains in the same position for 2 or 3 days permanent slight traction may be applied after administration of an appropiate drug, e.g. a "lytic cocktail". We call this procedure "trial loop" to indicate that extraction should not be forced and that repeated tries are possible.

The range of instrumental treatment is limited. If active treatment is still necessary operation should be considered. We feel that independent of the location of stones in the ureter a well performed ureterolithotomy is less hazardous than long lasting heroic extraction trials. They carry the risk not only of stenosis but also of torn ureter. The dangers of long lasting extraction trials are unavoidable urinary tract infection and prostatitis in the male, rendering him a permanent urological patient. They have so far not received appropiate consideration. In case of successful extraction complications are accepted with less concern. Unsuccessful trials with complications, however, are more than unsatisfactory. The impression that extraction of a stone carries no risk is wrong.

Renal Stones

a) Litholysis through Instruments

Chemical dissolution of renal calculi by local irrigation was introduced 1924 by Crowell and refined later experimentally and clinically by Suby. The reasons for increasing interest in this type of treatment are quite obvious: several years after the Second World War a rising stone wave was observed, leading to a growing number of problem cases due to the tendency of recurrences, especially of urate and phosphate calculi. The kidney not being amenable to as many operative interventions as might be wanted, the intensity of research into the practicability of instrumental litholysis is understandable. The problem of direct litholysis consists of finding a solvent that attacks the stone but not the renal parenchyma. In spite of considerable technical progress (Timmermann) the method has not been perfected to a point where is could be introduced into routine practice.

Application of the method depends on knowledge of indications, experience, and availability of optimal X-ray equipment (image amplifier).

After several years experience we feel certain to recommend the following *indications:*

Newly formed *recurring calculi in the renal pelvis* which lack the hard consistency of older stones. With younger stones it is possible to keep the duration of irrigation treatment within relatively short limits, i.e. several weeks.

The irrigation of staghorn stones is practicable only through a transrenal fistula following operative removal of the major part of the concrement which can usually be performed with ease (Fig. 1).

Little can be expected of irrigating stones in renal calyces because the solvent does not flow around the concrement.

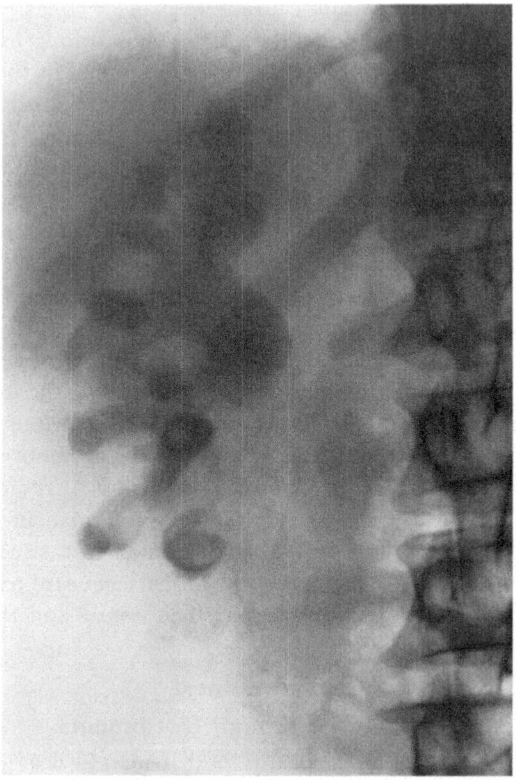

Fig. 1a

Fig. 1a and b. Solitary right kidney with large renal calculus (a) before and (b) after transrenal chemolitholysis

Several solvents are available today for different types of stones:

Table 1*

Type of stone	Solvent
Calcium oxalate	EDTA
Calcium phosphate	Renacidin
	citric acid citrate buffer
Calcium carbonate	Renacidin

* Uric acid calculi are not included in this table in view of their susceptibility to alkalizing drugs.

Patients who are inoperable due to concurring disease are not necessarily suitable for chemolysis because of possible complications of the method. They do not originate from the solvents used but their method of application. They will therefore hardly ever be diminished. The solvent must flow into the renal pelvis by constant drip for weeks or months through wide-bore double-lumen catheters. It has been shown that

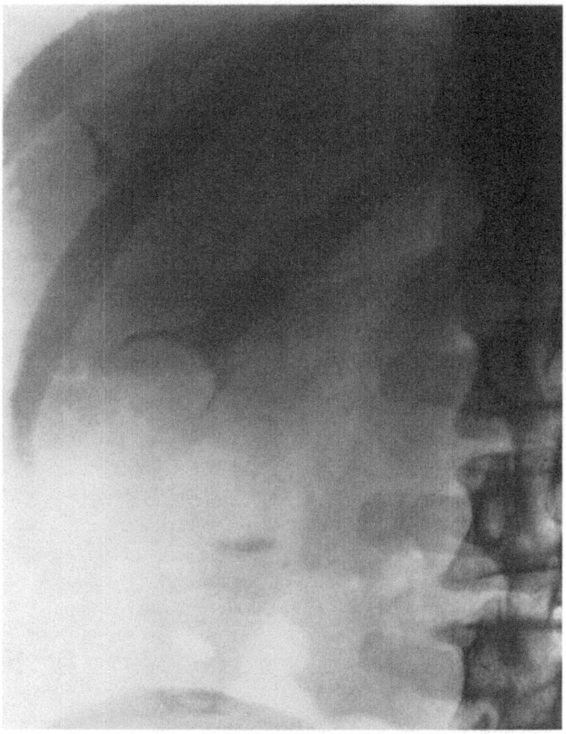

Fig. 1b

antibiotics added to the solvents or given parenterally cannot be relied upon to prevent an ascending and possibly abscess-forming pyelonephritis. Additional risks in the male: prostatitis and epididymitis.

A stone of about the size of a hazel nut needs to dissolve on the average 6 to 8 weeks. The result cannot be guaranteed, however. This considerable psychic and financial burden explains why for most patients instrumental litholysis is no rival method to operative treatment. Without doubt direct contact of solvent and stone favors therapeutic success. The application of the method demands narrow indications, however. Experience provided it offers a valuable addition to therapeutic possibilities.

b) Litholysis by Drugs

Man's old dream of dissolving stones by drugs has been partly realized in recent years. Among others a new concept was introduced into therapy by the discovery of solubility of *urate stones*. Operative interventions to remove urate calculi have become exceptional.

Carriers of urate stones characteristically show a narrow range of urine acidity around pH 5 except for patients with leucosis and following cytostatic treatment. At pH 5 uric acid and its salts have low solubility while above pH 6 no cristallization of uric acid is possible. Adjustment of urine pH at the desired level is best achieved by administration of a mixture of potassium-sodium citrate. Present experience indicates that failure or success of treatment depend on the reliability of the patient to follow his prescriptions. The urate stone carrier is comparable to a diabetic in this respect.

Alkalizing treatment will succeed in almost all instances in dissolving urate stones and preventing recurrences with considerable certainty. The therapy is not indifferent,

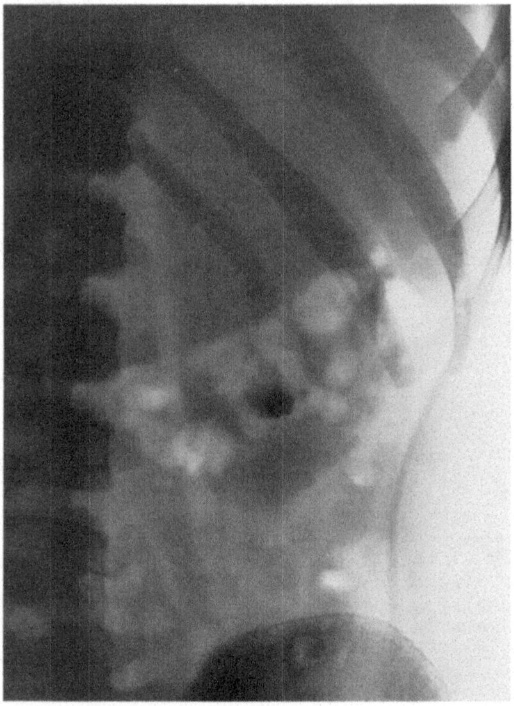

Fig. 2a

Fig. 2a and b. Disolution of a phosphatic calculus in a congenital solitary kidney by means of aluminium hydroxide, acidification of the urine and treatment of infection

however. Urine pH values above seven should be avoided because of the danger of phosphate cristallization. Overshooting of urine reaction into alkaline pH values is caused by overdosage of the drug of action of bacteria that metabolize urea. Simultaneous treatment of urinary tract infection and liberal fluid intake to achieve copious diuresis are therefore important for success. Diuresis should continue through the night because urine reaction varies and tends towards acidity during the night.

Alkalizing therapy today is standard treatment for urate stone carriers who are free of metabolic disturbances leading to elevated serum uric acid. Nowadays the latter can be treated successfully too. Urate stone diathesis is inhibited by administration of allopurinol which was originally introduced for gout. The drug reduces formation of uric acid from purines derived from food or intermediary metabolism. Both uric acid serum level and excretion are lowered.

In several European countries lemon juice is used as a household remedy against urinary stones. Its mode of action has not been explained scientifically, but the dissolving potential cannot be denied in a number of cases. It must be pointed out, however, that lemon treatment should be tried in case of urate stones only. Phosphate and oxalate stones have been found to enlarge during long term and high quantity lemon administration.

Phosphate stones are an indication for a trial of dissolution by aluminum hydroxide. The principle of aluminum hydroxide treatment is binding of soluble food phosphates, thus preventing their absorption. Here too the mode of action, which cannot

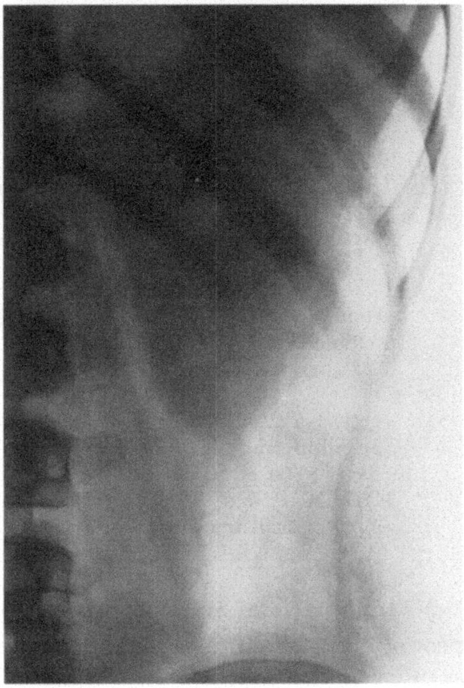

Fig. 2b

be denied (Fig. 2), is not completely clear. During treatment the urine concentration of a substance prone to stone formation doubtlessly is reduced. However, important additional factors are simultaneous treatment of urinary tract infection and acidification of the urine. It can be assumed that improved solubility in acid environment and simultaneous reduction of lithogenetic substances produce litholysis.

Cystine stones always indicate a congenital metabolic abnormality. Cystine, like uric acid, has low solubility in an acid environment. The principle of treatment therefore is, similar to urate stone diathesis, to increase the solubility of cystine by alkalizing the urine.

Alkalization can be carried out by a mixture of sodium-potassium citrate. Diuresis should amount to 3 l in 24 h because of considerable cystine production. In addition to this symptomatic treatment it has become possible recently to lower the fraction of cystine with low solubility. The amino acid D-penicillamine, used for years because of its complex formation with copper and lead in cases of poisoning, permits transforming cystine of low solubility into an easily soluble form preventing precipitation. According to present experience the lowering of urine cystine concentration with simultaneous increase in diuresis not only prevents recurrences but also dissolves stones in a considerable number of patients.

Treatment with D-penicillamine requires close observation of the patient. Daily substitution of B_6 is recommended because of an antagonism to this vitamin. To counteract the known tendency to form chelates with heavy metals the medication should be replaced by a mineral mixture once a week. In a few cases tubular damage with urea retention and albuminuria has been observed.

Oxalate stones at present are not amenable to dissolution by drugs.

Table 2. *Prophylaxis of stone formation*

General treatment
(1) 2000 to 3000 ml fluid daily
(2) Mixed diet
Drug treatment

Type of stone	Drug	Comment
Calcium oxalate	(1) Orthophosphate (2) Magnesium	Contraindicated with alkaline urine
Calcium phosphate Magnesium ammonium phosphate	Aluminium hydroxide plus Acidification	Treatment of infection
Urate	(1) K-Na-citrate (2) Allopurinol	Several urine pH determinations daily
Cystine	(1) K-Na-citrate (2) D-penicillamine	Test of urine pH

c) Prophylaxis of Stone Formation

Prophylactic treatment of urate, phosphate and cystine calculi is essentially identical with the principles of drug litholysis.

Prophylaxis of calcium oxalate stones is being tested clinically at present after identification by Fleisch of pyrophosphate as one of the most important cristalloid solutes. By oral administration of orthophosphates the excretion of pyrophosphates can be increased, reducing the cristallization of calcium in the urine. No side effects have been reported so far besides a laxative action.

Institution of treatment should take into account that this type of phosphate therapy is not without danger. In patients with ammoniacal decomposition of the urine due to bacterial infection phosphate therapy virtually has lithogenetic action. The alkaline urine reaction induces precipitation of phosphates and formation of fast growing phosphate stones (Fig. 3).

An alternative is the administration of magnesium which increases the solubility of calcium oxalate considerably. This treatment too is contraindicated in the presence of alkaline urine reaction with its inherent danger of formation of magnesium ammonium phosphate stones.

The dietary regimen is not overly important in any type of stone. There is growing reluctance towards rigid dietary rules since it is known that neither oxalate nor urate stone formation depends entirely on the oral intake of oxalic acid or purines respectively. At most it seems justified to avoid spinach, rhubarb and chocolate with oxalate stones, brain, liver and kidney with urate stone. Salt is not prohibited but recommended since it is an important cristalloid solute. Milk and dairy products should be reduced because of their calcium content. Besides this all stone carriers should follow the rule to take a normal mixed diet and to avoid all meticulous dietary rules that are impracticable and in general not adhered to. More important than complicated dietary prescriptions for all stone types and carriers is the rule to take 2 to 3 l of fluid daily, up to the late evening. Besides milk all kinds of fluid will do.

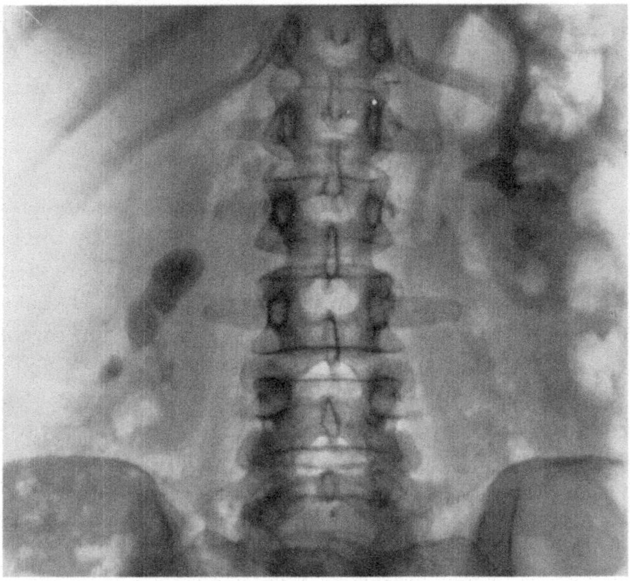

Fig. 3. Development of large phosphatic calculi under orthophosphate therapy with an alkaline urine

References

Brosig, W., H. Klosterhalfen, and J. Kaufmann: Z. Urol. **54**, 245 (1961).
Edwards, N. A., R. G. G. Russel, and A. Hodkinson: Brit. J. Urol. **37**, 390 (1965).
Fleisch, H.: Clin. Orthop. **32**, 170 (1964).
Gasser, G., and A. Preisinger: Klin. Wschr. **38**, 1130 (1960).
Gershoff, S. N.: Metabolism **13**, 875 (1964).
Gundlach, G., G. F. Hoppe-Seyler, H. Dörr, and M. Bressel: Urologe **7**, 56 (1968).
Hammersten, G.: Zit. nach E. Ljunggren: Z. Urol. **58**, 507 (1965).
Hauge, A., and R. Nagel: Urologe **7**, 52 (1968).
Horn, H. D.: Urologe **6**, 223 (1967).
Kollwitz, A. A., and B. Gesche: Urol. int. (Basel) **21**, 193 (1966).
—, and H. Kludas: Vorläuf. Mitt. Urologe **7**, 61 (1968).
—, R. Brauer, and H. Kracht: Urologe **6**, 228 (1967).
Lange, J., K. Freund, and H. Buechel: Arzneimittel-Forsch. (Drug Res.) **7**, 856 (1967).
Ljunggren, E.: Z. Urol. **58**, 507 (1965).
Rutishauser, G.: Dtsch. med. Wschr. **91**, 2302 (1966).
Suby, H.: J. Urol. (Baltimore) **68**, 96 (1952).
Timmermann, A.: Münch. med. Wschr. **104**, 797 (1962).
Zöllner, N.: Urologe **7**, 46 (1968).
—, and M. Schattenkirchner: Dtsch. med. Wschr. **92**, 654 (1967).

Surgical Management of Renal Stones

Walter S. Kerr Jr.

What I have to say about the surgical management of renal stones is not new. In the Massachusetts General Hospital whenever a surgeon — young or old — thought he had devised a new operation, the Residents would peruse a six volume Surgical Atlas which was very complete. Invariably, the operation had been described in the 19th century by a German surgeon.

For a number of years, I have been fortunate enough to work with Dr. Howard Suby, who was scheduled to have been on this program, and with Dr. Fuller Albright in caring for a large number of complicated stone problems. Today, I am going to stress the points which we have found helpful in the management of the complicated cases.

Indications for Operation

I believe that most urologists here would agree that if stones are left in the kidney, sooner or later they will cause damage either by infection or by obstruction. Thus, we feel that early operation on all stones should be advised. There are always exceptions to such a rule; and we have two. 1. Small, asymptomatic-calyceal stones unassociated with infection, bleeding, and non-progressive can be carefully followed 2. Asymptomatic stones of all kinds in very old people in poor general health are perhaps, best treated medically.

Once the operation has been decided upon, every possible step must be taken not only to insure the complete removal of the stones, but also to insure — if possible — that there will be no recurrences. Thus in addition to good surgical techniques, very thorough evaluation of all aspects are of the greatest importance.

Preoperative Evaluation

Infection

The presence and type of infection and sensitivities must be documented. If an infection is present, we try to save the strongest and most effective antibiotics for the day of the operation and the postoperative course. Thus, hoping, in this manner, to eradicate the bacteria.

Metabolic Causes

The need for evaluation of metabolic causes for stones is an obvious one. However, it is still surprising in the frequency with which patients with recurrent stones are referred without having been evaluated from this point of view. You have heard a good discussion of this aspect; and Dr. Cope will further enlighten you.

Drainage

In many cases, poor drainage of all or part of the kidney is a most important factor and one that the urologist is able to do something about. Causes of poor drainage are both physiological and structural. For example, a poorly draining calyx, kidney pelvis, or ureter may be due to congenital faulty innervation or obstruction of an infundibulum, a uretero-pelvis junction, or a ureter. It is important, if possible, to determine which is the case: for the treatment is different. Ureteral reflux must not be forgotten. The more one checks for reflux in adults, the more frequently it is found. Finally, a careful review of the bladder function and residual is mandatory.

Urograms

The number and type of urograms needed depends upon the complexity of the problem. A sufficient number must be done in each case to give the Urologist the best opportunity to remove all the stones and all the areas of obstruction and stasis: and thus, give the patient the best opportunity to avoid the formation of new ones.

Intravenous urograms, in many cases of single pelvic stones or a staghorn stone involving one infundibulum and one calyx, may be all that is necessary.

A request for oblique and lateral films will be helpful in identifying stones hidden by the obvious one.

When does one do retrograde pyelograms? This really depends upon how well the intravenous pyelogram has been done. If they are properly done, retrogrades are not often needed. Whenever there is a doubt as to the size and drainage pattern of the calyces, the size of the infundibula, the nature of the uretero-pelvic junction, or the funnelling of the pelvis, retrograde pyelograms should be performed.

Drainage films can be of great help in determining the area and degree of stasis and whether additional procedures, such as a lower pole nephrectomy may be indicated.

Unfortunately, not always do intravenous and retrograde studies give satisfactory information about the dynamic status of the drainage system. Cine infusion pyelograms can be and should be considered to complete the evaluation. They are, also, equally important in evaluating the postoperative results.

Cystograms are included in our preoperative work-up of all patients who have staghorn stones, all those with dilated ureters, all those with abnormal appearing ureteral orifices, and those patients with unusually large bladders to check on reflux. The more reflux is looked for, the more often it is found.

Renal angiograms are done in cases of horseshoe kidneys and partial nephrectomies. The nephrogram phase outline thickness of the cortex and can help in deciding if it is worthwhile to save kidney parenchyma.

Illustrative Cases

A 23 year old Greek female known to have bilateral staghorn stones for 3 years was referred for evaluation of decreasing creatinine clearances.

The KUB demonstrates a very large staghorn stone in the left kidney; and there was a smaller staghorn stone with eight smaller stones in the right kidney. Retrograde pyelograms were done in an effort to learn as much about the interior structure and drainage pattern as possible. Only a small amount of dye went up on either side. These films demonstrate that there was no stricture at the uretero-pelvic junction and that the ureters were normal. A cystogram demonstrated no reflux. A number of renograms were done over the past 3 years to check the renal function. A recent one shows no function on the left and impaired function on the right. A renal aortogram shows relatively good arterial pattern in the right kidney and a decreased arterial supply on the left. The nephrogram revealed good function; and it demonstrated dilated calyces in the lower and middle portion of the right kidney.

A selective renal angiogram on the left showed a surprising amount of cortical blood supply. The thickness of the cortex was demonstrated. To a large extent on the basis of this film, it was decided to make an effort to save the left kidney.

X-rays at the time of operation, as we all know, are essential in the complicated cases. The best pictures in our hospital are obtained by using a grid casette with the patient supine. Prior to starting the incision, films are taken to insure that they are going to be of good quality and all stones seen on the preoperative films are visible with the technique available in the operating room. This practice has saved us a lot of headaches. I highly recommend it to those of you who have difficulty getting good films taken at the time of operation.

Types of Incisions

The type of incision depends upon the size, the build of the patient, and the extent of the operation planned. In cases such as the one previously discussed, where there are many small stones and superior X-rays are needed, the patient is placed in a supine position and an anterior incision is made. Otherwise — in general, the incision is made through the bed of the eleventh rib without resecting it and with the patient in a semilateral position.

Types of Operation

There are so many types of operations which have been described by surgeons since the days of CZERNY; it is not possible to discuss them here. The aim is to most atraumatically remove all stones and provide optimum drainage.

What are the general considerations and general rules we follow?

1. Best possible exposure with freeing of entire kidney in complicated cases.

2. Evaluation and correction of all sites and causes of poor drainage.

3. Preservation of renal tissue.

a) When in doubt, do not remove it.

b) When possible, remove stone via pelvis, infundibulum, or calyx rather than through the cortex, for renal arteries are end arteries and a nephrotomy through thick cortex results in parenchymal destruction.

4. Value of clamping renal artery to soften the kidney and facilitate

a) Palpation of stones through cortex and

b) dissection of pelves, infundibula, and calyces.

5. Control of bleeding.

a) Clamp the renal artery 10 min at a time.

b) Exposure and control of segmental branch at its origin from renal artery.

c) Control of individual arterial bleeding by fulguration or ligature.

d) Avoidance of deep mattress sutures.

6. Indication for partial nephrectomy.

If tissue is so destroyed or scarred shut, prospect for good drainage and urine sterility are slight. Thus, a partial nephrectomy is done. Indigo carmine injected into the segmental artery is extremely helpful in outlining the site of incision. Ligate the segmental artery at its origin.

7. Calycealotomies, infundibulotomies, and pyelotomies are closed with very fine sutures.

8. Nephrostomy: Occasionally used when postoperative irrigations with Suby's solution is planned.

9. Nephrectomy.

In our era of conservatism, with every effort being spent to save kidney tissue, there still is a place for nephrectomy. Judgement from scan of symptoms, signs, laboratory studies, X-rays, and condition of other kidney will dictate the decision.

Illustrative Cases

Case 1. A very large stone was easily removed through a pyelotomy, for the pelvis was large and the infundibula and calyces were shallow. The point I would like to make in this patient is that there was a small vein running over the pelvis anteriorly which was ligated. We were chagrined to find that it was one of two unusually small renal veins and the remaining one was too small to empty the kidney. Before we were able to anastomose it, the patient developed severe unexplained hypotension; and a nephrectomy had to be done. Thus it is important before dividing a vessel, whether venous or arterial, to identify the other renal vessels to make sure no harm will result.

Case 2. The next patient had a very small intra-renal pelvis and an upper calyceal staghorn stone. Prior to my stimulation to do infundibulotomies, I would have done a pyelotomy; pushed the stone against the kidney cortex; and removed it through a nephrotomy. With renal artery clamping, the infundibulum was easily exposed and the stone removed.

Case 3. The final patient came to the Massachusetts General Hospital in 1943. He was found to have renal tubular acidosis. He was one of the first patients in the hospital to have a potassium determination. Dr. Fuller Albright instituted therapy. Over the years, he developed large stones. Ultimately, as a result disabling back pain thought to be related to the large calculi in his kidneys, it was decided to remove them.

On the right side, the calyces were markedly dilated. At operation, most of the calyces could easily be examined through very thin cortex and through the open pelvis. Dr. Suby and I were so confident that all stones had been removed, we unwisely did not obtain a film at the time of operation; and one stone was left. On the other side, through eleven nephrotomies, all of the stones were removed.

A film taken 8 years later showed that no other stones have formed; and the fragment on the right had not changed in size. Thus, we go from a very simple infundibulotomy to multiple nephrotomies. Again, we point out that the operation must be tailored to the need of the patient and the pathology.

Conclusion

The aim of a good renal calculus operation is that of removing the offending stone in toto, preserving renal tissues, providing a kidney with normal drainage, and free of infection.

The postoperative care is equally as important as the preoperative evaluation and the operation. Upon discharge from the hospital, the patient is provided with a hydrometer and instructions for keeping the specific gravity of the urine at 1.010 and with a clear understanding that he will have to be followed for years to come. These measures plus the effective antibiotics we have at the present time, result in a very low recurrence rate.

Kidney Stones and Hyperparathyroidism

M. Schwaiger

Albright and co-authors were the first to point out in 1934 that primary hyperparathyroidism (HPT) caused by an adenoma or hyperplasia of the parathyroid glands is not only found in osteodystrophia cystica (von Recklinghausen disease), but also in patients with urolithiasis with no or little involvement of the skeletal system. Today, after 30 years, this renal form of the disease and the renal mixed forms are clinically in the foreground. Our own material over the last 6 years comprises 87 cases of HPT consisting of 73 pure renal, 5 renal-osseous and altogether only 9 osseous or intestinal cases. These, our own figures, coincide with the general experience that the renal type represents over 80% of the surgical HPT cases.

The question, regarding the percentage of cases of urolithiasis caused by primary HPT, is of urological importance. Until recent years figures of the percentage incidence fluctuated widely from 0.7% to 22%. During the years 1962 to 1965 out of 978 patients suffering from urolithiasis we found primary HPT in 5.1% (35 men and 16 women). This figure tallies with information from comprehensive statistics in international literature, so that we may assume a primary HPT in about 5% of all cases of urolithiasis, and in patients with recurrences an incidence twice as high (10%). Although these percentage figures appear small, the absolute figures are high, owing to the frequency of urolithiasis. In the Federal Republic of Germany we thus must reckon approximately 13000 patients suffering from urinary calculi where primary HPT is the cause.

The following short preliminary remarks on the physiology or pathophysiology of the parathyroid glands will serve to explain the etiology of calculi. The parathyroid glands through their parathormone normally keep the level of serum calcium at 10 mg-% and the serum phosphorus level at 3.5 mg-%. The parathormone mainly acts on the bones by mobilizing calcium phosphate, also on the small bowel by increasing the reabsorption of calcium and lastly on the kidneys by inhibiting the reabsorption of phosphate in the proximal tubules of the kidneys. Our investigations showed that the reabsorption of calcium is less affected. If too much parathormone is poured out, e.g. through an adenoma of a parathyroid gland, hypercalcemia occurs through increased absorption of calcium from the intestines and especially through increased mobilization of calcium from the bones. Through this the glomerular calcium filtration is increased to a degree, that hypercalcuria results. The inhibition of tubular reabsorption of phosphate is increased, thus more phosphate is excreted (hyper-phosphaturia), the serum phosphorus level falls and hypophosphatemia results. The enormously increased passage of calcium through the kidney leads to nephrocalcinosis or nephrolithiasis. Nephrolithiasis may be present as solitary or multiple stones of various sizes and may be unilateral or bilateral. We observed stratified concrements up to the size of a hen's egg, while staghorn stones are very rare. While no infection exists, the stones consist mostly of pure calcium oxalate or a combination with calcium phosphate.

Nephrocalcinosis is generally discovered accidentally during X-ray examinations, as the characteristic symptoms of urolithiasis are absent. Marked forms (7.5 to 10.5%) are radiologically easily interpreted, it may, however, be difficult to distinguish nephrocalcinosis from very small concrements of the calyces. By a technically good excretion urogram, however, the calcium deposits can be localized and, perhaps, shown clearly to belong to the renal papillae.

There are no specific and typical urological criteria for the presence of HPT as the cause of stone formation. All carriers of urinary calculi may suffer from HPT, regardless of the position of the stone, and the length of the history and disease. There are, however, some indications for the experienced: The concentration power of the kidney is always limited and all patients thus show polyuria and polydypsia. More important still are general symptoms such as muscular hypotonia, tiredness, lumbar pains, constipation, meteorism and especially psychiatric disturbances like depressions and emotional forms of reactions.

Determination of the serum calcium is decisive for diagnosis and should be undertaken in every case of urolithiasis. Serum calcium levels above 10.5 mg-% are indicative of primary HPT. The determination must be undertaken repeatedly as in the purely renal form the values are often just above the normal range; furthermore inorganic serum phosphorus below 2.5 mg-%, 24 hourly urinecalcium in men above 300 mg, in women above 250 mg. The value of the renal phosphorus excretion in 24 h is only of little significance. It may be justified to conclude from the analysis of our cases that a certain correlation exists between the serum calcium level and the size of the adenoma (Fig. 1). In the renal cases we mostly find a small adenoma, often weighing less than 1 g, but a highly active endocrine gland, and accordingly the hypercalcaemic values are generally between 10.5 and 13 mg-%. Excessively high serum calcium values are mostly caused by an adenoma weighing several grams and this leads to HPT of the osseous, intestinal or mixed type. From the serum calcium level one may thus draw preoperative conclusions concerning the size of the adenoma. Thus hypercalcemia, hypercalcuria and diminished tubular phosphate reabsorption are the most important and best diagnostic criteria for primary HPT, which must lead to exploration of the parathyroid glands.

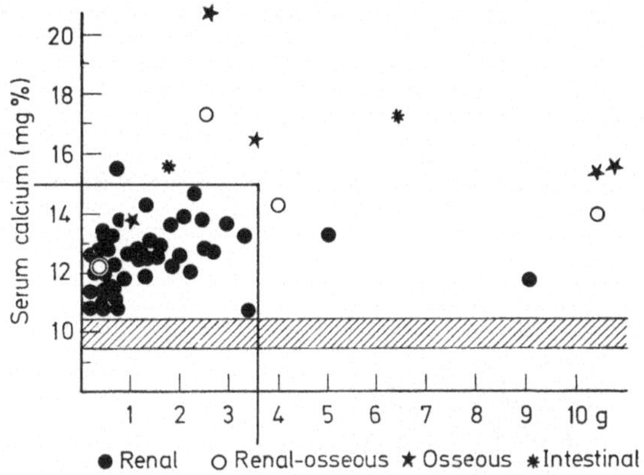

Fig. 1. Preoperative serum calcium and weight of the removed E.B. adenoma (in 60 HPT patients)

The fact that primary HPT is still too rarely remembered and that the simple causal diagnosis therefore is omitted, is shown by the anamnesis of our 78 patients with renal HPT: Before the establishment of the final diagnosis only 22 patients were not submitted to a urological operation, 56 patients were previously operated on, 29 of them underwent operations twice or more often (Fig. 2). Especially serious amongst them are six cases of nephrectomy; particularly as early diagnosis and early treatment protects against irreparable renal damage and also against the — however rare — change into acute HPT, the so called hypercalcemic crisis, which is particularly dangerous and has a high mortality rate.

In HPT the adenoma should, on principle, always be removed first while, if necessary, the kidney is treated in a second operation. This rule is, of course, not valid if urinary retention or a functional failure requires an immediate pyelo- or ureterolithotomy. (A relevant case report of our own will be given in the lecture.)

The decisive surgical-operative problem is to find the adenomata or the hyperplastic suprarenal glands. The number of the epithelial bodies is generally constant, their site, however, is variable. The abnormalities of their position result from the course or disturbance of the embryonic development, which already occurs from the 4th to the 8th embryonic week. Here I refer to the fundamental investigations by NORRIS/Detroit:

Both parts of the epithelial bodies (E.B.'s) originate from solid outgrowths of the dorsal epithelium of the 3rd and 4th branchial pouch. From the 3rd branchial pouch also originates the "anlage" of the thymus, from the 4th branchial pouch also originates the small lateral "anlage" of the thyroid gland. The larger medial thyroid gland-"anlage" proceeds downward from the floor of the mouth with the thyreoglossal tract. Medial and lateral thyroid gland "anlage" fuse and the four E.B.'s, after removal from their origin, lay alongside the thyroid gland "anlage". With the descent of the viscera in the neck during the 6th to 8th

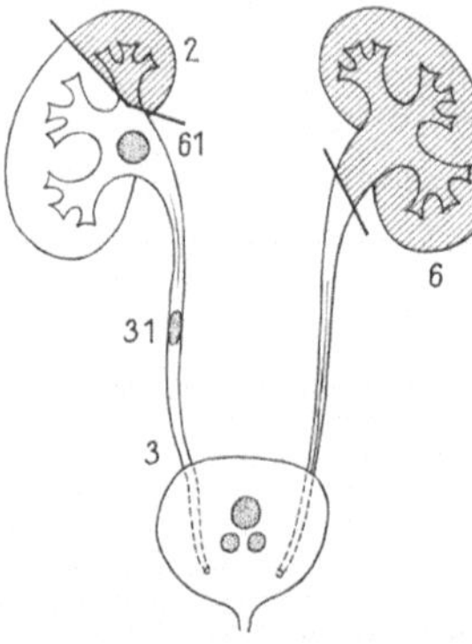

	No. of Operations	No. of Patients
	None	22
	One	27
	Two	15
	Three	10
	Four	4
Total	103	78

Fig. 2. Urological previous operations in 78 patients with primary HPT

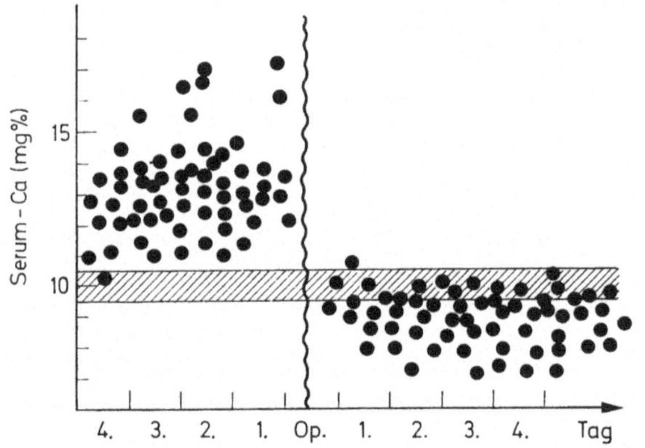

Fig. 3. Serum calcium in 61 HPT patients before and after operation for E.B. adenoma

embryonic week, the paired "anlage" of the thymus moves caudally. With it the epithelial bodies originating from the 3rd branchial pouch glide laterally past the thyroid gland. At the level of the lower pole of the thyroid gland they part company with the "anlage" of the thymus gland, which descends into the mediastinum. We thus see that the primarily higher situated E.B.'s originating from the 3rd branchial pouch become finally the caudal ones, while the primarily caudally situated pair finally becomes the cranial E.B.'s. If the caudal movement of an E.B. 3 is disturbed, it remains at the upper pole of the thyroid gland. If the E.B. 3 does not separate in good time from the thymus, it will be displaced into the anterior mediastinum. An E.B. 4 may be imbedded in the tissue of the thyroid gland if its separation from the lateral thyroid gland "anlage" is disturbed (the described course of development will be explained by a film). — Through enlargement of the lobes of the thyroid gland the E.B.'s normally adjoin the posterior aspect of the capsule of the thyroid gland. Hereby they come in close contact with the recurrent nerve and especially the inferior thyroid artery.

From their quite differing situation follow various possibilities of position, which can be enclosed by two overlapping areas.

The operation technique is in principle the same as for resection of a struma. (The typical procedure is demonstrated by a short film showing the operation.) The following general rules are important for operative treatment:

1. Even if, corresponding to the biochemical findings, a large adenoma is encountered, the remaining E.B.'s must always be exposed, in order to demonstrate a possible second adenoma or a primary hyperplasia.

2. Normal and apparently normal E.B.'s must never be removed, at the most one may remove a small biopsy specimen.

3. In cases of primary hyperplasia three hyperplastic E.B.'s must be totally removed, while a subtotal resection is performed on the 4th, leaving behind a remnant weighing approx. 100 to 150 mg.

4. Excised nodes and tissues must always be examined histologically during the operation. The operation can only be terminated when an unequivocal histological report is available.

5. If in spite of a careful search neither an adenoma nor hyperplastic E.B.'s are found, a typical bilateral subtotal thyroidectomy is performed, perhaps in order to include a dystopic intrathyroidal adenoma. If even after that an adenoma could not be verified histologically, the mediastinum must be revised in a second operation 2 to 3 weeks later (amongst my own cases mediastinotomy was performed in cases).

Unfortunately there still remain cases — 4 amongst our 87 — where in spite of an intensive search in several operations with accurate exploration the biochemically established adenoma could not be found. Here we will only succeed some day, when better preoperative localization methods are at our disposal.

The decisive criterion of the operative success is the prompt fall of the serum calcium values to the normal range (Figs. 3, 4a). Urine-calcium excretion becomes normal (Fig. 4b), tubular calcium reabsorption becomes increased (Fig. 4c), inorganic phosphorus in the serum rises (Fig. 4d), likewise the tubular reabsorption of phosphorus (Fig. 4e). The volume of urine and its specific gravity slowly return to normal. Also a marked change in the general condition is unmistakable, accompanied by a steadier frame of mind, increase of muscle tone, improved appetite, increased weight, etc.

In our experience postoperative complications are trivial and rare: we lost two patients who were in the worst possible general condition when we had to perform an emergency operation during a toxic crisis. Otherwise we had no operative mortality.

The urologist can make a tentative diagnosis of primary HPT with relatively few simple biochemical methods of investigation. If we succeeded in diagnosing HPT in 5.1% of our patients suffering from urolithiasis while other urologists and clinics over the years scarcely ever found a case of HPT, this is not because of a special selection, but only proves the accuracy of the old biblical saying "He that seeketh findeth". Many problems are, of course, still unsolved, to mention only the so called adaptation HPT or the significance of thyreocalcitonin. Nevertheless it is true today without reservation that in primary HPT, irrespective of how it manifests itself, timely, properly indicated and clinically accurately performed surgery of the E.B.'s achieves true prophylaxis or causal therapy of an otherwise irreparable damage or lethal outcome.

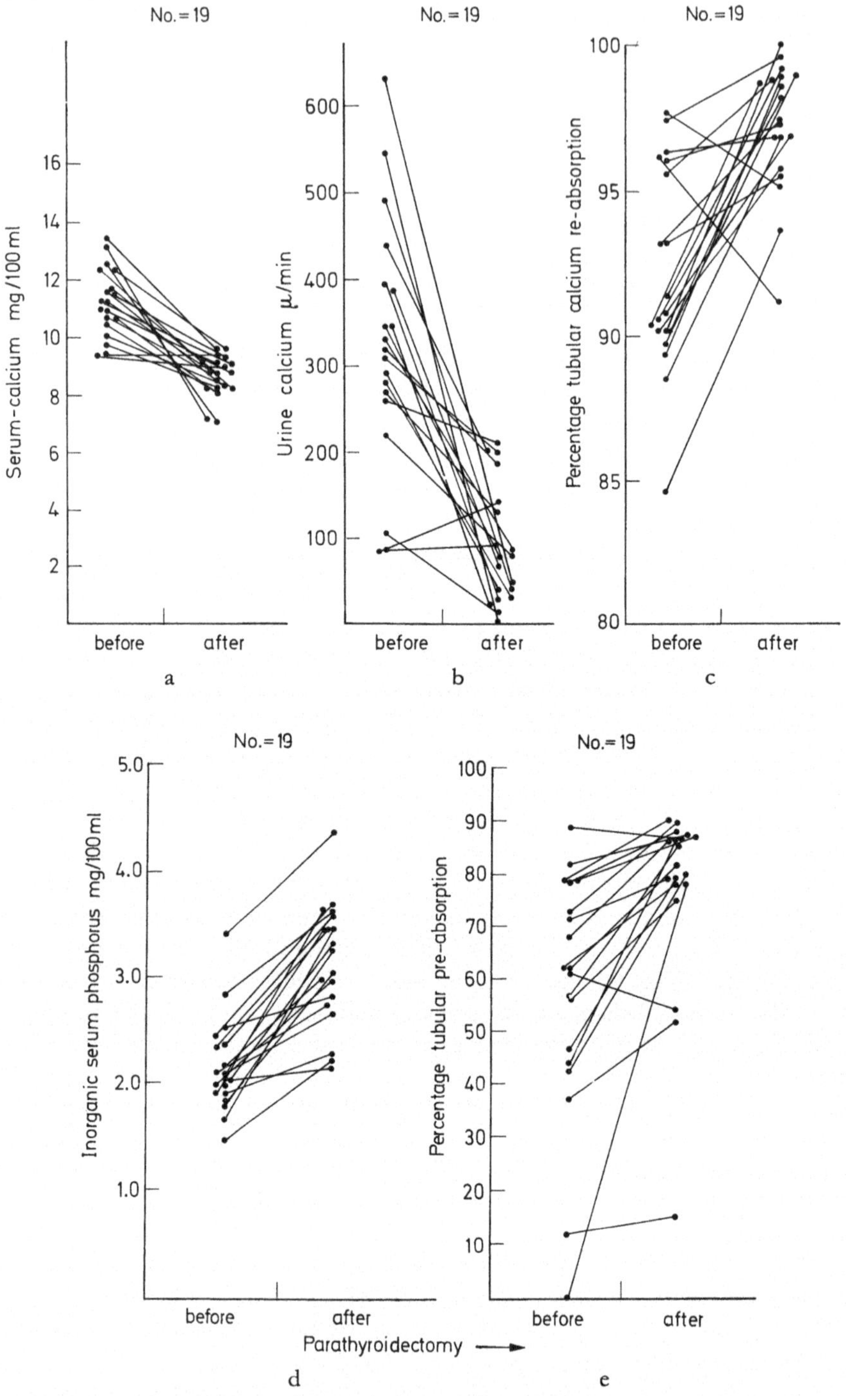

Fig. 4a—e. Biochemical investigations in 19 patients with primary renal HPT before and after operation for E.B. adenoma (according to investigations of Dr. D. Horn, formerly a coworker of the author). a Fall of the serum calcium level. b Fall of the urine calcium excretion. c Rise of the percentage of tubular calcium reabsorption. d Rise of the inorganic phosphorus in the serum. e Rise of the percentage of tubular phosphorus re-absorption

Surgery of the Parathyrods

Oliver Cope

The discovery of hyperparathyroidism by Mandl in Vienna in 1925 and its disclosure in Boston by Aub in 1926 came about independently and for different reasons. Each led to a somewhat different understanding of the primary disease. Now these differences are fast being reconciled, and the widespread nature of primary hyperparathyroidism is being more fully recognized.

In Vienna Mandl confirmed Schlagenhaufer's concept of the origin of von Recklinghausen's bone disease by finding and removing a parathyroid tumor. The parathyroid enlargement appeared, indeed, to be the primary cause of the bone disease, not the result as many pathologists had felt before then.

In America von Recklinghausen's disease was poorly recognized and the enlargement of the parathyroids unknown. The Sea Captain, Martel, was diagnosed as having hyperfunction of the parathyroid system because of the metabolic features which resembled those of dogs and patients with lead poisoning injected with parathormone. The American interest centered on the metabolic disorder.

The first several surgical attempts failed to disclose a parathyroid tumor in the Sea Captain's neck, and not until 1932 was an adenoma found and removed from the anterior mediastinum. In the interval from 1926 to 1932 he had been given a high calcium diet in an effort to improve his bones. His bones, indeed, were somewhat improved but his kidneys had been ruined. Not only did he develop bilateral renal stones but also nephrocalcinosis clearly visible by X-ray. There were also changes in the metabolic disorder. The blood calcium remained elevated at the same level, 14.0 mg-%. The serum phosphorus level, however, rose from the low level of 2.0 to the normal level of 4.0. His NPN rose from normal to 70 mg-%. The calcium excretion under a controlled low calcium intake which had been more than three times the normal amount in 1926 had fallen to the normal range, whereas the fecal excretion of calcium which had been subnormal in 1926 took over the excess which had previously been excreted through the kidney.

This evidence was in large measure responsible for the idea that hyperparathyroidism could well be a cause of renal stones. The idea was fortified by the reports of patients with von Recklinghausen's disease which had already appeared in the literature. 80% of these recorded cases had had renal stones.

In August of 1932 Albright started screening patients with renal stones for possible hyperparathyroidism. Within 2 weeks a women of 40 without any evidence of bone disease was found to have the metabolic characteristics of hyperparathyroidism. Operation disclosed a parathyroid adenoma; with correction of the hyperparathyroidism, the patient formed no further kidney stones. A new era in our understanding of renal stones had started. Every patient with renal stones entering the Massachusetts General Hospital from that time has been screened for possible hyperparathyroidism. The percentage of those having the endocrine disturbance has varied but is approximately 5 to 8% of the stone patients.

Since 1932, 380 patients with primary hyperparathyroidism have been operated upon at the Massachusetts General Hospital. Of these, the largest number by far were identified because of the presence or history of renal stones (see Table 1). A lesser number of patients in our country have been suspected of hyperparathyroidism because of the presence of bone disease. Other clues to hyperparathyroidism have turned out to be peptic ulcers, both duodenal and gastric, pancreatitis, fatigue, a group of curious neurological disorders and most recently pseudogout. Hyperparathyroidism has been found to appear, therefore, in a variety of forms, the most common being, and in the following order, renal stones, bone disease including simple osteoporosis, and peptic ulceration, both duodenal and gastric.

Our understanding of the endocrine disease is not as yet adequate to permit a medical therapy, and irradiation, though theoretically possible, has not helped,

Table 1. *Clues to diagnosis of hyperparathyroidism in the first 380 cases at M.G.H.*

	Cases
1. Bone disease	85
2. Renal stones	219
3. Peptic ulcer	30
4. Pancreatitis	11
5. Fatigue	11
6. Hypertension	6
7. Mental disturbance	3
8. Central nervous system signs	7
9. No symptoms	2
10. Lump in neck	1
11. Multiple endocrine	3
12. Pseudo-gout	2

Table 2. *Hyperparathyroidism — M.G.H. series 380 cases — 1930 to 1968*

	Cases
Neoplasia	
1. Single adenoma	295
2. Double adenoma	13
3. Carcinoma	17
Primary hyperplasia	
4. Clear cell	16
5. Chief cell	39

presumably because of the problem of localizing the site of the parathyroid enlargements. Surgical extirpation of the diseased parathyroid tissue, therefore, remains the sole effective treatment.

The surgical management of hyperparathyroidism has two principal problems — the isolation of the diseased parathyroid tissue and the identification of the nature of the parathyroid enlargement or enlargements. The parathyroid glands are usually four in number, but not infrequently there are supernumerary glands. Dr. C. A. Wang, in a painstaking anatomic study on postmortem cadavers, has found supernumerary glands in nearly 20% of normal people, usually 5 but occasionally 6 clearly identifiable glands. The glands are distributed from high in the neck down into the mediastinum. The lower pair are carried with their neighboring thymus tissue well down over the heart and sometimes on either side to the lung root. Glands enlarged in the neck may be displaced posteriorly and downwards into the posterior mediastinum. Thus, the surgeon's search may have to cover a wide area, and the disease may not be satisfactorily excluded by finding four normal glands. If the clinical and metabolic evidence is strongly in favor of hyperparathyroidism, the search needs to be continued for a 5th and possibly a 6th gland. We have now five cases in which a tumor in a supernumerary gland had to be sought.

When Mandl found the first parathyroid enlargement in his patient in 1925, he wondered whether the enlargement was hypertrophy or an adenoma. The pathologist decided the tumor was an adenoma. The disease in this patient recurred within 2 years, and one cannot help wondering whether Mandl's original speculation was not the correct one. An autopsy was not performed.

Mandl's original finding influenced surgeons and pathologists to conclude that hyperparathyroidism was always due to an adenoma and, indeed, to this date many are confused and consider "adenoma of the parathyroid" and "hyperparathyroidism" as synonymous. This is a grave trap for the surgeon to fall into.

Slowly over the years diffuse hyperplasia of all the parathyroid glands and carcinoma have been identified as causes of primary hyperparathyroidism in addition to the original idea of the adenoma (see Table 2). The first form of hyperplasia was the so-called wasserhelle cell or water clear cell hyperplasia. Dr. Churchill ran onto this entity in 1934. It gave considerable trouble in its identification. Later, by 1941, we surgeons suspected that there was another form of hyperplasia, namely of the chief cells, which was also a primary cause, but our pathologist colleagues at first considered this form to be secondary to the renal disease which was also found in some of the patients. Chief cell hyperplasia had been recognized by our pathologists in 1934 as a sequel to the renal disease. It was the pathologic form in secondary hyperparathyroidism. It was not until the early 1950's that we were able to convince our pathologists that the chief cell hyperplasia could also be a primary form of hyperparathyroidism, and it is now so established. Indeed, we now see it more frequently, and it has constituted nearly 25% of the last 150 cases in our series at the Massachusetts General Hospital. Looking at a single enlargement, it is difficult for the surgeon, and almost impossible for the pathologist, to tell on frozen or permanent section whether the enlargement is chief cell hyperplasia or a chief cell adenoma. Only if normal tissue can be seen either as a rim of the gland or in another gland can we be sure at operation that the tumor is an adenoma. Identification of a second parathyroid at operation has, therefore, become mandatory to know whether the first enlargement found is an adenoma or whether further search must be made to identify all glands presumably involved in hyperplasia. The pathologist is able to identify on frozen section the water clear cell hyperplasia because of the characteristic acinar-like arrangement of the large vacuolated cells.

Carcinoma has posed a special and stubborn problem. 17 of our series have proven to have a malignant hyperfunctioning tumor. 3 of these 17 were referred to us for further surgical care, the diagnosis already having been established. When these are excluded, the incidence is approximately 3%. With awareness and care, the surgeon can identify this type of the disease, and with a wide sweep it can be cured, for it is a sluggish growth. Surgical intrusion into the area of its spread, particularly violation of the thick reactive fibrous capsule, however, ends in widespread implants of tumor cells that grow locally to recreate the hyperparathyroidism. To get rid of these functioning implant metastases may become a major surgical endeavor.

The first problem of patients with renal stones is to make the diagnosis of the cause. There are other causes obviously for renal stones, and, indeed, in the patients with hyperparathyroidism, there are almost certainly several factors determining whether stones form and if so in which kidney. Many patients with proven hyperparathyroidism never form stones. Some form stones in only one kidney. There are, therefore, local reasons.

There are also metabolic reasons. Recently Dr. John Eager Howard, Professor of Medicine at Johns Hopkins, has identified a polypeptide in the urine and, indeed, in body fluids generally, which prevents precipitation of calcium phosphate. Its absence or relative absence is associated with calcification in the kidney and in the urinary tract. This substance may or may not be present in normal quantities in patients with hyperparathyroidism and is undoubtedly a factor or contingency in the patients under discussion. The amount of fluid and the dietary intake are also probably related factors. The diagnosis is made only by thinking of it and excluding it by metabolic measurement. Once the diagnosis is made, the surgical handling needs to be careful, precise and knowledgeable. Easy in the majority of cases, it may be taxing in the few.

Gynecology

Surgical Treatment of Defects of the Uterovaginal Tract

JOSEF ZANDER

According to ANTONII DE HAEN the first attempt of a surgical correction of a congenital absence of vagina was made in 1761 by an unknown surgeon. During this operation where he tried to create an opening between the bladder and rectum, the bladder and the urethra had been perforated. The 24 year old patient died 3 days later. Another attempt had been made about 150 years ago by DUPUYTREN (1817). [For historical review see SCHMID (1956) and STEINMETZ (1940).]

Since that time many operative techniques have been reported. They are compiled in Table 1. Larger series of operative construction of an artificial vagina, published in the world literature are summarized in Table 2. It can be estimated that about 1500 cases operated with different techniques have been reported until recently.

The principle of a simple reconstruction of the vagina was used by WELLS (1935), KANTER (1935), WHARTON (1938) and others (see Table 1). These methods were based on the tendency of the epithelium from the vestible to grow in, and line the vagina if the cavity is kept open. The disadvantages of this method were the slowness with which epithelialization proceeded particularly in the upper part of the created cavity, and its occasional total failure to produce skin. This led frequently to vaginal strictures.

Based on anatomical studies a modification of this method, the boring a double barreled canal, has been reported by SHEARES (1960). As a result islands of epithelium of the vestiges of the Müllerian ducts are surfaced and serve a secondary sources of squamous epithelium.

Methods using ileal transplants or rectal transplants were described by BALDWIN (1904) and MORI (1910) and by POPOFF (1910) and SCHUBERT (1911) respectively. Today they are used only in rare cases. The mortality rates in the preantibiotic period reached 10 to 20% and even more.

More satisfactory results were reported with methods using a portion of the sigmoid colon in the construction of a vagina by SCHMID (1956), SHIRODKAR (1960) and by ALEXANDROW and GIGOVSKIJ (cited by SCHMID, 1956) in Russia. SCHMID calculated for 311 collected cases of Rostock, Berlin, Moskau and some other places a mortality rate of 1.6%. Using this method a vagina with adequate lubrication and little tendency to contracture can be formed.

Flapp-swinging operations with labial and thigh grafts in different modifications have been also used for the formation of an artificial vagina. Disadvantages were the tendency of the vaginal cavity to contract down-ward, the distortion and deformity of the external genitalia, and finaly the formation of large scars on the thighs.

The transplantation devised by THIERSCH was tried by many surgeons and gynecologists. KIRCHNER and WAGNER (1930) used a rubber sponge prothesis covered with a THIERSCH graft. Among the modifications the so called McIndoe-Read technique, first described by MCINDOE and BANISTER (1937) is widely used. The graft-covered mould is inserted into the preformed cavity, and a perineal bridge is built beneath it so that it cannot slip out. The mould is left in place for 3 to 6 month and then renewed and replaced by a polythene dilator.

Table 1. *Methods of construction of an artificial vagina*

Method	Authors
Simple reconstruction (Wharton method)	KANTER (1935), WELLS (1935), SCHMIDT-ELMENDORFF (1937), using vernix caseosa, WHARTON (1938, 1940), COUNSELLER (1948), WORD (1951), BARROWS (1957), SHEARES (1960), EVANS (1967), CALI and PRATT (1968)
Fetal membranes (Burger method)	BRINDEAU (1934), BURGER (1937), RUNGE (1951)
Pedunculated grafts (Labial and tigh flaps)	BECK (1900), GRAVES (1921), FRANK and GEIST (1927), DAVIS and CRON (1928), FALLS (1940), BRADY (1945)
Free skin grafts (Kirschner-Wagner or McIndoe-Read method)	ABBE (1898), KIRSCHNER and WAGNER (1930), FLYNN and DUCKET (1936), MCINDOE and BANISTER (1938), COUNSELLER (1938), READ (1944), WHARTON (1946), COUNSELLER (1948), BRYAN et al. (1949), MCINDOE (1950), THOMPSON et al. (1957), TURUNEN (1957), COUNSELLER and FLOR (1957), JONES (1959), JACKSON (1965), EVANS (1967), CALI and PRATT (1968).
Intestinal transplantation	
Small intestine (Baldwin-Mori method)	BALDWIN (1904), MORI (1910), BRYAN et al. (1949), COUNSELLER and FLOR (1957)
Rectum (Popoff-Schubert method)	SNEGUIREFF (1904), POPOFF (1910), SCHUBERT (1911, 1933, 1936), SOUSTELLE et al. (1967)
Sigmoid (Schmid method)	SCHMID (1956), SHIRODKAR (1960), COUNSELLER and FLOR (1957)
Formation of large perineum with the inner sides of labia majora	WILLIAMS (1964)
Simple pressure (Frank method)	FRANK (1938), STEINMETZ (1940), HOLMES and WILLIAMS (1940)

According to MCINDOE (1950) the most important principles of inlay grafting are:

1. Careful preparation of the cavity,
2. Complete haemostasis and asepsis,
3. Thin split graft in one piece,
4. Continuous (not intermittent) dilatation until the contractile phase is overcome.

JACKSON (1965) described recently 128 cases operated with this technique within a 27 year period in the Chelsea Hospital for Women and in the Middlesex Hospital in London. The results were anatomically satisfactory in 85% of the cases and anatomically unsatisfactory in 5% of the cases. 10% were failures and these included 6 patients with rectal fistulas and 6 patients who refused to finish treatment.

In another recent study CALI and PRATT (1968) reported longterm results of 131 operations with the McIndoe technique within a 46 year period in the Mayo Clinic.

Of 113 traced patients 48 (42%) had some contraction of the vagina or stenosis. Yet 84 (90%) of 93 patients reporting on sexual function expressed satisfaction with function of the organ. There were 30 (22%) complete failures and 31 partial failures of the operative method. The total number of anatomic failures was 46,5% of 131 McIndoe operations.

Table 2. *Larger series of operative construction of an artificial vagina*

	Time period in years	Simple recon-struction	Free skin graft	Bowel trans-plants	Other methods
Chelsea Hospital for Women and Middlesex Hospital (JACKSON, 1965)	27		128[a]		
Johns Hopkins Hospital (THOMPSON, WHARTON, TELINDE, 1957)	14		32		
Mayo Clinic (CALI and PRATT, 1968)	46	25	123[b]	19[c]	8
Univ. of Malaya, Singapore (SHEARES, 1960)	5	18			
Univ. of Helsinki (TURUNEN, 1957)	20		47		
Univ.-Frauenklinik Kiel (SMOLKA, 1962)	15	30[d]			
Univ.-Frauenklinik Heidelberg, 1968	26	25[e]	20		
Wayne State Univ. and Univ. of Michigan (EVANS, 1967)		23	87[f]		
Collected cases of Rostock, Berlin and Moskau (SCHMID, 1956)				311[g]	

[a] 63 cases previously reported by MCINDOE (1950) and 39 cases reported by MCINDOE and SIMMONS (1959) are included in this series.

[b] Cases reported by BRYAN et al. (1949) and COUNSELLER and FLOR (1957) are included in this series.

[c] 13 cases with transplantation of small intestinum and 6 cases with transplantation of sigmoid.

[d] Cases performed with the Burger plastic using fetal membranes are included in this series.

[e] Performed with the Burger plastic using fetal membranes and previously described by RUNGE (1951) and by EBERLE (1959)

[f] 71 cases previously reported by MILLER et al. (1945) and by MILLER and STOUT (1957) are included in this series.

[g] Transplantation of sigmoid.

Turunen (1957) reported the results of 47 operations performed within a 20 year period in the Department of Obstetrics and Gynecology of the University of Helsinki using the Thiersch graft technique. Satisfactory results were obtained in 74% of the patients. According to a recent summary by Evans (1967) of 110 cases operated in the Departments of Obstetrics and Gynecology of the Wayne State University and the University of Michigan a good result was achieved in 75% of the cases. The fistula rate was about 5%.

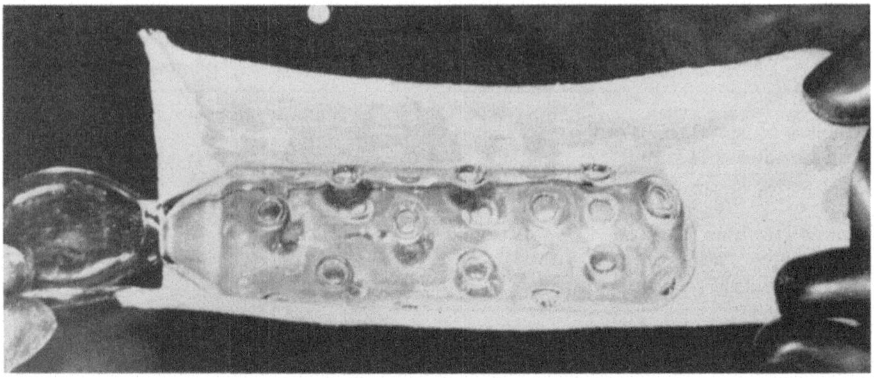

Fig. 1. The glass mould on the free skin graft. The small holes allow the irrigation of the vagina during the postoperative days

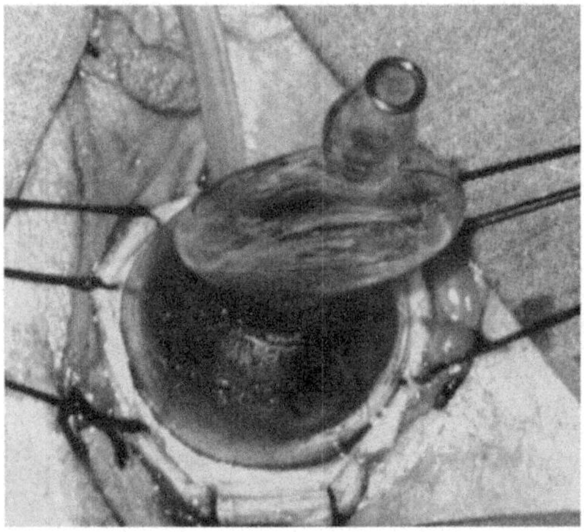

Fig. 2. The graft covered glass mould is inserted into the preformed cavity

At the Department of Obstetrics and Gynecology of the University of Heidelberg within a 26 year period 45 cases were operated. Until some years ago the so called Burger plastic (1937) using fetal membrans and first described by Brindeau (1934) has been used. The long-time results with this method were satisfactory in 64% of the cases (Runge, 1951; Eberle, 1959). Postoperative rectovaginal fistulas were observed in two cases. Since 1964 a free skin graft method has been the method of choice.

In the preparation of the cavity and the thin split graft we follow the principles of McIndoe (1950) as described above. A glass mould with small holes is used which allows the irrigation of the vagina during the postoperative days (Figs. 1 and 2). It is removed between the 12th and 14th day after the operation and immediately replaced by a Plexi glass mould. This prothesis as a general rule is worn at least for a period of 2 years continuously.

Selection of patients. Some authors believe that only those women who are married, or who are engaged should be accepted for surgical treatment. I can not agree with this general statement. An individual decision seems to be necessary in every case after careful psychologic exploration of the personality. In some cases the knowledge of the absence of the vagina can result in marked feeling of inferiority and this again can prevent a more intimate contact with the male sex. The patient can be protected against the premature contraction of the artificial vagina by the mould. Regular sexual intercourse is therefore not a factor necessary in the prevention of contractions.

The basal body temperature should be measured in every patient before operation. Today laparotomy is not indicated if biphasic temperatures are registrated and hematometra can be excluded.

Absence of ovarian function can not be regarded as a contraindication against the formation of an artificial vagina. However the genetic and endocrine diagnosis should be made before the operation is done.

It is well known, that abnormalities of the urinary tract (pelvic kidney, solitary kidney, horseshoe kidney, duplication of the ureters or renal pelvis) are frequently associated with congenital absence of the vagina. Urologic investigation including pyelogram is therefore essential in every patient before operation.

The mould. All sorts of material have been used to form the mould. We prefer an open glass mould with small holes for drainage which allows to irrigate the vagina after the operation. It is hold with a T-bandage. A few days before the patient is dismissed from the hospital she receives a plexi glass mould as long-time prothesis. This mould is formed according to the individual form of the vagina. The long-time mould is considered to be good, if after a while the women does not feel it any more.

Many different shapes have been designed for the mould. Mostly the cylindrical form is prefered. A remarkable modification has been recently described by STABLER (1966). Since normally at rest the front and back walls of the vagina are in contact, and only during coitus is the cylindrical form produced, a flattened form of mould was designed which maintains the physiological shape of the vagina during the whole of the postoperative period. This form may have indeed some advantages over the usual cylindrical shaped prothesis.

Special problems are involved in cases with a functional uterus, hematometra and congenital absence of the vagina, or vagina and cervix. FIKENTSCHER and SEMM (1966) have described a combined vaginal-intrauterine prothesis for those cases. We made successful use of this prothesis in a 13 year old girl 2 years ago. The patient is menstruating regularly. Today exstirpation of a functioning uterus should be avoided. Pregnancies and deliveries have been reported in many cases after the construction of an artificial vagina in cases where the uterus was functioning (WAGNER, 1923, 1927; WHITTMORE, 1942; READ, 1944; BAER, 1947; BAER and DE COSTA, 1947; POTOTSCHNIG, 1949; FAUVET, 1952; SOLOMONS, 1956; EVANS, 1967).

The contractile phase. According to MCINDOE the contractile phase is common to all forms of free grafted skin. Inlay grafts, which line concave surfaces, suffer from this phase more severely than any other type of free graft. The time period of the contractile phase seems to be different from case to case. During the contractile phase remarkable contraction of the upper third of the artificial vagina can occur if the prothesis is only removed for a night or a few days. Carefully controlled continuous dilatation is essential during the entire phase until healing and resolution are complete, and the tendency to contract has entirely ceased. CALI and PRATT recently reported that in 123 patients a vaginal mould was necessary for an average of about 2 years. In several instances moulds were utilized for more than 15 years. The early removal of the mould is particularly dangerous if epithelialization of the vagina is not complete. Too early removal of the mould is one of the major reasons for unsatisfactory results or failures. It is an advantage of the bowel methods that contraction seem to occur only to a minor extent.

Complications. Among the postoperative complications in the free graft techniques, vaginal and urinary infections have been observed primerally. Vaginal infections can prevent the healing of the graft. We have the impression that spong rubber moulds may favour vaginal infections. Since we irrigated the vagina postoperatively through the mould, vaginal infections were not observed any more. Urine cultures should be carried out routinely. Prophylactic use of antibiotics is necessary.

Rectovaginal, vesicovaginal and urethrovaginal fistulas can occur occasionally as serious complication during or after the operation. Rectovaginal fistulas have been more often observed than vesicovaginal fistulas, even several months after the operation. In some cases they healed spontaneously. Using the McIndoe technique, where the mould is left continuously in place for several months it has been observed that, in several cases the mould was passed per rectum. In repeated operations with extensive formation of scars the risk of damage of the rectum or bladder is significantly higher than in the first operation.

Other complications are haemorrhages, and seldom deep vein thrombosis.

The formation of vaginal granulation is a characteristic complication of the free skin graft methods. The granulation tissue is formed in areas where the graft has not survived. The granulation tissue is often found in the vault of the vagina. The granulation prevents epithelialization of this area and it is essential that these granulations be removed by currettage or cautery. In some cases a second graft is necessary. Since most of the patients have a ovulatory menstrual cycle, additional treatment with estrogens is not necessary. We have the impression that local treatment with estrogen ointment even stimulates the growth of granulation tissue.

References

ABBE, R.: Med. Rec. (N.Y.) **54**, 836 (1898).

ALEXANDROW, M. S.: Cited by H. H. SCHMID, Scheidenbildung aus dem S-förmigen Dickdarm. Jena: VEB Gustav Fischer 1956.

BALDWIN, J. F.: Ann. Surg **40**, 398 (1904).

BAER, J. L.: J. Mt Sinai Hosp. **14**, 244 (1947).

—, and J. DECOSTA: Amer. J. Obstet. Gynec. **54**, 696 (1947).

BARROWS, D. N.: Amer. J. Obstet. Gynec. **73**, 609 (1957).

BECK, C.: Ann. Surg. **32**, 572 (1900).

BRADY, L.: Ann. Surg. **121**, 518 (1945).

BRINDEAU, A.: Gynéc. et Obstét. **29**, 885 (1934).

BRYAN, A. L., I. A. NIGRO, and V. S. COUNSELLER: Surg. Gynec. Obstet. **88**, 79 (1949).

BURGER, K.: Zbl. Gynäc. **61**, 2437 (1937).

CALI, R. W., and J. H. PRATT: Amer. J. Obstet. Gynec. **100**, 752 (1968).

COUNSELLER, V. S.: Amer. J. Obstet. Gynec. **36**, 632 (1938).

— J. Amer. med. Ass. **136**, 861 (1948).

—, and F. S. FLOR: Surg. Clin. N. Amer. **37**, 1107 (1957).

Davis, C. H., and R. S. Cron: Amer. J. Obstet. Gynec. **15**, 196 (1928).
DeHaen, A.: Cit. by B. Word. Sth. med. J. (Bgham. Ala.) **44**, 375 (1951).
Eberle, H.: Medizinische **8**, 332 (1959).
Evans, T. N.: Amer. J. Obstet. Gynec. **99**, 944 (1967).
Falls, F. H.: Amer. J. Obstet. Gynec. **40**, 906 (1940).
Fauvet, E.: Geburtsh. u. Frauenheilk. **12**, 897 (1952).
Fikentscher, R., u. K. Semm: Geburtsh. u. Frauenheilk. **26**, 132 (1966).
Flynn, C. W., and J. W. Ducket: Surg. Gynec. Obstet. **62**, 753 (1936).
Frank, R. T.: Amer. J. Obstet. Gynec. **35**, 1053 (1938).
—, and S. H. Geist: Amer. J. Obstet. Gynec. **14**, 712 (1927).
Gigowskij, E. E.: Cited by H. H. Schmid, Scheidenbildung aus dem S-förmigen Dickdarm. Jena: VEB Gustav Fischer 1956.
Graves, W. P.: Surg. Clin. N. Amer. **1**, 611 (1921).
Holmes, W. R., and G. A. Williams: Amer. J. Obstet. Gynec. **39**, 145 (1940).
Jackson, J.: J. Obstet. Gynaec. Brit. Cwlth **72**, 336 (1965).
Jones, H. W.: Clin. Obstet. Gynec. **2**, 1053 (1959).
Kanter, A. E.: Amer. J. Surg. **30**, 314 (1935).
Kirschner, M., and G. A. Wagner: Zbl. Gynäk. **43**, 2690 (1930).
McIndoe, A. H.: Brit. J. plast. Surg. **2**, 254 (1950).
—, and J. B. Banister: J. Obstet. Gynaec. Brit. Emp. **45**, 490 (1938).
—, and C. A. Simmons: Proc. roy. Soc. Med. **52**, 952 (1959).
Miller, N. F., and W. Stout: Obstet. and Gynec. **9**, 48 (1957).
—, J. R. Willson, and J. Collins: Amer. J. Obstet. Gynec. **50**, 735 (1945).
Mori, M.: Zbl. Gynäk. **33**, 172 (1909); **34**, 11 (1910).
Popoff, D. D.: Russk. Vrach. St. Petersb. **60**, 1512 (1910); Cited by McIndoe, Brit. J. plast. Surg. **2**, 254 (1950).
Pototschnig, G.: Zbl. Gynäk. **71**, 792 (1949).
Read, C. D.: Irish J. med. Sci. **6**, 52 (1944).
Runge, H.: Zbl. Gynäk. **73**, 599 (1951).
Schmid, H. H.: Die Scheidenbildung aus dem S-förmigen Dickdarm. Jena: VEB Gustav Fischer 1956.
Schmidt-Elmendorff, H. R.: Zbl. Gynäk. **45**, 2602 (1937).
Schubert, G.: Ber. ges. Gynäk. Geburtsh. **23**, 241 (1933).
— Die künstliche Scheidenbildung aus dem Mastdarm nach Schubert. Stuttgart: Enke 1936.
— Zbl. Gynäk. **35**, 1017 (1911).
Sheares, B. H.: J. Obstet. Gynaec. Brit. Emp. **67**, 24 (1960).
Shirodkar, V. N.: Contributions to Obstet. and Gynec. Edinburgh: E. and S. Livingstone Ltd. 1960.
Smolka, H.: Geburtsh. u. Frauenheilk. **22**, 1187 (1962).
Sneguireff, W. F.: Zbl. Gynäk. **28**, 772 (1904).
Solomons, E.: Obstet. and Gynec. **7**, 329 (1956).
Soustelle, J., H. Villiers et P. Vuillard: Traitement chirurgical de l'aplasie vaginale. Lyon: S.I.M.E.P. Editions 1967.
Stabler, F.: J. Obstet. Gynaec. Brit. Cwlth **73**, 463 (1966).
Steinmetz, E. P.: West. J. Surg. **48**, 169 (1940).
Thompson, J. D., L. R. Wharton, and R. W. TeLinde: Amer. J. Obstet. Gynec. **74**, 397 (1957).
Turunen, A.: Ann. Chir. Gynaec. Fenn. **46**, 121 (1957).
—, and C. E. Unnérus: Acta obstet. gynec. scand. **46**, 99 (1967).
Wagner, G. A.: Arch. Gynäk. **120**, 136 (1923).
— Zbl. Gynäk. **51**, 1302 (1927).
Wells, W. F.: Amer. J. Surg. **29**, 253 (1935).
Wharton, L. R.: Ann. Surg. **107**, 842 (1938).
— Ann. Surg. **111**, 1010 (1940).
— Amer. J. Obstet. Gynec. **51**, 866 (1946).
Whittmore, W. S.: Amer. J. Obstet. Gynec. **44**, 516 (1942).
Williams, E. A.: J. Obstet. Gynaec. Brit. Cwlth **71**, 511 (1964).
Word, B.: Sth. Med. J. (Bgham. Ala.) **44**, 375 (1951).

Polycystic Ovarian Disease

Michael L. Leventhal

Polycystic ovarian disease is an entity in which the anovulatory ovary can be converted into an ovulatory one. Wedge resection of the ovaries, often producing a dramatic and irreversible return of hormonal homeostasis, has been the treatment of choice for many years. First performed in 1895, wedge resection of the ovaries was frequently done in the first part of this century for a wide spectrum of menstrual disorders with varying results. In 1935 Stein and Leventhal brought some order out of chaos by defining a syndrome of polycystic ovaries in which wedge resection, in properly selected cases, was very successful. Since 1950 their results have been confirmed by many observers throughout the world.

Concomitant with the widespread use of wedge resection, other modalities of treatment began to appear and to challenge the surgical approach in the treatment of polycystic ovaries. The ability of some types of polycystic ovary to respond to medications that restore a normal hypothalamo-pituitary-ovarian relationship, even though temporarily, is evidence of the dysfunctional nature of the disease. However, the establishment of prolonged normal function by wedge resection following failure of medical treatment lends support to the view that an organic component (grossly thickened capsules) may have to be removed before proper ovulation can be restored in some patients. It is perhaps these cases, rare in occurrence, which comprise the segment in the broad spectrum of anovulation known as the Stein-Leventhal syndrome.

The important non-surgical modalities in the treatment of polycystic ovarian disease include corticosteroids, clomiphene citrate, human pituitary gonadotropin (HPG) and human menopausal gonadotropin (HMG). Thus, a discussion of the surgical treatment of polycystic ovaries must attempt a comparison of the results of wedge resection with the results of medical treatment.

Corticosteroids

The polycystic ovaries typical of the Stein-Leventhal syndrome have been shown to be an important source of abnormal androgen, producing an increase of plasma testosterone levels. Androgens from this ovarian source contribute little towards an increment of total urinary 17-ketosteroids and are usually associated with normal or, at most, slightly elevated values. They are not however, responsive to corticosteroid suppressive therapy. If regular menstruation does follow suppressive therapy, it is likely that the anovulation is due to a type of mild postpubertal or borderline adrenocortical syndrome. Patients with this condition are indistinguishable clinically from patients with the Stein-Leventhal syndrome. Enlarged polycystic ovaries are present in about 50% of these patients but wedge resection notoriously fails; and, it is in these failures that subsequent corticosteroid therapy may be effective. When the typical polycystic ovary is associated with secondarily induced adrenocortical hyperfunction, corticosteroids may induce ovulation. However, after 1 or 2 menstrual periods, amenorrhea usually recurs in spite of continued therapy. Such patients then often respond to wedge resection. Markedly increased excretion of 17-ketosteroids, as a rule, eliminates the ovary as the source of abnormal androgen and should direct attention to the adrenal gland itself.

Gonadotropins

Anovulatory patients with low urinary gonadotropins and little or no detectable estrogen activity have the worst prognosis for the return of homeostatic hormonal activity, but are best treated with pituitary gonadotropins in conjunction with human chorionic gonadotropin (HCG). Even though this situation does not exist with typical polycystic ovaries (in which urinary gonadotropins are normal and there is good evidence of endogenous estrogen activity), gonadotropins have been used with some success in patients with the syndrome as well as in patients with other types of anovulation, Pergonal (HMG) is the one most available for clinical use. Gonadotropin prepared from postmortem human pituitaries, used in a few select research centers, is not available commercially for clinical studies. The biologic activity of the two is predominantly that of FSH, and is identical. At the present time there is difficulty in assaying the concentration of FSH and LH in human gonadotropin, and although proper dosage schedules have not been definitely determined, excellent results have been obtained by TAYMOR et al. (1967) and others by monitoring the gonadotropin dose with daily estrogen excretion levels. Gonadotropins have been used successfully after clomiphene and wedge resection failures in some patients in whom the anovulation was based on a presumed diagnosis of the Stein-Leventhal syndrome. These are probably patients who have low estrogen secretion as manifested by vaginal smear and atrophic endometrium, and perhaps should have been treated by gonadotropins initially. They require human pituitary gonadotropins plus sequential HCG in order to achieve follicular maturation and ovulation. In retrospect they should not have been included in the category of the syndrome.

Patients with the syndrome should be treated with gonadotropins, if at all, only with great care and experience and only after failure of clomiphene, clomiphene-HCG and wedge resection. The possibility of dangerous overstimulation of the extremely responsive follicles in the polycystic ovary is real, requiring frequent pelvic examinations and careful titering of the gonadotropin dose to the patient's level of total estrogen. As with clomiphene, the number of pregnancies is relatively low compared to the high percentage of apparent ovulations. GEMZELL reported an 80% ovulation rate, a 40% pregnancy rate of which 44% were multiple, and an abortion rate of 25% in his series of patients with secondary amenorrhea treated with HPG. TAYMOR et al. (1967), using HMG in a selected group of patients who failed to ovulate with clomiphene, reported a 63% pregnancy rate in 24 amenorrheic patients. In a larger series of cases of anovulation treated with HMG, he reported an overall ovulation rate of 72% and a pregnancy rate of 26%. The abortion rate was 25% and there were only 10% multiple pregnancies compared to 44% reported with HPG. It is obvious that even ready availability of human gonadotropins, which is not likely, will not make the more effective and safer modalities of treatment of polycystic ovaries, such as clomiphene and wedge resection, obsolete.

Clomiphene Citrate

It has been well established that clomiphene citrate is capable of inducing ovulation in a wide spectrum of menstrual disturbances associated with anovulation. Included in the spectrum is a segment occupied by an endocrine disturbance characterized by *enlarged* ovaries, with varying degrees of *thickening of the capsule* and with small subcapsular cysts. These ovaries may produce abnormal amounts of androgen. When these patients exhibit urinary gonadotropins in the normal range, show evidence of endogenous estrogen activity, and have essentially normal 17-ketosteroids, a therapeutic course of clomiphene, if otherwise not contraindicated, is very often rewarding in inducing ovulation. However, since pregnancy is the only irrefutable evidence of ovulation, the results of treatment of anovulation by any modality is best analyzed from the standpoint of the pregnancy rate. In a group of 24 patients with the Stein-Leventhal syndrome, COHEN reported an 80% ovulation rate but only 35% became pregnant. 6 of the patients were considered to be clomiphene failures, and 5 of these conceived promptly following subsequent wedge resection. SCOMMEGNA treated 18 patients with a presumed diagnosis of Stein-Leventhal syndrome, of whom 17 ovulated (90%). Pregnancy was desired in 11 of the ovulators, and of these only 4 or 36% conceived. 1 patient failed to respond to clomiphene, but conceived promptly following wedge resection. According to KISTNER (1965) who analyzed large numbers of reports, about 75% of infertile polycystic ovary syndrome patients will respond to clomiphene with ovulation, but only 40 to 45% will conceive. Thus there appears to be a discrepancy between the ovulatory rate and the expected number of pregnancies.

Why is there such a discrepancy? It should first be acknowledged that such a difference could be more apparent than real. There are no reports in which clomiphene-induced and normal pregnancy rates are compared with regard to length of exposure while ovulating, patient's age, and coital frequency. In many, only infrequent mention is made of investigation of male factors. However, assuming that this discrepancy *is* a real one, is it possible to postulate a reason on an ovarian basis? It is well known that the tunica albuginea in the typical polycystic ovary is invariably thickened, stands out in marked contrast to the underlying stroma, and contains no primordial follicles. The thick fibrous capsule is due to hyperplasia and hypertrophy of collagen fibers, which may increase the diameter of the layer 2 to 6 fold. A study of some wedges from enlarged ovaries due to overstimulation with clomiphene revealed luteinization of cystic follicles and corpora lutea under a thickened capsule. Progesterone secreted from these structures would produce clinical and laboratory findings typical of ovulation without the occurrence of external ovulation. In one ovary we have observed rupture of an ovum from a mature follicle into an adjacent cystic follicle, under a thickened tunic. This patient became pregnant after wedge resection and continued to have regular ovulatory cycles. PEREZ-PELAEZ described a patient who had evidence of ovulation after extensive treatment with clomiphene. Resected wedges from her ovaries revealed several corpora lutea inside the parenchyma of the ovaries. There is evidence to suggest that patients with *prolonged* amenorrhea associated with *large* ovaries are less likely to become pregnant following clomiphene therapy than patients with the syndrome of shorter duration and perhaps smaller ovaries. FERRIMAN et al., in comparing *ovulatory response* in relation to *ovarian size* showed that patients with large polycystic ovaries fare better than those with normal sized ovaries. However, their conception rate was lower. He stated that "perhaps the thickened capsules of the polycystic ovaries interfere with the release of ova; or, the increased production of androgen by these ovaries impairs nidation". He also showed that ovulatory response was better when the estrogen excretion level exceeded 21 µg/24 h. This correlates well with the better response obtained in patients with marked proliferative or hyperplastic endometrium.

Is it possible that when the typical polycystic ovary is treated medically, the extremely thickened capsule prevents external ovulation? It would be pertinent to the above proposal to know whether patients becoming pregnant on clomiphene have a thin capsule and if the failures have a thick one. Perhaps the latter are the ones that require wedge resection. Since it is impossible to know this before surgery, it is logical that clomiphene should be tried as the initial form of therapy.

Cases meeting all the criteria for the Stein-Leventhal syndrome are rare. STEIN (1966) collected 108 cases in 35 years of active practice. INGERSOLL collected only 21 cases of typical polycystic ovaries (with ovarian enlargement of 2 to 5 times) in 27 years. In the widely quoted article by GOLDZIEHER and AXELROD, close scrutiny of the large numbers of cases of presumed Stein-Leventhal syndrome that they collected from the literature makes it obvious that the inclusion of many reported cases into the syndrome is not substantiated.

Wedge Resection of the Ovaries

That favorable results are obtained with wedge resection in patients with the typical Stein-Leventhal syndrome is indisputable. It is possible that infertile patients with prolonged amenorrhea, who have enlarged ovaries with marked capsular thickening are more likely to become pregnant following wedge resection than by medical treatment. It is my impression from personal experience that this is so. It is important to rule out all other causes of anovulation and to filter out these select cases for surgical treatment. This may be difficult because the etiology in a majority of these patients is often obscure. It would therefore be prudent to treat all patients whose anovulation appears to be the basis of their infertility and who show evidence of adequate endogenous estrogen, initially with clomiphene citrate. If such a course fails to induce ovulation within no less than 6 months, then clomiphene plus sequential HCG should be used. This combination has been shown to increase the ovulation percentage by 20% over clomiphene alone, and also to increase the pregnancy rate. Following failure with this, wedge resection may produce a beneficial result. Since most patients with the Stein-Leventhal syndrome exhibit an apparent ovulatory response to clomiphene (80 to 90%), but only 40 to 50% of these become pregnant, the surgical treatment of polycystic ovaries must remain an important modality of treatment. STEIN (1964) reported a pregnancy rate as high as 85% in his private series. Pregnancy rates following wedge resection vary widely in reported series. Having reviewed the literature, I feel that a higher pregnancy rate than the 40 to 50% reported for clomiphene might have been obtained by a more careful selection of cases for wedge resection. The restoration of ovulation following wedge resection may be permanent, as compared to the temporary restoration of function following clomiphene treatment, which most often is limited to the treatment cycle. One potential complication of wedge resection is the formation of peritubal and periovarian adhesions as reported by KISTNER (1968). If it occurs, and its occurrence obviously has to do with surgical technique as well as host response, it may in itself prevent pregnancy even though ovulation is established.

The polycystic ovary syndrome should be treated at all ages when accurately diagnosed. In the young unmarried patients, including late teen-agers, it is not necessary to establish ovulatory cycles. If hirsuitism is a disturbing symptom, suppression of the ovary by cyclic therapy with estrogen-progestin combinations is valuable in reducing the abnormal androgen production. Cyclic progesterone may also be used. It will cause regular monthly bleedings and oppose the prolonged uninterrupted estrogen stimulation of the endometrium, thus preventing hyperplastic and anaplastic changes. Wedge resection may be rarely indicated in the young unmarried woman who has developed a neurosis about her abnormal menstrual function and defeminization. If medical therapy is unsuccessful in married infertile women with the syndrome, wedge resection may be effective. Long term results from wedge resection seem to continue to justify its place in the treatment of the polycystic ovary syndrome. Correct diagnosis and proper selection of cases for surgery is often a difficult task. The ultimate treatment of the syndrome will probably have to await an exact delineation of the basic metabolic defect.

References

COHEN, M. R.: Fertil. and Steril. **17**, 765 (1966).

FERRIMAN, D., A. W. PURDIE, and M. CORNS: Brit. med. J. **4**, 444 (1967).

GEMZELL, C.: Clin. Obstet. Gynec. **10**, 401 (1967).

GOLDZIEHER, J. W., and L. R. AXELROD: Fert. and Steril. **14**, 631 (1963).

INGERSOLL, F. M.: Some anovulation still needs surgery. Obstet. Gynec. digest. 1968.

KISTNER, R. W.: Obstet. gynec. Surv. **20**, 873 (1965).

— Peri-tubal and peri-ovarian adhesions subsequent to wedge resection of the ovaries. Presented at the annual meeting of the American Fertility Society, March 29, 1968. Fertil. and Steril. (in press).

PEREZ-PELAEZ, M.: Personal communication.

SCOMMEGNA, A.: Investigator's report on clomiphene. Wm. S. Merrill Co., Cincinnati, Ohio. Personal communication.

STEIN, I. F.: West. J. Surg. **78**, 237 (1964).

— In: Ovulation, ed. by R. B. GREENBLATT. Philadelphia: J. B. Lippincott Co. 1966.

—, and M. L. LEVENTHAL: Amer. J. Obstet. Gynec. **29**, 181 (1935).

TAYMOR, M. L.: Clin. Obstet. Gynec. **10**, 685 (1967).

—, S. H. STURGIS, D. P. GOLDSTEIN, and B.LIEBERMAN: Fertil. and Steril. **18**, 181 (1967).

The Role of Fallopian Tubes in Physiology of Conception

WILLIAM J. MULLIGAN

Proper assessment of the role of the Fallopian tubes in physiology of conception requires much more than the time allotted me. It is as though one were compressing a book into a page, and, I, perforce, may dwell only on the highlights with proper consideration of the dynamic and complex role of the oviduct in transport, nuture and the consummation of the mechanism of fertility.

The adult human Fallopian tube is 8 to 15 cm in length and is divided into four zones.

1. An intramural portion actually in the wall of the uterine fundus.

2. The isthmus — about 3 cm in length with lumen averaging 300 micra in diameter and lying distal to the fundus uteri.

3. The ampulla — averaging 7 cm in length with gradually increasing lumenal diameter up to 2 cm at the distal end.

4. The infundibulum, consisting of numerous longitudinal folds of mucous membranes subdividing an ever increasing diameter and terminating in the fimbrial ostium.

The inner mucosa varies from a simple pattern at the isthmus to the longitudinal folds of the ampulla. The projections of mucous membranes at the ampulla float freely in one lumen under normal conditions.

In accordance with the parameso-nephric system, the mucosal cells exhibit varying patterns of activity. The columnar epithelial cells are in part ciliated with the prevailing current directed toward the uterus. Numerous secretory cells are recognized and a "peg-like" supporting cell is present. Even though numerous extensive investigations have been carried out, one may only conclude that the various ciliated and secretory cells are most important in the transport and sustenance of the fertilized ovum.

In passing, it may be noted that the so-called lamina propria of the tube is almost identical in appearance and in cyclic variations with endometrial stroma.

During the growth of the follicle and subsequent rupture, estrogen and progesterone, in ever varying proportions appear to sensitize the entire oviduct to ideally affect maximum fertility. In optimum circumstances the egg or eggs should be quickly transferred to ampulla and subsequent fertilization. BLANDAU has shown this effective mechanism in the rat in a brilliant cinema production of the closed ovisac. Man, the less efficient breeder, presents the end of the oviduct as an open funnel.

We are indebted to WESTMAN for original observations regarding ovum transfer. These observations have been confirmed by many of us through culdoscopy and laparotomy at the time of ovulation. At the time of ovulation approaches the fimbriae contract at an ever increasing rate. The ovary is drawn into a recess in the posterior aspect of the broad ligament. The tubo-ovarian ligament is shortened, bringing the ostium into a position embracing the ovary. Thus a physiologic ovisac is created, and in the absence of pathologic disturbances, the juxta-position facilitates the pick-up mechanism of the tubal ostium.

The ciliary mechanism of the tube sustains a steady stream of fluid from the abdominal cavity to cervix and vagina. This, then, is an initiating factor in transport of the egg into the potentially fertilizing atmosphere of the infundibulum.

Tubal musculature consists of a central circular layer, and an outer-longitudinal layer interspersed with the musculature of serosal vessels and the typical pattern of the isthmus in which inner longitudinal bundles are not clearly defined. As may be expected, the tubo-ovarian ligament exhibits muscular layers beneath the peritoneum. This pattern contributes, of course, to the previously described pick-up mechanism.

According to RADECKI, amular contractions occur without propagation along the tube, and in the gestational tube afford a segmental "to and fro movement" of intratubal contents — thus more or less recapitulating smooth muscle activity in the intestinal tract.

All mammals, according to HARTMAN, require the same time for transport of eggs from ovary to uterus, namely, 3.5 to 4 days. One simple explanation as demonstrated by CHANG, is that this delay affords maturation of eggs and implantation of the fertilized egg into the properly prepared endometrium.

Apparently, as has so brilliantly been demonstrated by Blandau's photography, peristaltic and segmental muscular contractions of the tube results in the egg being rolled back and forth in a single loop for some time and apparently demonstrating peristaltic reaction complexes to ovum sized particles.

Influences on peristalsis are mainly estrogens and progesterone. Estrogen apparently increases the rate, tonus and amplitude of tubal contractions. Most observers agree that the pattern of contractions is modified by progesterone. The role of pituitary extracts, epinephrine, and the prostaglandins has not been properly assessed. But it is increasingly evident from adequate research that priming of the tube with estrogen, as has been demonstrated in the endometrial pattern, is an essential initial step, perhaps providing the "locking mechanism" attributed to the isthmic segment and insuring the release eventually of a maturated ovum available for implantation. Indeed the response of the tubal isthmus and that of the cervical isthmus, under the influence of estrogen and progesterone during pregnancy, invite the prospectus that these are special target tissues, apparently histologically identical with adjacent tissues but possessing unique characteristic response. Perhaps in the presence of adequate estrogen-progesterone balance on the isthmic target tissue, the isthmic block opens and the mature ovum enters the endometrial cavity to seek its destiny.

Roentgenographic and Other Techniques in the Diagnosis of Uterotubal Factors in Sterility and Infertility*

JOHN W. HUFFMAN

WILLIAM ROENTGEN of Würzburg, discoverer of the X-ray, paved the way for those who subsequently developed hysterosalpingographic techniques. LUDLOW (1909) reported calcified fibromyomata of the uterus which had been diagnosed roentgenologically. The first hysterosalpingogram was obtained by RINDFLEISCH (1910) who filled the uterine cavity with a barium paste and then made a roentgenogram which demonstrated the endometrial cavity and the left tube. RUBIN (1914) and CAREY (1914) pioneered in the evolution of uterosalpingography. HEUSER (1925) and STEIN and ARENS (1927) demonstrated the value of hysterosalpingography combined with pneumoperitoneum. It is fitting that we should acknowledge the help which these and many other investigators have given us.

The determination of tubal patency by insufflation, salpingoroentgenography or perfusion is an indispensable part of most infertility studies. In addition, the clinician seeks to determine, when possible, whether there are partial obstructions of the tubes by intratubal disease or extratubal factors and whether there are functional disturbances in tubal motility.

The diagnosis of tubal obstructions by uterotubal insufflation was first made by RUBIN in 1920. His work gave impetus to the interest in infertility which has continued to the present. The investigations of SIEGLER of New York have added immensely to the practical application of uterosalpingography.

The relative merits of insufflation and hysterosalpingography are sometimes debated. Actually, they supplement each other. Insufflation is simpler because it requires relatively inexpensive equipment, can be done in the clinic and is attended by minimal hazards when carbon dioxide is used. It is hoped that air insufflation with its hazard of embolism will soon be abandoned. A kymograph used in conjunction with insufflation will record tubal spasm not easily recorded by hysterosalpingography.

Hysterosalpingography, on the other hand, gives visual evidence of many tubal disorders in addition to obstruction which are related to infertility and sterility. By

* From the Department of Obstetrics and Gynecology, Northwestern University Medical School and the Department of Obstetrics and Gynecology, Passavant Memorial Hospital, Chicago, Illinois.

means of hysterosalpingography it is possible to diagnose tubal diverticula (Fig. 1), tubal tuberculosis, partial tubal occlusion and certain tubal anomalies. Again, it is hoped that rapidly absorbing, non-irritating media, which do not produce foreign body reactions, will soon completely replace oily preparations in the performance of hysterosalpingography.

Inasmuch as tubal spasm may create a false impression of tubal occlusion on either hysterosalpingography or insufflation it is advisable to repeat either or both procedures when there is unexplained tubal blockage.

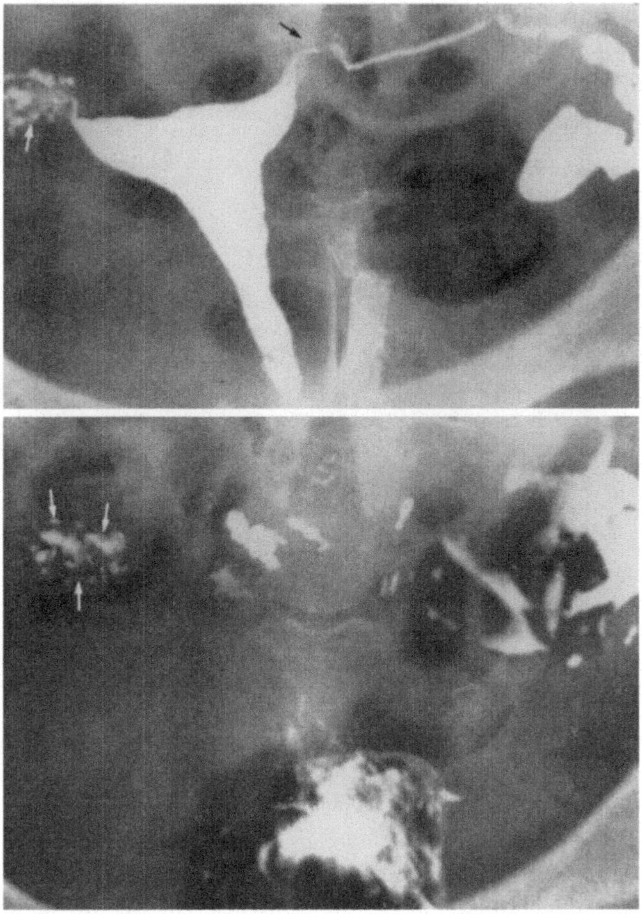

Fig. 1. *Top*, Trabeculation is present in left tubal isthmus (white arrow) with slight, similar changes in the right tube (black arrow). *Bottom*, In a delayed film, taken 1 h later, the medium persists in extraluminal channels (arrows). From SIEGLER, A.: *Hysterosalpingography*. New York: Hoeber Medical Division, Harper and Row, Publishers 1968

There is little doubt that 8 or 16 mm cineuterosalpingography would be a valuable tool for the diagnostician. Cineroentgenography has been of great help in the study of other areas of the body and has been used a few times in the diagnosis of infertility. However, the amount of radiation the ovaries receive during the process of making even a short film is large enough to make its application undesirable. Instead, the uterus and tubes are studied fluoroscopically during the injection of the media and serial films, exposed at significant times, are able to satisfactorily identify abnormalities of uterine and tubal structure and the location of tubal stenoses or obstructions.

It is a moot question whether or not the conceptus is nourished by the tubal secretions. It is known that the tubal mucosa does elaborate monosaccharides during the period the fertilized egg is in the tube. At present we know of no way to evaluate this physiologic component of the reproductive process.

I will not discuss tubal perfusion because I note that Dr. FIKENTSCHER is going to talk about that subject.

Abnormalities of the uterine corpus which interfere with conception are rare. They are much more likely to prevent nidation or to cause abortion. Lesser degrees of uterine growth failure with hypoplasia or persistence of an adolescent cervico-corporeal structural relationship are encountered in infertile women but they are, most often, signs of impaired ovarian function rather than a fault of uterine growth. The role of imperfect paramesonephric duct fusion in the etiology of abortion is well known.

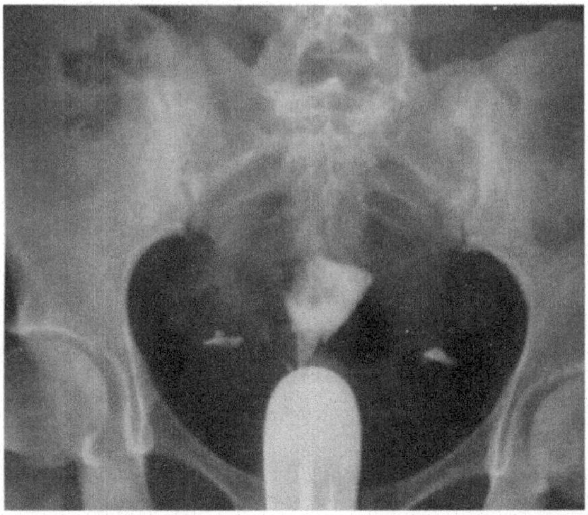

Fig. 2. Hysterogram demonstrates an oval defect in the corpus. A submucus myoma was found at hysterotomy. The patient had had hypermenorrhea and had been infertile for 6 years. Myomectomy was followed by two normal pregnancies

It has often been said that uterine myomas are associated with decreased fecundity but a really satisfactory explanation as to why intramural and subserous tumors interfere with reproduction has never been offered. It is easy to understand why a submucous tumor may do so. The endometrium over such a neoplasm is often so distorted that no self-respecting conceptus would ever consider implanting on it; or the tumor may, perhaps, act as an intrauterine device. Be that as it may, the diagnosis of lesser uterine anomalies, of endometrial synechiae and of uterine tumors, particularly submucous myomas, are essential considerations in infertility cases of obscure etiology. The value of hysteroroentgenography in the diagnosis of such problems (Fig. 2) is undisputed.

The technique of hysteroroentgenography is too well known to require discussion here. It may be well to emphasize, however, that overdistention of the uterus by the injected media or air bubbles in the uterine cavity may lead to erroneous diagnoses.

Hysterotomy may be required to confirm the roentgenographic diagnosis when there is a small submucous myoma that cannot be palpated manually.

The secretory activity of the endometrium is the mechanism which supplies the young conceptus with the nutritive substances it must have before and immediately after implantation. These substances are contained in the endometrial extracellular fluid and, presumably, the free fluid on the surface of the endometrium. Nutrients, vitamins and enzymes have been identified. The metabolism of some of these substances has been studied. That of the carbohydrates has been explored, particularly by EDWARD HUGHES. Alkaline phosphatase and glycogen in the endometrium and the secretion within the endometrial glands in the postovulatory phase apparently are responses to normal ovarian hormonal activity. HUGHES and his coworkers demonstrated aberrations in carbohydrate metabolism in the endometrium of patients with

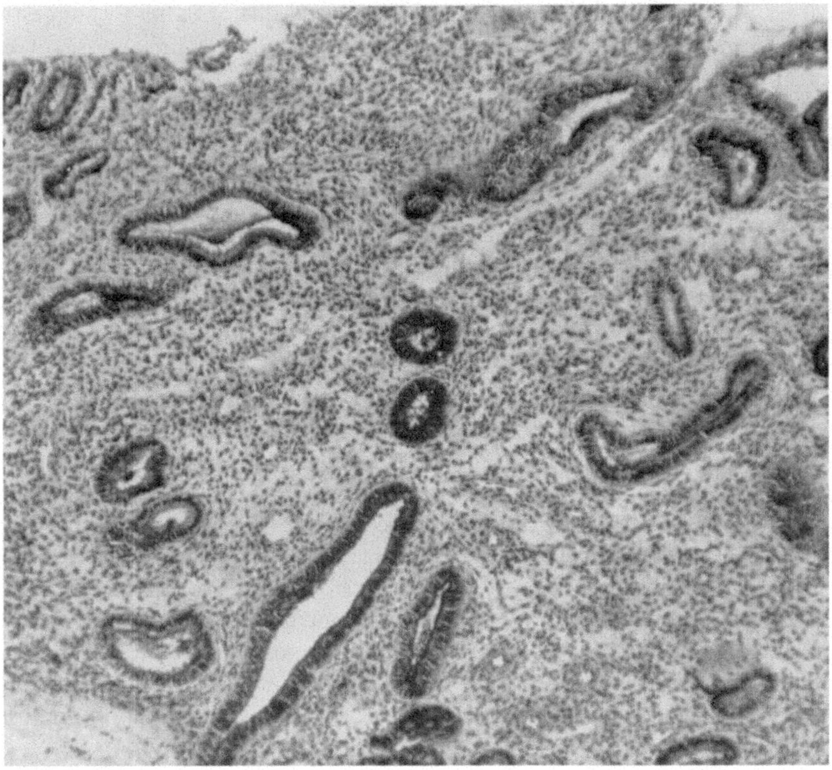

Fig. 3. The presence of alkaline phosphatase is indicated by dark granules in the epithelium and lumens of the endometrial glands (Gomori stain). From HUFFMAN, J.: Gynecology and Obstetrics. Philadelphia: W. B. Saunders Company 1962

histories of infertility and abortion. They found that the endometrium of women who were infertile contained an adequate amount of alkaline phosphatase but no glycogen. It is interesting to note that 84% of HUGHES' patients who were infertile showed a deficiency in endometrial glycogenesis although it did reveal secretory changes.

Studies of the histochemical reactions of the endometrium would therefore seem worthwhile in obscure problems of infertility. Endometrium for alkaline phosphatase and glycogen studies is obtained by biopsy on the 10. or 12. postovulatory day. The tissues are fixed in 95% alcohol. The Gomori technique is used to stain the sections to be examined for alkaline phosphatase (Fig. 3).

At the present time we have no way of determining the effect of the uterine secretions on the spermatozoa which migrate through the uterus on their way to the uterine tube. Presumably they are in a salutary environment. Nevertheless, relatively few male cells live to reach the uterine tube. The possibility that in some cases the secretions from the endometrial glands may have a deleterious effect on spermatozoa warrants consideration and would be a worthwhile subject for investigation.

The competency of the internal cervical os usually is not considered to be a necessary part of an infertility diagnostic study. It is not until the patient has suffered several late abortions or premature labors that incompetency of the internal os is suspected. The demonstration of a thin area in the upper portion of the anterior cervical wall by digital palpation over an intracervical dilator is highly suggestive. I also wish to mention the value of hysterography in making the diagnosis of an incompetent internal os (Fig. 4).

We have made relatively little progress in the diagnosis of cervical factors in infertility since J. Marion Sims (1866) first described the examination of postcoital cervical secretion. The identification of appreciable numbers of motile spermatozoa in cervical mucus for a number of hours after coitus is proof not only that there is no cervical barrier to sperm migration but that the sperm themselves are viable and, presumably, fertile. The value of the Sims-Huhner test as an index of the husband's fecundity, ideally performed after 4 days of continence, is not sufficiently appreciated. Furthermore, the admonition that one negative test may be misleading is not always kept in mind.

In vitro study of the penetration of the cervical secretions by the spermatozoa is of value when repeated Sims-Huhner tests are unsatisfactory. The simple procedure consists of placing a drop of the husband's seminal fluid inside a ring of cervical mucus. Microscopic examination of the preparation will give some idea of the interaction between the sperm and the cervical secretion. Failure of penetration by the spermatozoa presumably may be caused by hostile factors in the cervical mucus or the spermatozoa may be weak. The test does not differentiate between the two. Control preparations can be made using the husband's sperm and the cervical secretion from a women who is known to be fertile or by using the wife's secretion and seminal fluid from a fertile man. Such tests are not conclusive; they are helpful in those unusual instances where a cervical factor is thought to be responsible for the patient's infertility.

The presence of glairy, crystalline cervical mucus demonstrating *Spinnbarkeit* during the ovulatory phase of the cycle (Fig. 5) is an obvious indicator of cervical normalcy. The formation of fern-like patterns in the dried mucus at the time of ovulation, as demonstrated by La Paz, is a further indicator that the cervical secretions are normal. Such secretions presumably favor sperm migration. On the other hand, the cervical canal, when filled with a thick, viscid secretion at midcycle, may be a barrier instead of a passageway for the spermatozoa. Obviously, study of the cervical mucus and evaluation of the cervical secretions are important parts of the examination of the infertile women.

The possibility that clear, crystalline cervical mucus could, of itself, be hostile to spermatozoa would seem inconceivable yet there are patients who seem to exhibit such a state. Although its chemical composition is not precisely known, cervical mucus exhibits several specific characteristics. Those characteristics which are best understood have to do with its physical rheological properties. But these are not specific. *Spinnbarkeit* varies from patient to patient and from cycle to cycle. Fern

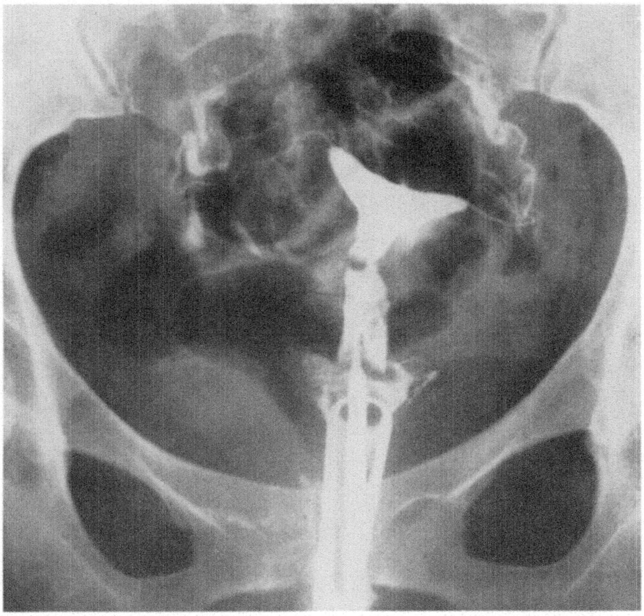

Fig. 4. Incompetent internal cervical os. Patient had had four late abortions. The isthmic canal measures more than 1 cm in width. An incompetent os was demonstrated surgically. Following cervicoplasty she had an uneventful term pregnancy

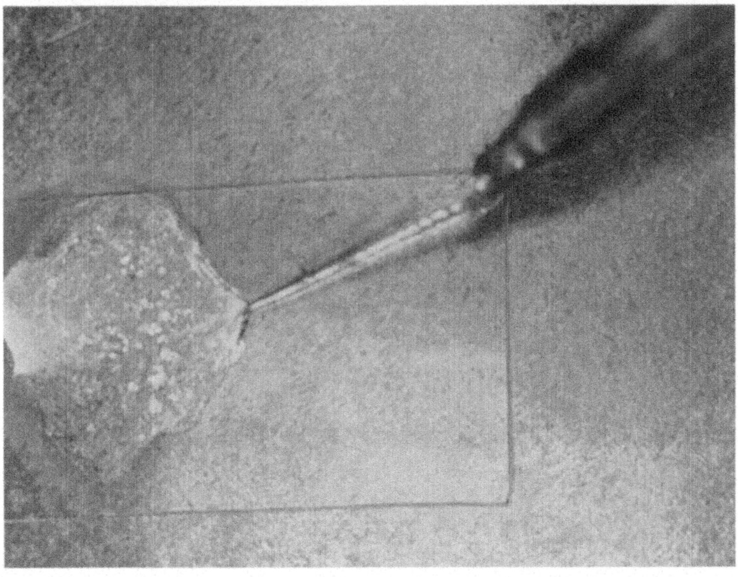

Fig. 5. *Spinnbarkeit* is demonstrated by lifting a thread of cervical secretion from a glass slide with a pipet

formation depends on electrolyte concentration and is not necessarily an indicator of specific organic events. It occurs, however, under the influence of estrogen and often does not occur in mucus from infected glands. We have yet to develop the sophisticated techniques which are needed to determine the chemical, enzymatic and immuno-

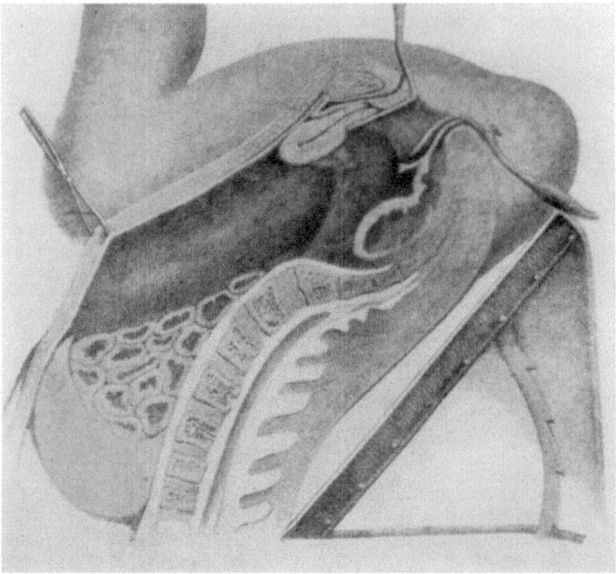

A

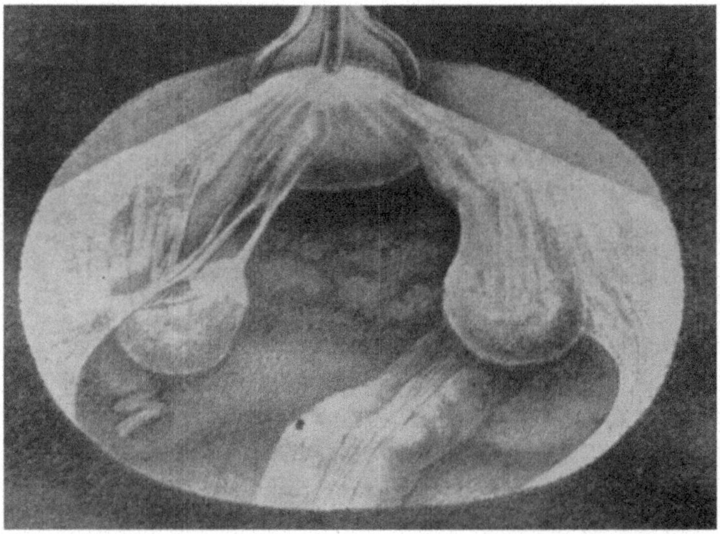

B

Fig. 6. A—B. Colpotomy for visualization of the pelvic viscera was first described by von Ott (1903). A Illustration from von Ott's original paper showing wide colpotomy incision, use of long vaginal retractors and patient's pelvis markedly elevated. B An illustration from von Ott's paper demonstrating the ease with which the pelvis could be visualized; there are adhesions about the uterine tubes and ovaries logical reactions of the cervical mucus. We will not be able to deal competently with cervical factors in infertility until the exact composition of normal and pathological cervical mucus is known as well as the process for their biosynthesis.

Many things may alter normal cervical secretions and interfere with sperm migration. Most often the absence of crystalline midcycle secretion indicates defective hormonal stimulation. The role of chronic endocervicitis in the interference of sperm migration merits emphasis. Chronic infections, whether they are secondary to partial obstruction and poor drainage or are residues of specific disease, may cause a persistent mucopurulent discharge which blocks the cervical canal. The inflammatory reactions interfere with the normal alterations in the cervical secretion. Conization or other surgery on the cervix and excessive electrical and chemical cauterization may destroy the cervical mucosa with the loss of necessary cervical secretion.

I find it difficult to accept the thesis that cervical polyps, a small cervical os or a nabothian follicle cyst will block a cervical canal to the point where the spermatozoa cannot find a passageway. Admittedly, the long, narrow, adolescent type of cervix with a pin-point os which is characteristic of uterine hypoplasia may be inimical to sperm transport but such a structure, in most cases, is the result of ovarian hypofunction rather than failure of cervical development.

There are, in addition, occasional instances when the diagnosis of uterotubal factors which adversely affect reproduction may not be evident by insufflation or hysterosalpingography. In these diagnostic problems culdoscopy, devised by DECKER, and colpotomy are of value. Culdoscopy has the advantage of simplicity, of returning the patient to her normal activities within a short time and of safety. Use of fiber optic sources has improved the clarity and extent of visualization and tubal and ovarian disease can be diagnosed with considerable accuracy.

Colpotomy, first described by VON OTT (1903), has the disadvantage of being a surgical procedure which requires several days' hospitalization. It is, however, associated with a minimal degree of surgical risk and gives the operator not only excellent visualization of the internal genitalia (Fig. 6) but also the opportunity to perform necessary corrective procedures.

There are cases in which every diagnostic procedure has been performed without uncovering a reason for the patient's infertility. Exploratory laparotomy merits consideration in carefully selected cases of this type because unsuspected uterine, tubal or ovarian pathology will be uncovered in an appreciable number of them.

Conclusion

The physician, when he considers the role of uterotubal factors in infertility and sterility, needs to know whether the patient's cervical canal affords a friendly environment for the passage of spermatozoa, whether the region of the internal os is competent to retain a conceptus within the uterine cavity, whether the endometrium offers a favorable environment for its growth and whether the uterine tubes not only are unobstructed avenues for the transport of the zygote but also have the necessary peristalic movements to propel the ovum on its way. He has available a number of roentgenographic and other techniques to help him assess the patient's reproductive potential. This has been a brief and necessarily panoramic review of those techniques. The procedures mentioned included: Sims-Huhner postcoital test; in vitro study of cervical-seminal hostility; study of the rheological and physical characteristics of the cervical secretions; roentgenographic study of cervical competency; hysterography;

histochemical study of endometrium; endometrial culture; uterotubal insufflation; uterotubal perfusion; hysterosalpingography; culdoscopy; colpotomy and laparatomy.

References

BANG, J.: Acta obstet. gynec. scand. **29**, 383 (1950).
BÉCLÈRE, C., et G. FAYOLLE: L'Hystérosalpingographie. Paris: Masson et Cie 1961.
BUXTON, C. L., and L. MASTROIANNI: Fertil. and Steril. **14**, 284 (1963).
CAREY, W. H.: Amer. J. Obstet. Dis. Wom. **69**, 462 (1914).
COHEN, M. R., I. F. STEIN, and B. M. KAYE: Fertil. and Steril. **3**, 201 (1952).
DECKER, A.: Culdoscopy. Philadelphia: F. A. DAVIS: 1967.
—, and T. CHERRY: Amer. J. Surg. **64**, 40 (1944).
DE PAZ, A. C., JR.: Fertil. and Steril. **4**, 137 (1953).
GOLDBERT, B., and H. W. JONES: Proc. Soc. exp. Biol. (N.Y.) **83**, 45 (1953).
HEUSER, C.: Lancet **1925 II,** 1111.
HUGHES, E. C.: Amer. J. Obstet. Gynec. **49**, 10 (1945).
JEFFCOATE, T. N. A., and J. K. WETSON: N. Y. St. J. Med. **56**, 680 (1956).
JOHNSTONE, J. W.: J. Obstet. Gynec. Brit. Emp. **65**, 208 (1958).
LASH, A. F., and S. R. LASH: Amer. J. Obstet. Gynec. **59**, 68 (1950).
LUDLOW, I.: Cleveland med. J. **8**, 398 (1909).
PALMER, R., et M. LACOMME: Gynéc. et Obstét. **47**, 905 (1948).
PLATT, H. A.: Ann. N.Y. Acad. Sci. **130**, 925 (1966).
POMMERENKE, W. T.: Amer. J. Obstet. Gynec. **52**, 1032 (1946).
POCHER, P., et J. VARANGOT: Bull. Fed. Gynéc. Obstrt. franç. **7**, 44 (1955).
PULLMAN, I., and J. S. LAUGHLIN: Gonadal dose produced by the medical use of X-rays. National Acad. Sci., Nat. Research Council, Washington 1957.
RINDFLEISCH, W.: Klin. Wschr. **47**, 780 (1910).
RÖNTGEN, W. C.: S.-B. physik. med. Ges. Wurzburg **137**, 132 (1895).
RUBIN, I. C.: Zbl. Gynäk. **38**, 658 (1914).
— Amer. J. Obstet. Gynec. **14**, 557 (1927).
RUBOVITS, F. G., N. R. COOPERMAN, and A. F. LASH: Amer. J. Obstet. Gynec. **66**, 269 (1953).
SIEGLER, A. M.: Fertil. and Steril. **6**, 432 (1955).
— Hysterosalpingography. New York: Haeber Medical Division, Harper and Row, Publishers 1967.
STALLWORTHY, J.: Fertil. and Steril. **14**, 284 (1963).
STEIN, I. F.: Surg. Gynec. Obstet. **42**, 83 (1926).
—, and R. A. ARENS: Amer. J. Obstet. Gynec. **18**, 130 (1929).
TOMPKINS, P. T.: Amer. J. Obstet. Gynec. **83**, 1599 (1962).
VON OTT, D.: Mschr. Geburtsh. Gynäk. **18**, 645 (1903).

Utero-tubal Insufflation and Perfusion

R. FIKENTSCHER

The diagnostic grasp of the tubal factor as the cause of female sterility presents many problems today. We have to keep in mind that the present available methods of examination may discover the impassibility of the tubes. But in no way can they show us other disorders of the physiological functions of the tubes which may be important in the occurrance of pregnancy. In other words we can discover very well the different forms of mechanical obstructions in the medium of transportation which the tubes represent. We cannot say with certainty anything about the finer functions of the tubes; for example, whether they are capable enough to transport and nourish the eggs. (Their importance was presented in the report of Dr. MULLIGAN.)

Of course the discovery, the prognostic judgement and the possible elimination of the mechanical obstructions in the tubes play a dominant role in the treatment of sterility. In the following we will show the diagnostic procedure of the Second Frauenklinik of the University of Munich and how we are endeavouring to expand the therapeutic possibilities with hydropertubation.

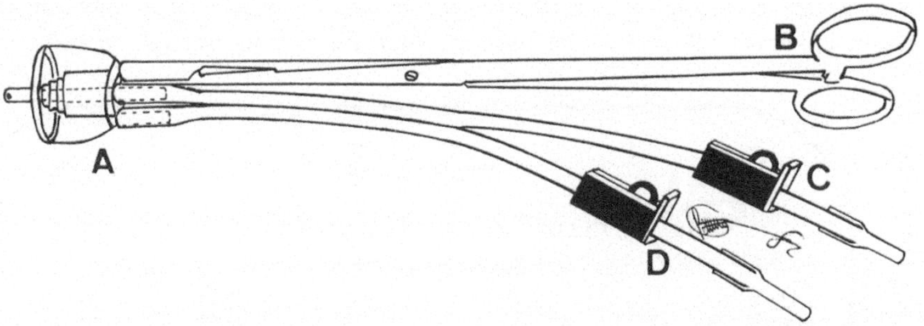

Fig. 1 A—D. Cervix Adapter according to FIKENTSCHER and SEMM for insufflation of carbon-dioxide gas, hysterosalpingography or hydropertubation (flexible disposable instrument made of transparent plastic). A Cervix Adapter bell, B forceps to direct the Cervix Adapter into the vagina, C insufflation tube with "roll-on" clamp, D Vacuum tube with "roll-on" clamp

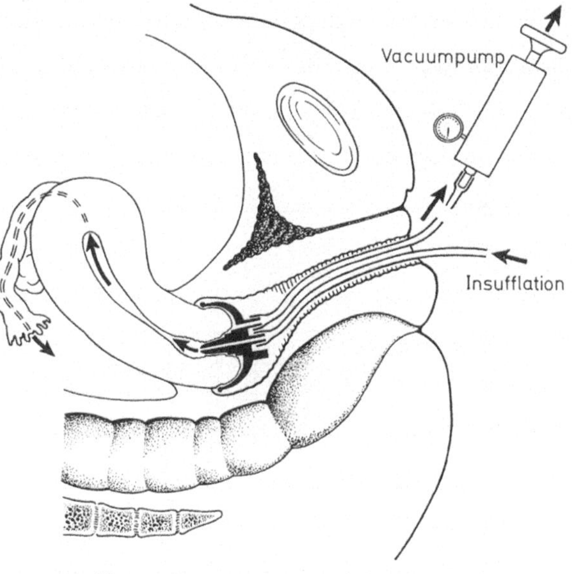

Fig. 2. Cervix Adapter according to FIKENTSCHER and SEMM in situ. The flexible instrument seals the cervical canal by suction and is used for carbon-dioxide gas pertubation, hysterosalpingography and hydropertubation

For the patency test of the tubes *the utero-tubal insufflation* is of primary importance in our clinic:

After sealing the cervical canal, carbon dioxide gas is blown through the uterus and the tubes. The pressure and the quantity of the carbon dioxide gas are precisely controlled by an apparatus (Fig. 1).

Our cervix-adapter serves as the sealing instrument. Together with its flexible tubes it forms a handy system and seals the cervical canal through suction (Fig. 2).

The low pressure is produced by a little vacuum pump and controlled with a manometer. The cervix-adapter is a disposable instrument.

The suction on the portio causes neither tissue damage nor pain. The examination can be performed without narcosis. The flexible tubes present no change in the topographical position of the uterus and the adnexes.

The necessary pressure for persufflation of the tubes is produced by our universal pertubation apparatus (Fig. 3). The pressure increase is fractionated, starting with

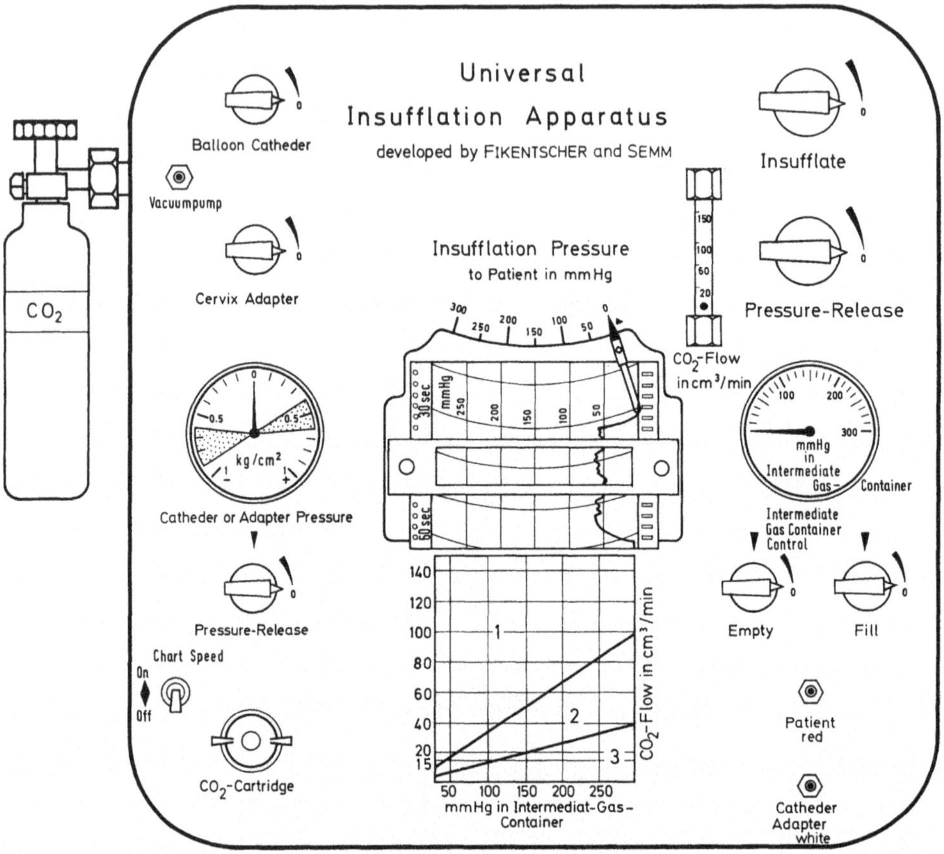

Fig. 3. Universal Pertubation Apparatus according to Fikentscher and Semm with graphic registration of the pressure values during the carbon dioxide gas insufflation; atraumatic sealing of the cervical canal by double-balloon-catheter or Cervix Adapter

50 mm of mercury. The suspension height of the ball in the flow meter (Fig. 4) indicates how many ccm of carbon dioxide gas flow through the tubes into the abdomen. Corresponding to the suspension height of the ball we are able to infer from our diagram the following degrees of patency:

1. normal patency,
2. difficult patency,
3. and stenosed patency.

The comparison of the obtained oscillogram with its characteristic curve traces makes a broad diagnostic possible (Fig. 5).

Consequently, there are specific curve pictures which are very typical of the different morphological and functional changes of the tubes. The characteristic oscillogram:

by normal bilateral tubal patency,
by unilateral tubal patency,
by tubal or uteral spasm,
by tubal stenosis,
by unilateral or bilateral hydrosalpinx,
by intramural occlusion.

The eventual occurrence of pain during the insufflation together with such oscillograms are important differential diagnostic hints: If the insufflation of carbon dioxide gas up to 300 mm of mercury is possible without any special reference of pain on the part of the patient, it is highly probable that the occlusion is intramural. The gas in the uterus is only felt as dull pressure. However, if the patient complains of pain at a pressure of 100 to 150 mm of mercury, the occlusion is without a doubt

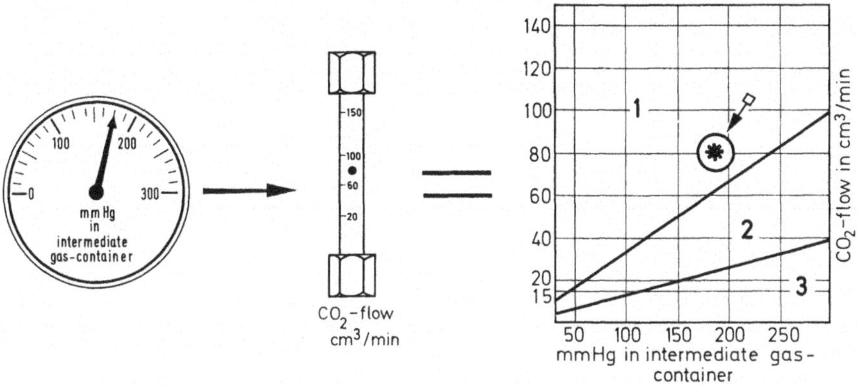

Fig. 4. Determination of the degree of tubal patency by two values: insufflation pressure (in this case the manometer shows 180 mm of mercury) and gas flow (in this case 80 ml/min). The diagram shows the first degree of tubal patency for both values

peripheral. Peritoneal pain develops from tubal inflation. We observe these peritoneal pains from hydrosalpinx, from peripheral occlusions and from peritubal adhesions. These different tubal changes show different diagrams.

The diagrammatic indications and the degree of persufflation in connection with the pain diagnostic are very valuable.

The presented technique of a utero-tubal insufflation represents the smallest degree of a surgical procedure necessary to clarify the tubal factor. This technique makes it possible for us to acquire essential information about the tubal situation and, therefore, in our clinic it is the first diagnostic stage in the clarification of the tubal factor.

Surely the utero-tubal insufflation is not able to give definite information relative to some questions, for instance concerning the relationships of the tubal ostia to the ovary and the eventually existing obstructions there. In spite of these obstructions, sometimes almost normal diagrams are obtained.

As a further diagnosis of utero-tubal patency *the hysterosalpingography* is at our disposal. We are again using our flexible cervix-adapter which even for this purpose does not change the topographical situation. In addition it also makes possible a

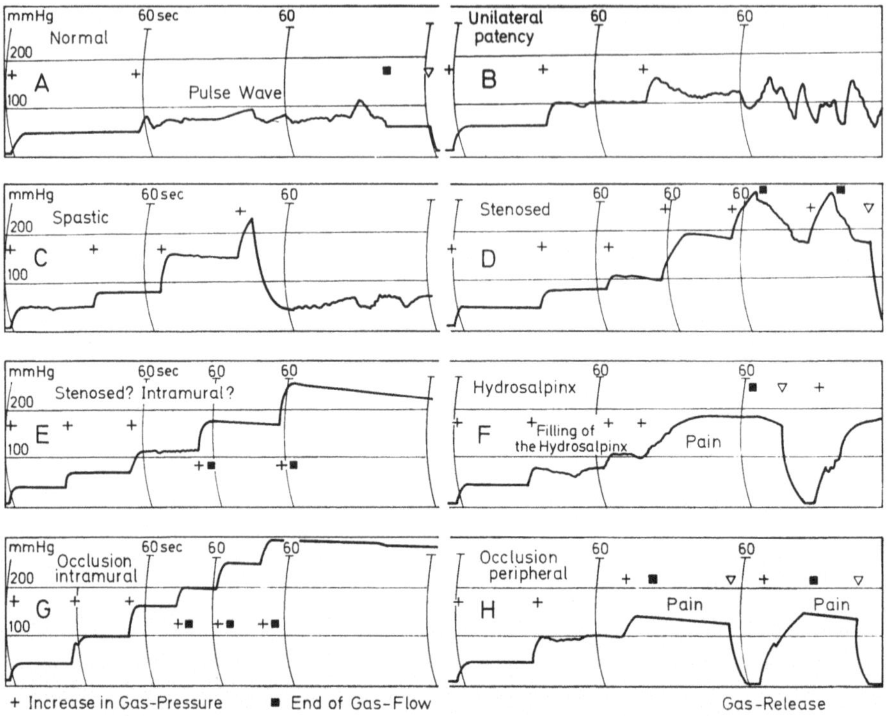

Fig. 5 A—H. Curve-traces obtained by pertubation of the tubes with the Universal Insufflation Apparatus by Fikentscher and Semm. A Normal bilateral patency of the tubes. After increase in pressure step by step for 1 min from 50 mm Hg to 75—100 mm Hgthe graph shows shallow oscillations modulated by oscillations of a higher frequency equal to the pulse frequency. Flow is 120 ml per min at 300 mm Hg in the intercontainer. B Unilateral patency of the tubes. The gas passage is set at 100 mm Hg. After a gradual increase of the pressure to 110 mm Hg the graph shows high amplitudes, which are also modulated by pulse-waves. Flow is 100 ml per min at 300 mm Hg in the intercontainer. C Spasm of the tubes or the uterus. With spastic patients the pressure can be painlessly increased to 200 to 250 mm Hg step by step in intervals of 1 min each. A sudden decrease of the pressure graph and flow, as in A, is typical. D, E Peripheral or intramural stenosis. During gradual increase of the pressure the graph already shows a slight gas flow at 100 mm Hg. After the gas is stopped, the flow graph slopes down at an angle of about 45 degrees. Flow is less than 40 ml per min at 300 mm Hg in the intercontainer. F Unilateral or bilateral hydrosalpinx. After a graduated increase of pressure the graph at first is normal. The trace, however, soon flattens out. In most cases the insufflation has to be stopped at 150 mm Hg because the pain becomes unbearable. If insufflation is repeated, a sudden increase of pressure causes pain as the tubes are still filled with gas. G Intramural occlusion of the tubes. After each increase of pressure the graph shows a straight trace in the same pressure range. The slight pressure decrease after the gas flow is stopped is caused by the gas resorption by the endometrium. H Peripheral occlusion of the tubes. After a graduated increase of the pressure to about 100 mm Hg a further increase of pressure to 150 mm Hg or at most 200 mm Hg causes unbearable pain. This can be repeatedly reproduced by releasing the gas and then increasing the pressure to 150 or 200 mm Hg. A and F Peritubal intergrowths. If the pain already starts during procedure A after 1.5 to 2 min or earlier and is unilateral or bilateral without a decrease in the flowing gas volume (as in F), the diagnosis is peritubal intergrowths. This phenomenon will be observed in most cases after an insufflated gas volume of 150 cc. In these cases the shoulder pain will be observed to be delayed or will not occur at all

clear observation of the cervical canal and the configuration of the entire uterus cavity in the contrast picture. The course of the tubes and their patency are diagnosed either immediately with the X-ray screen or in the X-ray picture (through the first or later pictures after 30 to 60 min).

The type of spreading of the contrast substance in the lesser or true pelvis gives valuable hints. Sharp straight lined shadows of the contrast substance indicate perisalpingitic adhesions (Fig. 6).

Even the HSG cannot give definite information about the anatomic-functional connections of the tubes, especially their ampulla ends to the ovaries and the other neighboring organs. Therefore, and because of possible actinogene injuries, we normally use it only in cases for the necessary clarification of the cervix and uterus cavity situation in the form of a hysterography.

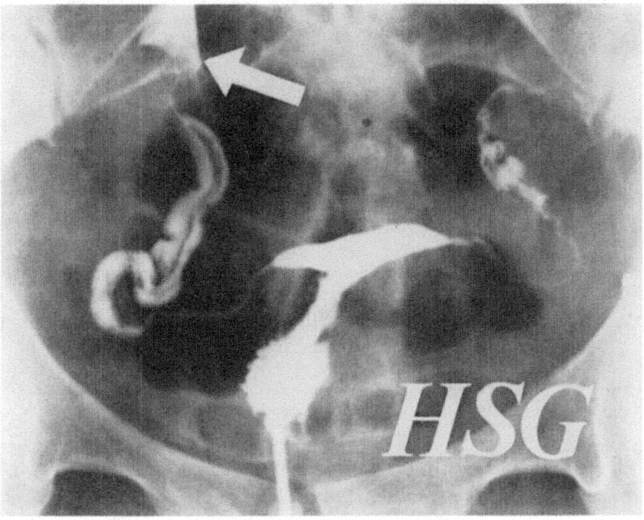

Fig. 6. Hysterosalpingography of 32 year old woman. The hysterosalpingogram gives a precise picture of the lumina of cervix, uterus and tubes. The straightlined shadows (mark) indicate perisalpingitic adhesions. An exact diagnosis of these adhesions, however, can not be made by hysterosalpingography

In view of the prognosis and the assessment of the chances of success of surgical treatment of a tubal factor, we regard *the gynecological pelviscopy* as the best diagnostic method.

In association with our carbon dioxide persufflation or a chromopertubation we are in the position to answer the above mentioned questions.

The gynecological pelviscopy, still widely regarded as very severe, relatively dangerous and technically difficult, has become a routine method today due to the essential improvement of the instruments.

The technique developed by Semm in my clinic makes use of the following:

1. The navel pit is the portal of entry for the carbon dioxide gas and for the pelviscope (Fig. 7).

2. Three technical improvements:

a) The cold light, in spite of its high illumination, does not endanger the body cavity.

b) The optic with its extremely small systems makes it possible to construct very thin pelviscopes.

c) Through the automatisation of the gas filling process, a false inflow of the gas is immediately indicated on the apparatus.

3. A newly developed inflexible perforated vacuum intrauterine sound by SEMM (Fig. 8) is sucked by means of low pressure on to the portio vaginalis. The instrument

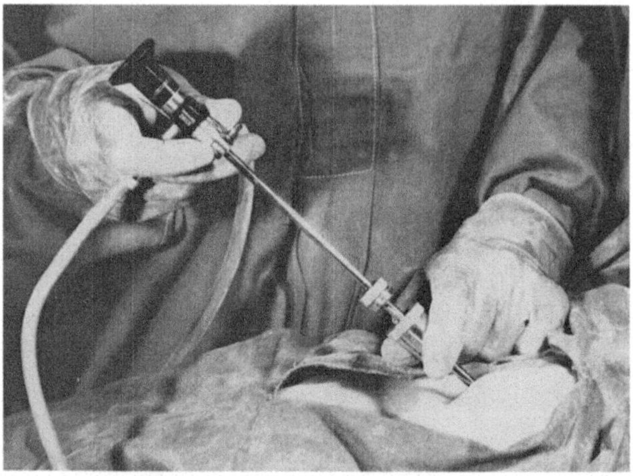

Fig. 7. Introduction of a 4 mm Hopkins-endoscope through the navel pit for "Gynecological Pelviscopy". The abdominal cavity is filled with carbon-dioxide gas, using the CO_2-Pneu-Automatic according to SEMM

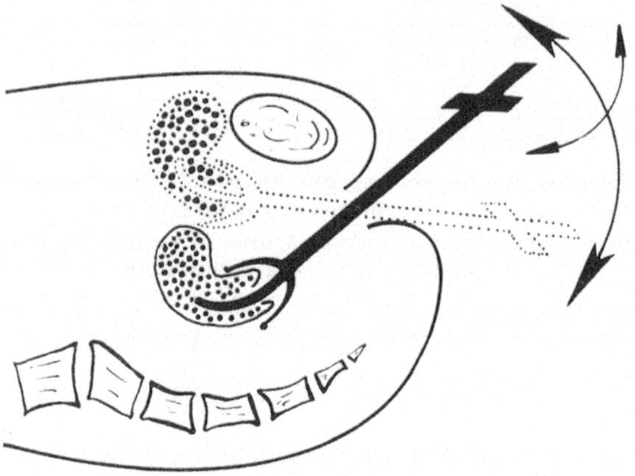

Fig. 8. Vacuum intrauterine sound developed by SEMM, permitting the three-dimensional movement of the uterus during the "Gynecological Pelviscopy". Carbon-dioxide gas or indigocarmine solution can be brought into the uterine cavity by the multiperforated intrauterine sound

permits the movement of the uterus in different directions during endoscopic observation and simultaneously insufflates gas or blue colored solution as a test of tubal patency. The mobility of the uterus by means of the sound, for example by elevating it and the additional chromopertubation (Fig. 9), permit an exhaustive observation with the pelviscope.

The perfusion of liquids through Müller's ducts has been used for many years as the only or additional diagnostic method. Hydropertubation (perfusion) as a remedy has become increasingly important in latter times. We obtain an essential improvement through "*repeated long acting-hydropertubation*". Considering that the instilled solutions with the generally used techniques of hydropertubation remain only a short time in the genital tract, we developed a special method. In principle the instilled

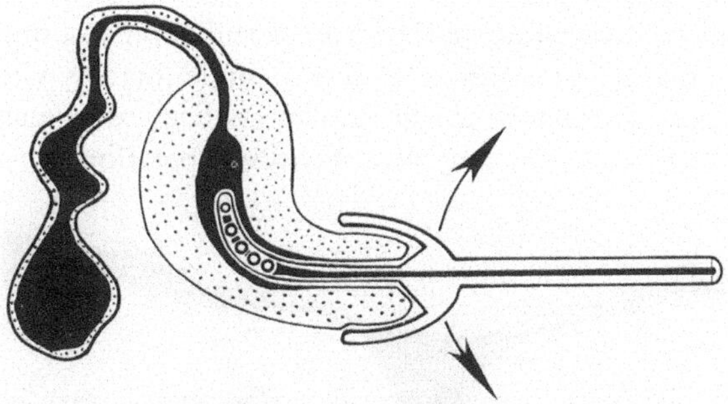

Fig. 9. Chromopertubation: The uterine cavity and the sactosalpinx are filled with blue solution at a pressure of 150 mm mercury. The endoscopic observation shows a thick blue tube. The "Gynecological Pelviscopy" in connection with the Chromopertubation allow a perfect diagnostic evaluation of the Fallopian tubes

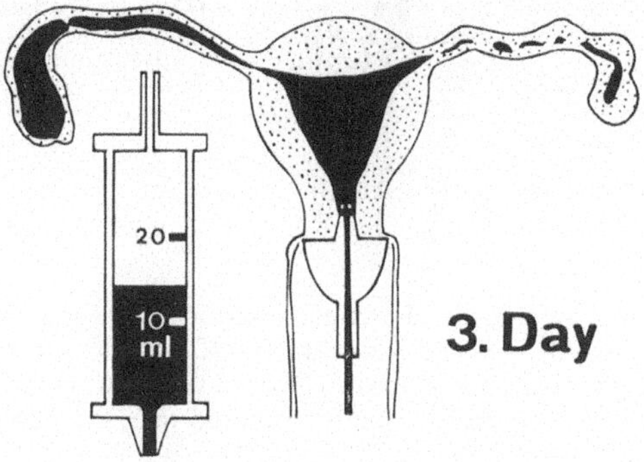

Fig. 10. Repeated Long-acting Hydropertubation: situation on the third day: 7 ml are instilled. The liquid has reached the ampullary end of the right tube, the left tube shows only a slightly filled lumen

solution *remains* for several hours (on the average 6 to 8 h) in those places where the therapeutic effects are desired (Fig. 10) and a *repetition* of such instillations is performed 6 or 8 days in the first half of the cycle.

Again we use our flexible disposable cervix-adapter which by means of low pressure is sucked onto the portio vaginalis. The instillation of the solution succeeds under a controlled pressure of 100 to 200 mm of mercury. The reflux of the solution is prevented as long as the adapter is not removed (Fig. 11).

The following instillation solution consisting of a mixture of 0.4 g of streptomycin-sulfate, 0.01 g of hydrocortison-acetate and 0.04 g of procaine-hydrochloride with the addition of 10 ml of distilled water has been approved by us.

In addition 25 C.Hb.E. α-chymotrypsin are dissolved in 5 ml of distilled water. Consequently this mixture has a combined antibacterial, antiphlogistic and fibrinolytic effect.

Especially, we want to mention that a repeated long acting-hydropertubation with our technique is well tolerated:

1. The procedure causes no special pains, as the instilled solution contains procaine and the vacuum fixating the adapter is decreased after the instillation.

2. We never observed a new or recurrent adnexitis.

3. Furthermore, by often repeated long acting-hydropertubation we found no evidence of local or general injury.

We perform our repeated long acting-hydropertubation as a preoperative as well as a postoperative measure, sometimes even as a single therapy without any surgical procedure. In one case we start the instillation immediately after menstruation, and in the other case the first or second day after the tubal operation.

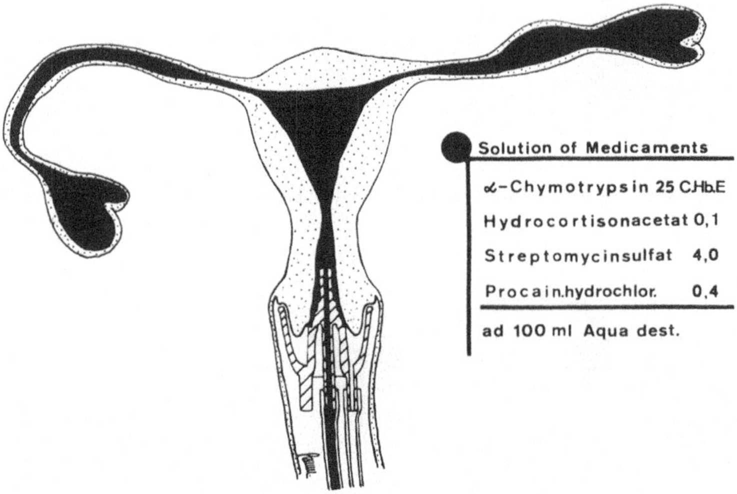

Fig. 11. Principle of the Long-acting Hydropertubation: Liquid is instilled into the tubes and the uterine cavity using the Cervix Adapter. The Cervix Adapter prevents the reflux of the solution for 6 to 8 h. During this procedure the vacuum for fixing the Cervix Adapter to the portio vaginalis is being lowered to —0.1 kg/cm²

The success of hydropertubation series on the obstructed tubes can be proved by the daily increasing quantity of the instillation. Usually the break through of the therapy solution into the free abdominal cavity occurs on the 5th or 6th day.

By the introduction of repeated long acting-hydropertubation the rate of postoperative tubes remaining open has increased considerably. In our operative material by the test of tubal patency with carbon dioxide gas after the third to fifth postoperative cycle the rate of re-occluded tubes decreased from 25% to nearly 10%. After we began to treat every tubal sterility operation with repeated long acting-hydropertubation the frequency of open tubes increased from 76% to 90%.

Our reported diagnostic method of utero-tubal insufflation and the repeated long acting hydropertubation is further illustrated in our films "The tubal diagnostic" and "The hydropertubation therapy".

References

FIKENTSCHER, R.: Geburtsh. u. Frauenheilk. **26**, 686 (1966).
— Z. Geburtsh. Gynäk. Suppl. **168**, 168 (1968).
—, u. K. SEMM: Geburtsh. u. Frauenheilk. **15**, 313 (1955).

— — Présentation d'un Appareil Universel pour I.U.T. et H.S.G. In: Société nationale pour l'étude de la Stérilité et de la Fécondité. La Fonction tubaire et ses Troubles, p. 65. Paris: Masson et Cie. 1956.
— — Arch. Gynäk. **188**, 184 (1956).
— — Gynéc. prat. **9**, 413 (1958).
— — Geburtsh. u. Frauenheilk. **18**, 161 (1958).
— — Beitrag zur Deutung der bei der utero-tubaren Persufflation erhaltenen Oscillationen. Proceedings of the IV. World Congress on Fertility and Sterility Vol. I., p. 949. Neapel 1958.
— — Geburtsh. u. Frauenheilk. **19**, 868 (1959).
— — Z. Geburtsh. Gynäk. **155**, 215 (1960).
Mohr, A. R., e J. Gomes da Silveira: Rev. Assoc. méd. Rio Gr. Sul **4**, 111 (1960).
Semm, K.: Prüfung der Tubendurchgängigkeit. In: Friedberg, V. F., K. G. Ober, K. Thomsen und J. Zander, Gynäkologie und Geburtshilfe, Vol. 1, p. 272. Stuttgart: Thieme 1968.
— Geburtsh. u. Frauenheilk. **27**, 1029 (1967).
— Diagnostic methods. In: Behrman, S. J., and R. Kistner, Progress in infertility, chapt. X/39. Boston/Mass.: Little Brown & Comp. 1968.

Restorative Surgery of the Tubes

(a study of 600 personal cases)

Raoul Palmer

Organic obstruction of the tubes is still in France the most frequent factor of persistent sterility (around 40%). *Pelvic adhesions* are also an important factor, isolated in 5 to 10%, associated with organic obstruction in 25% at least.

Statistical Evaluation of Results

My *personal global statistic* from 1942 to 1961, published in Vienna in 1964, included 489 tuboplasties, 306 with patency (62%), 105 with uterine pregnancy (21%) and 30 with extra-uterine pregnancy (6%).

Results by category of operation are much more difficult to establish, because quite often a different operation has been done on the right and the left side, and, if a uterine pregnancy occurs, it is difficult to assess which operation was successful. Therefore, we have selected, from our personal statistics until 1965, 600 unequivocal cases, where the same operation has been done on both sides (or on one side, the other tube being removed).

Pre-Operative Explorations

A recent hysterosalpingography with hydrosolubles is compulsory to visualize perfectly a) *the interstitial part of the tube* (especially in cases of proximal occlusion); b) *the folds of the ampulla* (if they are very irregular, the danger of tubal pregnancy is great).

A search for signs of latent tuberculosis is very important (we find in France 16% proved and 20% probable tuberculosis, and the results among 110 such cases operated by me, are: 2 tubal and *no* uterine pregnancy).

Laparoscopy is compulsory in cases of proximal occlusion (as more than 60% are associated with distal pathology); it is also very useful in distal occlusion, as it is the only way (besides laparotomy) to know the state of fimbria and ovary and the extension and density of adhesions. In most cases, we perform the laparotomy *just before* the operation.

Absolute contra-indications to tuboplasty were:

1. the known tuberculous origin of the obstruction; 2. other important and persistant factors in man or women; 3. tubes with narrow ampulla or multiple strictions at salpingography; 4. very dense adhesions at laparoscopy; 5. age above 37.

Temporary contra-indications were:

1. Subacute inflammation; 2. tubal pregnancy: in such cases we postpone tuboplasty for some months.

Tuboplasty must be as atraumatic as possible; the mucosa should never be caught with a forceps; any distension or traction should be avoided; atraumatic needles with 0000 nylon, or other non-reactive material, should be used. The instruments we use are those designed for ophthalmologic surgery. Gentleness and minutia are compulsory.

Operation is done just after menstruation, through a low Pfannenstiel incision; the uterus is anchored with two catguts placed in cross on the top.

Salpingolysis

Salpingolysis (the operative liberation of adhesions) is the first, and very important step. It should always be done under *total visual control* (changing side when necessary), and by section or resection with Knife or Scissors and never with the fingers.

It must be carried out methodically:

1. *The omentum* should first be separated completely from abdominal wall, bladder, uterus, tube and ovary;

2. *The intestines* should then be dissected cautiously, with immediate repair, if any injury;

3. *The adnexa* should be separated from the uterus and ligamentum latum progressively, with maximal caution at the inferior pole, where the end of the tube is often imbedded in dense adhesions.

Then, the whole adnexa can be brought upwards and the careful separation of the tube from the ovary is performed. Then the ovary is thoroughly "cleaned" from adhesive remnants. Adhesions between tubal loops are mostly respected, except when there is compression by a true fibrous band (v.i.).

Salpingolysis may sometimes be the whole operation.

In 26 cases of *bilateral* operative Salpingolysis for sterility of more than 3 years duration, we had 14 uterine pregnancies (56%) — most of them in the year.

Per-operative Exploration

Thorough per-operative exploration of the tubes includes:

1. *Inspection* of the distal end, to see what remains of the infundibulum; 2. *palpation*, to locate the indurated or thickened areas; 3. exploration of the infundibulum and ampulla with a No. 10 Nelaton catheter.

True study of patency should only be performed if doubt persists between *organic* or *spasmodic* stenosis or occlusion of the proximal portion of the tube. In such cases, we perform hydrotubation with Shirodkar's technique, but using blue dye and manometric control. If any doubt about spasm persists, I amp. hydergin is injected intra-venously.

A *tubal biopsy* should be done every time the operation is not confined to blunt separation of agglutinated fimbria, either by sending the resected parts, or taking a strip on the margin of section. The tubal biopsy is very important for the management of postoperative treatment, as it may show unsuspected tuberculosis, inflammatory active sclerosis, endometriosis, etc. *The importance of inflammatory sclerosis* must be emphazised: in a series of 108 ampullar salpin gostomies (in a study presented at Stockholm with JEAN DE BRUX in 1966) this pathology was present in 28 cases, with 22 re-occlusions, 1 E.U.P. (extra-uterine pregnancy) and only 1 U.P. (uterine pregnancy). On the contrary, 45 cases with simple sclerosis, gave only 14 re-occlusions, 9 U.P. and 6 E.U.P.

Codonolysis

Codonolysis (or fimbriolysis) consists in the blunt separation of agglutinated fimbriae, leading to the reshapening of the original ostium. It is the operation which gives the best results, everytime it is possible.

Sometimes, we find only *phimosis* of the infundibulum, and one can introduce into it a very fine Leriche forceps, and open it in various diameters, to de-agglutinate the fimbrial folds.

On other occasions, the peritoneal cover is continuous, but, after distension of the ampulla with hydrotubation, a slight depression, or a blue spot marks the site of the preexisting ostium. In such cases, Shirodkar's technique consists of crucial incision of the peritoneum alone (1 cm for each branch) and then the *codonolysis* as above described. Four stitches may help persistent extroversion of the fimbriae.

Our results with true codonolysis are, among 56 cases, 41 with patency (75%), 16 U.P. (29%) and 5 E.U.P. (9%).

Salpingostomy

Salpingostomy is the creation of a new opening in the tube, with or without resection of a part of it. It may be terminal, ampullar or isthmic.

Some facts should be remembered:

1. Persistence of a well patent ostium is a sine qua non condition of success.

2. There should also be some substitute to the fimbriae, that is some exterior mucous surface, with ciliated cells, to help the capture of the ovum.

3. It should preferably be in a position facilitating this capture.

4. The preserved portion of the ampulla should be sane.

But one should, cut away only the very dilated parts (more than the thumb), or the very thickened or sclerotic ones.

Terminal salpingostomy is done when the distal part of the tube is neither thickened nor too much distended. In most cases, we use a variant of Bonney's cuff technique: after vertical incision of the tubal end we put Bonney's clamp, and a cuff is easily obtained, and fixed with 5 or 6 well anchored stitches of nylon 0000 (Fig. 1).

When the cuff is impossible, we use Pollosson's technique, longitudinal dorsal incision, 25 to 30 mm long, and eversion of the mucosa by 8 to 12 stitches; the most distal stitch fixes the racket-shaped new ostium to the surface of the ovary (Fig. 2).

Among 123 cases of terminal salpingostomy of our 51 to 65 private patient series, we find 94 patencies (77%), 34 U.P. (27%) and 16 U.E.P. (13%). The results are about the same with the two varients.

Ampullar salpingostomy, though avoided when possible, is frequent in our series (148 cases).

Here too, we perform, when possible, a variant of *Bonney's cuff operation*, which we described in London in 1959: clamping of the ampulla as distally as possible; section and hemostasis of the meso salpinx; circular section of the peritoneum 2 cm from the clamp; section of the tube just besides the clamp; removal of the peritoneal cylinder; placing of Bonney's or Caplier's tubal clamp; making the cuff, and fixing it with

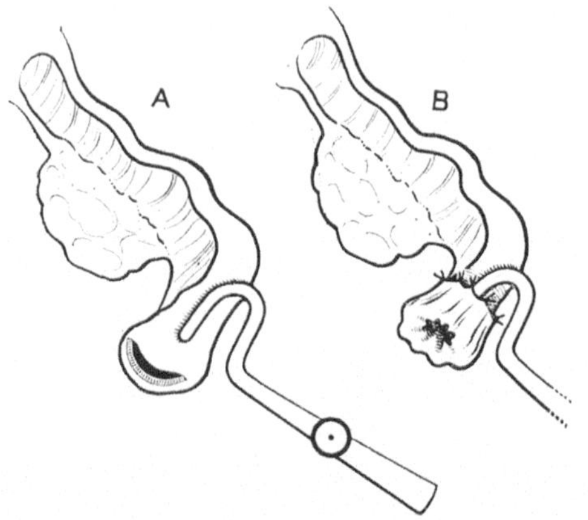

Fig. 1. Terminal salpingostomy by Bonney's cuff technique

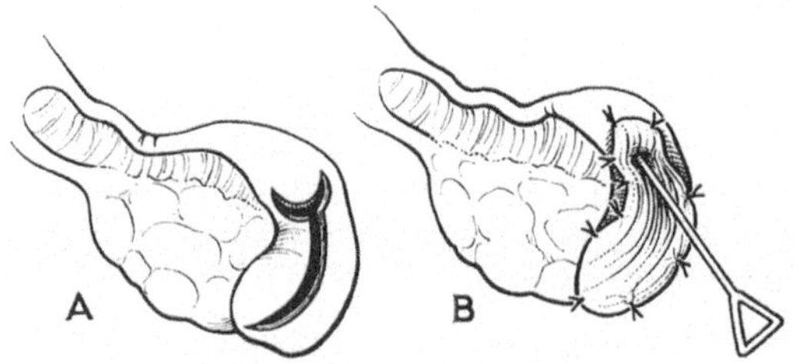

Fig. 2. Terminal salpingostomy ny Pollosson's racket technique

5 to 6 stitches of nylon 0000. Reconstruction of the tubo-ovarian ligament. The reason to remove the peritoneal cylinder is that it is the peritoneum which prevents the easy formation of the cuff, and good maintainance of it after operation (Fig. 3).

If the cuff is not possible, we use a variant of Dudley's operation, *Pollosson's racket-like salpingostomy*: after resection of the diseased distal part, a dorsal longitudinal incision, 25 to 35 mm long is performed. The extremity is anchored to the ovary by one solid silk stitch. Then the mucosa is everted by several fine silk sutures.

The 3 last years, we have also several times performed a *bivalve variant*, which gives a well-looking fimbria, and the results are encouraging (Fig. 4).

Among 148 cases of ampullar salpingostomy, we have obtained: 75 patencies (50%), 20 U.P. (13%) and 9 U.E.P. (6%).

If we differenciate between techniques, we find:

— for the cuff: 57 cases, 25 reocclusions (43%), 32 patencies (57%), 13 U.P. (23%), 4 E.U.P. (7%).

— for the racket-type: 71 cases, 42 re-obstructions (59%) only 29 patencies (41%), 3 U.P. (4%) and 3 E.U.P. (4%).

— for the bivalve: 20 cases, 6 re-obstructions (30%), 14 patencies (70%), 4 U.P. (20%) and 2 E.U.P. (10%).

These figures suggest that the cuff and the bivalve are better that the racket, but it is necessary to stress that the last was done only when the cuff was not possible, that is in the worst cases.

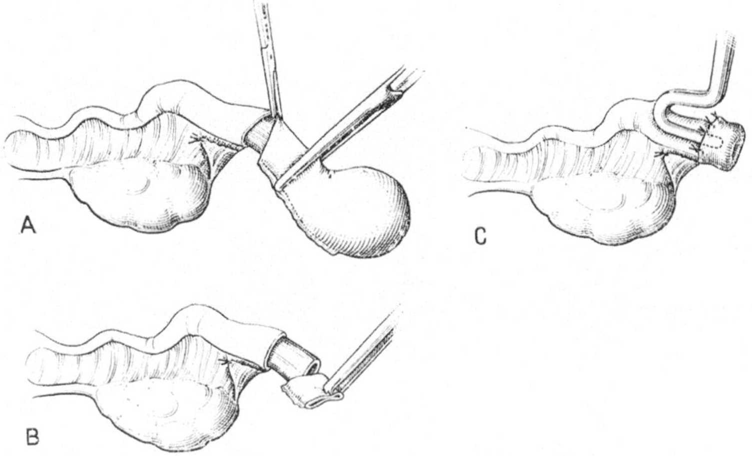

Fig. 3. Ampullar salpingostomy by the Bonney-Palmer cuff technique

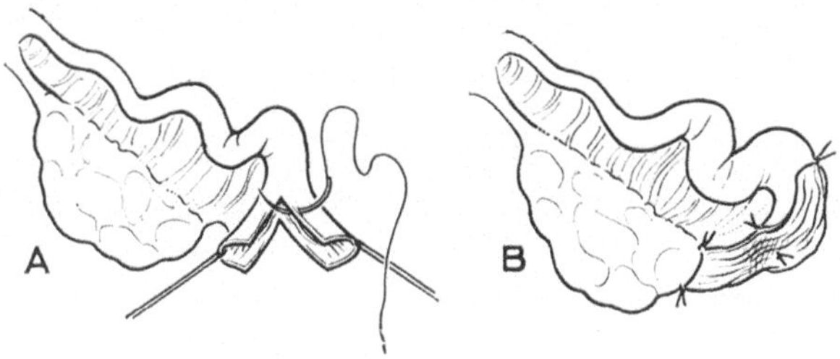

Fig. 4. Ampullar salpingostomy by the Palmer bivalve technique

Isthmic salpingostomy, either transversal or longitudinal, has never given any success in our hands in 29 cases and in most cases rapid reocclusion could be found.

An alternative to it should be subtotal linear salpingotomy, as advocated by CHALIER (1938).

We used this technique in 8 cases between 1938 and 1948, with three persistent patencies, and regret not to have tempted it in many cases, where we performed ovaro-uterine implantation.

Many types of prosthesis have been neggested, to avoid re-occlusion of the neostomy, including allantoid (GEPFERT 43) amnion (SNAITH 49) cholesterol (WESTMAN) polyethylene and silastic lubing and hoods (MULLIGAN 47, 53, 66).

Poly-ethylene tubing has never been used in our series. We have been favourably impressed by the results published with *Mulligan's silastic hoods*, claiming, in his last series of 45 cases, 81% patency, 27% U.P. and 8% E.U.P., but we have not yet used them, partly because of the necessity of a second operation after 3 months to remove the hoods.

Tubo-uterine Implantation

Tubo-uterine implantation was for us until recently the operation of choice for all proximal occlusions.

The section of the tube may be through the isthmus, or the proximal part of the ampulla. In a first period (until 1951) we advocated the ampullo-uterine implantation, because it was much more easy to carry out correctly, with a rather good rate of patencies and pregnancies. Later, we discovered some disadvantages. Most of them

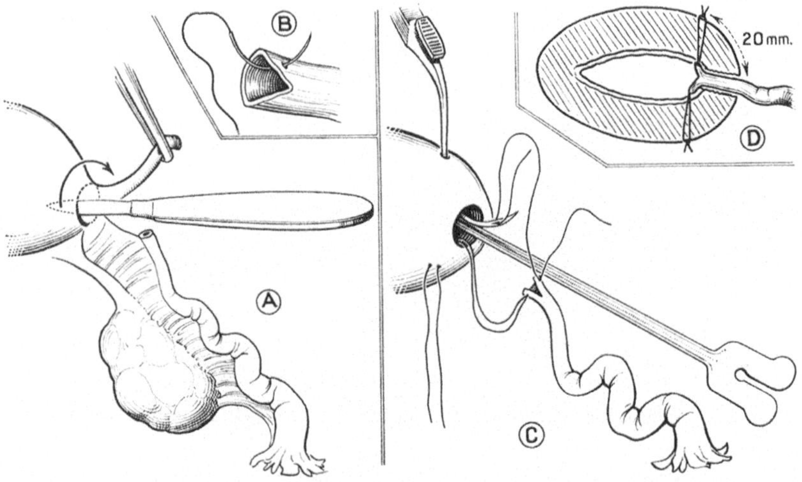

Fig. 5. Isthmo-uterine implantation by Palmer's technique

were explained by *tubal incontinence*; which might cause reflux of menstrual blood, with dysmenorrhea and sometimes secondary peri-tubal adhesions and phimosis, and even endometriosis. It was also felt that the difference between patency rate (75%) and pregnancy rate (32%) could be explained by the excessive shortening of the tube.

Therefore, mostly since 1960, we have used as often as possible the *isthmo-uterine implantation*, the isthmus being cut at first near the cornu, then, if it was too narrow, re-cut 1 cm more distally, and so on until it fits for good implantation.

Our technique is as follows (Fig. 5).

A Kocher forceps seizes the isthmus just outside the occlusion site; the tube is sectioned, and also the meso salpinx just below the tube until the uterine angle; a knife with narrow blade creates a tunnel, 5 to 7 mm of diameter, by a circular incision which, after 2 or 3 turns around the interstitial portion of the tube, penetrates the uterine cavity.

The tubal stump is then prepared for implantation: a dorsal incision 8 mm long is done on the stump, and 2 nylon 0000 stitches are put on each side of the incision at 4 mm from the angle, taking mucosa *and serosa*. Then, a grooved probe is introduced through the tunnel into the uterine cavity, and Reverdin's needle (third of circle, with a cord of 4 cm) penetrates the anterior surface of the uterus at 25 mm from the entry of the tunnel in the direction of the endometrial angle; the grooved probe is there to lead the needle toward the entry of the tunnel. The needle seizes one of the threads of the anterior flap, and then the other, by a second travel 1 mm apart from the first. Same on the posterior surface. The threads are then pulled, and the tube enters in the tunnel; they are tied cautiously (to avoid breaking) but firmly.

Our results, among 93 cases of *ampullo-uterine implantation*, are 73 patencies (78%), 31 U.P. (33%) and 8 E.U.P. (8.5%), and among 26 cases of *isthmo-uterine implantation*, performed between 1953 and 1963, are: 20 patencies (74%) 10 U.P. (43%) and 2 E.U.P. (8%).

After isthmo-uterine implantation, complete tubal incontinence is rare; in most cases, the insufflation curve is above 30 mm Hg and presents characteristic oscillations. Dysmenorrhea also is rare. Re-occlusion is a little more frequent (26% instead of 22%), but *pregnancy rate is higher* (43% instead of 33%).

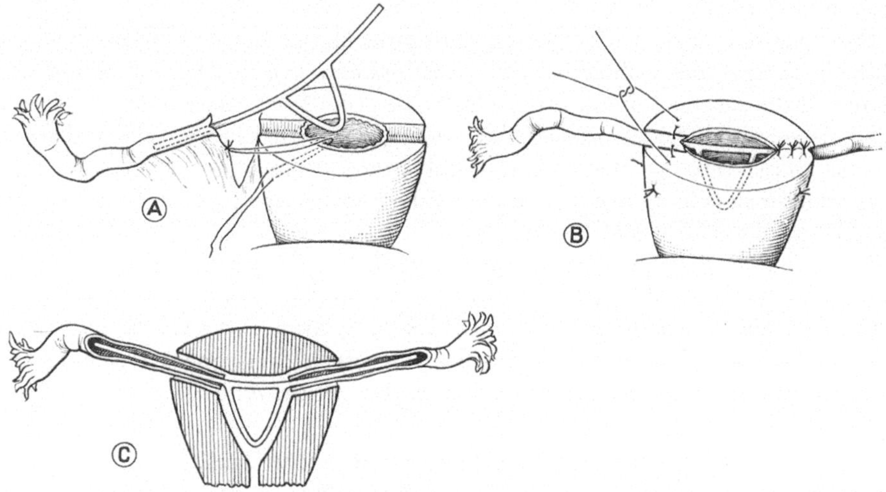

Fig. 6. Tubo-uterine implantation by Shirodkar's technique

I must confess that some collegues, after having used my technique, had re-occlusions, I feel that their failures are due to the fact that the tube was not implanted far enough so that a part of the tunnel is ready for coalescence of its walls. With the above described technique, *without poly-ethylene tubing*, the result depends entirely on the exact evaluation of the site of the endometrial angle, and the stump must really protrude a little in the uterine cavity.

Two ways to avoid the coalescence of the walls of the tunnel are possible, and may be associated:

a) One is the implantation under complete visual control — by frontal incision of the whole fundus, as advocated by SHIRODKAR, 1966.

b) The other is the use of poly-ethylene tubing, or the new Shirodkar's device (Fig. 6), but all the authors who use one or the other agree to let it stay in place at least 3 months.

In conclusion, although I still personally persist in doing implantations without intubation, I feel that the beginner in tubo-plasty should preferably use intubation or the Shirodkar's device.

Tubal Anastomosis

Tubal anastomosis, after resection of a segment of the tube, may be on the free portion of the tube or intra-mural.

Tubal anastomosis on the free portion of the tube is mostly indicated after tubal sterilization, or mid-tubal occlusions.

It is generally done with poly-ethylene tubing, and the best way to avoid expulsion of the tubing by uterine contractions, is, after a shirt median anterior hysterotomy, to insert Shirodkar's device, or to construct its equivalent with poly-ethylene tubing; four total stitches with nylon 000 are enough.

Our personal series is short: 3 cases, with 2 U.P. and 1 E.U.P.

Intra-mural anastomosis has been advocated by EHRLER (1966) as a substitute for tubal implantation, because it would avoid the risk of tubal incontinence, and preserve the true tubo-uterine junction, which seems to control the migration of the egg. He states that, in most cases of proximal occlusion, its site is not at the ostium, but 10 to 20 mm more laterally.

The indurated segment is first resected, then the uterine angle cut perpendicularly, and the interstitial tube catheterized, or visualized by retrograde hydrotubation with blue dye. If the passage is poor, the uterine angle is cut 1 or 2 more times, until good patency is evident. Then a poly-ethylene tubing is inserted in the tube and passes into the uterus through the preserved tubo-uterine junction. (A short anterior hysterotomy may help to make a ring with the intra-uterine part of the tube). The tubing be removed after 8 to 10 days.

EHRLER, among 29 personal cases, has 12 U.P. (41%) and 2 E.U.P. (6.8%), which compares favourably with the results of the implantations.

The intra-mural anastomosis is now advocated by SHIRODKAR (1968), and I have done recently two of them, and shall probably use it everytime a recent H.S.G. demonstrates a preserved normal interstitial portion of the tube.

Combined Operations on the Same Tube

Combined operations on the same tube (Implantation + Salpingostomy) may be the only solution for some cases with bipolar occlusion, if the situation has not been diagnosed before the operation through laparoscopy. I have done it in 87 private cases between 1956 and 1965, with 2 U.P. (2.2%), 4 E.U.P. (4.5%) and 46 re-occlusions (53%), most of them at the fimbria. 25 of them (29%) were latent tuberculosis; 4 of them had to submit to ulterior salpingectomy.

Some complementary operative steps

Some complementary operative steps seem to us very important in the *prevention of new adhesions*. They are:

1. *Subtotal omentectomy*, advocated by EHRLER, which we perform when the omental adhesions are extensive or dense.

2. *Uterine suspension*, mostly by the Pellanda ligamentopexy technique, to avoid postoperative retroversion and prolapse of the adnexae at the site of previous adhesions.

3. *Ovarian temporary suspension* by one stitch of catgut fixing the lateral pole of the ovary to the peritoneum of fossa iliaca, just outside the iliac artery.

4. *Perfect hemostasis* and final meticulous removal of all clots.

5. *Perfect peritonisation*, eventually with a peritoneal flap, resected from the vesico-uterine fold.

6. Any other useful operations on uterus (myomectomy, etc.) or ovaries (resection of foci of endometriosis, wedge resection for poly cystic ovary) etc. But we *avoid appendicectomy*, especially if we intend to use high dosage cortisone therapy.

Perioperative Care

Perioperative care, to suppress the normal inflammatory reaction to the surgical trauma, consists of:

a) *High dosage intra-muscular dexamethazone* (16 mg every 4 h, beginning 4 h before the operation, until the next morning), as advocated by Horne (1966).

b) *High dosage intra-peritoneal hydrocortisone acetate* (1000 mg in 20 ml of saline, injected in the pelvic cavity, just before closing the peritoneum).

This association has been studied by Swolin in animal experiment and in the human, with systematical laparoscopic control 6 months after the operation.

We are using it for the last 2 years, without any trouble, and find a better patency rate, but it is too early to make definite conclusions.

We do often also a *hydrotubation on the third postoperative day* with 500 mg of hydrocortisone acetate in 20 ml of saline, in order to wash away fibrin clots which may tend to agglutinate the fimbria, and give a new dose of the drug, the action of which lasts about 4 days.

Antibiotics are given routinely for 5 days — either penicillin-streptomycin, once a day — or penicillin-colimycin, twice a day — or some other combination.

Early mobilisation is advocated by Miss Moore-White, with frequent positional modifications, to avoid the pelvic organs to stay in immobile contact.

We give *dexamethazone* per os for 3 or 4 more weeks, 6 tablets (of 0.5 mg) a day the first week, 3 tablets the next 3 weeks.

An *insufflation* is generally done 1 month after the operation, and repeated each second month, 2 or 3 times.

Control hysterosalpingography is generally done after 6 to 8 months.

Control laparoscopy is performed, if pregnancy has not occurred after 12 to 18 months; it was several times possible, at this occasion, to suppress, with the biopsy forceps of the special operative Wolf laparoscope, adhesions around the fimbria or the ovary, and 5 times a pregnancy occurred in the 3 next months.

References

Complete bibliography until 1964 may be found in Marchesi, Albano, Cittadini's book "Le Salpingoplastiche" universo editors, Rome 1965.

More recent important publications are:

Horne, P. H.: Int. J. Fertil. **11**, 271 (1966).

Mulligan, W.: Int. J. Fertil. **11**, 385 (1966).

Palmer, R.: Chirurgie restauratrice tubaire dans la stérilité. Encyclopedie Medico Chirurgicale, techniques Chirurgicales. Gynécologie **41**, 550—565 (1967).

—, J. de Brux, M. Cognat, J. Cohen, M. Gordji, J. Noel et J. Vinourd: Le traitement chirurgical des stérilités tubaires. Congrès de la Fédération des Sociétés de Gynécologie et d'Obst. de langue française, Paris 1968, Bull. Fed. Soc. Gynéc. Obstet. franç. 1968.

Pasetto, N.: La Chirurgia funzionale della tuba 52. Congresso Nazionale della Società italiana di Ostetr. Ginec. Rome 1966.

Shirodkar, V.: Vth World Congress on Fertility, Stockholm 1966. Excerpta Medica editors, pp. 230—353.

Swolin, K.: Beträge zur operativen Behandlung der weiblichen Sterilität, vol. 1. Göteborg: Elanders édit. 1967.

Histopathology and Biology of Carcinoma in Situ

H. HAMPERL

"Cancer of the cervix is now regarded as a preventable disease" — so ran the statement in one of the publications of WHO (1964); a well known pathologist chimed in by saying: "We see the day ahead when there will be no more invasive carcinoma of the cervix and many of us, we hope, will live to see this day". These highflying statements, hopes and predictions are based on two assumptions:

I. Every invasive carcinoma (i. ca.) of the cervix evolves through a preparatory stage called carcinoma in situ (ca.i.s.).

II. Every ca.i.s., after some duration turns into an i.ca.; this transition can be prevented by recognition and adequate treatment of the ca.i.s.

Considering the immense practical implications of these statements it seems worth while to look closer into the evidence, on which they are based.

I.

It was a great scientific achievement, when the combined efforts of gynecologists and pathologists succeeded in establishing the following fact: in contrast to the old classical belief, that the i.ca. of the cervix originates from normal squamous epithelium, there is in many cases to be found an intermediate stage which is now generally called ca.i.s. (Table 1). It is intermediate in two aspects: clinically, as the lesion antecedes the i.ca. and morphologically, as the lesion holds a middle position between normal and cancerous epithelium.

Let us first discuss the purley histological aspects of the problem! It soon became clear that *two boundaries were difficult for the histologists to establish.*

Table 1

Normal Epithelium
Carcinoma in situ
Invasive carcinoma

Table 2

Normal Epithelium
Dysplasia
Carcinoma in situ
Invasive carcinoma

The histological picture of the ca.i.s. is frequently not easy to separate from a lesion commonly called *dysplasia* (Table 2); this lesion in turn fades morphologically into the normal squamous epithelium. We have to admit that practically all efforts to establish a clear-cut boundary between dysplasia and ca.i.s. have failed. This statement should, however, not obscure the fact that typical cases of ca.i.s. and dysplasia are nowadays easily and uniformly diagnosed by all competent histologists. It is only the boundary-region between these two lesions, where discrepancies in the evaluation of the histological picture many occur as several tests have shown (SIEGLER, 1956; GOVAR et al., 1966; HOLMQUIST et al., 1967). I, therefore, would prefer not to put all lesions between typical ca.i.s. and normal epithelium under the heading "boundary-lesions" (KOSS et al., 1963), but to reserve this term for cases not falling unequivocally into the category of dysplasia or ca.i.s. By following this concept one can hope to reach a higher consensus between the diagnoses of different histologists.

An other area of uncertainty we encounter at the boundary between ca.i.s. and i.ca. At the first glance no diagnostic doubts seem to exist about ca.i.s. and the smallest i.ca., the microcarcinoma (Table 3). The latter shows all the histological qualities of the classic i.ca. and differs from it only by the smaller size and, therefore, remains clinically occult, as a "preclinical" carcinoma. Most characteristic is, in our opinion, the netlike arrangement of the epithelial strands infiltrating only the superficial layer of the stroma. There are, however, cases of ca.i.s. where single protrusions of the surface epithelium seem to project into the stroma. As they often show a pointed end they have been likened to the claws of a crayfish. This picture is usually to be found at many places in a given case of ca.i.s. and is known as "*early stromal invasion*" (Fennell, 1955; Friedell et al., 1958) — with the silent understanding that a "late stromal invasion" would already be a (micro-)invasive ca. Many authors do not hesitate to put the diagnosis "carcinoma" on this picture although with the complementing adjectiv "micro-invasive" or "superficially invasive" (Dilworth and Maxwell, 1962). They regard the destruction of the basal membrane as evidence for

Table 3

Normal epithelium

///////////////////

Dysplasia

///////////////////

Carcinoma in situ

///////////////////

Carcinoma in situ with early stromal invasion (carcinoma with microinvasion)

///////////////////

Microcarcinoma
Preclinical carcinoma
Invasive carcinoma

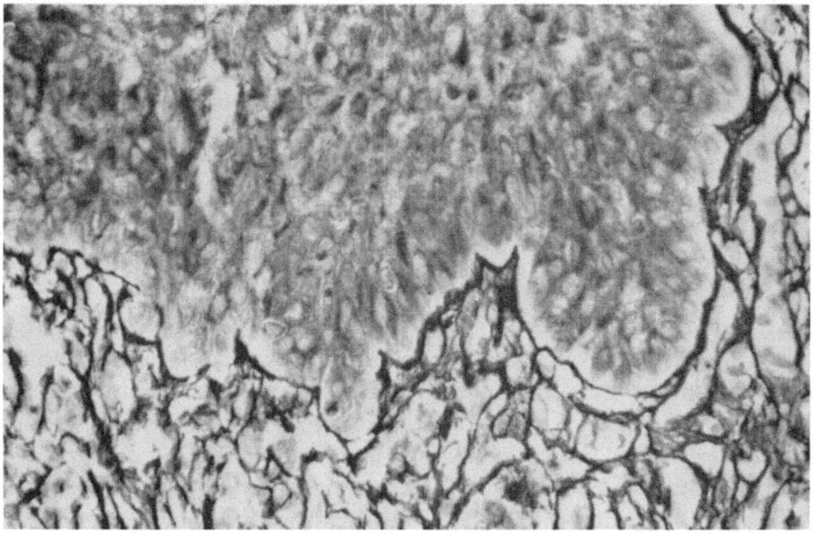

Fig. 1. Ca.i.s. with beginning stromal invasion. The basal membrane not interrupted but pushed downwards. Reticulin-stain with silver. (From Hamperl, 1966)

malignancy. By systematically studying this "microinvasion" I found (1966) that it may proceed in two ways; either the intact basal membrane is pushed downwards and accompanies the epithelial outgrowth as an uninterrupted layer (Fig. 1 u. 3/I), or the basal membrane is disappearing through the action of invading migrant cells, predominantly lymphocytes (Fig. 3/IIa). The epithelium then only uses these breaks to grow into the stroma (Fig. 2 u. 3/IIb) but does not by itself produce the breaks in the basal membrane.

As one can see not only the boundary between ca.i.s. and dysplasia but also between ca.i.s. and i.ca. seems to be somewhat blurred, depending upon whether we put a lesion with early stromal invasion (microinvasion) into the category of ca.i.s. or microcarcinoma. Generally the latter is done in order to be on the safe side when treating patient. The question is however not finally settled from the point of view of the pathologist. For him it is only clear, that there is a very strict biological dividing-line between all kind of precancerous lesions and real cancer as manifested by a

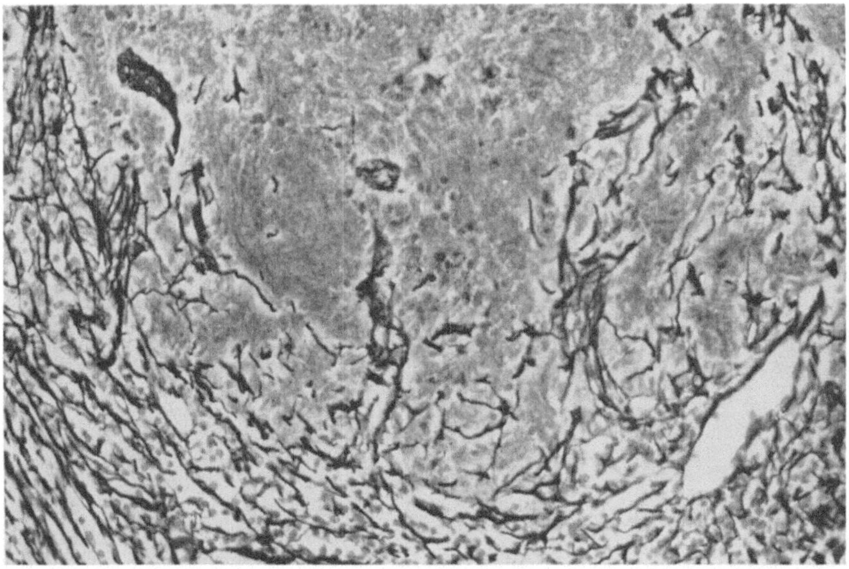

Fig. 2. Ca.i.s. with early stromal invasion. The epithelial masses growing downwards into the spaces between the reticulin fibers. Reticulin-stain with silver. (From HAMPERL, 1966)

fundamentally different pattern of chromosomes, grade of ploidy and DNA-content of the nuclei (KIRKLAND et al., 1967; AUERSPERG et al., 1967).

Finally, some *subdivisions* have been suggested even *in the area of unquestionable ca.i.s.* (Table 4). There are cases where the epithelium of the ca.i.s. simply replaces the normal epithelium on the surface (Fig. 4), in others the pathological epithelium is extending downwards into the cervical glands or clefts (Fig. 4), displacing and replacing the normal cylindrical epithelium, and finally converting the gland into a solid epithelial mass by entirely filling the lumen. As pointed out by HILLEMANNS (1964, 1968) another variety is due to the fact that the epithelium sometimes pushes downwards into the stroma through bulky outgrowth (Fig. 5) sometimes accompanied by a crowding of cells. The same author regards areas of cellmaturation either located inside the surface epithelium or peripherally towards the stroma as a special sign of impending infiltration. Many other authors including myself (1959) have tried to classify ca.i.s. into subgroups (NESBITT and STEIN, 1958; FLUHMANN, 1960; NIEBURGS, 1963; TITKIN, 1963; BURGHARDT, 1964; ATKIN, 1964; OLD et al., 1965;

Wielenga et al., 1965) but none of these classifications has till now been generally accepted.

It is very tempting to arrange all these somehow related pictures into a row, and by so doing, succumb to the very suggestive assumption that they represent not

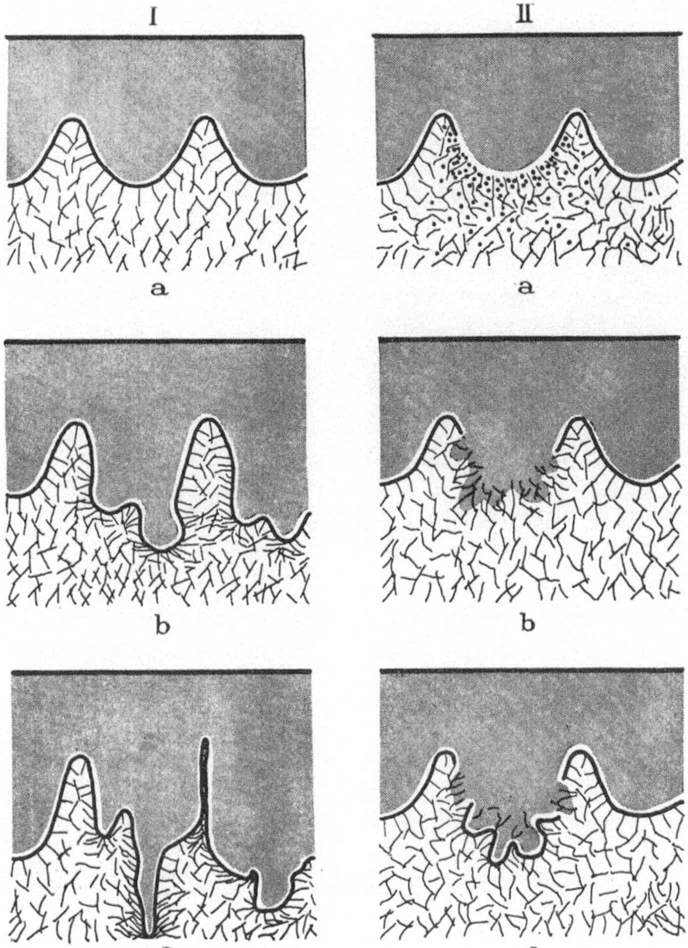

Fig. 3. The different behaviour of the basal membrane and the reticulin fibers in ca.i.s. (grey). I/a—c: The intact basal membrane is pushed downwards as in Fig. 1; II/a: The basal membrane is dissolved while lymphocytes emigrate; II/b: The ca.i.s. uses these breaks to infiltrate into the spaces between the reticulin fibers as in Fig. 2; II/c: At some places a new basal membrane is formed. (From Hamperl, 1966)

Table 4. *Carcinoma in situ*

Symply replacing normal epithelium
Infiltrating cervical glands
Preinvasive crowding of cells (bulky outgrowth)
With intraepithelial areas of maturation
Large-cell type
Small-cell type

merely a pathohistologic fiction but the natural course of events leading eventually to i.ca. (Table 3, arrows at left). There are in fact some indications that this may be so: HERTIG, FIDLER and BOYD (1960), DUNN and PURVIS (1967) and others, pointed to the different age groups affected by the different lesions: the dysplasia and ca.i.s.

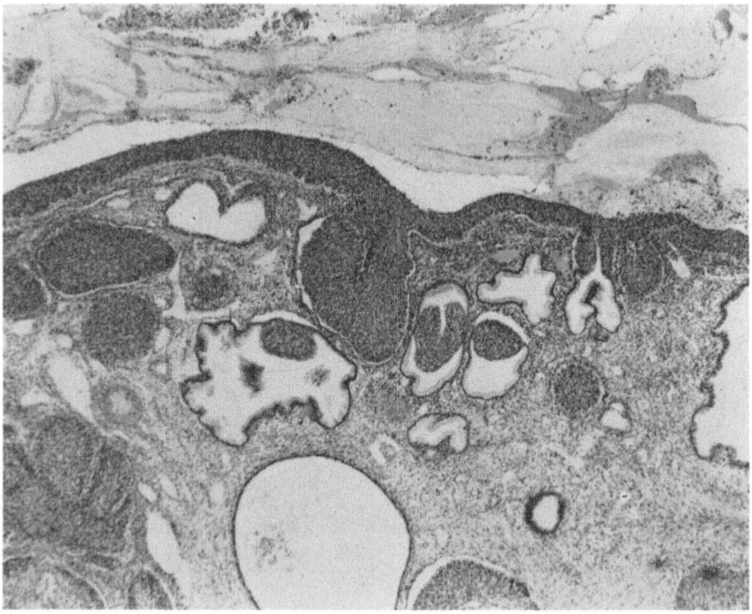

Fig. 4. Ca.i.s. with simple replacing growth on the surface and filling the lumina of the cervical glands

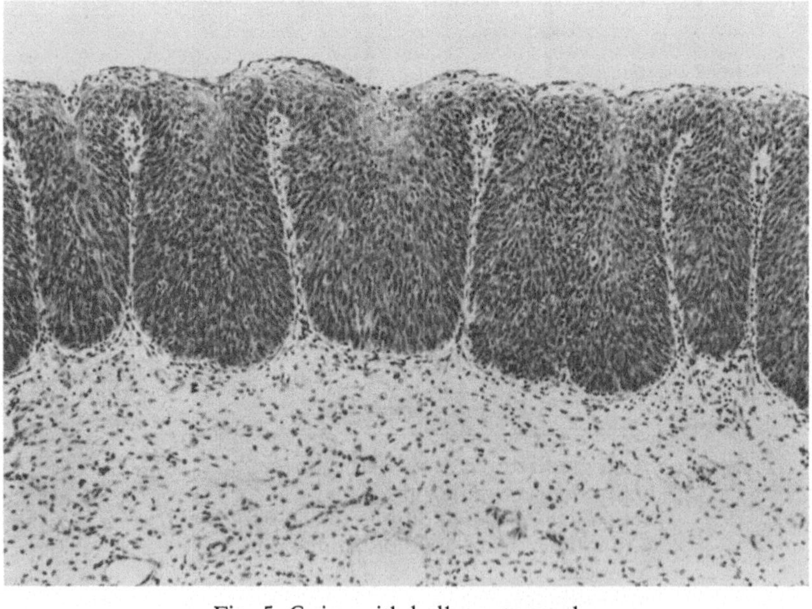

Fig. 5. Ca.i.s. with bulky outgrowth

occuring at a younger age than the i.ca. It was even calculated that ca.i.s. needed an average of 5 to 8 years in order to progress to an i.ca. The strongest argument in favor of the theory of a slow progression from bad to worse came from the clinical observation of untreated cases of ca.i.s. developing into i.ca. after several years duration.

It remains, however, still questionable whether in these cases the progression runs through all the histological patterns so neatly arranged by the pathologist. There exist, indeed, several reports indicating other possibilities (Table 3, arrows at right): BURGHARDT (1967) has recently published four cases, in which he felt reasonably sure that an i.ca. developed immediately from/or in a normal epithelium; SCHILLER et al., spoke of a "spray-carcinoma" as early as 1953; in screening programs cases have turned up where there was only evidence of a previous dysplasia and not of ca.i.s., before the appearance of i.ca. (KOSS et al., 1963; BANGLE et al., 1963; DUNN and PURVIS, 1967).

It seems even doubtful whether the "microinvasion" ever develops into real i.ca., since the microinvasion occurs at many places in a given ca.i.s., where as the i.ca., also in its microcarcinoma-form originates at only one definite spot (FENNELL, 1954).

On the basis of all the known facts we may, therefore, formulate the answer to our first question, whether every i.ca. of the cervix is preceeded by a ca.i.s.: *many, probably even the majority of i.ca., develop from a precancerous lesion, the ca.i.s., but by no means all of them.*

II.

The second question, whether every ca.i.s. eventually progresses into i.ca., is almost equally important from the point of view of prevention of i.ca. The problem consists in establishing to what extent the ca.i.s. is a progredient, or a stationary lesion, or even is able to regress completely. The differences in the answers in the current literature are mainly due to the lack of a clear distinction between ca.i.s. and i.ca. on one hand and dysplasia on the other, as explained earlier. If one includes in ones classification of ca.i.s. lesions, another pathologist would rather diagnose as dysplasias, one would quite correctly come to the conclusion that regression is possible. On the other hand, a narrower definition of the term ca.i.s. may lead to just the opposite conclusion.

The simple way of establishing the presence of a ca.i.s. in one of its forms and then waiting to see what happens is, unfortunately, not feasible because the inflammatory reaction following a diagnistic excision of a ca.i.s. is able to destroy the remaining parts of the lesion. The problem amounts to the impossibility of having ones cake and eating it at the same time. To rely only on cytologic evidence is open to criticism, since the method, the achievements of the cytologists not withstanding, is scarcely able to distinguish between the whole spectrum of the pertaining lesions with desirable accuracy. There are, however, cases on record with the cytological findings of ca.i.s. over many years, even decades, without any inclination towards i.ca. We can, therefore, only assume that the possibility of regression of a ca.i.s. most probably diminishes as it approaches the i.ca. BURGHARDT (1966) tried to illustrate this in a schematic drawing (Fig. 6). We, therefore, may answer our second question by the statement that *a part of the ca.i.s. in a strict sense may inevitably progress into i.ca., but by no means all ca.i.s.*

It would be of paramount interest to know how big this part is. KIRKLAND et al. (1967) think that only half or one third of all preinvasive lesions reach the stage of i.ca. BOYES et al. (1964) came on the basis of their mass-screening to the conclusion that only about 60% of all ca.i.s. become eventually i.ca. MEYER (1965) found even in about barely $^1/_{10}$ of all cases of early i.ca. (including microcarcinoma) traces of ca.i.s. Also on statistical grounds it is improbable that all ca.i.s. would progress into i.ca., as too many ca.i.s. were found compared with the lower incidence of i.ca.

As you see my answer to both initial questions is not a simple "yes" or "no" due to the fact that i.ca. may arise without a preceding ca.i.s. and a ca.i.s. may remain stationary or even regress and never develop into an i.ca. Unfortunately, even after examining our cytological and histological preparations, we are not able at present, to say exactly how frequently this occurs or when the point of no return is reached. A screening program embracing a whole population may succeed in early recognizing and consecutively weeding out all ca.i.s., but if not all these lesions would have progressed into cancer the whole action may seem, at least partly, a very costly luxury,

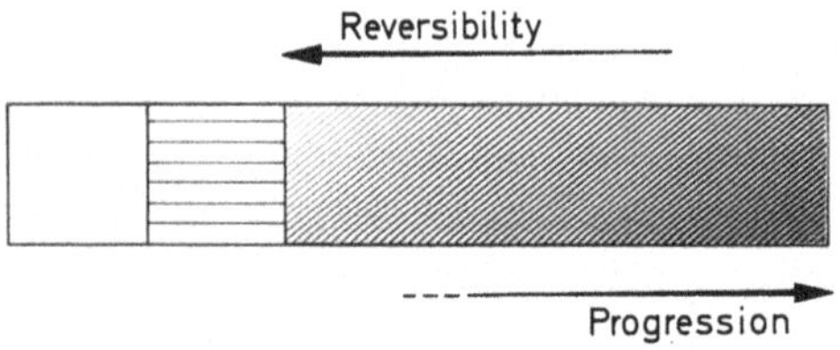

Fig. 6. The decreasing reversibility of ca.i.s. as it approaches invasiveness (right hand end of the drawing: normal epithelium at left). (From BURGHARDT, 1964)

the more so if i.ca. may be able to evade the screening by hiding in the cervical canal or by developing rapidly without previous warning. The real test for the usefullness of mass screening will, therefore, be a significant lowering of the death rate of i.ca. of the cervix. The pertinent statistics are still controversial in this respect (see GREEN, 1966) to say the least. Let us, however, hope that the optimistic statements I mentioned at the beginning of my exposé may be supported by solid facts in the future.

References

ATKIN, N. B.: Nature (Lond.) **202**, 201 (1964).
AUERSPERG, N., M. J. COREY, and A. WORTH: Cancer Res. **27**, 1394—1401 (1967).
BANGLE, R., JR., M. BERGER, and M. LEVIN: Cancer (Philad.) **16**, 1151—1159 (1963).
BOYES, D. A., H. K. FIDLER, and D. R. LOCK: Brit. med. J. **1962** I, 203—205.
BURGHARDT, E.: Verh. dtsch. Ges. Path. **1964**, 12—33.
— Geburth. u. Frauenheilk. **27**, 1170—1180 (1967).
DILWORTH, E. E., and G. E. MAXWELL: Amer. J. Obstet. Gynec. **84**, 83—88 (1962).
DUNN, J. E. M., and L. PURVIS: Cancer (Philad.) **20**, 1899—1906 (1967).
FENNELL, R. H.: Amer. J. Path. **3**, No. 178, 623—624 (1954).
FENNELL, R. F., JR.: Cancer (Philad.) **8**, 302—309 (1955).
FIDLER, H. K., and J. R. BOYD: Cancer (Philad.) **13**, 764—771 (1960).
FLUHMANN, C. F.: Amer. J. Obstet. Gynec. **16**, 424—437 (1960).
FRIEDELL, G. J., A. T. HERTIG, and P. A. YOUNGE: Arch. Path. **66**, 494—503 (1958).
GOVAN, A. D. T., R. M. HAINES, F. A. LANGLEY, C. W. TAYLOR, and A. S. WOODCOCK: J. Obstet. Gynaec. Brit. Cwlth, N.S. **73**, 883—896 (1966).
GREEN, G. H.: Amer. J. Obstet. Gynec. **94**, 1009—1022 (1966).
HAMPERL, H.: Virchows Arch. path. Anat. **340**, 185—205 (1966).
— Definition and classification of the socalled carcinoma in situ. Symposium CIBA Foundation study group No. 3:2. London: Churchill 1959.
HILLEMANNS, H. G.: Arch. Gynäk. **191**, 235—270 (1958).
— Entstehung und Wachstum des Zervixkarzinoms. Basel/New York: S. Karger 1964.

—, B. Sixtus-Klug und E. Prestel: Arch. Gynäk. **206,** 82—97 (1968).
Holmquist, N. D., C. A. McMahan, and O. D. Williams: Arch. Path. **84,** 334—345 (1967).
Kirkland, J. A., M. A. Stanley, and M. K. Cellier: Cancer (Philad.) **20,** 1934—1952 (1967).
Koss, L. G., F. W. Steward, F. W. Foote, M. J. Jordan, G. M. Bader, and E. Day: Cancer (Philad.) **16,** 1160—1210 (1963).
Meyer, P. C.: J. clin. Path. **18,** 414—423 (1965).
Nesbitt, R. E. L., Jr., and A. A. Stein: Surg. Gynec. Obstet. **107,** 161—168 (1958).
Nieburgs, H. E.: Cancer (Philad.) **16,** No. 2, 141—159 (1963).
Old, J. W., G. Wielenga, and E. v. Haam: Cancer (Philad.) **18,** 1598—1611 (1965).
Schiller, W., A. F. Daro, H. A. Gollin, and N. P. Primiario: Amer. J. Obstet. Gynec. **65,** 1088—1098 (1953).
Siegler, E. E.: Cancer (Philad.) **9,** 463—469 (1956).
Titkin, K. D.: Acta Un. int. Cancer **19,** 1377—1378 (1963).
Wielenga, G., J. W. Old, and E. v. Haam: Cancer (Philad.) **18,** 1612—1621 (1965).
World Health Organization: Technical Report Series Nr. 276, 1964.

Early Detection and Cytology of Carcinoma in Situ*

Günther Kern

Great numbers of the so called carcinoma in situ have been detected by cytodiagnosis of exfoliated cells of the cervix uteri. With increasing experience the intraepithelial malignant lesion was no longer understood as real cancer, but as a precancerous lesion, which precedes cervical cancer.

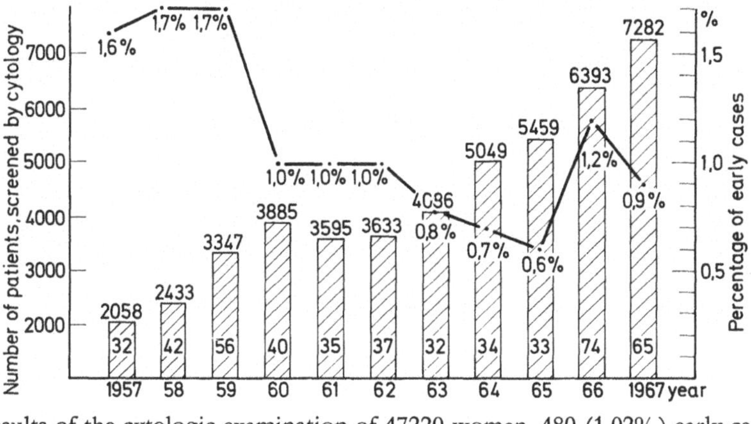

Fig. 1. Results of the cytologic examination of 47220 women. 480 (1.02%) early cases have been detected. (Dysplasia: 67, carcinoma in situ: 364, microcarcinoma: 49)

The clinical consequence was the limitation of the therapeutical approach. Today the excision of the area concerned the so called conization is the method of choice.

Younge in 1957 expressed the opinion, that cervical cancer is a preventable disease, if every women had adequate precautious examinations. The World Health Organization recently also came to the same opinion. Before discussing the part of cytolo gy in reaching this objective, I should like to point out some important aspects in our experience with the cytodiagnosis of carcinoma in situ.

* From the University Hospital of Gynecology and Obstetrics Cologne (Direktor: Prof. Dr. C. Kaufmann).

1. Without doubt the detection of premalignant epithelial atypias is most successfully accomplished by means of cytology. The carcinoma in situ is neither detectable by inspection with the naked eye, nor by gynecological palpation. The inspection of

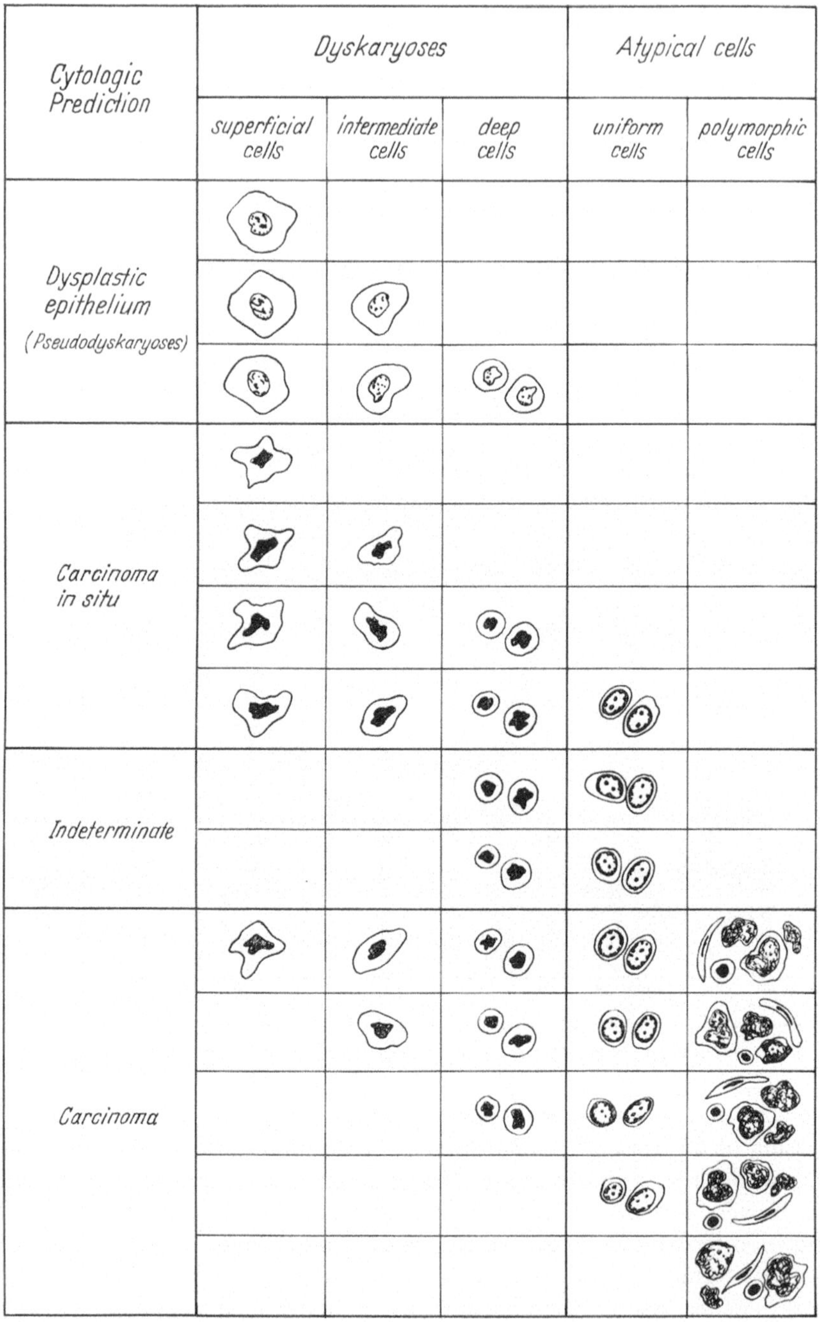

Fig. 2. Partly schematic representation of cellular types in the cytologic smear, from which a prediction can be made about the histologic change. (KERN, 1962)

the cervical surface with a magnifying glass called colposcopy also has many disadvantages in comparison with cytology. Fig. 1 shows the number of patients examined cytologically in the past 11 years as well as the numbers and percentages of the detected and treated early cases. We investigated 47220 mostly out-patients in the University Hospital of Gynecology and Obstetrics in Cologne.

We found 480, this means 1.02% carcinoma in situ. This figure does not include cytologically detected but clinically still asymptomatic invasive cancers. Mass-screening programs of presumably healthy women usually arrive at a percentage of around 0.5.

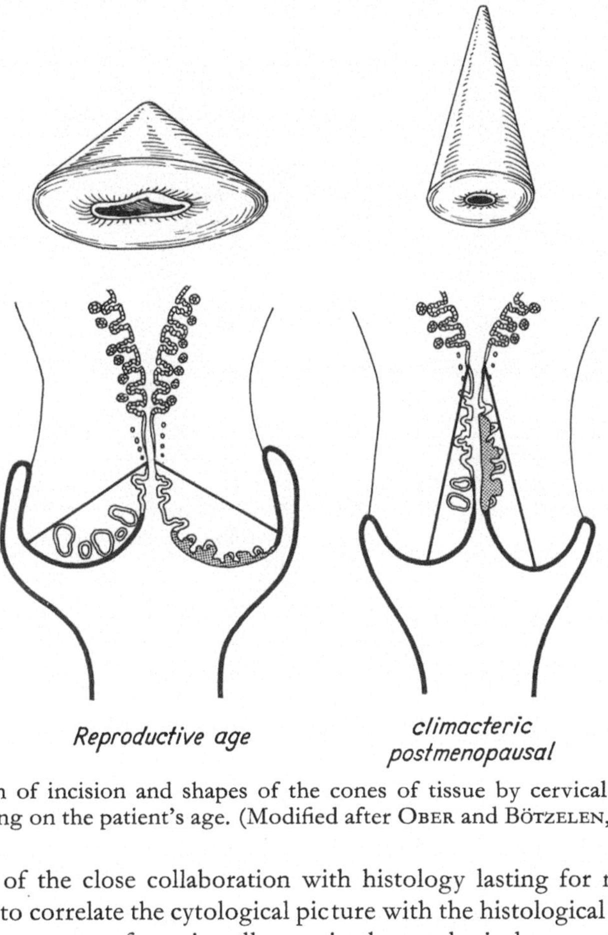

Fig. 3. Direction of incision and shapes of the cones of tissue by cervical conization, depending on the patient's age. (Modified after OBER and BÖTZELEN, 1959)

2. Because of the close collaboration with histology lasting for many years we have been able to correlate the cytological picture with the histological lesion (Fig. 2).

From the appearance of certain cell-types in the cytological smear, which I cannot discuss in detail in this presentation we reach a prediction of the histological epithelial atypia with an accuracy of around 90%. For the clinician the cytological prediction has the following consequences: If the smear indicates a dysplasia, the patient is scheduled for cytological controls in regular intervals. A treatment is not yet indicated. If the cytological prediction indicates a carcinoma in situ, or — in a very small group — a prediction is not possible, the patient is diagnosed and treated by conization in one procedure (Fig. 3). In elderly women we also consider a hysterectomy. If so called polymorphic atypical cells appear in the smear our experience indicates an invasive cancer. After the usual methods of biopsies the patient is treated by radical operation or radiationtherapy. The presentation of Prof. HAMPERL has shown, that the transition between dysplasia and carcinoma in situ in the same case may be not well defined. But also histologically it may be difficult to decide, if one still deals with a dysplasia or already with a carcinoma in situ. It is obvious that this kind of diagnosis is even more difficult from single cells in the smear no longer in contact with the epithelium.

I stress this point, because internationally a variable diagnostic value is attached to both lesions. Therefore some doubts were recently expressed about the biological significance of carcinoma in situ as a precancerous lesion.

Results of prospective cytology	Number of cases	%	Observation time → histologic diagnosis	Type of histologic change
Stationary	6 16	(7.4) (19.8)	3—5 years 2—8 years	Dysplasia Carcinoma in situ
Progression normal → Dysplasia → carcinoma in situ	30	(37.0)	2—9 years	Carcinoma in situ
normal → dysplacia → carcinoma in situ → invasive carcinoma	3	(3.7)	4—9 years	invasive cancer
Regression Dysplasia → normal	26	(32.1)	2—11 years (Cytological observation time)	normal epithelium (only six patients had a curettage)
	81	(100.0)		

Fig. 4. Long period observations with prospective cytology

3. As I already mentioned, we do not treat but control patients with a dysplasia. Women with more severe lesions are always scheduled for treatment. Nevertheless 81 patients during 11 years declined treatment, but they came for cytological controls. In this cases we could do long-term observation by means of prospective cytology. We investigated whether the lesion behaved stationary, progressive or regressive, without having been able to disturb the development of the lesion by biopsies.

It was first pointed out by PAPANICOLAOU in 1949 that only observation-periods with the smear method may give an answer about the development of intraepithelial changes, because any kind of biopsy may excise totally, or damage or miss the lesion. Fig. 4 gives a general survey about the 81 cases. In 22 patients the cytological smears were *stationary* and did not change within 2 to 8 years indicating a dysplasia or a carcinoma in situ. The observation time was terminated with the treatment of the patient. However the beginning of the epithelial atypia is still unknown.

33 patients showed a *progression* within 2 to 9 years. The cytological smears had been unsuspicious for several months and changed afterwards to dysplasia or carcinoma in situ. Of special interest are three patients, where the step to the invasive cancer could exactly be recognized in the cytological smears. Fig. 5 shows an example. The third group behaved *regressively*, that means, the pathological celltypes could be recognized for several months up to 3 and 4 years and disappeared afterwards. In this group it is of special importance that we observed a regression only in those cases, which indicated cytologically a dysplasia. In women with cytological findings indicating a carcinoma in situ we never found a regressive tendency.

I should like to summarize briefly:

1. Premalignant epithelial atypies at the cervix uteri are best detected by means of cytology.
2. It is possible to correlate the cytological picture with the histological lesion.
3. Long-term-observation periods demonstrated, that a carcinoma in situ may be stationary over many years. Our material shows in no case a tendency of regression.

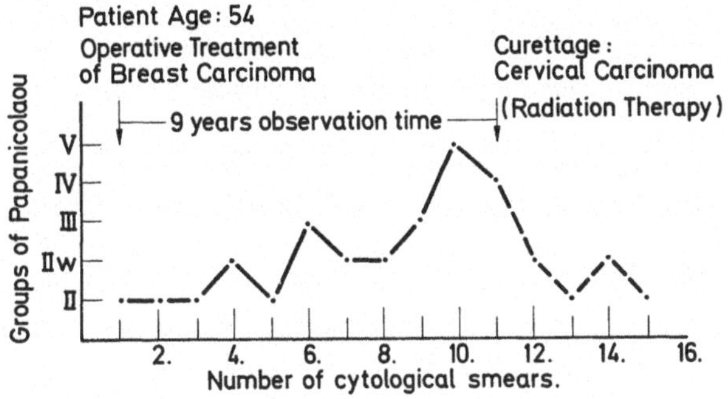

Fig. 5. Cell types in the smears changed from normal cells up to polymorphic tumor cells over a period of 9 years. In this patient a progression of the epithelial atypia could be observed by means of cytology

However dysplasia may be regressive in a very high percentage. The step from carcinoma in situ to invasive cancer seems to proceed rather quickly.

May I finally come back to the question whether we have reached the objective of preventing cervical cancer.

Unfortunately this aim still is far away. Countries with a high population are only able to screen a very small percentage of all females. In Cologne, which has a very good screening program, we estimate that it includes about 10% of all women in 1 year. If a higher percentage took part in, we would not have enough cytologically trained people, to examine such mass-material. An excessive work load for the doctors and technicians and other factors would lead to an increase of false negative cytological results, which would give the patients a false feeling of security. If a women returns to a cytological examination in yearly intervals in 1 to 2% a precancerous lesion may be detected and in some cases even an invasive cancer.

The cytodiagnosis of the cervix uteri is the most reliable method to recognize premalignant lesions. However, a significant prevention of cervical cancer has not yet been achieved despite all efforts.

Surgical Treatment of Carcinoma in Situ of the Cervix Uteri*

WOODARD D. BEACHAM, and EDWIN HUGH LAWSON JR.

At the Congress of the International Federation of Gynecology and Obstetrics held in Vienna in 1961 the Cancer Committee under the chairmanship of Kottmeier defined stage 0, carcinoma of the cervix as preinvasive carcinoma, so-called carcinoma in situ. In 1964 the American College of Obstetricians and Gynecologists distributed *Clinical Staging System for Carcinoma of the Cervix* by the American Joint Committee for Cancer Staging and End Results Reporting. This Committee is sponsored by the American College of Surgeons, the American College of Radiology, the College of American Pathologists, the American College of Physicians, the American Cancer Society, and the National Cancer Institute. The brochure contained the above definition and designated the clinical stage as TO carcinoma in situ (intraepithelial). Its detection and eradication offer marvelous opportunity to prevent the havoc caused by invasive cancer. The advantages of treating any disease in its asymptomatic state is obvious.

In 1965 HAMPERL [1965 (1)] discussed what is meant by the term "carcinoma in situ". In the same year he [1965 (2)] described the prestages and early stages of cervical carcinoma.

In an editorial in the February 1968 issue of *Obstetrics and Gynecology* DEMIN of the Cancer Unit of WHO discusses "some aspects of carcinoma in situ of the uterine cervix". He presents various viewpoints hoping "to provoke more discussions on this important subject and to obtain views and guidance to clarify the definition, limits, and proper use of this term of so great importance to pathologists, gynecologists, and oncologists". GREEN has presented his views regarding the significance of cervical carcinoma in situ which are at variance to those generally held by contributors to the literature. ASHLEY thinks there is strong evidence for the existence of two forms of cervical carcinoma. JONES et al. used a direct squash technic to study the chromosomes of tissue from the cervix from patients with atypia, carcinoma in situ, and invasive epidermoid carcinoma of the cervix. They concluded: "The findings are not inconsistent with the concept that aneuploidy is concurrent with cancer, but further study will be required to unequivocally establish this possibility and to demonstrate the diagnostic role of chromosome determination in early cancer of the cervix". At the recent meeting of the American Gynecological Society his subject was "The Value of the Assay of Chromosomes in the Diagnosis of Neoplasia". An abstract of his dissertation is as follows: "It now seems well established that most invasive epidermoid carcinomas and intraepithelial carcinomas of the cervix are composed of cells displaying aneuploidy. In lesions which are less severe than unequivocal carcinoma, it is important to determine when cytogenetic abnormalities first appear in relation to abnormalities revealed by other diagnostic methods, such as colposcopy, cytopathology and histopathology. The present study correlates the assay of chromosomes with findings of other diagnostic studies on more than 20 patients with early cervical neoplasia. From these data an estimate may be made of the value of karyotype analysis in the management of patients with squamous atypia of the cervix".

* From the Department of Obstetrics and Gynecology, Tulane University School of Medicine, Tulane Unit, Charity Hospital of Louisiana at New Orleans, and Southern Baptist Hospital, New Orleans.

68 years ago CULLEN's monograph on Cancer of the Uterus appeared. 8 years later SCHAUENSTEIN published his histologic studies of the cervix. 2 years threeafter RUBIN wrote on the pathological diagnosis of incipient carcinoma of the uterus. This was followed by SCHOTTLANDER and KERMAUNER's volume *Zur Kenntnis des Uteruscarcinoms.* To MEYER and SCHILLER must go credit in the recognition of the work on carcinoma in situ of the cervix. HINSELMANN's classic article in *Zbl. Gynäk.* appeared in 1927. The popularity of the colposcope in European clinics resulted in frequent cervical biopsy and study of cervical lesions earlier than in the United States of America. However, it must be said that PEMBERTON and SMITH reported their series under the title of the early diagnosis and prevention of carcinoma of the cervix in 1929. In 1928 at the Third Race Betterment Conference PAPANICOLAOU presented "new cancer diagnosis through the recognition of exfoliated cancer cells". 5 years later SCHILLER wrote in the Official Scientific Journal of the American College of Surgeons on the early diagnosis of carcinoma of the cervix. In 1943 the volume entitled *Diagnosis of Uterine Cancer by the Vaginal Smear* by PAPANICOLAOU and TRAUT resulted in the acceptance and appreciation of this excellent diagnostic procedure. DOUGLAS informs us that PAPANICOLAOU graduated at the University of Athens Medical School and went to Vienna to study philosophy. Disenchantment followed and he enrolled at Hertig's Institute for Experimental Biology at the University of Munich. In 1949 YOUNGE et al. reported 135 cases of carcinoma in situ. Since then substantial series have been reported by those authors shown in Table 1 and others. In 1963 FUNNELL and MERRILL reported a recurrence rate of 8.1% in 74 cases. Published tables compiled from reported cases regarding vaginal recurrencies and/or invasive carcinoma must be analyzed taking into consideration the thoroughness of the surgical procedure in each case, the total number of patients treated, and the time interval since treatment. Undoubtedly there have been cases in which areas of carcinoma in situ in the upper vagina have not been excised. Some so-called "recurrences" are attributable to field cancerization for embryologic reasons. Others are explainable by the multicentric origin of cancer in the genital tract. The reader is referred to articles by MARCUS, NEWMAN and CROMER, HALLGRIMISSON, LAUCHLAN, and STAHMANN.

It would probably be startlingly interesting to know the number of women whose cervical carcinoma in situ has been cured by postpartum electric cauterization. The senior author has been and continues to be a strong advocate of the procedure in cases where there are eversions, erosions and/or cysts provided PAPANICOLAOU smears are negative.

Given a patient with a proved diagnosis of carcinoma in situ of the cervix one must consider the following. Is she pregnant? If so, what is the duration of gestation? What are her age, gravidity, parity, and number of living children? Does she desire additional progeny? What is her general condition? What signs and symptoms are present or elicitable? What is her attitude toward her uterus? What is her husband's attitude toward it? Time explaining the function of the uterus may prevent unhappiness to all concerned. Ignorance causes uncertainty. In *Maxims in Prose* JOHANN WOLFGANG GOETHE said, "What we do not understand we do not possess".

In surgically treating each patient it is essential to individualize the patient. She must not be treated as a statistic.

It is generally agreed that if a cervical lesion is present, punch biopsy is indicated. TE LINDE and others have been strong advocates of multiple punch biopsies. If this procedure reveals some condition less severe than invasive carcinoma or the cervix presents a homogeneous appearance, multiple sections must be examined by the pathologist so that he can properly report on the condition of the cervix. Most of the workers agree that this is best accomplished by submitting a cold knife cone specimen to the pathologist. If his final analysis confirms the presence of cervical carcinoma in situ the definitive treatment recommended is total hysterectomy with adequate excision of the vaginal cuff. The type of hysterectomy will depend upon the case. Inasmuch as patients with carcinoma in situ frequently present a history of multiparity and findings of pelvic relaxation, hysterectomy is often performed by the vaginal route with the indicated reparative procedures.

Writing on the evaluation of biopsy, cone and hysterectomy sequence in intraepithelial carcinoma of the cervix SILBAR and WOODRUFF stated: "In a series of 124 cases in which biopsy, cone and hysterectomy specimens were available, there were three instances in which invasive cervical cancer was not discovered on biopsy but recognized in the cone, an incidence of 2.4%. In an additional 61 cases, 8 instances of invasive carcinoma were not recognized in biopsy material but discovered in the cone specimen. The overall error in the 195 cases was 5.94%. Biopsy is an important step in the planned diagnostic study of cervical disease. It is imperative that the biopsy be adequate and that the pathologist's report include a statement as to its adequacy. The more widespread use of such diagnostic tools as colposcopy in association with the directed biopsy...may lead to refinement in diagnosis of cervical disease and reduction in percentage error in tissue study".

If childbearing function is to be preserved, cervical conization is the treatment advised. If that operation reveals no evidence of invasion, the patient is seen for examination and PAPANICOLAOU smears every 3 months for 1 year and every 6 months thereafter. If the cervical and vaginal smears continue to be normal the patient is advised to become pregnant. If the smears again show cytologic abnormality further investigation is indicated and definitive therapy may be necessary. If the smear during pregnancy indicates the necessity for re-evaluation and it is necessary to perform a cervical conization to rule out invasive carcinoma, it is advised that the procedure be done during the second trimester of pregnancy. If only carcinoma in situ is proved by conization during pregnancy the patient should be allowed to deliver vaginally unless there are obstetric indications for cesarean section.

Cervical Conization

In 1955 SCHIFFER et al. reported 210 cervical conizations. In a discussion of their technic they mention that a 1:100,000 Neosynephrine solution is injected submucosally and into the body of the cervix. In their summary they state: "The extended cone biopsy may be used as the definitive treatment for carcinoma in situ in selected patients. Cytologic follow-up of patients having had this procedure is an intrinsic part of the procedure".

In 1960 HESTER and READ evaluated 155 cervical conizations listing the indications and complications. They stressed the reliability of this procedure for diagnostic purposes. They concluded: "The high percentage of residual abnormal cervical epithelium in the uterus following conization re-emphasizes total hysterectomy as the treatment of choice in carcinoma in situ".

At the 1966 meeting of the Central Association of Obstetricians and Gynecologists ROGERS and WILLIAMS evaluated the impact of the suspicious PAPANICOLAOU smear on the outcome of pregnancy. They stated: "102 pregnant patients who were found to have suspicious smears were studied. Over 40% were found to have carcinoma in situ but none had frank invasive carcinoma. Of the patients subjected to conization, $^1/_3$ had postoperative complications. There were significant and related perinatal problems in approximately $^1/_5$. The immediate routine conization biopsy when the repeated suspicious PAPANICOLAOU smear is found in a pregnant patient is a rule of therapy which should be challenged, studied, and revised. This conclusion is at odds with the opinions of a majority of the chiefs of approved Obstetrics and Gynecology residency programs whose views were surveyed." This was a study of nationwide attitudes and maternal and perinatal complications.

In 1967 ANDERSON and LINTON presented the results of a retrospective survey of 415 cervical conizations comparing the diagnostic accuracy of cervical biopsy and cervical conizations. They wrote: "Conization of the cervix is recommended as the diagnostic procedure of choice after an abnormal cytologic smear because of its greater accuracy."

In 1967 ADELMAN and HAJDU reviewed a series of 100 cone biopsy specimens diagnosed as carcinoma in situ followed by hysterectomy. They stated: "The purpose of the study was to determine when the cone biopsy in itself may constitute the final therapy for carcinoma in situ. The data, although statistically insignificant, suggest that such a predictable relationship does exist and that hysterectomy can be bypassed in certain patients provided that a close follow-up is assured." They concluded: "An undeniable risk is associated with conservative therapy of carcinoma in situ and this must be weighed against the equally undeniable risk associated with overtreatment to determine the proper course of action in individual patients."

In 1968 CRISP et al. discussed shallow conization of the cervix, having performed it in 232 patients for diagnostic purposes. They found carcinoma in 41% of the specimens. The chief advantage of the method is the relative freedom from complications. In a discussion of their technic they mention the use of Ioprep[1]. They stated that this stains the cervix like Schiller's solution. They suggest the use of scissors after the incision is carried around the circumference of the cervical os to a depth of approximately 1.5 to 2 cm. After removal of the cone with the scissors the cervical canal is dilated and a fractional curettage is done. A Surgicel[2] pack is placed in the conization site. Only 4 of 227 nonpregnant patients required later suturing of the cervix according to their report.

At the 1967 meeting of District VII of the American College of Obstetricians and Gynecologists MCCANN et al. presented their analysis of the records of all patients undergoing sharp conization on the Louisiana State University Unit at Charity Hospital in New Orleans from January 1, 1949 through 1964. During that time there were 431 conizations performed on 400 patients. There were no conization operative deaths or hysterectomies required for control of bleeding. Of the 114 patients with diagnosis of carcinoma in situ in the conization specimen, 29 had residual carcinoma in situ in the hysterectomy specimen.

Obviously, a candidate for cervical conization is entitled to complete preoperative evaluation. It is mandatory that she not have any disturbances in her bleeding and coagulation mechanisms. The type of anesthesia will be selected in each case. Although FLEMING and others have devised special conization instruments the use of the scalpel

[1] Arbrook, Somerville, N.J.

[2] Surgicel, Johnson & Johnson, New Brunswick, N.J.

blade is most common. Over 20 years ago CROSSEN advocated extensive conization using an electrode but this method had a destructive effect on the tissues to be examined. Technics for cervical conization and/or hysterectomy have been described by MARTIUS, TE LINDE, BALL, LYON et al., TOPEK, KAPLAN and KAUFMAN, and many others.

After arrival in the operating room the patient's urinary bladder is emptied by catheterization. (If hysterectomy is contemplated as the definitive procedure, a No. 14 or 16 Foley catheter is left indwelling.) The vagina is sponged dry. For many years operators have been scrubbing the vulva and vagina with soap and water prior to painting the cervix and vagina with Lugol's solution. It has been pointed out by numerous writers that the scrubbing and use of detergents should be discontinued.

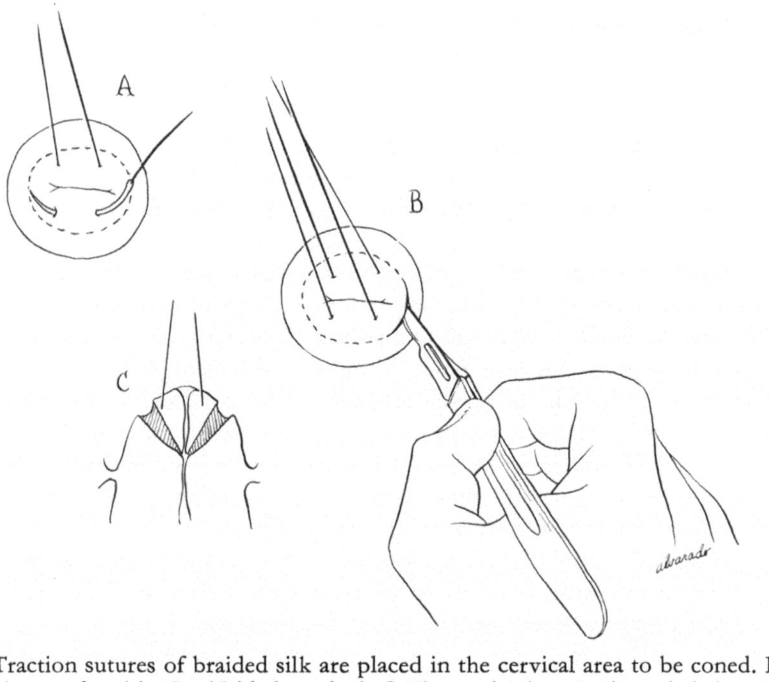

Fig. 1. A Traction sutures of braided silk are placed in the cervical area to be coned. B Incision is being made with No. 15 blade scalpel. C The conization specimen is being pulled away from the cervix. It should be conical, not cylindrical

At the present time we are of the opinion that 1% aqueous solution of toluidine blue dye applied to the cervix and vagina followed by destaining with 3% acetic acid as described by RICHART is more accurate than the Schiller test. One notes "the confluent areas of blue-staining epithelium adjacent to the squamocolumnar junction lying in the transformation zone". As a result, areas of nuclear concentration are thereby demonstrated. A figure of eight 0 chromic catgut suture is placed bilaterally at the cervicovaginal junction. When tied, these sutures serve for purposes of hemostasis and traction. Two sutures of braided silk are placed in the base of the cone to be removed as shown in Fig. 1 and as described by TWOMBLY at the last Clinical Meeting of the American Association of Obstetricians and Gynecologists.

Depending upon the results of the staining test a circular incision is made with a No. 15 scalpel blade. The mucous membrane peripheral to this incision is then freed for several millimeters. A cone of tissue is removed, care being taken to stay below the internal cervical os. The remaining portion of the cervical canal and the internal os are dilated and uterine curettage performed. Two or more figure of eight sutures may be required laterally to secure hemostasis.

Fig. 2 illustrates the overlapping of catgut sutures placed just below the cervicovaginal junction as advocated by TOPEK et al. in pregnant patients. He points out that the tying of the sutures results in constriction of the cervix. They state: "As a result, the cervix is somewhat puckered and everted; therefore, the scalpel should be directed to obtain what appears to be a very shallow cone. However, the cone will be adequate and sufficiently deep. Further hemostasis and correction of the defect of the cervix can then be accomplished by figure of eight or Sturmdorf type sutures

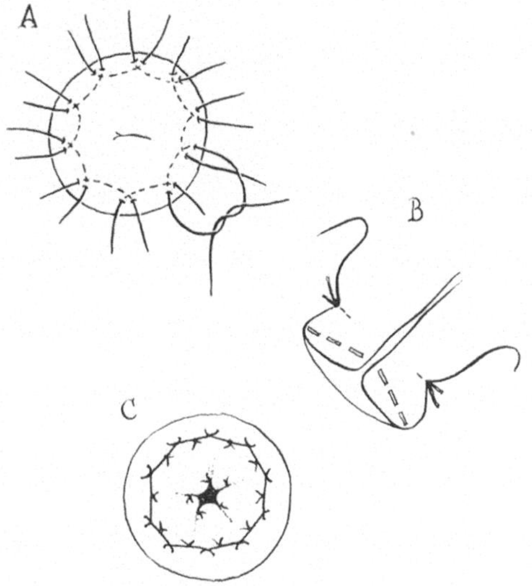

Fig. 2. A Overlapping 0 chromic catgut sutures in the cervix of pregnancy. B Lateral sutures have been tied. C Sturmdorf and Fig. 8 sutures are used for tissue approximation and for hemostasis

again employing atraumatic 0 chromic catgut. He also describes in considerable detail technic for hysterectomy with vaginal cuff, stating, "To date we have accomplished this procedure in 42 patients. 32 of them had epidermoid carcinoma in situ of the cervix".

Hysterectomy with Vaginal Cuff Excision

When definitive treatment for carcinoma in situ of the cervix is required, a hysterectomy with removal of approximately 2.5 cm of vaginal cuff is advisable. As pointed out by PARKER et al. vaginal hysterectomy has been performed in preference to abdominal hysterectomy in recent years for the reason that the necessary margin of vaginal cuff can be delineated under direct vision and the hysterectomy may be combined with colpoplastic repair when indicated. Furthermore, as LASH has stated, the extracervical lesions disclosed by the Schiller test can be excised. The use of braided silk traction sutures placed in the four quadrants at the cervicovaginal junction is advocated. The vaginal cuff is developed posteriorly beginning in the midline about 2.5 cm from the cervicovaginal junction. In extending the incision laterally one should follow a ruga. This also facilitates removing a satisfactory amount of tissue in all directions. Anteriorly the mucous membrane is freed by dissection from the bladder, laterally from the ligaments and posteriorly from the peritoneum

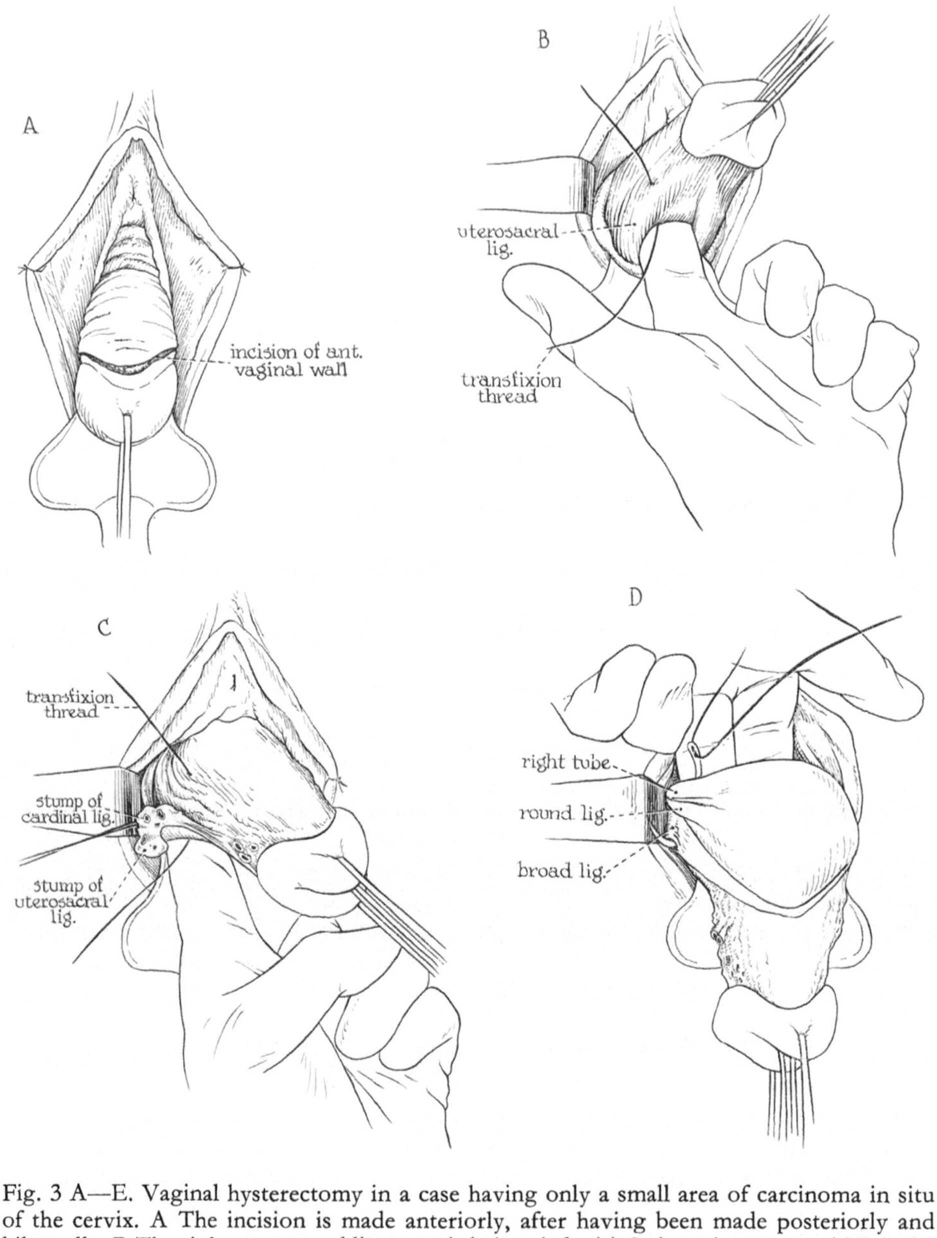

Fig. 3 A—E. Vaginal hysterectomy in a case having only a small area of carcinoma in situ of the cervix. A The incision is made anteriorly, after having been made posteriorly and bilaterally. B The right uterosacral ligament is being tied with 0 chromic catgut, which is the suture material to be used throughout the operation. C The uterosacral and cardinal ligaments have been ligated with transfixion sutures and a similar suture is being placed to ligate the uterine blood vessels. D The salpinx, the top of the broad ligament, and the round and utero-ovarian ligaments are being ligated. E The peritoneum of the cul-de-sac of Douglas is ready for closure. A pursestring suture will be used

of the cul-de-sac of DOUGLAS. The cuff should be adequate to cover a 7.5 × 7.5 cm 12 ply gauze sponge. The cuff is sutured and the cul-de-sac of DOUGLAS is entered. The supravaginal septum is cut and the vesicouterine fold of peritoneum opened. Hysterectomy is performed by modified Martius technic (see Fig. 3). The tubes and ovaries are inspected and palpated. In the absence of disease they are left in situ. If the patient has an enterocele it is corrected. If she has stress urinary incontinence a urethrocystopexy is done. If there is a rectocele and/or perineal relaxation repair is done. If the patient is a candidate for an abdominal rather than a vaginal hysterectomy we favor development of the cuff vaginally as described. We suture it over the previously mentioned sponge prior to placing the patient in the usual position for laparotomy. Upon opening the abdomen the tubes and ovaries are carefully inspected and palpated. Their removal will be predicated upon their condition and not on the age of the patient. If the appendix vermiformis is in view it will be removed prior to packing off the intestines; otherwise, its extirpation will be done subsequent to the hysterectomy and exploration of the peritoneal cavity.

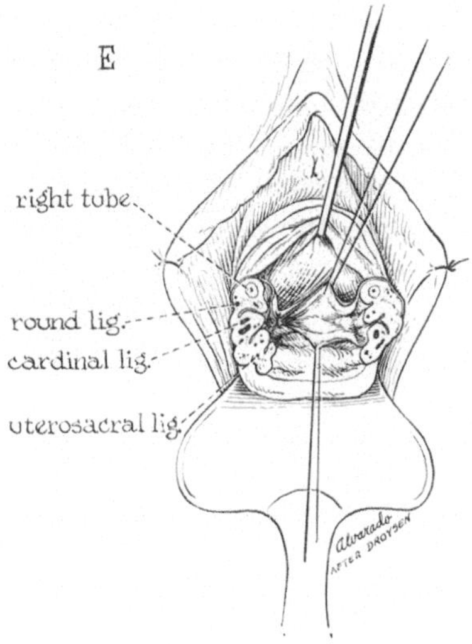

Fig. 3E

Patients treated by hysterectomy and vaginal cuff excision should be followed at regular intervals by examination and cytologic studies to detect the occasional recurrence of intraepithelial cancer or the development of an invasive lesion in the vagina.

OSOBA, CAVANAGH and RUTLEDGE, RUTLEDGE and IBANEZ, and MALINAK et al. have studied the conization-hysterectomy time interval. They concluded: "Hysterectomy should be postponed for at least 3 weeks and probably longer after conization, unless the conization specimen can be accurately studied immediately so that a definitive operation may be carried out without delay." In 1962 KAUFMAN et al. discussed "use of the refrigerated microtome for rapid diagnosis of cervical conization specimens". In this and subsequent articles they have demonstrated the accuracy of frozen section study and enumerated the advantage of the cryostat method. Among these is definitive surgery, including hysterectomy, which can be performed while the patient is still on the operating table. If she proves to have invasive carcinoma she can be treated definitively by the application of radium or by the indicated surgery. Immediate complications of conization such as bleeding and infection while the patient waits for the surgery are eliminated when the hysterectomy is promptly done.

The morbidity rate associated with the delay in performing hysterectomy following conization is markedly decreased; furthermore, the hospital stay is definitely shortened. At the Southern Baptist Hospital we have been impressed by the advantages of the cryostat technic. In cases of carcinoma in situ of the cervix requiring hysterectomy the cone has been obtained and hysterectomy done under the same anesthetic upon receipt of the pathologist's report. As KAUFMAN states: "The psychologic advantages for the patient when immediate hysterectomy is performed are quite obvious. The prospect of having to return to the operating room for a second operative procedure or having to delay surgery for 6 or more weeks, is not a pleasant one for most patients."

Carcinoma in Situ During Pregnancy

Greene and Peckham have proved that physiologic gestational cervical epithelium does not mimic carcinoma in situ. Mussey and Decker, Walters and Reagan, and Wright have written convincingly regarding the accuracy of cytologic diagnosis of cervical conditions during pregnancy. At the present time one might surmise that the incidence of cervical carcinoma in situ in pregnancy is about 1 in 333 gestations. The hazards of bleeding, infection, abortion, premature labor, and malfunction of the cervix during labor are discussed in articles on cervical carcinoma during pregnancy by many contributors.

Table 1. *Reported recurrence of carcinoma in situ of cervix uteri*

Author	Years	Pts.	Pts. treated	Recurr.
Friedell et al.	1926—52	235	232	0
Fennell	1927—53	118	106	3
Gusberg and Marshall	1927—59	327	310	6
Mussey and Soule	1932—47	842	838	5
Parker et al.	1947—53	485	361	2
Cox	1955—59	146	146	3
Devereux and Edwards	1960—64	632	630	6
		2785	2623	25

The number of pregnant patients included in the series of the authors listed in Table 1 are as follows: Parker et al. 64, Devereux and Edwards 19, Mussey and Soule 14, Cox 7. In 1960 Beecham and Andros reported a series of 26 conization biopsies of the cervix during pregnancy. Indications, technics, and complications were discussed. In the same year Ferguson and Brown reported 50 cases. In 1964 Boutselis and Uliery discussed 69 cases of intraepithelial carcinoma of the cervix in pregnancy. The incidence of complications following diagnostic conization was 14.5%. They stated: "Definitive therapy for carcinoma in situ at our institution consists of total hysterectomy, resection of 1 to 2 cm of upper vaginal cuff and preservation of the ovaries during the childbearing years." Williams and Turnbull reported on 76 cases, 52 of whom were treated by modified Wertheim hysterectomy, 10 had conizations of the cervix alone. In 1966 Moore et al. discuss the diagnosis and management of 42 cases with carcinoma in situ of the cervix during pregnancy. They included "not only cancer confined to the surface epithelium and/or the endocervical glands but also microscopic stromal invasion — i.e. that limited to the outer 2 to 3 mm of subepithelial tissue". 29 patients were subjected to cervical conization and this was the definitive treatment in 25% of the patients. At the time of the report they had not observed any recurrences after definitive treatment (conization or hysterectomy). Four cesarean hysterectomies were performed.

In a review of 60 cases of pregnancy following the conservative treatment of 50 patients with cervical carcinoma in situ GREEN stated: "Whilst the number of patients with abortion, premature labour, or cervical dystocia was not greatly increased it is considered that cervical conization tends to cause these complications and should be replaced by a ring-type biopsy when future childbearing is important."

FESTE et al. reported 13 cesarean section hysterectomies with abnormal cervicovaginal smears detected late in pregnancy. They stated: "Cervical conization with cryostat frozen section evaluation followed by immediate cesarean section hysterectomy was carried out on 9 patients. 4 patients had cesarean section hysterectomy performed at term because of a prior conization during pregnancy revealing squamous cell carcinoma in situ." Among their conclusions we find: "Cesarean section hysterectomy with removal of 2 to 3 cm of vaginal cuff is advocated at or near term as treatment for those patients diagnosed as having squamous cell carcinoma in situ of the cervix during pregnancy when no further childbearing is desired. When more children are desired, vaginal delivery is allowed."

MUSSEY and DECKER gave a case analysis of 95 patients who were pregnant either when intraepithelial carcinoma was proved or within the previous year. Of the 37 patients having intraepithelial carcinoma during pregnancy gestation was interrupted in 12 instances by hysterectomy. Four additional patients had carcinoma in situ in association with incomplete abortion and the remaining 21 women were allowed to complete their pregnancies after the malignancy had been proved. Their final comment is: "Cancer of the cervix in association with pregnancy need no longer be a tragic situation, difficult to manage, if adequate cytologic screening of the cervix of the young women becomes an integral part of the practice of every physician managing prenatal care. Conization, although not as extensive as in the nonpregnant patient, can and should include adequate tissue for examination by means of the frozen section technic, permitting prompt and accurate evaluation by the pathologist as to the inclusion of a margin of normal epithelium and the exclusion of microinvasion. Iodine staining of the cervix prior to conization also helps delineate the size of the cone. We conclude that cauterization should be used for hemostasis after conization since there is a much lower incidence of residual intraepithelial carcinoma in cervices thus treated."

At the 1967 meeting of the Pacific Coast Obstetrical and Gynecological Society, JONES et al. reported the results of 5 years of cytodetection of the cervix during pregnancy in the Prenatal Clinics of the City and County of Los Angeles, stating: "Patients with carcinoma in situ, regardless of age, were urged to have a hysterectomy. Women desirous of having children and willing to continue cytologic examinations every 3 months, were treated by the diagnostic conization. Only half of these patients have honored their commitment to appear regularly for cytologic follow-up".

Carcinoma in Situ at Charity Hospital at New Orleans

Table 2 bearing the caption Charity Hospital of Louisiana at New Orleans concerns an institution of over 2400 beds which are divided in two Medical School Services called Units.

TORRES states that on the Louisiana State University Unit of Charity Hospital at New Orleans the number of carcinoma in situ of the cervix cases were as follows: 1960 — 33, 1961 — 23, 1962 — 32, 1963 — 51, 1964 — 50, 1965 — 71, 1966 — 42, 1967 — 25. He stated: "As you may know, in 1963 we extended our cytology screening program in our clinics and the increased number of cases diagnosed from 1963 through 1965 I believe is a reflection of the efficacy of this program. The drop that has occurred in 1966 and 1967 I believe is due to the fact that we are reaching a prevalence figure in our static clinic population which is approaching the figure for new case incidence per year." The total number of cases diagnosed during pregnancy for the years 1956 through 1966 was 34. In an article published in 1964 TORRES et al.

Table 2. *Charity Hospital of Louisiana at New Orleans*

	1963	1964	1965	1966	1967	Total
Births	8983	8785	8925	8741	8444	43878
Cesareans	439	382	333	315	312	1781
C. Hysterectomies	100	94	86	92	77	449
Gyn. Admits.	2471	2467	2669	2603	2298	12508
Abd. Hysterectomies	469	543	311	401	317	2041
Vag. Hysterectomies	451	332	774	620	408	2585

Table 3. *Charity Hospital of Louisiana at New Orleans. Tulane unit*

	1963	1964	1965	1966	1967	Total
Births	4432	4361	4481	4345	4244	21863
Cesareans	131	118	124	150	137	660
C. Hysterectomies	44	54	49	49	63	259
Gyn. Admits.	1236	1209	1250	1066	1127	5888
Abd. Hysterectomies	143	148	145	151	215	802
Vag. Hysterectomies	265	275	298	285	216	1339

Table 4. *Cervical carcinoma in situ at New Orleans Charity Hospital. Tulane unit*

	1960	1961	1962	1963	1964	1965	Total
Cases	14	39	22	21	31	15	142
White/nonwhite	2/12	7/32	2/20	7/14	9/22	0/15	27/115
Conization only	1[a]	2	1[a]	0	1	1	6
Wide cuff hysterectomy	10	28	17	17	23	11	106
Abd. hysterectomy	2	5	2	2	3	3	17
Vag. hysterectomy	1	2	0	1	2	0	6
Cesarean hysterectomy	0	1	0	0	1	1	3
Residual tumor in hyst. specimen	0	0	0	9	12	7	28

[a] Pregnant.

stated: "It is possible that dysplasia may precede the appearance of carcinoma in situ. For this reason it is necessary to follow patients with dysplasia carefully, since an unknown number of these women may develop carcinoma".

Table 3 provides some data concerning the Tulane University Unit at Charity Hospital. During the last 5 years for which records were available 142 proved cases of cervical carcinoma in situ were tabulated. See Table 4. Of these 27 were white and 115 nonwhite. The oldest patient was 82 and the youngest 15. As shown, wide cuff hysterectomy was the most often employed type of treatment. Most of these were done by the vaginal route. The 17 patients who had abdominal hysterectomy without wide cuff excision included such emergency cases as ruptured tubo-ovarian abscesses and ectopic pregnancies. A number of the hysterectomies were for myomas. There were 3 cesarean hysterectomies. Residual tumor was found in 28 hysterectomy specimens. In 1963 a patient who had a recurrence after wide cuff vaginal hysterectomy was given the benefit of exenteration. She is alive today.

Carcinoma in Situ at Southern Baptist Hospital

The Southern Baptist Hospital is a private institution of approximately 475 beds. In contrast to Charity Hospital where the patient population is overwhelmingly non-white the patients at this institution are white. Table 5 shows that there were 21,008 births there during the past 5 years. This exceeds the number of white births at Charity Hospital during the same time. Records of 87 patients having cervical carcinoma in situ from January 1, 1963 through 1967 were available for perusal. Treatment of 73 patients was by 27 obstetricians-gynecologists. 5 patients were treated by general surgeons, the same number by general practitioners, and 3 were operated upon by Residents in Obstetrics and Gynecology. 1 patient deserted after histologic diagnosis had been made but before hysterectomy with wide cuff excision could be performed.

Table 5. *Southern Baptist Hospital, New Orleans*

	1963	1964	1965	1966	1967	Total
Births	4426	4417	4121	4106	3938	21008
Cesareans	283	238	228	224	183	1156
C. hysterectomies	32	26	42	46	33	179
Gyn. admits.	1888	1707	1776	1859	1852	9082
Abd. hysterectomies	353	514	576	613	652	2708
Vag. hysterectomies	343	342	364	365	319	1733

Table 6. *Southern Baptist Hospital. Carcinoma in situ of cervix uteri*

	1963	1964	1965	1966	1967	Total
Patients	9	12	19	25	22	87
Conization only	1	2	3	4	4	14
Conization and hysterectomy	1	4	6	7	5	23
Conization, hysterectomy later	5	5	6	7	11	34
Abdominal hysterectomy	7	7	10	7	13	44
Vaginal hysterectomy	0	2	5	11	5	23
Excision cervical stump	0	0	0	1	0	1
Cesarean hysterectomy	1	0	0	1	0	2
Residual tumor in hyst. specimen	4	8	5	10	8	35

1966 1 case radio-therapy.
1964 and 1965 1 case D and C and cervical biopsy.

In Table 6 it will be noticed that 23 patients were given the benefit of hysterectomy as soon as the pathologist reported on examination of the conization specimen by the cryostat method. As previously stated, this is a time and money-saving procedure. Even more important, it prevents complications and dangers inherent in a second stage procedure, also anxiety. Two of the patients had cesarean hysterectomy. 35 hysterectomy specimens showed residual tumor. During the last few years more of the operators have been employing the wide cuff hysterectomy technic. Fig. 4 shows the age distribution of the patients. The youngest patient was 20 and the oldest was 65. HAJDU et al. reported the case of a 15 year old Negress who had two babies. He mentioned the 16 year old patient of FERGUSON.

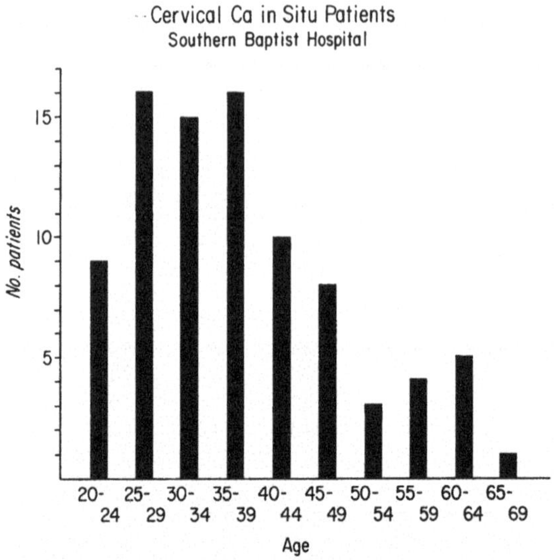

Fig. 4. Most of the patients in the Southern Baptist Hospital series were in the 25 through 39 years age groups

References

ADELMAN, H. C., and S. J. HAJDU: Amer. J. Obstet. Gynec. **98**, 173—179 (1967).
ANDERSON, S. G., and E. B. LINTON: Amer. J. Obstet. Gynec. **98**, 113—116 (1967).
ASHLEY, D. J. B.: J. Obstet. Gynaec. Brit. Cwlth **73**, 382—389 (1966).
— J. Obstet. Gynaec. Brit. Cwlth **73**, 372—381 (1966).
BALL, T. W.: Gynecologic surgery and urology, 2nd. ed. St. Louis, Mo.: C. V. Mosby Co. 1963.
BEECHAM, C. T., and G. J. ANDROS: Obstet. and Gynec. **16**, 521—526 (1960).
BOUTSELIS, J. G., and J. C. ULLERY: Amer. J. Obstet. Gynec. **90**, 593—609 (1964).
CAVANAGH, D., and F. RUTLEDGE: Amer. J. Obstet. Gynec. **80**, 53—59 (1960).
COX, B. S.: J. Obstet. Gynaec. Brit. Cwlth **74**, 723—727 (1967).
CRISP, W. E., H. SHALAUTA, and W. A. BENNETT: Obstet. and Gynec. **31**, 755—758 (1968).
CROSSEN, H. S., and R. J. CROSSEN: Operative gynecology, 6th ed. St. Louis, Mo.: C. V. Mosby Co. 1948.
CULLEN, T. S.: Cancer of the uterus. New York: Appleton 1900
DEMIN, V. N.: Obstet. and Gynec. **31**, 288—292 (1968).
DEVEREUX, W. P., and C. L. EDWARDS: Amer. J. Obstet. Gynec. **98**, 497—508 (1967).
DOUGLAS, R. G., GEORGE N. PAPANICOLAOU: Trans. Amer. gynec. Soc. **85**, 185—187 (1962).
FENNELL, R. H., JR.: Cancer (Philad.) **9**, 374—384 (1956).
FERGUSON, J. H., and G. C. BROWN: Surg. Gynec. Obstet. **111**, 603—606 (1960).
FESTE, J. R., R. H. KAUFMAN, H. L. SKOGLAND, and N. H. TOPEK: Amer. J. Obstet. Gynec. **95**, 763—768 (1966).
FRIEDELL, G. H., A. T. HERTIG, and P. A. YOUNGE: Carcinoma in situ of uterine cervix: A study of 235 cases from the Free Hospital for Women. Springfield: Thomas 1960.
FUNNELL, J. D., and J. A. MERRILL: Surg. Gynec. Obstet. **117**, 15—19 (1963).

GREEN, G. H.: Amer. J. Obstet. Gynec. **94**, 1009—1022 (1966).
— Obstet. Gynaec. Brit. Cwlth **73**, 897—902 (1966).
— Int. Surg. **47**, 511—517 (1967).
GREENE, R. R., and B. B. PECKHAM: Amer. J. Obstet. Gynec. **75**, 551—564 (1948).
GUSBERG, S. G., and D. MARSHALL: Obstet. and Gynec. **19**, 713—720 (1962).
HAJDU, S. I., J. SO-BOSITA, and A. B. LITTLE: Amer. J. Obstet. Gynec. **100**, 1154—1155 (1968).
HALLGRIMISSON, J. T.: Acta obstet. gynec. scand. **46**, 268—272 (1967).
HAMPERL, H.: (1) Med. Welt (Stuttg.) **20**, 1098—1100 (1965).
— (2) Geburtsh. u. Frauenheilk. **25/2**, 105—111 (1965).
HESTER, L. L., and R. A. READ: Amer. J. Obstet. Gynec. **80**, 715—721 (1960).
HINSELMANN, H.: Zbl. Gynäk. **51**, 901—903 (1927).
JONES, E. G., C. P. SCHWINN, W. K. BULLOCK, A. VARGA, J. E. DUNN, H. FRIEDMAN JR., and J. WEIR: Amer. J. Obstet. Gynec. **101**, 298—306 (1968).
JONES, H. W., JR., K. P. KATAYAMA, A. STAFL, and H. J. DAVIS: Obstet. and Gynec. **30**, 790—805 (1967).
KAPLAN, A. L., and R. H. KAUFMAN: Clin. Obstet. Gynec. **10**, 871—878 (1967).
KAUFMAN, R. H.: Clin. Obstet. Gynec. **10**, 838—852 (1967).
—, J. T. ABBOTT, and W. C. SCHEIHING: Amer. J. Obstet. Gynec. **84**, 107—112 (1962).
—, O. G. JANES, and H. A. COX: Amer. J. Obstet. Gynec. **92**, 71—77 (1965).
—, W. A. JOHNSON, J. J. SPJUT, and A. SMITH: Acta cytol. (Philad.) **11**, 272—278 (1967).
KOTTMEIER, H. L.: Official classification of certain pelvic malignancies approved. A.C.O.G. Newsletter, p. 11—12, Feb. 1963.
LASH, A. F.: Int. Surg. **47**, 518—527 (1967).
LAUCHLAN, S. C., and D. W. PENNER: Cancer (Philad.) **20**, 2250—2254 (1967).
LYON, J. B., S. HAJJAR, and J. D. THOMPSON: Sth. med. J. (Bgham, Ala.) **58**, 937—944 (1965).
MALINAK, L. R., R. A. JEFFREY JR., and W. J. DUNN: Obstet. and Gynec. **23**, 317—329 (1964).
MARCUS, S. L.: Amer. J. Obstet. Gynec. **80**, 802—812 (1960).
MARTIUS, H.: Martius' gynecological operations, 7th. ed. Translation by MCCALL, M. L., and K. A. BOLTEN. Boston: Little, Brown & Co. 1956.
MCCANN, S. W., A. MICKAL, and J. T. CRAPANZANO: Personal communication.
MEYER, R.: Zbl. Gynäk. **47**, 946—960 (1923).
MOORE, J. G., R. G. WELLS, and D. G. MORTON: Obstet. and Gynec. **27**, 307—318 (1966).
MUSSEY, E., and D. G. DECKER: Amer. J. Obstet. Gynec. **97**, 30—38 (1967).
—, and E. H. SOULE: Amer. J. Obstet. Gynec. **77**, 957—972 (1959).
NEWMAN, W., and J. K. CROMER: Surg. Gynec. Obstet. **108**, 273—281 (1959).
OSOBA, D.: Canad. med. Ass. J. **79**, 805—809 (1958).
PAPANICOLAOU, G. N.: Proc. Third Race Betterment Conference, 1928.
—, and H. F. TRAUT: Diagnosis of uterine cancer by the vaginal smear. Cambridge: Commonwealth Fund, Harvard Univ. Press 1943.
PARKER, R. T., W. K. CUYLER, L. A. KAUFMAN, B. CARTER, W. L. THOMAS, R. N. CREADICK, V. H. TURNER, C. H. PEETE JR., and W. B. CHERNEY: Amer. J. Obstet. Gynec. **80**, 693—710 (1960).
PEMBERTON, F. A., and G. V. S. SMITH: Amer. J. Obstet. Gynec. **17**, 165—176 (1929).
RICHART, R. M.: Amer. J. Obstet. Gynec. **86**, 703—712 (1963).
ROGERS, R. S., and J. H. WILLIAMS: Amer. J. Obstet. Gynec. **98**, 488—494 (1967).
RUBIN, I.: Amer. J. Obstet. Gynec. **62**, 668—676 (1910).
RUTLEDGE, R., and M. L. IBANEZ: Amer. J. Obstet. Gynec. **83**, 1208—1213 (1961).
SCHIFFER, M. A., J. J. GREENE, W. POMERANCE, and A. MOLTZ: Amer. J. Obstet. Gynec. **93**, 889—895 (1965).
SCHILLER, W.: Surg. Gynec. Obstet. **56**, 210—222 (1933).
SCHAUENSTEIN, W.: Arch. Gynäk. **85**, 576—616 (1908).
SCHOTTLANDER, J., and F. KERMAUNER: Zur Kenntnis des Uteruskarzinoms. Berlin: Karger 1912.
SILBAR, E. L., and J. D. WOODRUFF: Obstet. and Gynec. **27**, 89—97 (1966).
STAHMANN, F. S.: S. Dak. J. Med. Pharm. **17**, 19—21 (1964).

TE LINDE, R. W.: Operative gynecology, 3rd. ed. Philadelphia (Pa.): J. B. Lippincott Co. 1962.
—, G. A. GLAVIN, and H. W. JONES JR.: Amer. J. Obstet. Gynec. **74**, 792—803 (1957).
TORRES, J. E.: Personal communication.
— Acta cytol. (Philad.) **8**, 284—287 (1964).
TOPEK, N. H.: Clin. Obstet. Gynec. **10**, 853—870 (1967).
TWOMBLY, G. H.: Personal communication.
WALTERS, W. D., and J. W. REAGAN: Amer. J. clin. Path. **26**, 1314—1325 (1956).
WILLIAMS, T. J., and K. E. TURNBULL: Obstet. and Gynec. **24**, 857—864 (1964).
WRIGHT, L.: J. Obstet. Gynaec. Brit. Cwlth **68**, 771—777 (1961).
YOUNGE, P. A., A. T. HERTIG, and D. ARMSTRONG: Amer. J. Obstet. Gynec. **58**, 867—895 (1949).

Tendencies of Growth and Spread of Squamous Cell Cancer of the Cervix

K. G. OBER

HENRIKSEN (1960) one time compared the spread of carcinoma of the cervix with a roulette. While the ball is rolling, nobody knows where it is going to stop. The probability, however, which will promise success to repeated putting in, may be small or great. Therefore the stakes are limited.

In selecting an operation for cancer most surgeons are considering different point of views. Among them are evaluation of the disease and its potential spread in the individual case.

We evaluated specimens of 379[1] abdominal operations for squamous cell carcinomas using identical techniques. The *continuous* growth of the primary tumor we use to catch by histologic giant sections of the cervix in two directions (MATUSCHKA, 1962; OBER and HUHN, 1962) in different blocks and between 100 and 300 micron in thickness (Figs. 1, 2, 4). For evaluating the *discontinuous* growth, which in most of the cases is lymph node involvement, during operation the lymph nodes are fixed in different containers with alcoholic Bouin's fluid. After a careful count the lymph nodes also are worked up by step sections (HUHN, 1964; OBER and HUHN, 1962; VOGT-HOERNER and GÉRARD-MARCHANT, 1958). In individual operations between 9 and 54 lymph nodes were removed, in the average 20.7. Altogether 7845 nodes were examined.

Extensive abdominal surgery for cancer with lymphadenectomy we carry out for those tumors almost exclusively which already can be seen with the naked eyes or palpated with the fingers. Figs. 1a—c show typically those squamous cell carcinomas which I want to talk about. Adenocarcinomas, cancers of the mesonephric duct, mucoepidermoids, mixed tumors — that are neoplasms which represent approximately 5 to 6% of all cervical cancers — are left out. Ignored are also carcinomas of the vagina (Fig. 1d) which at occasion unfoundedly may have been called cervical

[1] Part of these observations had been reported by the author together with HUHN in 1962 from the University-Women-Hospital in Cologne. Professor Dr. C. KAUFMANN was kind enough to place at our disposal another 110 specimens, which were obtained by the same surgical technique since 1962.

cancers. Quite frequently we operate the large, extensive tumors of the cervix where we still can find a dissection plane against the pelvic wall (Figs. 1b and c).

Fairly scarce among our specimens are the small, clinically easily detectable carcinomas (Fig. 1a). They can be operated well. Therefore these cases are probably treated more often outside of the large hospitals. Our material contains a relatively

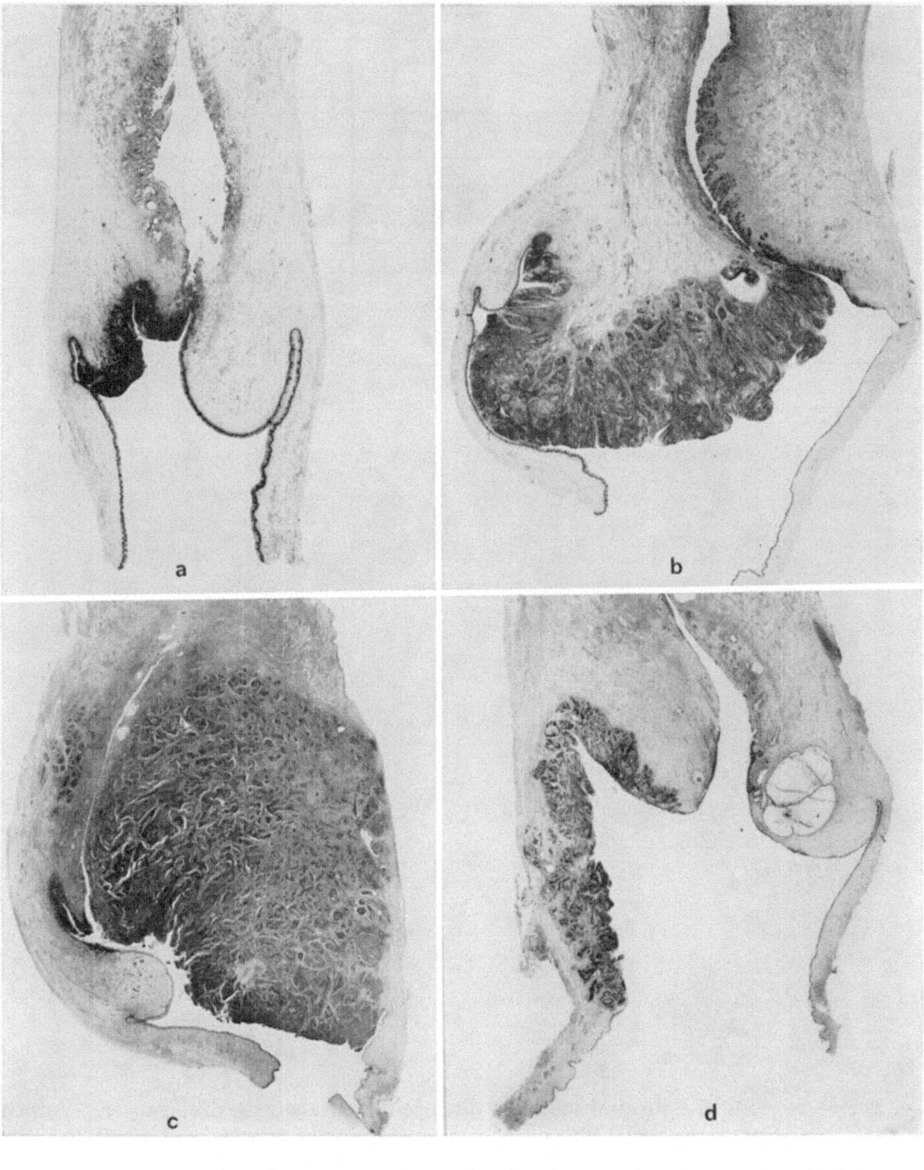

Fig. 1. Three different forms of typical carcinomas (a, b, c) compared with a high-located carcinoma of the vagina (d). b and c represent typically exophytic and endophytic growth. The carcinoma in situ which can be seen in d just above the cervical glands does not justify a classification as cervical carcinoma. The major portion of the cornified squamous cell carcinoma most likely has derived from the upper part of the vagina

small group of early cancers (Table 1)[2]. We also did not evaluate specimens of women who had received irradiation treatment prior to surgery or of others who required some type of evisceration procedure after a previous operation or curative radiation treatment had failed.

Furthermore our cases are selected from another point of view: I consider the fact that one can avoid castration to be one of the great advantages of the surgical

Table 1. *Relation of continuous growth of the primary tumor to involvement of lymph nodes of pelvic wall*

Continuous growth of the primary tumor	Cases	Lymph node involvement	
		Tumor cell emboli	Metastases
Microcarcinomata	25	—	—
Strictly confined to the cervix	207	12	35
Laterally still within the cervix, but involvement of the vagina	24	1	13
Involvement of the boundary zone(s)	70	3	24
Involvement of the boundary zone(s) and the vagina	19	—	10
Involvement of the paratissues	34	2	21
Total	379	18	103

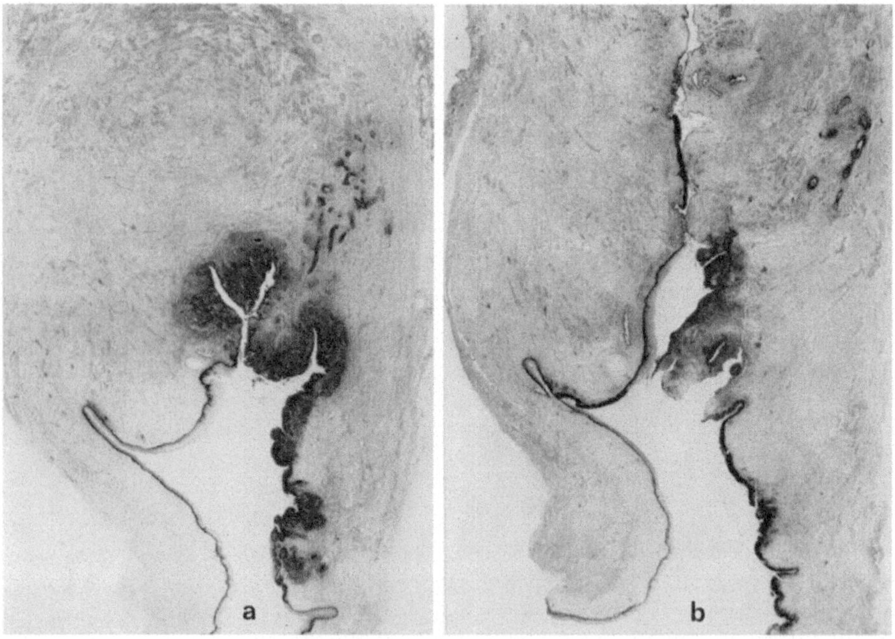

Fig. 2. Step sections of a surgical specimen disclose that a relatively small cancer — which indeed is extending to the upper fifth of the vagina — continuously makes a breach towards the paratissues. The boundary zone of the cervix has not been crossed yet. There is no case in our material showing this type of spread into the paracervical tissues

[2] 21 of the so-called microcarcinomata are coming from the hospital in Cologne. The special problems of this group were brought to attention by Kaufmann, Ober and Huhn on hand of 130 observations in 1965.

approach. Therefore in Erlangen we almost never use irradiation treatment following surgery. Quite independent of the surgical risk we predominantly operate on women under 50 years of age — even in relatively advanced carcinomas.

Since beginning of this century one was concerned with the problem of growth and spread of carcinoma of the cervix. Until about 10 years ago the investigations of BRUNET (1905), KUNDRAT (1903) and SCHEIB (1909) carried great weight. Even today they are the fundament of the international classification of stages. It is certain that cervical cancers have the special feature of remaining within the pelvis for a relatively long period of time. But the assumption that rather seldom tumors are reaching the paracervical, the paravaginal and occasionally even the parametrial tissue by continuous growth — without leading to metastases to the regional lymph nodes — today is not valid any more.

The definition of the *continuous* growth is obvious: The most advanced proliferations of the tumor still will have to be in cellular connection with the primary growth (Figs. 2a and b). The term *discontinuous* spread we apply for metastases (HAMPERL, 1960). The latter don't have direct contact with the primary tumor anymore (Figs. 3b and c, as well as Figs. 4b and c).

In regard to the *continuous* spread of cervical cancers the following suggestion appears necessary: There does not exist a distinct boundary line between the cervix and the paracervical tissues, which in the beginning of this century caused investigators to register a transgression of the cervix by the tumor for 1 or 2 mm. Cervix and paracervical tissues cannot be separated accurately from each other. A *boundary zone* (Fig. 4a) up to 5 mm in depth is located in between (OBER and HUHN, 1962; OBER and MEINRENKEN, 1964). Not before this zone has been exceeded by the cancer one is allowed to call it a *continuous* spread into the paracervical tissues. The surgeon is not able to recognize this boundary zone during the operation. A simple hysterectomy will always take place within this zone. Only operations which take along a portion of the paravaginal and paracervical tissues, will include the boundary zone too.

The diagnosis of metastases to the lymph nodes may be a problem. One will have to reckon with entirely different interpretations. A metastasis exists in that case only when a conglomerate of tumor cells has become firmly adherent to the lymph node (Figs. 3c, 5c; HAMPERL, 1960; HUHN, 1967). Not unusually seen are pictures of cell complexes which are found to be free within the marginal sinus (Figs. 3a, partly 3b). These should not be called metastases. This term should be used even less for the rather varying pictures of epithelial complexes, which at times assume more solid, more frequently, however, glandular forms. These so-called "gland inclusions", which HUHN had observed in 1962 in more than 40% of all women who had radical abdominal surgery because of a cervical cancer were partly interpreted as cancer metastases early this century.

Tables 1 and 2 show a classification of the 379 observations in regard to the *continuous* as well as the *discontinuous* spread. Most of our observations are referring to tumors which histologically clearly were limited to the cervix (207 of 379). $^1/_6$ of them (35 of 207) showed metastases of the lymph nodes. $^1/_4$ of the cancers (89 of 379) had proliferated continuously up to the boundary zone. A good $^1/_3$ of those showed involvement of lymph nodes (34 of 89). About $^1/_{10}$ (34 of 379) of the surgical specimens showed the *continuous* penetration of the boundary zone into the paravaginal, paracervical and parauterine tissues. 21 of these 34 cases showed *discontinuous* involvement of the lymph nodes.

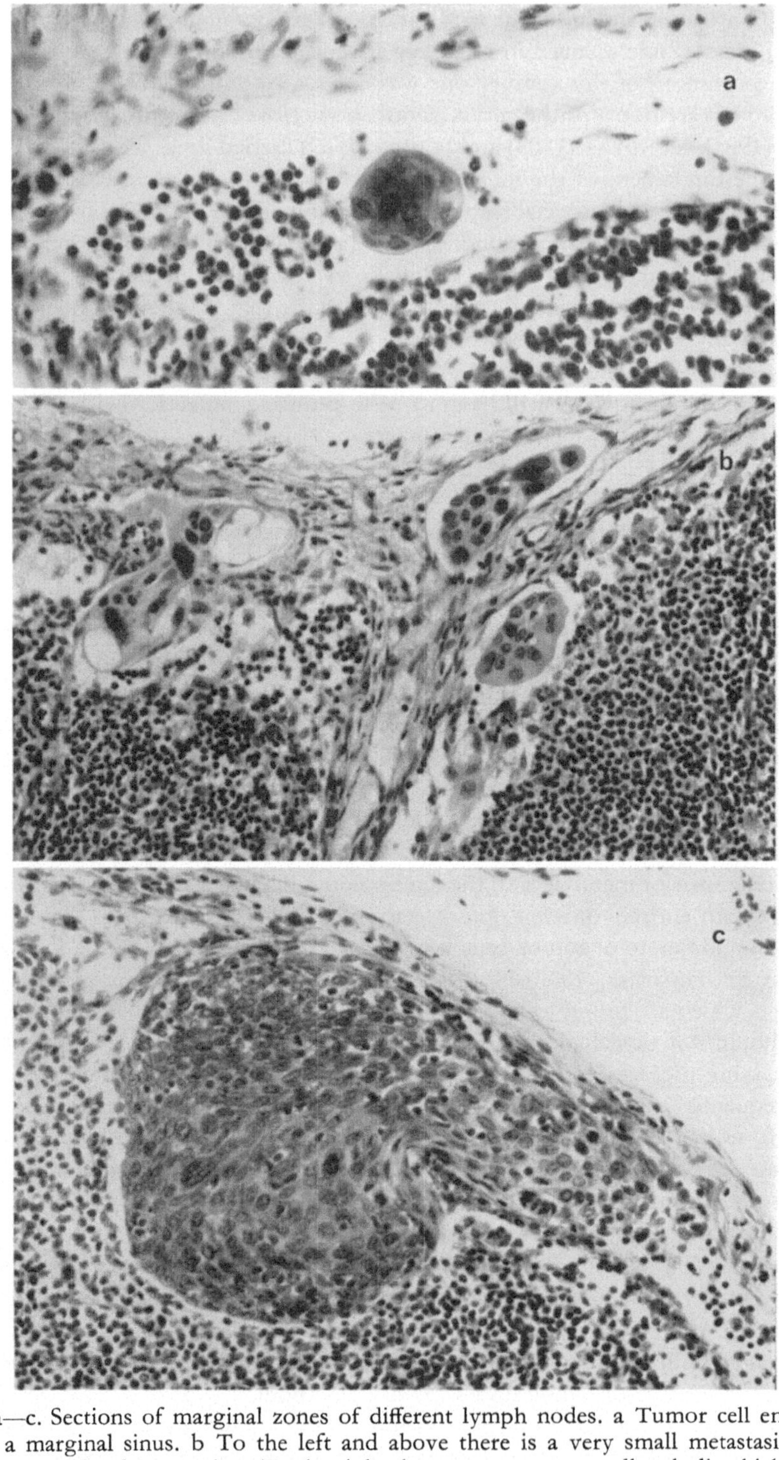

Fig. 3a—c. Sections of marginal zones of different lymph nodes. a Tumor cell embolism within a marginal sinus. b To the left and above there is a very small metastasis partly showing vacuolar degeneration. To the right there are two tumor cell emboli, which cannot be interpreted as metastases for certain from this section. c Small metastasis

It happens extremely seldom that small cancers having the size of a lentil or a pea already have metastasized. The metastasis of the smallest carcinoma which we discovered with our technique is shown in Fig. 5. The probability of metastatic spread of these carcinomas may be in the range of 1:50 up to 1:100. These estimations are supported, however, by additional 112 observations of women with microcarcinomata, which were not treated with lymphadenectomy (compare with page 582).

The quantitative correlation between size of tumor and involvement of lymph nodes was secured by HUHN in 1964 through careful measurements.

Table 1 points out to an observation which at first surprised us very much. Tumors which have not reached the boundary zone, but which have expanded with an infiltrative growing pattern towards the vagina — which frequently occurs beneath the vaginal epithelium — show metastases of the lymph nodes in approximately half of the cases (13 of 24). The same relationship exists in tumors which have proliferated into the boundary zone and at the same time into the vagina (10 of 19). Our numbers are small. One will have to watch this problem in the future more carefully. A short remark regarding the stage grouping appears important at this point. Stage IIa usually can be diagnosed easily. Many patients of our entire patient collective would have been grouped stage II b or even stage III by other colleagues. With this point in mind our observation in regard to the involvement of the vagina appears to be important.

Table 2. *The relation of continuous growth of the primary tumor to its discontinuous spread to the paratissues*

Continuous growth of the primary tumor	Cases	Involvement of paratissues by discontinuous spread
Microcarcinomata	25	—
Strictly confined to the cervix	207	14 (+ 1 TE)[a]
Laterally still within the cervix, but involvement of the vagina	24	2 (+ 2 TE)
Involvement of the boundary zone(s)	70	11 (+ 1 TE)
Involvement of the boundary zone(s) and the vagina	19	4
Involvement of the paratissues	34	4
Total	379	35 (+ 4 TE)

[a] TE = tumor cell emboli only.

Table 2 shows a survey of the correlation of the *continuous* spread to the *discontinuous* metastazising into the parametria. Tables 3 and 4 points out that with ignoring the involvement of the boundary zone two thirds (46 of 64) of the women with involvement of the parametria had metastases to the lymph nodes of the pelvic wall. For considerations in respect to surgical techniques this appears to be important.

One could discuss the question, whether involvement of the parametrial lymph nodes better ought to be added to involvement of the nodes of the pelvic wall. From the pathologic-anatomical point of view it would appear reasonable to include

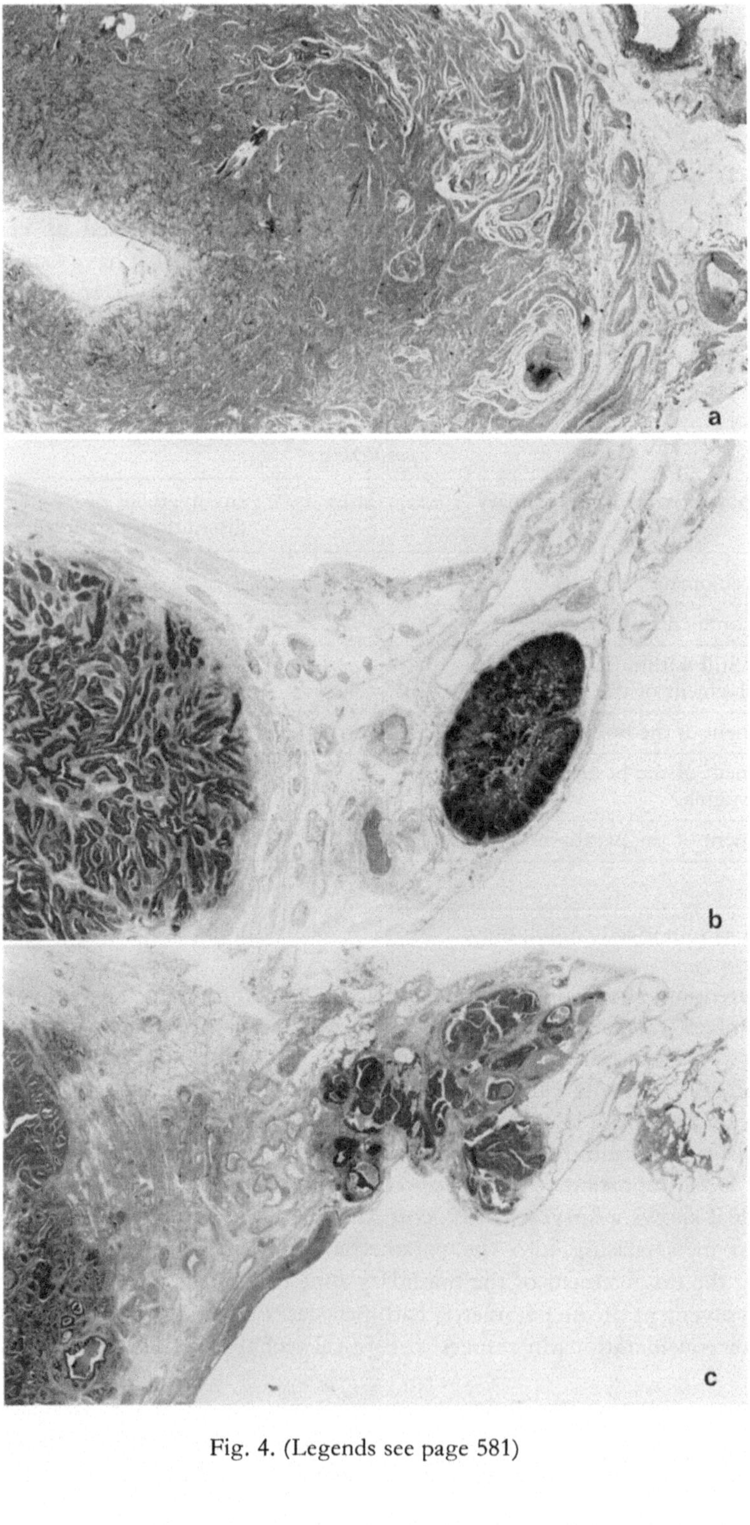

Fig. 4. (Legends see page 581)

Table 3. *Coincidence of discontinuous involvement of the paratissues and the lymph nodes of pelvic wall*

Continuous growth of the primary tumor	Paratissues			Lymph nodes	
	Strictly confined to lymph node(s)		TE[a]	TE[a]	Metastases
Strictly confined to the cervix	9	5	1	—	13
Laterally still within the cervix, but infiltration of the vagina	1	1	2	—	3
Involvement of the lateral boundary zone(s)	7	4	1	1	6
Involvement of the lateral boundary zone(s) and the vagina	1	3	—	—	3
Involvement of the paratissues	1	3	—	1	3
Total	19	16	4	2	28

[a] TE = tumor cell emboli only.

Table 4. *Coincidence of cancer involvement of the paratissues (contin. a./or discontin.) and lymph nodes of pelvic wall*

Continuous growth of the primary tumor	Paratissues	Lymph nodes
Strictly confined to the cervix	14 (+ 1 TE)[a]	13
Laterally still within the cervix, but infiltration of the vagina	2 (+ 2 TE)	3
Involvement of the lateral boundary zone(s)	11 (+ 1 TE)	6 (+ 1 TE)
Involvement of the lateral boundary zone(s) and the vagina	4	3
Involvement of the paratissues	33	21 (+ 2 TE)
Total	64 (+ 4 TE)	46 (+ 3 TE)

[a] TE = tumor cell emboli only.

lymph nodes of the paratissues to those of the pelvic wall. However, surgeons usually should class them as belonging to the paratissues since the deciding difference between vaginal and abdominal operations is the fact that the vaginal approach will not permit removal of lymph nodes of the pelvic wall while lymph nodes of the paratissues can be taken along. One may also ask, whether once in a while the *discontinuous* involvement of the parametrial tissues may have happened retrogradely. The latter we were not able to prove for certain in operable cases. Sometimes metastases in the parametrial tissues will develop apparently in spite of progressively more dilating vessels (Fig. 4c).

Fig. 4. a Boundary zone between cervix and paracervical tissues. One cannot draw an exact boundary line between cervix and supporting tissues. There is a vascular boundary zone, which may be up to 5 mm in depth in the non-magnified specimen. b A lymph node in the paracervical tissues filled out with cancer in a tumor which did not yet invade the boundary zone for certain. c A metastasis in the paracervical tissues which developed by discontinuous growth obviously without relation to lymph nodes. This metastasis has derived from a tumor which had invaded the boundary zone

In regard to the side localization of the continuous and discontinuous spread of cancer our material did not reveal any significant differences (Table 5). The preference of one side does not appear to play a role, neither in continuous growth nor in development of metastases. The relationship of left to right is in *unilateral* spread with involvement of the boundary zone 43:34, with penetration of the boundary zone 11:9, with the *discontinuous* involvement of parametrium 15:15 and with the involvement of the lymph nodes of the pelvic wall 31:37.

It does not make any difference whether the tumors are extending to both sides or to one side only: The involvement of the lymph nodes of the pelvic wall shows approximately twice as frequently metastazising to the lymph nodes around the common iliac vessels and to lymph nodes of the so-called vessel triangle between the external and internal iliac vessels than to the lymph nodes of the paravesical and pararectal area. Involvement of the inguinal lymph nodes we did not yet observe in operable cases.

Table 5. *Localization of unilateral continuous and discontinuous spread of cancer*

	Continuous spread		Discontinuous spread	
	Left	Right	Left	Right
Boundary zone	43	34		
Paratissues	11	9	15	15
Lymph nodes of pelvic wall			31	37

Usually we don't resect the hypogastric vein together with its branches. The 3 or 4 gluteal lymph nodes therefore are not removed. I cannot tell much about their involvement, but I want to stress this point: Among 148 women who were observed at least for 3 years and who did not have metastases of the lymph nodes when examined with our method, there were four women until now who showed a recurrence in the pelvis.

There appear to be physicians who carry out the vaginal cancer operation taking along the paravaginal, paracervical and parametrial tissues assuming that very small cancers are able to make a breach by growing continuously into the paratissues without involving the lymph nodes of the pelvic wall (Fig. 6). We did never see this type of picture although we have removed in healthy tissues additional 112 microcarcinomas by simple hysterectomy or conization beside the 25 microcancers mentioned in Table 1. We have observed these cases now for at least 3* years (Kaufmann et al., 1965; Ober, 1965). So it has to be very rare. Figs. 2a and b demonstrate this type of expansion in an extreme manner *within* the cervix and without involving the boundary zone and the paracervical tissues. This type of infiltration is a very rare one. Only 3% of the tumors are growing this way; more than 90% have a shallow front of invasion (Ober and Huhn, 1962). The typical manner a cervical cancer encroaches is shown by the Figs. 4b and c. The *discontinuous* spread within the paracervical or paravaginal tissues (Figs. 4b and c) very often goes along with involving lymph nodes of the pelvic wall (28 of 34 cases; Table 3).

To the question regarding metastazising into the ovaries we can contribute just a little, as we don't castrate most of our patients — no matter how big the primary tumor may be. None of these women later on did run a course indicating that we had

* 4 years in May 1969.

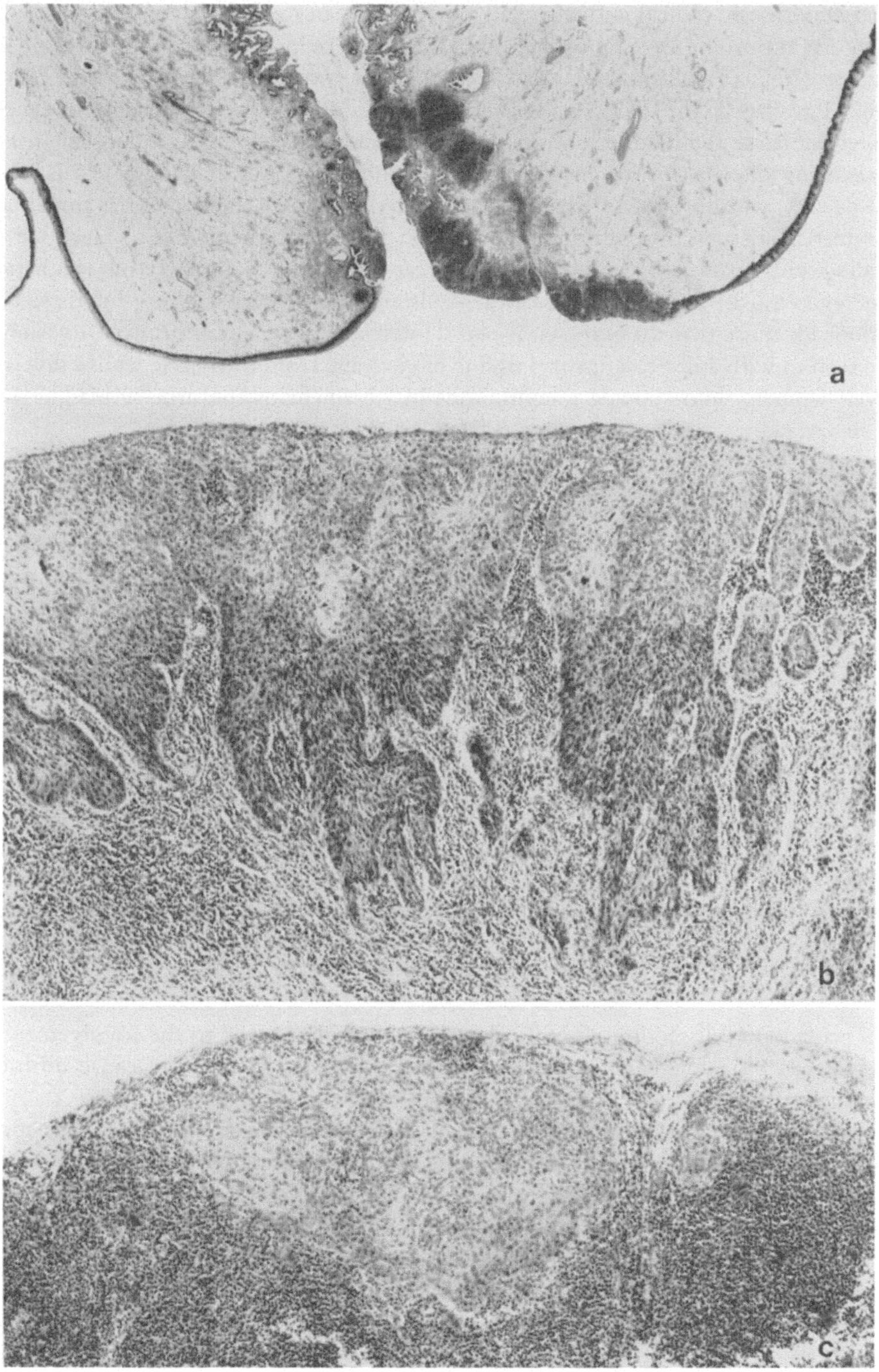

Fig. 5. a Pocket-lens magnification of the smallest cancer we observed with metastases to the lymph nodes of the pelvic wall. b Low magnification of the border section of this tumor. c Low magnification of the metastasis within a lymph node of the pelvic wall

left a metastasis behind. Twice only we had to deal with patients, which could not be operated grossly radical and who had already ovarian metastases.

Very important appears to be another question which has been a matter of discussion lately (FRIEDELL and PARSONS, 1961; HENRIKSEN, 1960; OBER and HUHN, 1962; PARSONS et al., 1959; PARSONS et al., 1960): What is the significance of cancers which infiltrate the bladder continuously or invade the rectum as a consequence of preexisting disease (for instance peritonitis within the pelvis or endometriosis in the cul-de-sac) without already having penetrated the paracervical, paravaginal and parametrial tissues by continuous expansion up to the pelvic wall? Here we are dealing with those cases which one could treat operatively without trying irradiation. One even must operate in these cases — ultraradically! I am looking for these conditions for more than 10 years with special interest. I never saw a primary invasion of the rectum with still present surgical line of cleavage from the pelvic wall. I saw only seven women, who showed a continuous involvement of the urinary bladder who

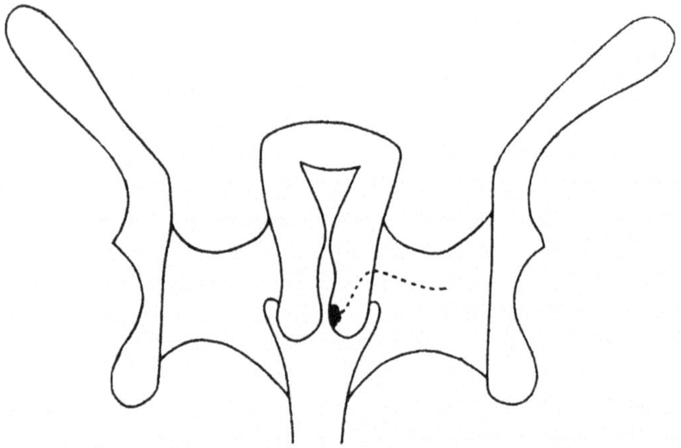

Fig. 6. The idea of the continuous manner of expansion of a very small carcinoma of the cervix which that physician should have in mind who would use in this case the vaginal operation described by SCHUCHARDT-SCHAUTA-AMREICH. (After OBER, 1965)

still presented a dissection plane to the pelvic wall. In regard to the involvement of the rectum I could imagine that high-located vaginal cancers may cause misinterpretations (Fig. 1 d).

As a gynecologist, who is doing the surgery and who uses to evaluate the specimens histologically himself, I should emphazise therapeutic points of view, of course.

Cervical cancers, which an experienced gynecologist can recognize clinically, always should be operated in conjunction with lymphadenectomy. The metastatic spread to lymph nodes of the pelvic wall plays a much greater role than one thought in earlier times. If a simple hysterectomy is not be sufficient, one will have to remove the paravaginal and paracervical tissues and the lymph nodes of the pelvic wall as well. If one considers an involvement of the paratissues, consequently one will have to lymphadenectomize.

In very small cancers (microcarcinomata) one does not have to consider a spread into the paravaginal, paracervical or parametrial tissues. The probability of metastazising into the lymph nodes is extremely small. In cases of great surgical risk or those cases of increased risk to irradiation this knowledge will facilitate the choice of treatment.

Provided one should not find any metastases of lymph nodes following extensive surgery and most thorough examination of the specimens, the probability of a so-called "recurrence" is extremely small. This knowledge may at times be of great help for answering the question of castration during an operation or for making the decision of irradiation treatment following an operation.

References

Brunet, G.: Z. Geburtsh. Gynäk. **56**, 1 (1905).
Friedell, G. H., and J. B. Graham: Surg. Gynec. Obstet. **108**, 513 (1959).
—, and L. Parsons: Cancer (Philad.) **14**, 42 (1961).
Hamperl, H.: Langenbecks Arch. klin. Chir. **295**, 22 (1960).
Henriksen, E.: Amer. J. Obstet. Gynec. **80**, 1919 (1960).
Huhn, F. O.: Geburtsh. u. Frauenheilk. **22**, 335 (1962).
— Virchows Arch. path. Anat. **325**, 84 (1962).
— Die Lymphknotenveränderungen beim Cervixcarcinom und die Beziehungen Tumorgröße und lymphogene Ausbreitung. Habil.-Schrift, Köln 1964.
— Morphologie der Tumormetastasierung, Krebsforschung und Krebsbekämpfung, VI, p. 238 (1967).
Kaufmann, C., K. G. Ober und F. O. Huhn: Geburtsh. u. Frauenheilk. **25**, 112 (1965).
Kundrat, R.: Arch. Gynäk. **69**, 355 (1903).
Matuschka, M.: Geburtsh. u. Frauenheilk. **22**, 497 (1962).
Ober, K. G.: Geburtsh. u. Frauenheilk. **25**, 464 (1965).
—, u. F. O. Huhn: Arch. Gynäk. **197**, 262 (1962).
—, u. H. Meinrenken: Gynäkologische Operationen. In: Guleke u. Zenker, Allgemeine und spezielle chirurgische Operationslehre, Band IX. Berlin-Göttingen-Heidelberg-New York: Springer 1964.
Parsons, L., F. Cesare, and G. H. Friedell: Surg. Gynec. Obstet. **109**, 279 (1959).
— — — Ann. Surg. **151**, 961 (1960).
Scheib, A.: Arch. Gynäk. **87**, 241 (1909).
Vogt-Hoerner, G., et R. Gerard-Marchant: Bull. Cancer **45**, 446 (1958).

Individualization of Treatment for Cancer of the Cervix*

S. B. Gusberg, and John Rudolph

If one is to take the position that we should individualize treatment for cancer of the cervix as we do for other diseases according to the patient's age, general health and outlook one must choose between the two excellent modalities of treatment available to us: radical surgery and radiotherapy, or elect combinations thereof. In order to make this choice dependent upon patient factors rather than therapist factors, by which I mean the training, temperament, departmental policy or other variables related to the physician in charge, we must utilize the biological parameters clinically available for this decision.

If we assume that all other factors are equal, we might start with the premise that radiation will give as good a cure rate in Stage I or Stage II ("the operable stages") as will radical surgery, with a lesser rate of therapeutic mortality and a greater rate of

* From The Department of Obstetrics and Gynecology of The Mount Sinai School of Medicine and Hospital. — This work was supported in part by The American Cancer Society: Grant No. T-7F. and by the U.S.P.H.S.

Table 1. *Mean survival rate in cancer of the cervix*[a]

Modality		No. of patients	5year survival rate
Stage I	Radiation	7,133	72.0%
	Combined	4,621	78.2%
	Surgery	391	71.8%
	Selected surgery	2,052	74.0%
Stage II	Radiation	12,120	53.8%
	Combined	6,407	55.7%
	Surgery	601	52.5%
	Selected surgery	2,523	50.6%

[a] From 14th Annual Report, Stockholm.

Table 2. *Radiation therapy — selected*

Stage I with 80% + survival:

Institution	% 5year survival	No. of patients
Erlangen, Germany	80.4	97
Munich I, Germany	83.8	290
Munich II, Germany	93.8	64
Warsaw, Poland	80.7	378
Stockholm, Sweden	86.4	471
Houston, USA	86.6	216
San Francisco, USA	83.9	143
Leningrad, USSR	82.6	161
	Mean 84.8	1,820/7,133

% of total number subjected to Rx in clinics with this high cure rate = 25.5%. Rx = treatment

Table 3. *Radiation therapy — selected*

Stage II with 60% + survival:

Institution	% 5year survival	No. of patients
Innsbruck, Austria	70.6	126
Brno, Czechoslovakia	67.0	91
Brno II, Czechoslovakia	67.8	118
Aarhus, Denmark	65.1	338
Erlangen, Germany	66.1	230
Munich I, Germany	69.9	1,002
Munich II, Germany	66.3	187
Tubingen, Germany	63.5	348
Wurzburg, Germany	67.5	114
Rotterdam, Netherlands	64.4	149
Stockholm, Sweden	60.0	1,094
Houston, USA	69.9	382
	Mean 66.5	4,179/12,120

% of total number subjected to Rx in clinics with this high cure rate were = 34.4%.

applicability. However, we must acknowledge that "all other factors" are not equal and that experience with the management and follow-up of these patients forces one to the conclusion that some patients will benefit more from surgical treatment in an era when the morbidity from such surgery is small and early, whereas the morbidity from radiotherapeutic treatment may be commulative and late, when the life expectancy of the "cured" young patient (and we see more of these with early lesions) may be 30 to 40 years, when there are simple observations to be made that suggest that the requirement of radiation for a particular tumor of low sensitivity will be of such an intensity as to increase the tissue damage over that usually seen under skilled treatment. This message of individualization will not influence those wedded to a technical rather than a biological concept of cancer treatment.

To make a comparison between the survival rates following surgery and irradiation treatments in Stages I and II carcinoma of the cervix we have analyzed the tabulations in the 14th Annual Report compiled in Stockholm in an effort to seek out data

Table 4. *Combined treatment — selected*

Stage I with 80% + survival:		
Institution	% 5year survival	No. of patients
Frankfurt, Germany	80.8	271
Kiel, Germany	88.0	133
Wuppertal, Germany	82.1	240
Kumamoto, Japan	83.8	111
Okayama, Japan	85.6	299
Tokyo, Japan	85.0	333
Bucharest, Rumania	81.3	252
Zurich, Switzerland	88.0	125
Moscow, USSR	90.6	159
Ljubljana, Yogoslavia	84.2	330
Zagreb, Yugoslavia	80.8	266
	Mean 84.6	2,519/4,621

% of total number of patients subjected to Rx in clinics with this high cure rate = 54.5%.

that could influence our choice of treatment. One quickly finds that there is little difference in the "cure" rate of surgery or irradiation in either the average group or those selected for superiority of reported result (Tables 1 to 7).

The criteria used for the selection of clinics and the definition of treatment groups are outlined below:

1. Each clinic must have had at least 100 patients in Stage I and Stage II or a combined total of at least 200 patients (1956 to 1960).

2. *Radiation:* The majority of the patients (greater than 70%) with Stage I and II lesions must have received primary radiotherapy.

3. *Surgery:* The majority of the patients (greater than 50%) in Stages I and II must have had primary surgery.

4. *Combined:* The majority of the patients (greater than 50%) in Stages I and II received surgery and planned pre or postoperative radiotherapy.

5. *Selected surgery:* A group wherein more than 30%, but less than 50%, of Stage I and II lesions received primary surgery. The remainder received radiotherapy.

Table 5. *Combined treatment — selected*

Stage II with 60% + survival:		
Institution	% 5year survival	No. of patients
Vienna, Austria	61.5	122
Frankfurt, Germany	64.9	245
Okayama, Japan	68.4	820
Tokyo, Japan	69.9	530
Amsterdam, Netherlands	62.2	193
Zurich, Switzerland	63.8	130
Zagreb, Yugoslavia	62.2	429
	Mean 64.7	2,469/6,407

% of total number of patients subjected to Rx in clinics with this high cure rate = 38.3%.

Table 6. *Surgical treatment in selected clinics*

Stage I with survival rate 80% +:		
Institution	% 5year survival	No. of patients
Nagasaki, Japan	86.0	50
Heidelberg, Germany	80.4	184
Boston, USA	80.3	132
Col.-Presby., N.Y., USA	80.6	139
	Mean 81.3	505/2,443

% of total number of patients subjected to Rx in clinics with this high cure rate = 20.6%.

Stage II with survival rate 60% +:		
Institution	% 5year survival	No. of patients
Nagasaki, Japan	70.1	137
Paris, Inst. G-Roussy	61.9	202
	Mean 66.0	339/3,124

% of total number of patients subjected to Rx in clinics with this high cure rate = 10.8%.

Table 7. *Selected superior survival rates*

	Stage I survival	% applicable	Stage II survival	% applicable
Radiation	84.8	25.5	66.5	34.4
Combined	84.6	54.5	64.7	38.3
Surgery	81.3	20.6	66.0	10.8

Selection of clinics reporting 80% + survival in Stage I and 60% + in Stage II.

It is noteworthy that the clinics reporting a combined treatment of planned radiotherapy and surgery, showed some superiority both in survival rate and the percentage of patients to whom the superior treatment was being offered, but it is difficult to assay the role of selection in these figures.

Furthermore when the rate of major injury from each modality was inspected in the literature, there was little to choose between radiotherapy and surgery, though here once more the combined treatment seemed to show a higher rate. One must quickly add that the rates of injury shown here (Tables 8 to 12) are high for modern

Table 8. *Criteria for major injury in Rx of carcinoma of cervix*

Surgery	Radiation
Fistula	Fistula
Rectal	Rectal
Ureteral	Ureteral
Vesical	Vesical
Intestinal obstruction stricture	Stricture
Ureteral	Ureteral
	Rectal
Thromboembolic hemorrhage	Persistent proctitis and cystitis

Table 9. *A comparison of % injuries in relation to mode of treatment*

Mode	% injury
Surgery	13.1
Combined	16.9
Radiation	11.6

Table 10. *Surgical injury in operable carcinoma of the cervix*

Senior author	% injury
Calame	13.0
Brunschwig	22.4
Masterson	5.0
Meigs	11.0
Yagi	2.1
Symmonds	4.0
Green	20.3
Louros	2.8
Graham	17.0
	Mean 13.1

Table 11. *Combined treatment in carcinoma of the cervix*

Senior author	% injury
Talbert	15.0
Hurteau	16.9
Crawford	13.0
Stallworthy	0.0
Greiss	22.2
Graham	34.0
	Mean 16.9

Table 12. *Radiation injury in carcinoma of the cervix*

Senior author	% injury
Kottmeier	3.9
Sherman	17.0
Hurteau	7.5
Crawford	20.0
Graham	6.0
Calame	16.3
Greiss	9.1
	Mean 11.6

treatment and they are declining for all modalities, as greater therapeutic precision and more careful selection of mode has prevailed.

If then, we cannot depend upon survival rate or injury rate for the selection of treatment in an operable patient with carcinoma of the cervix in those clinics where treatment by either mode is available we must turn to a more careful analysis of the patient and her tumor for help in this decision; we have chosen a radiosensitivity test based on a test dose technique.

Radiosensitivity and the Test Dose Technique

Three factors concerned with the cure of tumors by radiation are: (1) Excellence of treatment, (2) Radiation sensitivity and (3) Virulence of the tumor. As Gynecologists perhaps we are not privileged to discuss publicly the excellence of any radiotherapeutic treatment. However, I shall briefly refer to our study of these other factors as they influence our choice of treatment.

We have described before our Test Dose Technique with the administration of a provocative quantity of radiation, small enough so that it does not interfere with later surgical treatment or the precise planning of the geometry of radiotherapeutic treatment yet large enough to produce a spectrum of response. We have used in the past several experimental approaches to this test, including 3,000 R (250 KV, 15ma, 43 cm target-skin distance, half value layer 2 mm Cu) in 500 R daily exposures, via transvaginal cone, or 800 r $\times$ 2, 24 h apart, or external irradiation of 1,600 rads by supervoltage (Cobalt 60 or Betatron) but we have now standardized our test by giving 400 Rads $\times$ 3 in 3 days with external irradiation via parallel opposing fields (Betatron, whole pelvis technique) and continuation of treatment to 2000 Rads while awaiting the proper interval for the response biopsies. Control biopsies are taken in quadrants in healthy sectors of tumors and repeated on the 11th day after the onset of the test dose, i.e. 1 week after the test dose is concluded. The continuation of irradiation in the interval permits continuity of treatment if radiotherapeutic treatment is elected; this interval of 1 week may be used in addition for the general work-up required of patients with cervix cancer.

Tissue sections and tissue smears are made from these biopsies and stained by the previously described techniques for histologic, cytomorphologic and cytochemical reactions and, in addition, fixed in osmic acid for electron microscopic study.

There are three types of tumor cell reaction indicating responsiveness to irradiation: 1. death and dissolution of cells; 2. increased differentiation of cells; 3. radiocytologic reactions indicating the probability of irreversible cell injury such as (a) enlargement of cells and cell nuclei, (b) enlargement of nucleoli (RNA) and (c) alteration in chromatin material (DNA) with an apparent early increase followed by relative decline. As you know our testing studies are based in general upon the sensitivity of the reproductive apparatus of the cell to injury by irradiation while the organelles, more directly or more secondarily related to protein synthesis, seem to carry on with less sensitivity to the time of virtual explosion or dissolution of the cell.

The method is relatively simple and reproduceable and can be used in any laboratory where there is a pathologist available who will study radiation change in cells and tissues. We have used more elaborate quantitative methods but at present they are still too laborious for clinical application.

Response and Result

The incidence of good response in our series is close to 70%, in this analysis 68.1% without significant variation from stage to stage.

You have perhaps been accustomed to the philosophy that tumors that shrink early recur early, in this way prohibiting early prognosis of healing under radiation. We do not find this to be true. Indeed you will note that the initial response of these tumors to the test dose, i.e. 1 week following the administration of this relatively small amount of irradiation, enabled us to make a reasonably good estimate of the final response. In this group of patients, for example, where the radiotherapeutic mode was chosen without respect to the outcome of radiosensitivity testing, you will note that the relative cure rate in Stage I and II (excluding small Stage I's — Stage I-b and microcarcinomas — Stage I-a) was 72.1% whereas the relative cure rate for those with poor radiosensitivity testing declined to 32.5%; those of Stage II extent appeared to show the widest disparity. That the factors of radiosensitivity and virulence are intertwined may be seen from the following table wherein we have shown the result attained by the clinical use of radiosensitivity testing. In this group patients of Stage I and II extent with poor radiosensitivity testing were subjected to radical hysterectomy and we were able to bring the relative cure rate to 56% (Table 13).

Table 13. *CA cervix — Stages I and II. Response and treatment*

	No.	Cure
RST good-radiation	123	72.1%
RST poor-radiation	47	32.5% [a]
RST poor-surgery	28	56.0% [a]

[a] Significant at .05 level.

This appears to be a significantly better result for these individuals than that to be expected with continuation of radiotherapy but not as good as that for those with a good radiosensitivity testing response treated in the radiotherapeutic group above described.

As a relatively modest approach to the problem of virulence by the use of a parameter readily available to clinical study before treatment we investigated the presence or absence of lymphatic invasion in the control biopsy. This proved to be a valuable index for in the "good" radiosensitivity testing group we found an 86% relative cure rate in those without lymphatic invasion, but a 39.4% cure rate only in those with good radiosensitivity testing with positive lymphatic invasion. Expressed in another way those with good response who were living and well showed a 14.9% incidence of lymphatic invasion in the control biopsies, whereas those who recurred showed a 72.8% incidence (almost five times greater). This virulence factor has not been applied clinically as yet, but it could persuade us to use combinations of surgery and radiotherapy for this group. We have some small, statistically insignificant evidence that the lymphatic invasion factor did not effect the outcome in those patients treated surgically as much as it did those treated radiotherapeutically, which we shall pursue.

Discussion

It may be that we can raise our cure rate by this radiosensitivity testing program but our purpose may be more properly expressed as an effort to find the parameters that will enable us to choose between two relatively good forms of treatment or combinations thereof most suited to the needs of the individual patient. It is clear that most of the factors in tumor healing, like those of tumor growth, are as yet unknown. At the same time I believe we have wasted much time and energy in polemic displays suggesting that our modalities of treatment are competitive rather than complementary. We should get on with further biological studies now possible by more sophisticated techniques to assay the response to radiation and the areas where surgery may be more efficiently utilized with the premise that tumors of greater resistence or higher virulence may require an intensity of radiotherapy that makes the cost in normal tissue damage prohibitive and we may then alter our radiation approach or substitute surgery or combine it with surgery, in a manner that will most suit the nature of the tumor and its host.

References

Annual Report Vol. 14 — Stockholm. Ed. Hans L. Kottmeier.

Brunschwig, A., and H. R. K. Barber: Obstet. and Gynec. **27**, 21—29 (1966).

Calame, R., and R. Wallach: Surg. Gynec. Obstet. **125**, 39—44 (1967).

Crawford, E., L. S. Robinson, and J. Vaught: Amer. J. Obstet. Gynec. **91**, 480—485 (1965).

Graham, J., R. Graham, and M. Schulz: Amer. J. Obstet. Gynec. **89**, 421—431 (1964).

Green, T. H.: Progress in the management and prevention of the urologic complications of radical Wertheim hysterectomy. In: Meigs, J. V., and S. H. Sturgis, Ed., Progress in gynecology, p. 646—659. New York: Grune and Stratton, Publishers 1963.

—, J. V. Meigs, H. Ulfelder, and R. Curtin: Obstet. and Gynec. **20**, 293—312 (1962).

Greiss, F. C.: Combined radiation and surgical treatment for carcinoma of the uterine cervix. In: Lewis, G. C., W. B. Wentz, and R. M. Jaffe, Ed., New concepts in gynecological oncology, p. 133—141. F. A. Davis Co., Publishers 1966.

—, D. D. Blake, and F. R. Lock: Obstet. and Gynec. **18**, 417—427 (1961).

Gusberg, S. B.: Amer. J. Obstet. Gynec. **72**, 804 (1956).

—, and G. G. Herman: Amer. J. Obstet. Gynec. **100**, 627 (1968).

— — Amer. J. Obstet. Gynec. **87**, 60 (1962).

Hurteau, G. D., J. Morris, and C. H. Chang: Amer. J. Obstet. Gynec. **95**, 696—705 (1966).

Kottmeier, H. L.: Amer. J. Obstet. Gynec. **88**, 854—866 (1964).

Liu, W., and J. V. Meigs: Amer. J. Obstet. Gynec. **69**, 1—32 (1955).

Louros, N. C.: Amer. J. Obstet. Gynec. **89**, 432—438 (1964).

Masterson, J.: Clin. Obstet. Gynec. **10**, 927—939 (1968).

Sherman, A. I., and H. M. Camel: Amer. J. Obstet. Gynec. **89**, 439—452 (1964).

Stallworthy, J.: J. Amer. med. Ass. **195**, 465—470 (1966).

Symmonds, R. E.: Amer. J. Obstet. Gynec. **94**, 663—678 (1966).

Talbert, L. M., L. Palumbo, H. Shingleton, C. A. Bream, and J. A. McGee: Sth. med. J. (Bgham, Ala.) **58**, 11—17 (1965).

Yagi, H.: Amer. J. Obstet. Gynec. **69**, 32—47 (1955).

Abdominal Operations for Cervical Cancer

Langdon Parsons

Nearly 30 years after the resurgence of abdominal surgery for cervical cancer in the United States it is appropriate to review the experience and attempt to delineate the role it should play as the sole definitive mode of therapy.

Modern surgery makes it possible for us to adapt our therapy to the individual needs of the patient. We are aware of the fact that cancer of the cervix may be treated by either radiation or surgery. For Stages I and II we speak of having a choice in our selection of therapy. The choice does exist but only if there is equal competence in both fields.

A large portion of radiation therapy for cancer of the cervix is given by radiologists whose primary interest and training is in diagnosis rather than therapy. Similarly a great deal of surgery is performed by men who have limited knowledge of the life history of cervical cancer or the problems that they may encounter.

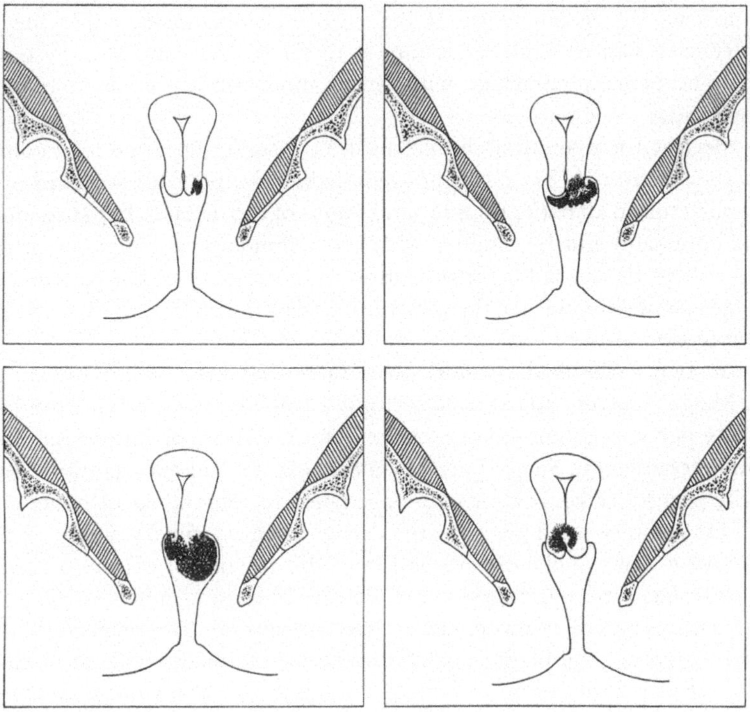

Fig. 1. Stage I cancer of the cervix. The lesion is confined to the cervix. It may be ulcerating or exfoliating

Unfortunately, despite the fact that radiation has improved and surgery has become more extensive, we still are not doing as well as we should for invasive cancer of the cervix. The most recent statistics, recounting the world experience as published in the 14th volume of the Annual Report on the results of treatment in carcinoma of the uterus and vagina, suggest that approximately 50% of all women with cervical cancer fail to survive the 5 year period.

It is my firm belief that cancer of the cervix is basically a local disease. We should be able to cure more patients than we do. It is possible to do so provided the therapy is well conceived and vigorously carried out.

The problem is not whether radiation or surgery will offer the highest percentage of cure in all cases seen but what is best for the individual. Within the scope of individualization abdominal surgery has a logical place in the management of cervical cancer.

The primary aim of surgery is to encompass all the tumor at the primary site and the areas to which it may be expected to extend, including the regional nodal areas. The indications for the abdominal surgical approach would seem to be well defined, but in the United States at least they appear to be much misunderstood and are variously interpreted. A considerable amount of confusion still exists as to (1) when to offer the patient surgery, (2) what the limitations of surgery are, and (3) how extensive the operation should be to be considered adequate.

In my opinion there would be less uncertainty of the role abdominal surgery should play if we had a better understanding of what it is that we are trying to accomplish. To have such understanding we must have a workable knowledge of the life history of the tumor we are dealing with. It has been well documented that the growth pattern of cervical cancer tends to confine it to the primary site and the immediate paracervical and paravaginal areas, with only a moderate degree of involvement of the regional nodes.

To be effective the operation chosen must have sufficient scope to encompass all the disease the patient may have. It is not reasonable to expect one standard operation will accomplish this in all patients and for all stages of the disease. The surgeon should have at his command and be familiar with the techniques of a number of different procedures so that he can tailor his operation to the amount of the patient's disease. It is no longer justifiable to force the patient to accept the only procedure the surgeon knows how to do.

There are two abdominal surgical procedures that may be employed. (1) The Wertheim Meigs' type of radical hysterectomy combined with pelvic lymphadenectomy. (2) The pelvic exenteration operations. The Wertheim operation is done as the sole definitive treatment in Stages I and II cervical cancer. The exenteration operations are primarily performed on patient who have failed to respond to adequate radiation therapy. There is, however, a place for the exenteration as primary definitive therapy. We are all aware that the clinical evaluation of the amount of disease present, since it is done with the examining finger alone, may be in error as much as 20%. In most instances this is on the side of more, rather than less, disease. The surgeon then should be prepared to remove the bladder or rectum and occasionally both, if he finds that he has underestimated the amount of disease and there is actually more cancer present than he anticipated. The only other alternative available to the surgeon is to discontinue the operation, mark the gross extent of the tumor with dura clips so that the radiologist has some idea of the amount and location of the disease and submit the patient to radiation therapy. It is not in the best interest of the patient to persist in continuing with a Wertheim procedure that is doomed to failure from the beginning.

This is one of the reasons why I prefer the abdominal rather than the vaginal surgical approach in cervical cancer. The radical Schauta Amreich procedure does not permit the flexibility present in the Wertheim Meigs' hysterectomy when the patients found to have more disease than was originally anticipated.

How well does the Wertheim Meigs' hysterectomy with pelvic node dissection meet the requirements of encompassing all of the cancer at the primary site and in the areas to which it may logically spread? It is my impression that in my own country too much of the surgery that is performed as definitive therapy is less than adequate. I believe this is so for two reasons. (1) The Wertheim type of hysterectomy with pelvic node dissection is performed on too many patients who have too much disease to hope that the operation will encompass all of their disease. (2) The Wertheim hysterectomy and node dissection or radical hysterectomy and node dissection as it is inadvisably named in the United States, focuses too much attention on the regional nodes and not enough on the primary tumor and the immediate extensions from it.

Let me first discuss the contention that too often the surgeon tries to make the Wertheim operation accomplish more than it is designed to do. It is generally agreed

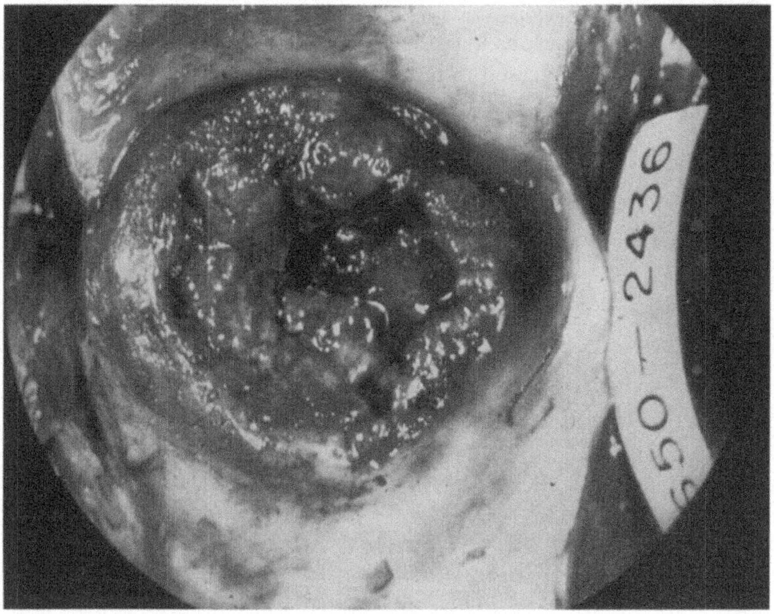

Fig. 2. Stage I. An example of the ulcerating type

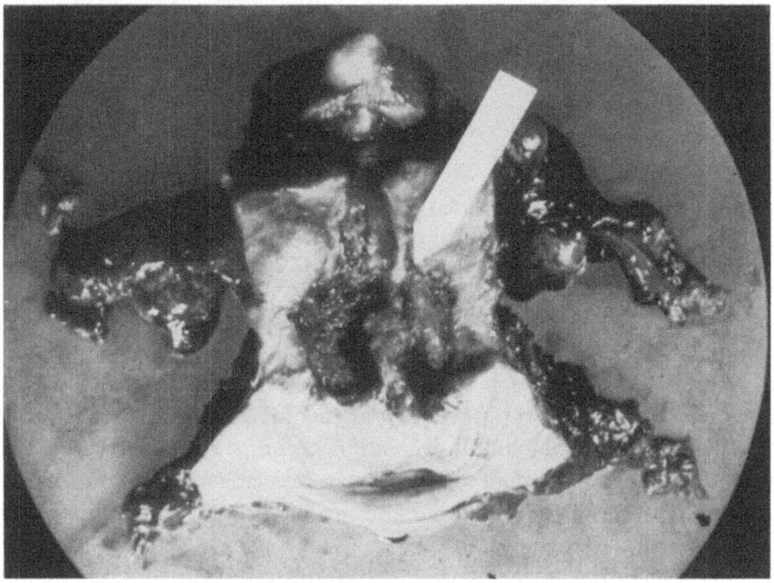

Fig. 3. Stage I. The lesion involves the endocervix

that this surgical procedure is an adequate operation for patients with the amount of disease that would place them in the categories of either Stage I or II cervical cancer. I would take issue with this statement.

In my opinion the Wertheim with pelvic node dissection gives the best results when it is restricted to patients with Stage I and IIA. The 5 year survival statistics will be less regarding when the operation is performed in patients classified as Stage IIB or III.

In evaluating my own results in patients in Stage II where the Wertheim and node dissection was done I was pleased to note a salvage rate of 67%. The 14th volume of the Annual Report notes a 53% survival for Stage II. My pleasure was short lived,

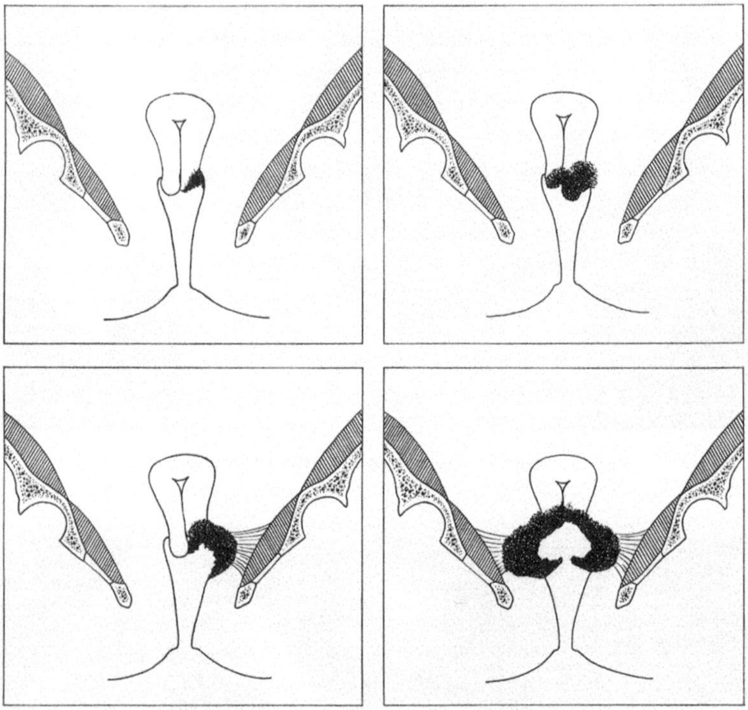

Fig. 4. Stage II. The upper portion shows the extent of the disease in the IIA classification. The lower portion shows the IIB staging

however, when closer analysis breaking down Stage II into Stage IIa and IIb that the results continued to be satisfactory in Stage IIa at 80% but fell to 43% in Stage IIb. This is what I mean about the operation being offered to patients who have too much disease to expect the Wertheim procedure will encompass all the disease and cure the patient. In my opinion if the clinical evaluation suggests more and varied disease in the IIb category that these patients should be treated by radiation, not surgery. It is not a question of technique, but rather the life history of cervical cancer and the nature of its growth pattern.

It would appear then that the Wertheim hysterectomy and pelvic node dissection has a logical but restricted place in the treatment of cervical cancer.

The next subject for consideration is the observation that some of the radical abdominal surgery is less than adequate because the emphasis in the excision is placed on the node dissection rather than on the primary tumor and its environs. In general the radical nature of the operation is judged by the extent of the node dissection. In my opinion this is in error.

No one will deny that the presence or absence of nodal metastases has a direct bearing on prognosis. We also know that patients with positive nodes can be salvaged.

In recent years there has been a tendency to shift the emphasis in therapy from the primary tumor to the regional nodes. This has been true of both surgery and radiation. The radiologist sets up arbitrary reference points at A, near the cervix and

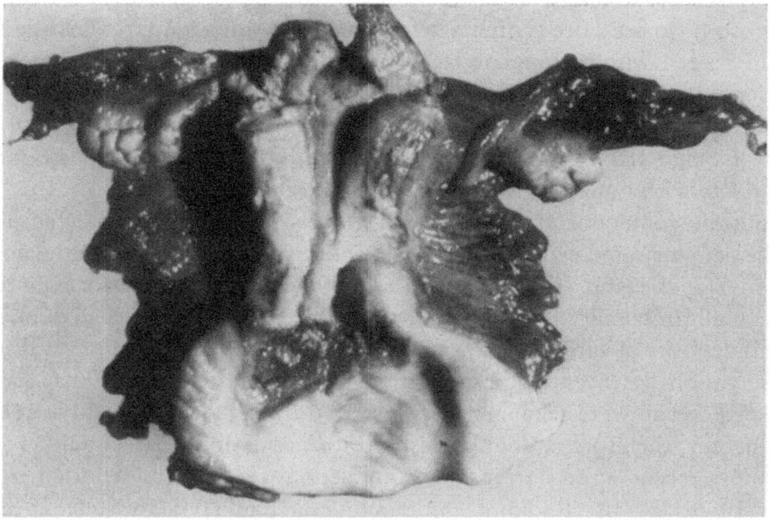

Fig. 5. Stage IIA. The cancer has left the cervix and extended to the wall of the vagina. The specimen shows the extent of the paravaginal and paracervical dissection

B, on the pelvic wall and develops elaborate dosage tables to enable him to balance the effect of the local radium and external radiation. Proper use of the tables helps him to deliver uniform without undue destruction of normal tissue or injury to bladder and rectum. Because of the doubt cast about the ability of radiation to cure metastatic nodes he concentrates on delivering radiation to the lateral areas.

The surgeon in turn, realizing that the prognosis is directly related to the extent of nodal involvement, places his emphasis on the nodal dissection and is less concerned with the vital paracervical and paravaginal area. Too much of the surgery for cancer of the cervix done in the United States today is little more than an extension of the type of hysterectomy done for benign disease with a lymphadenectomy added.

It is my contention that the success or failure of the surgical treatment of cervical cancer will depend on how well you treat the local disease and the spread to adjacent areas. The salvage figures will not improve by doing an extensive and beautiful node dissection but an inadequate excision of the tissues around the cervix.

To truly evaluate the impact of the nodal dissection on patient survival we must first have some idea of (1) how often the nodes are involved, and (2) how often the patient can be cured if they are.

How often are the nodes involved? This type of information is now becoming available as the result of the increasing experience with *Radical Surgery*. From a review of this experience it would seem to be true that the nodes are actually not involved as frequently as we have become accustomed to believe. In many instances, even when there is an extensive amount of tumor present such as we find in Stages III and IV, the patient will have no node involvement. The percentage of nodal metastases increases as the local disease becomes more advanced, but not as much as we might expect. It would be incorrect, for example, to assume that because a patient was classified as Stage III that she would certainly have positive nodes. In our experience the nodes were involved in Stage I in 14%. In Stage II the percentage of regional node metatsases was 22%. In the more advanced cases in Stages III and IV metastatic nodes were present in 36%.

How often do we cure patients with positive nodes? Approximately 50% of patients in Stage I with regional nodal involvement will survive for 5 or more years. If all patients in Stage II are included the 5 year end results will be around 35%. The chance of improving the salvage figures by the node dissection falls off sharply in the category of Stage IIb or more advanced disease. You will be fortunate indeed if 1 of 5 patients with nodal metastases survives 5 years.

It is not my contention that the regional nodes should not be dissected. In addition to the demonstrated proof that long term survival is possible when the nodes are positive in Stages I and IIa, there is an additional reason for performing a nodal excision. In all probability the patient who is reported as having negative nodes will have small deposits of carcinoma in small nodes that the pathologist never discovers. This observation has been made in relation to breast carcinoma. When the nodes were cleaned and all were examined serially a 33% higher yield of positive nodes was found. There is, therefore, a double reason for doing a node dissection.

The most recent figures from the compilation of statistics reported from the World institutes by the Radiumhemmet suggests that approximately 25% of all cervical carcinoma is in Stage I and 37% in Stage II. Only 15% of patients in Stage I have positive nodes and we salvage one half of them. Similarly 25% of Stage II cancer of the cervix will have positive nodes and the expected salvage is one in five. It would seem obvious then that the impact of the nodal dissection on the total salvage in cervical cancer is not great. The node dissections should be done, but the emphasis in therapy should be on the local tumor and the extensions from it rather than on the nodes.

Complications. If we are to shift the emphasis in treatment from the nodal and concentrate our therapy on the local area we pose problems for both the surgeon and the radiologist. Both are concerned with proper function of the bladder and intestine in the post treatment period. There is an impression that only the surgeons have complications. Recent reports in the literature suggest that serious bladder and bowel injuries have increased in number as the radiologists attempt to deliver larger doses from super voltage machines. The damage from radiation is apt to be permanent and progressive in contrast to the ureteral and vesical injuries that follow surgical intervention.

A certain number of fistulae will heal spontaneously. The remainder may pose more serious problems and require transplantation of the ureter into the bladder dome, or at times a nephrectomy. If meticulous dissections are done around the bladder the surgeon runs the risk of interrupting the blood supply to the bladder and lower ureter. In addition dissections of this magnitude impair the nerve supply to the bladder which produces the troublesome complication of bladder atony. This is more of a nuisance than a serious complication.

Fistula formation and bladder atony are technical problems inherent in any operation designed to remove all of the carcinoma. We should not fall into the trap of performing a less extensive dissection to avoid the complications and leave potential disease behind.

In past years my own fistula rate has been as high as 10%. Recently we have materially reduced the incidence of fistula formation as well as the pelvic sepsis that occasionally occurs by closing the vaginal apex and instituting catheter drainage.

The morbidity from the abdominal surgical procedures for cancer of the cervix tends to be high while the morbidity is relatively low in the neighborhood of 1%.

What about the combined use of radiation and radical abdominal surgery? The combination of radiation and surgery is being tried in a number of clinics in the United States. By combining modalities the surgeon hopes to preserve the best features of both while minimizing the complications. Such therapy may be employed in a number of different ways.

1. A preliminary trial dose of radiation is given followed by radical hysterectomy when either biopsies or vaginal smears suggest that the radiation response is unsatisfactory. If the smears and biopsies will pinpoint the radiation resistant case this will be a major contribution in the treatment of cervical cancer. Our hopes for the future rest on our ability to select the proper treatment for the individual case. As of the present time we do not have satisfactory method of making the selection although we badly need such a test.

2. In some clinics local radium therapy is routinely followed by radical abdominal surgery. In my own opinion it would appear to be more logical to carry out definitive therapy by either surgery or radiation rather than use them in combination according to a standardized plan.

3. A full course of radiation is followed by a radical abdominal hysterectomy and node dissection as part of a regular treatment program in certain clinics.

In my own experience with this approach I have found that the technical phases of the operation are not necessarily increased but there have been far too many serious injuries to the bladder. They do not appear immediately but are prone to occur after 2 or 3 weeks. It is reasonable to expect that they might for radiation has jeopardized the blood supply and surgery has added further insult. If the therapist gives less radiation or the surgeon does less of a dissection in order to minimize the damage he reduces the chance of cure. It is possible that combination therapy of this magnitude may also act as a disservice to the patient. It would seem to be unwise to have the patient go through a dangerous operation which may be unnecessary if the radiation has destroyed the tumor.

Rather than employ combination treatment in any form I would prefer to select the type of therapy which I felt best suited the needs of the patient and give it to the best of my ability.

Vaginal Surgery of Cervical Carcinoma*

E. NAVRATIL

The use of the two basic methods, surgery and radiotherapy, either alone or in various combinations at our disposal for the treatment of epidermoid carcinoma of the cervix of the uterus enabled the introduction of a selective therapy. This form of treatment can only take into account the many individual variations of patients. One of the greatest advantages of surgery consists in the possibility of choosing one of the several types of operations providing different degrees of radicality proportionate to the stage of disease and to the individual case. Such a procedure corresponds to the aim of our treatment to make every possible effort to achieve optimal results with minimal risk to the patient. Accordingly different types of operations have been used by us when operative treatment was considered. Disregarding conizations and simple hysterectomies in the period from 1946 through 1967 without preoperative irradiation 564 Wertheim's, 989 Schauta-Amreich's operations and 56 Schauta-Amreich's operations with bilateral extraperitoneal lymphadenectomy (extended radical vaginal operation) have been performed. After preoperative irradiation 52 patients underwent the abdominal, 23 patients the radical vaginal operation and one case the extended radical vaginal operation (Table 1).

Table 1. *Epidermoid carcinoma of the cervix of the uterus. Types of radical operations. Performed 1946 to 1967 incl.*

Without preoperative irradiation			1609
Schauta-Amreich's operation	989	61.5%	
Schauta-Amreich's operation with bilateral extraperitoneal lymphadenectomy	56	3.5%	
Wertheim's operation	564	35.1%	
With preoperative irradiation			76
Schauta-Amreich's operation	23	30.3%	
Schauta-Amreich's operation with bilateral extraperitoneal lymphadenectomy	1	1.3%	
Wertheim's operation	52	68.4%	
Total			1685

Having been asked to discuss radical vaginal surgery only, some preliminary comments may be made. The following widely accepted factors are valid reasons for the selective use of this operative procedure:

1. Patients withstand the operation much better than the Wertheim operation. Therefore the operation is rarely contraindicated on general medical grounds or advanced age. Thus the vaginal approach is used even by those operators, who generally are not in favour of it, in cases in which the Wertheim's operation is contraindicated or in cases with extreme stoutness or an associated prolapse.

* From the Department of Obstetrics and Gynecology, University of Graz, Graz, Austria.

2. A very low postoperative mortality and a very low incidence of postoperative complications can be claimed as one of the great advantages of the radical vaginal operation. Uretero-vaginal fistulae especially are extremely rare.

3. Follow-up examination of the patients show that late complications of the urinary tract are relatively rare.

The main argument advanced against the use of the radical vaginal operation is that it does not allow a lymphnode dissection. However, experience has proved that the end results by the Schauta operation achieved are satisfactory. In discussing the value of this procedure SHAW for instance stated, that "it is one of the puzzling features of gynecological surgery that such good figures are obtained when pelvic lymphatic glands are left undisturbed". These good results can be explained by the different incidence of lymphnode involvement in the various histological and clinical stages and by the statement again advanced by LANGDON PARSONS, CESARE and FRIEDELL that "the problem of successful management rests largely on the adequacy with which the local spread of the disease is treated. The emphasis should not be primarily on the node dissection but on the adequate excision of the paravaginal and paracervical tissue". If the vaginal operation would not satisfy this last postulate, the reported end results could not be understood. On the other hand there seems to be till now no agreement regarding the necessity of the surgical removal of the lymph-field and in regard to the therapeutic value of lymphadenectomy. Like the other advocates of the radical vaginal operation MCCLURE BROWNE believes that if the nodes are involved there is no point in the dissection and if they are not involved there is no need for it. Furthermore neither GRAHAM nor RAUSCHER and SPURNY found good evidence that the surgical removal of the lymphnodes significantly increases the 5-year survival rates. These statement would logically speak in favour of the vaginal operation. However, we do not agree to these arguments unconditionally. Our attitude towards the lymphnode problem is based on the assumption that lymphadenectomy is of great importance in cases, in which in the light of our informations the incidence of lymphnode metastases can be expected to be high. That applies especially to cases of progressed Stage I and to the cases of Stage II. The same is valid for cases of all stages of disease regardless of the histologic grade of stromal invasion, if on a biopsy or on the extirpated uterus a carcinomatous lymph- or bloodvessel invasion can be demonstrated. Therefore the vaginal approach was used selectively.

The efficiency of the vaginal operation has already been substantiated by numerous reports. However, in general, they do not seem to have attracted much attention. Within the brief period still at my disposal it is therefore my intention to present our immediate postoperative results and survival rates, achieved by the Schauta-Amreich operation in cases without preoperative irradiation. Postoperative X-ray treatment was applied to the majority of cases of clinical stages, whereas in preclinical cases this treatment was omitted.

The distribution of stages and ages respectively of the 989 patients is presented in Table 2. According to our indications for the Schauta-Amreich operation the majority of cases belonged to Stage I. However, more than one third have been cases of early Stage II and some of Stage III (vagina). 10% of the patients have been older than 60 years.

In the discussion of the complications it seems justified to subdivide the whole period in the years 1947 through 1951 and 1952 through 1967, as the first 5 years represent the postwar time with various well-known difficulties. Besides that the method of the isolation of the ureter was changed in 1949. Thus for assessing actual results reference must be made to the 756 operations performed in the last 15 years.

Regarding the injuries to bladder, ureter and rectum it must be pointed out that no distinction is made between avoidable and unavoidable ones according to the spread of the carcinoma. Thus their total incidence is presented in Table 3. The majority of these lesions occurred in the first 5 years. As our experience increased their incidence was reduced considerably. The isolation of the ureter is generally considered as the crucial point of the operation. Accordingly it may be emphasized that one ureter was lacerated in only five cases (0.5%) during the course of its isolation. Among the first 233 operations a damage to one ureter occured twice (0.9%) and among the last 756 operations three times (0.4%). The bladder was injured in 16 cases (1.6%) and the rectum in one case (0.1%). In the light of these results it can be stated that the incidence of injuries to ureter, bladder and rectum is very low, providing that the vaginal approach is correctly indicated and that a satisfactory operative technique is followed. However, it can not be expected that avoidable injuries can ever be eliminated completely.

Table 2. *Schauta-Amreich operation. No preoperative irradiation. Epidermoid carcinoma 1947 to 1967 incl. Ages of 989 patients*

Age	Stage							
	I		II		III		Total	
	No. of cases	%	No. of cases	%	No. of cases	%	No. of cases	%
21—30	41	4.1	6	0.6	—	—	47	4.8
31—40	203	20.5	61	6.2	3	0.3	267	27.0
41—50	206	20.8	120	12.1	6	0.6	332	33.6
51—60	111	11.2	123	12.4	6	0.6	240	24.3
61—70	45	4.6	56	5.7	1	0.1	102	10.3
71—80	1	0.1	—	—	—	—	1	0.1
	607	61.4	366	37.0	16	1.6	989	100.0

For the evaluation of all radical hysterectomies the development of secondary fistulae, especially of the urinary tract, is of great importance. The incidence in our cases is presented in Table 4. The majority of uretero-vaginal fistulae was observed in the first 5 years. Whereas among 233 operations performed during this period seven unilateral uretero-vaginal fistulae (3.0%) developed, among the following 756 operations only one fistula (0.1%) was observed. This improvement is in our opinion due to the modified method in the isolation of the ureters described by us in the year 1949. As the incidence of other fistulas is also extremely low it can be postulated that the problem of fistulae can be practically disregarded.

Using a 30 day follow-up suggested by BRUNSCHWIG to estimate postoperative mortality, our mortality for the first 5 years was relatively high (3.4%), but for the following period only 0.8%. Thus as of today it can be assumed to be approximately 1%.

In conclusion it can be stated that the immediate results are satisfactory. However, it must be emphasized particularly that they can be evaluated correctly only in

Table 3. *Schauta-Amreich operation. No preoperative irradiation. Epidermoid carcinoma. Incidence of injuries. 1947 to 1967 incl.*

Period	No. of cases	Bladder		Ureter		Rectum		Bladder and Rectum		Total	
		No. of cases	%	No. of cases	%	No. of cases	%	No. of cases	%	No. of cases	%
1947—1951	233	7	3.0	2	0.9	—	—	—	—	9	3.9
1952—1967	756	9	1.2	3	0.4	1	0.1	1	0.1	14	1.8
1947—1967	989	16	1.6	5	0.5	1	0.1	1	0.1	23	2.3

Table 4. *Schauta-Amreich operation. No preoperative irradiation. Epidermoid carcinoma. Incidence of postoperative fistulae. 1947 to 1967 incl.*

Period	No. of cases	Bladder		Ureter		Rectum		Bladder and Rectum		Intestines		Total	
		No. of cases	%	No. of cases	%	No. of cases	%	No. of cases	%	No. of cases	%	No. of cases	%
1947—1951	233	1	0.4	7	3.0	1	0.4	—	—	—	—	9	3.9
1952—1967	756	2	0.3	1	0.1	2	0.3	—	—	2	0.3	7	0.9
1947—1967	989	3	0.3	8	0.8	3	0.3	—	—	2	0.2	16	1.6

relation to the end results achieved. The 5-year cure rate has been generally accepted for estimating the therapeutic results although this does not mean freedom from recurrence 5 years after initial treatment. Accordingly in the Annual Report the results of various institutions after periods of 7 and 10 years are published too. Thus our survival rates will be presented not only after 5 years, but also after 10 and even after 15 years. In doing so there remains to be mentioned that no distinction is made between death from carcinoma or from other disease because not every case had a postmortem examination.

The 5-year survival rates for 823 patients operated upon in the years 1947 through 1962 are summarized in Table 5. Of these cases 611 or 74.2% survived 5 years. The survival rate in 502 cases Stage I disease was 86.3%, in 306 cases Stage II 55.9% and in 15 cases Stage III (vagina) 46.7%. One case of Stage III formerly missed is living after 5 years. The survival rates for the last 10 years are presented in Table 6. They demonstrate the results achieved by our present indication for the Schauta-Amreich operation.

Table 5. *Schauta-Amreich operation. No preoperative irradiation. Epidermoid carcinoma. 5-year survival 1947 to 1962 incl.*

Stage	No. of cases	5-year survival		
		No. of cases	%	Lost sight of
I	502	433	86.3	4
II	306	171	55.9	—
III	15	7	(46.7)	—
I—III	823	611	74.2	4

For the evaluation of the 10-year cure rates 568 cases operated upon during the period 1947 through 1957 are at our disposal (Table 7). The 10-year cure rate was for these cases 63.0%. Of 323 cases of Stage I 77.1%, of 231 cases of Stage II 44.6% and of 14 cases of Stage III (vagina) 42.9% are living after 10 years.

The 15-year cure rates refer to 294 patients who had been operated upon in the years 1947 through 1952 (Table 8). Of these cases 142 or 48.3% have reached the 15-year survival date. The survival rate in 132 cases Stage I disease was 66.7%, in 151 cases Stage II 33.8% and in 11 cases Stage III 27.3%. It must be assumed that these results will be improved in the future because they are now based on operations performed in their majority in the post-war time.

Summarizing it can be expected that the reported results and the survival rates should be accepted as a proof of the efficiency of the radical vaginal operation in a selective treatment for epidermoid cervical carcinoma. There is no question, that in surgical treatment of cervical cancer the Schauta-operation will maintain its ground because there will always be cases, which are operated better by the vaginal than by the abdominal procedure and because more and more early cases will be detected, in which the dissection of the lymphnode bearing areas is unnecessary. In closing, I hope that this presentation will stimulate interest in this operative procedure and will lead to its further use.

Table 6. *Schauta-Amreich operation. No preoperative irradiation. Epidermoid carcinoma. 5 year survival. 1947 to 1952 incl. and 1953 to 1962 incl.*

Period	Stage											
	I			II			III			I—III		
	No. of cases	%	Lost sight of	No. of cases	%	Lost sight of	No. of cases	%	Lost sight of	No. of cases	%	Lost sight of
1947—1952	132/105	79.5	1	151/74	49.0	—	11/4	(36.4)	—	294/183	62.2	1
1953—1962	370/328	88.6	3	155/97	62.6	—	4/3	(75.0)	—	529/428	80.9	3

Table 8. *Schauta-Amreich operation. No preoperatioe irradiation. Epidermoid carcinoma. 5-, 10- and 15-year survival. 1947 to 1952 incl.*

Stage	No. of cases	Living at 5 years			Living at 10 years			Living at 15 years		
		No. of cases	%	Lost sight of	No. of cases	%	Lost sight of	No. of cases	%	Lost sight of
I	132	105	79.5	1	95	72.0	2	88	66.7	4
II	151	74	49.0	—	60	39.7	—	51	33.8	2
III	11	4	(36.4)	—	4	(36.4)	—	3	(27.3)	1
I—III	294	183	62.2	1	159	54.1	2	142	48.3	7

Table 7. *Schauta-Amreich operation. No preoperative irradiation. Epidermoid carcinoma. 5- and 10-year survival 1947 to 1957 incl.*

Stage	No. of cases	Living at 5 years			Living at 10 years		
		No. of cases	%	Lost sight of	No. of cases	%	Lost sight of
I	323	275	85.1	2	249	77.1	8
II	231	124	53.7	—	103	44.6	2
III	14	6	(42.9)	—	6	(42.9)	—
I—III	568	405	71.3	2	358	63.0	10

References

GRAHAM, J. B., L. S. J. SOTTO, and F. P. PALOUCEK: Carcinoma of the cervix. Philadelphia: W. B. Saunders Co. 1962.

MAYER, H. G. K.: Geburtsh. u. Frauenheilk. **28**, 338 (1968).

McCLURE BROWNE, J. C.: Discussion. J. Obstet. Gynaec. Brit. Emp. **67**, 724 (1960).

NAVRATIL, E.: The Schauta-Amreich operation. In: MEIGS, J. V., and S. H. STURGIS, Progress in gynecology, Vol. IV. New York, London: Grune and Stratton 1963.

— Amer. J. Obstet. Gynec. **86**, 141 (1963).

— Radical vaginal hysterectomy (Schauta-Amreich operation). In: Clin. Obstet. Gynec. Vol. 8, No. 3. New York: Hoeber Med. Division. Harper and Row Publ. 1965.

PARSONS LANGDON, and G. H. FRIEDELL: The evaluation of pelvic lymphadenectomy in the treatment of cervical cancer. In: MEIGS, J. V., and S. H. STURGIS, Progress in Gynecology, Vol. IV. New York, London: Grune and Stratton 1963.

—, F. CESARE, and G. H. FRIEDELL: Surg. Gynec. Obstet. **109**, 279 (1959).

RAUSCHER, H., u. J. SPURNY: Geburtsh. u. Frauenheilk. **19**, 651 (1959).

Evaluation of Different Methods of Treatment of Cervical Carcinoma*

O. KÄSER and A. CASTAÑO Y ALMENDRAL

Cure of cancer of the cervix depends first on the nature and extent of the tumor, second to a lesser degree on the skill and experience of the therapist, and third to some extent on the modalities of treatment [*21*].

This could explain why the results of different methods of treatment — radiotherapy, surgery and various combinations — do not differ materially. The question then arises as to whether the different therapeutic regimes cure the same tumors and fail to do so with the others, or if their therapeutic spectrum is different thereby enabling a selective therapy to produce better results. A definitive answer cannot be given at the present time. However, experience has shown that a few persistent or recurrent carcinomas after radiotherapy can be cured by surgery and vice-versa [*5, 28*]. The number of these cases, however, is too small to alter the apparent 5 year recovery rate significantly. The number of cures would most likely be increased if the diagnosis of a persistent or recurrent carcinoma could be made earlier than it is possible by the now available methods.

It is well known that at the present time in most institutions about one third to one half of all cases are beyond cure at the beginning of primary therapy [*27*]. This

* Herrn Dr. H. J. WESPI, Chefarzt der Frauenklinik Aarau (CH) zum 60. Geburtstag in Freundschaft gewidmet.

situation can only be changed by earlier detection of cancer with a broad scale screening program [*29*, *37*].

Another question which cannot be answered satisfactorily is the difference in terms of cure rates between what we consider an optimal and an inadequate surgical or radiotherapeutic treatment of cancer of the cervix. It is true that the Annual Reports [*27*] show improving apparent recovery rates which are probably due in part to better treatment. But it is also well known that cases have been cured after insufficient treatment, and that failures occur after seemingly adequate therapy.

Table 1 shows the 5 year apparent recovery rates of the four most important therapeutic regimes:

1. Surgery with minimal selection and so called "tailored procedures".
2. Surgery, mostly abdominal, different degrees of selection with or without pre- and/or postoperative radiotherapy.

Table 1. *5-years apparent cure rate*
(14th annual report and other sources)

	Stage I %	Stage IV %	Stage I—IV %
Surgery[a] (minimal selection)	79	20	57.4
Surgery[b] (mostly abdominal ± heavy selection)	73—84	0—5	44—64
Surgery[c] (vaginal and abdominal ± heavy selection)	72—82	0—9	54—63
Radiotherapy[d] (minimal selection)	69—86	5—12	42—59

[a] Memorial Hospital and James Ewing Hospital New York.
[b] Frankfurt, Graz, Ljubljana, St. Louis.
[c] Amsterdam, Hannover, Jena, Wuppertal.
[d] Copenhagen, Manchester, München, Stockholm.

3. Surgery, mostly vaginal or partly vaginal partly abdominal, with different degrees of selection with or without irradiation and
4. radiotherapy exclusively or with only occasional surgery.

The results shown are those of a few institutions with large numbers of cases chosen arbitrarily in the 14th Annual Report [*27*] or the literature [*4*, *19*, *48*]. The 5 year results for League of Nations Stage I, Stage IV and all stages combined for these four therapeutic regimes do not differ significantly. This is true also for two additional methods; the first systematic preoperative radiation [*16*, *17*, *45*], and the second systematic postradiological lymphadenectomy in advanced cases. This second method has never gained wide acceptance and has now mostly been abandoned because of a prohibitive morbidity [*38*].

There are of course a few "high fliers" in the literature with better results [*27*] but smaller numbers of patients. This fact does not prove a superiority of treatment, as it is well known, and has repeatedly been pointed out by KOTTMEIER, that results depend on many other factors [*27*].

The recovery rates by BRUNSCHWIG and his collaborators [*47*] with different surgical procedures according to stage of disease and condition of patients and minimal selection are impressive especially in Stage IV cases; but they are not superior to those with other therapeutic regimes [*11, 27*]. Also few other institutions have the facilities to repeat Brunschwig's surgical experiment.

We therefore come to the conclusion that presently available data and especially the lack of controlled studies do not prove the superiority of anyone of the above mentioned methods. Also according to some authors [*13, 42*] there is no statistically significant difference between the abdominal operation with and without lymphadenectomy.

If the data about recovery rates are inconclusive, there is, however, little doubt that for many and perhaps most cases of carcinoma of the cervix radiotherapy is the best or often the only possible form of treatment because of the size of the tumor and/or the condition of the patient. The two advantages of radiotherapy are a lower mortality — generally below 0.5% — and morbidity especially early morbidity [*2, 6, 8, 10—12, 23, 24, 26, 35, 36, 40, 44*]. The number of fistulas in Stages I and II is very small [*26, 47*].

An additional reason to favor radiotherapy has recently been given by BADIB and collaborators [*3*]. These authors found in autopsy cases of cancer of the cervix that modern radiotherapy had cured cancer of the cervix spreading beyond this organ more often than surgery. After radiotherapy significantly more women showed only distant metastasis and no residual cancer in the pelvis. After both methods — modern surgery and modern radiotherapy — the women survived much longer than they would have formerly. Again the number of cases is too small and the groups are not comparable statistically to prove a point.

Both methods of treatment have a significant morbidity which is higher however after surgery (and most probably higher after abdominal than after vaginal operations) than after radiotherapy. Surgical mortality has been cut down to less than 1% in many institutions [*15, 24, 29, 30, 44*].

In Frankfurt three patients were lost in 667 radical abdominal operations giving a primary or hospital mortality of 0.45%. The morbidity of our abdominal operations is high if asymptomatic bacteriuria is included. The rate of severe complications is not excessive however and the number of fistulas which has been lowered as in many institutions [*2, 15, 24*] is acceptable.

In our hospital 78% of all patients showed one or more complications (Table 2) the most frequent being bacteriuria. The number of ureteric fistulas was 21 or 3%, in the last 150 cases there were 3 or 2%. Six patients had rectal or bladder fistulas. We feel that the measures listed in Table 3 are important in order to prevent ureteric fistulas.

What then are the advantages and indications for surgery? Two important advantages are the possibility of preserving the ovaries and a functional vagina in younger women. Preservation of these structures probably does not constitute a risk for the patient and preserving these organs is becoming more important as an increasing number of young women with early lesions are being treated. For these cases (carcinoma in situ and early invasive cancer) surgery is probably the best form of treatment because its radicality can be adapted to the individual patient. After surgery these patients can be followed by cytology which is more difficult or impossible after radiotherapy.

For many authors diagnostic conization or hysterectomy in certain cases in an adequate treatment for carcinoma in situ localized to the cervix [*1*, *29*, *37*, *49*]. Hysterectomy may even be adequate for early invasive cancer. The question then arises for which size of the tumor and for which additional qualities of early carcinomas — infiltration of blood or lymph vessels, histologic type, inflammation etc. — full cancer therapy — radiologic or surgical — is mandatory. This question cannot

Table 2. *Complications (% of total) in 667 Wertheim operations for cancer of the cervix (1950 to April 1968)*

Mortality	(3)	.45
Intestinal obstruction		1.6
Thrombo-embolism		4.5
Pneumonitis		2.0
Urinary tract infection		45.5[a]
Pyelonephritis		7.3
Febrile course (48 h <)		29.0
Lesions of ureter	(8)	1.2[b]
Fistulas ureter	(21)	3.0
Fistulas bladder/rectum	(6)	.9
Wound infection		
abdominal		3.5
vaginal		3.0
Wound disrupture	(2)	.3
No complications		22.0

[a] 80% with urine culture.
[b] 2 intentional sections.

Table 3. *Prevention of urinary tract damage*

1. Pre- and postoperative urography.
2. Preservation of mesureter.
3. Limited dissection of ureterovesical angle.
4. Preservation of umbilical artery.
5. Extraperitoneal suction drainage.
6. Double layer peritonealization.
7. Closed system bladder drainage.
8. No routine irradiation.

be answered satisfactorily, but it is reasonable to assume that with a tumor of less than 0.5 to 1 cm the advantages in terms of 5-year cure rates of a conservative approach; i.e. smaller mortality and of course morbidity, may outweigh its disadvantages; i.e. the possibility of lymphatic spread. It has been shown in many institutions including Frankfurt that with microcarcinomas of the cervix positive regional lymph nodes are found only very exceptionally, i.e. in less than 1 to 2% [*22*, *50*]. Even with tumors of up to 1 cm in diameter positive nodes seem still to be rare [*49*, *50*].

An important concern of many authors at present is the search for a "minimal effective and safe treatment" [*29*, *37*] of the early stages of cancer of the cervix. The dangers of overtreatment of these cases are considerable at least in many European countries.

The other indications for surgery are listed in Table 4. The indications 1 to 5 are widely accepted. Radioresistent and recurrent carcinomas after radiotherapy are only exceptionally cured by a second course of ionizing agents, and the results of chemotherapy are equivocal and palliative at best [*25*, *41*]. Therefore surgery is often the only hope of cure.

The indications 6 to 10 are not generally accepted. Probably the 5-year recovery rates of surgery and radiotherapy in these cases are more or less identical. It is possible, however, that by individualizing therapy and selecting patients for one or the other form of treatment results might be improved. But this depends on a close cooperation of the radiotherapist and the gynecologic surgeon.

The success of operative treatment of cancer of the cervix depends largely on the experience and skill of the surgeon. These qualities cannot be gained by operating the

Table 4. *Indications and possible indications for surgery in operable cases of invasive cancer of the cervix*

1. Early lesion, Stage Ia.
2. Radioresistant or recurrent tumors
3. Ca cervix and fibromyomas or ovarian tumor.
4. Ca cervix and p. i. d.
5. Ca cervix, unfavourable local conditions for radiotherapy.
6. Stage Ib to IIa cases.
7. Stage IV cases (exceptional).
8. Ca cervix and pregnancy.
9. Adenocarcinoma.
10. Ca cervix and positive nodes (lymphangiography).

exceptional radioresistant cases only. This is therefore an additional reason why surgery of primary cases should be continued.

In summarizing I would say that radiotherapy is the best form of treatment for the majority of cases examined in most institutions at the present time. On the other hand, surgery still holds an important place in treating cancer of the cervix because of its advantages, especially in younger women and in early lesions. The results of the two methods in operable cases are comparable and the complication rate of surgery is not prohibitive.

References

1. Adelman, H. C., and S. I. Hajdu: Amer. J. Obstet. Gynec. **98**, 173 (1967).
2. Antoine, T.: Med. Coll. Virg. Quart. **3**, 56 (1967).
3. Badib, A. O.: Cancer (Philad.) **21**, 434 (1968).
4. Barber, H. R. K.: Results of the surgical treatment of cancer of the cervix at the Memorial-James Ewing Hospital, New York. In: Marcus, S. L., and C. C. Marcus, Advances in obstetrics and gynecology, Vol. 1, p. 622. Baltimore: The Williams and Wilkins Company 1967.
5. —, and A. Brunschwig: Results of the surgical treatment of recurrent cancer of the cervix. In: G. C. Lewis, New concepts in gynecological oncology. Philadelphia: F. A. Davis Company 1966.

6. Bickenbach, W.: Med. Coll. Virg. Quart. **3**, 35 (1967).
7. Brunschwig, A.: The operations for cancer of the cervix. In: Marcus, S. L., and C. C. Marcus, Advances in obstetrics and gynecology, Vol. 1, p. 608. Baltimore: The Williams and Wilkins Company 1967.
8. Colpitts, R. V.: Urologic complications encountered in the treatment of patients with squamous carcinoma of the cervix. In: Carcinoma of the uterine cervix, endometrium and ovary, p. 175. Chicago: Year Book Publ. 1962.
9. Cuccia, C. A.: Amer. J. Roentgenol. **99**, 3711 (1967).
10. Deddisch, M. R.: Med. Coll. Virg. Quart. **3**, 54 (1967).
11. Fletcher, G. H.: Radiotherapy of cancer of the cervix uteri. In: Carcinoma of the uterine cervix, endometrium and ovary, p. 69. Chicago: Year Book Publ. 1962.
12. Friedman, E. A., and H. C. Taylor Jr.: Amer. J. Obstet. Gynec. **93**, 758 (1965).
13. Froewis, J.: Wien. klin. Wschr. **74**, 357 (1962).
14. Graham, I.: Surg. Gynec. Obstet. **126**, 799 (1968).
15. Green, T. H.: Obstet. and Gynec. **28**, 1 (1966).
16. Greiss, F. C., Jr.: J. Amer. med. Ass. **193**, 1105 (1965).
17. Greiss, F. C.: Combined radiation and surgical treatment for carcinoma of the uterine cervix. In: G. C. Lewis, New concepts in gynecological oncology, p. 133. Philadelphia: F. A. Davis Company 1966.
18. —, and D. D. Blake: Clin. Obstet. Gynec. **10**, 567 (1967).
19. Gorys, H. P.: Zbl. Gynäk. **82**, 1561 (1960).
20. Guttmann, R.: J. Amer. med. Ass. **193**, 1104 (1965).
21. Hahn, G. A.: Amer. J. Obstet. Gynec. **96**, 631 (1967).
22. Hillemanns, H. G., u. T. Kröpelin: Arch. Gynäk. **204**, 42 (1967).
23. Holzaepfel, I. H., and T. C. Pomeroy: Amer. J. Obstet. Gynec. **97**, 625 (1967).
24. Käser, O.: Med. Coll. Virg. Quart. **3**, 42 (1967).
25. Karnofsky, D. A.: Chemotherapy of recurrent cervical cancer. In: G. C. Lewis, New concepts in gynecological oncology, p. 171. Philadelphia: F. A. Davis Company 1966.
26. Kottmeier, H. L.: Complications of radiotherapy of carcinoma of the cervix. In: Marcus, S. L., and C. C. Marcus, Advances in obstetrics and gynecology, p. 633. Baltimore: The Williams and Wilkins Company 1967.
27.— Annual report on the results of treatment in carcinoma of the uterus and vagina. 14th Vol. Stockholm 1967.
28. — Evaluation of treatment of recurrences after surgery and radiotherapy of carcinoma of the cervix. In: G. C. Lewis, New concepts in gynecological oncology, p. 161. Philadelphia: F. A. Davis Company 1966.
29. Latour, I. P. A.: Amer. J. Obstet. Gynec. **97**, 631 (1967).
30. O'Leary, I. A., and R. E. Symmonds: Obstet. and Gynec. **28**, 745 (1967).
31. Louros, N. A.: Med. Coll. Virg. Quart. **3**, 40 (1967).
32. Lucci, I. A.: Carcinoma of the cervix and pregnancy. In: Carcinoma of the uterine cervix, endometrium and ovary, p. 217. Chicago: Year Book Publ. 1962.
33. Nolan, J. F.: Megavoltage radiation therapy in recurrent cancer of the uterine cervix. In: G. C. Lewis, New concepts on gynecological oncology, p. 157. Philadelphia: F. A. Davis Company 1966.
35. Parker, R. T.: Amer. J. Obstet. Gynec. **99**, 933 (1967).
36. Rogge, U.: Zbl. Gynäk. **90**, 487 (1968).
37. Roman, T. N., and I. P. A. Latour: Amer. J. Obstet. Gynec. **97**, 739 (1967).
38. Rutledge, F.: Experience with pelvic lymphadenectomy. In: Carcinoma of the uterine cervix, endometrium and ovary, p. 175. Chicago: Year Book Publ. 1962.
39. — J. Amer. med. Ass. **193**, 1102 (1965).
40. — The role of surgical resection in the management of cervical carcinoma. In: Carcinoma of the uterine cervix, endometrium and ovary, p. 149. Chicago: Year Book Publ. 1962.
41. Smith, I. P., and F. Rutledge: Amer. J. Obstet. Gynec. **97**, 800 (1967).
42. Spurny, J.: Krebsarzt **13**, 401 (1958).
43. Symmonds, R. E.: Carcinoma of the cervix and pregnancy. In: G. C. Lewis, New concepts in gynecological oncology, p. 181. Philadelphia: F. A. Davis Company 1966.
44. — Amer. J. Obstet. Gynec. **94**, 633 (1966).

45. Stallworthy, I. A.: Med. Coll. Virg. Quart. **3**, 45 (1967).
46. Truelsen, F.: Cancer of the cervix. London: Lewis 1949.
47. Weise, W., u. G. Reichel: Zbl. Gynäk. **83**, 1561 (1960).
48. Anselmino, K. I.: Geburtsh. u. Frauenheilk. **21**, 120 (1961).
49. Ober, K. G., u. H. Meinrenken: Gynäkologische Operationen. In: Guleke, N., u. R. Zenker, Hrsg., Allg. und spez. Chirurg. Operationslehre. 2. Aufl., Bd. IX. Berlin-Göttingen-Heidelberg-New York: Springer 1964.
50. Reiffenstuhl, G.: Das Lymphknotenproblem beim Carcinoma colli uteri etc. München-Berlin-Wien: Urban und Schwarzenberg 1967.

Diagnosis of Recurrent Carcinoma of the Cervix

Joseph H. Pratt

Nearly half of the patients with carcinoma of the cervix will eventually die of persistent or recurrent disease. If patients who do not respond to initial therapy could be identified early and positively, many of them could be cured or the course of their disease so modified as to offer significant palliation. However, for the purpose of this discussion, we must distinguish between persistent and recurrent cervical cancer. Persistent cancer is that which never disappears, and all cases should be diagnosed during the first 3 months after treatment. Recurrent tumors are those that initially heal after radiotherapy and subsequently recur locally or elsewhere. When the primary treatment involves surgical extirpation of the lesion and the margins of the wound seem to be free of tumor, any reappearance — other than immediate local reappearance — is considered a recurrence.

Our problem is to diagnose recurrences as early as possible. Since additional treatment not only carries a considerable risk but may be mutilating, the diagnosis must be as nearly unequivocal as we can establish it. This, of course, means pathologic identification of viable tumor cells. However, most carcinomas of the cervix are treated primarily with radiotherapy, and surgical meddling with vigorously irradiated tissue may lead to necrosis, complications, or the breakdown of tissue barriers. Therefore, indiscriminate or "routine" biopsies should be avoided. Only when the radiologist, clinician, or surgeon believes a lesion is not responding satisfactorily should the patient be subjected to additional biopsies.

The majority of recurrences and deaths from cervical cancer take place in the first 3 years, and this is the critical time for care and diagnosis of recurrent tumor. But even after 5 years, 3% to 5% or more of the patients will die of recurrences. The first step in a program to diagnose recurrent cancer is in the routine care of all patients after primary treatment. Gary et al. (1964), on the basis of their studies, advise examinations monthly during the first 3 months, every 2 months from 3 to 27 months, and biannually thereafter. Breen goes even further and sees his patients every 2 weeks for 3 months and every month for 2 years. At the Mayo Clinic, where our patients come from a wide geographic area, we have advised routine examination every 3 months for 1 year, twice a year for 5 years, and once 1 year thereafter. Suit et al. (1967) rather pessimistically expressed the opinion that radiation doses necessary to kill all tumor cells would have to be in excess of the amounts used clinically; thus, since there is no natural mortality of tumor cells, recurrences would be found in almost all cases, if the tumor sites were examined long enough. In a recently reported case, recurrence did appear after 30 years (Howkins and Andrews, 1955).

Our base line for the evaluation of a patient is her general health and the local pelvic findings at the conclusion of her initial course of therapy. From this point on she should improve; if she does not, then more extensive investigations rather than routine examinations are indicated. Unexplained loss of weight is significant, as is a general deterioration of strength, vitality, or physical well-being. Since the administration of radiation therapy is subject to variation and since tissue response to irradiation varies considerably, each patient must be judged on the basis of the course of her own illness, including physical findings and laboratory data.

The cervix and upper part of the vagina receive the maximal doses of radiation and are therefore less likely to be sites of *recurrent* cancer than are other parts of the vagina or the lateral pelvic tissues. Furthermore, if the upper part of the vaginal tract is free and pliable, if there is no ulceration, and if there is no induration, then there is no *local* or *central* recurrence. Any area of ulceration, of course, should be biopsied. Vaginal smears are not as satisfactory after radiation as one could wish but are helpful, and they are very good after primary surgical treatment. If a smear is positive *and the cervix and vaginal vault seem normal*, then Schiller's iodine test may help one pick a spot to biopsy. A test involving the use of a hematoporphyrin derivative may point out a precise spot to biopsy (LIPSON et al., 1964), if the necessary materials are available and if one has had sufficient experience with it. Solitary suburethral metastasis is uncommon from a cervical lesion, yet PAUNIER et al. (1967) reported 17 cases in a series of 965 in which the patients were known to have died of recurrent cervical malignancy. Biopsy and diagnosis of such lesions present no problem.

There is always some change in the pelvis after irradiation or operation. An experienced radiologist or surgeon can, hopefully, distinguish the nodular, wooden-hard, fixed tissues of recurrent cancer from the smoother lesions of radiation fibrosis. Yet mistakes can be made, either in observing the malignant tissue too long or in assuming that everything palpable is malignant. KAPLAN et al. (1965) have reported several such cases. We recently had a case which illustrates the problem. The patient, a 44 year old women with a Stage III lesion, had been treated with an adequate course of radium and X-rays. 4 months later — primarily because of a nonfunctioning left kidney but also because of a large ulcerating hemorrhagic fixed pelvic mass, anemia, and a high erythrocyte sedimentation rate — definitive operation was thought to be contraindicated. Because of brisk hemorrhage 1 month later, she was operated on, and bilateral ligation of the internal iliac arteries was done. The patient was sent home for terminal care, but she subsequently came to the Mayo Clinic. Reexploration was thought advisable, and it turned out that, after resection of the left ureter and its reimplantation into the bladder, a Wertheim type hysterectomy and node dissection were possible. Most of the pelvic fixation proved to be the result of radiation changes, necrosis, and ulceration, only an occasional clump of tumor cells being found near the ureter. One positive node was found. This patient lived comfortably and well for more than 2 years. While such cases are unusual, far too often a patient with a questionably recurrent cancer is observed until the lesion is so large and so characteristic that it has become truly unresectable and the patient is beyond hope of surgical extirpation of the cancer.

If, during a routine examination, the physician finds a palpable change in the pelvis, either a distinct nodule, a noticeable increase in fibrosis or fixation, or a lateral mass, he must obtain biopsy specimens of the responsible tissue. Sometimes this may be accomplished by means of needle biopsy through the vaginal vault, rarely transrectally. Frequently, it is necessary to make a small incision in the vault to reach the suspicious region. This should be done in an operating theater, as bleeding may be excessive. Also, a pathologist should be available to give a diagnosis based on examination of a frozen section. More often than not, the first specimen or two is inflammatory, but a deeper one may show malignant cells.

Another patient, a 32 year old women, had had a simple vaginal hysterectomy for what was apparently a Stage I lesion. On examination here 1 year later, a 4 cm mass was found behind the vault. The ovaries could not be identified per se. Needle biopsy through the vault confirmed recurrence of cancer. Thus, a lesion was discovered at a time when it was resectable, and a Wertheim hysterectomy was carried out. The patient has survived 10 years.

Lateral pelvic masses are most often confused with lymphocysts. The latter are rounded, hemispherical, smooth, generally nontender, and discrete; but they do *not* feel cystic on palpation. They are present early, by the third month postoperatively, they do not change in size, and they contain clear fluid. They can be explored extraperitoneally and unroofed for biopsy. Lymphocysts should not cause ureteral obstruction; therefore, if obstruction is present, the retroperitoneal tissues should be explored further.

If the uterus remains, as after radiation therapy, and there is any change in vaginal discharge, or if the uterus seems to become larger on subsequent bimanual examinations, then dilatation and curettage of the endocervical region, as well as the fundus, is indicated to rule out spread of the malignant disease into the body of the uterus. A diagnostic Wertheim hysterectomy may be the procedure of choice if the post-treatment vagina and cervix are completely stenotic.

The patient with pelvic metastasis may develop signs or symptoms suggesting a deeper or higher recurrence. Unilateral edema frequently is the first hint of recurrence along the pelvic wall, involving the iliac or obturator region and extending behind the iliac artery and vein onto the muscles and fascia. These regions are high enough in the pelvis that pelvic examination of even a thin patient may reveal very little. Persistent sciatica, with some progression of pain, not particularly related to activities or position but present at night as well as in the daytime, is a poor prognostic symptom. In fact, after treatment for cancer of the cervix, any persistent, newly developing, localized, and not easily explained ache should alert the physician to the necessity of obtaining roentgenograms of the bones in the region of pain or even a bone scan of the pelvis and spine. Hydronephrosis and hydro-ureter also suggest recurrence of tumor. Ureteral obstruction low in the pelvis may be due to radiation fibrosis, but high ureteral obstruction, at the pelvic brim, is due almost always to recurrent cancer. The triad of edema, sciatica, and hydronephrosis must be considered as due to malignant disease, not fibrosis.

Persistent urinary tract symptoms or repeated urinary tract infections require excretory urograms and cystoscopic studies. The symptoms may result from radiation cystitis, but active cancer occasionally is found. If bullous edema is seen, the probability is great that cancer is invading the bladder wall.

Proctoscopic examinations are helpful. They permit one to observe changes in the bowel and, particularly if ulceration is present in the rectovaginal septum, to carefully obtain biopsy specimens to exclude malignant ulceration.

We do not use lymphangiograms, as they have not proven as accurate as we would like in picking out metastatically involved nodes. Ultrasonic waves may eventually prove helpful but are not diagnostic. Venography as reported by DALALI et al. (1954) is more diagnostic, especially when one is trying to distinguish between edema due to lymphatic obstruction and that due to venous obstruction. It can be attributed to venous obstruction only in the absence of adequate collaterals.

If there is a suggestion of recurrence or if the patient's symptoms are suspicious, laparotomy may be necessary to prove or disprove the diagnosis. When possible, of course, such a diagnostic procedure should be continued as definitive treatment. Unfortunately, at times even laparotomy does not answer the question conclusively, and then one can only treat the patient conservatively and optimistically. If there still is a suggestion of a central recurrence though not confirmed by biopsy and the tissues could be extirpated surgically, then the surgeon will have to decide whether to go ahead with a Wertheim or exenterative operation or to persist in further observation.

The diagnostic laparotomy is, hopefully, to exclude cancer or, if it is present, to determine its extent. The first tissues to be checked, therefore, should be the liver, the peritoneal surfaces of the upper part of the abdomen, and the omentum. Metastasis in these regions precludes definitive or radical pelvic operation. The aortic nodes should then be palpated; and, if enlarged nodes are present, one or more should be removed for diagnosis. Only then should the surgeon take the time and energy to look for recurrent cancer in the pelvic region. Retroperitoneal exploration of the iliac and obturator regions is not difficult, nor is it difficult to explore the ureters at the pelvic brim and to obtain biopsy specimens from near the ureters or even from behind the great vessels. However, when sciatica is the presenting symptom, it is extremely hard to dissect along the obturator nerve, into the iliopsoas muscle, or close enough to the sacral plexus to really exclude a deeply metastasizing cancer. When recurrent cancer has been identified, yet is unresectable, silver clips can be used to outline the extent of the recurrence.

Cervical cancer does tend to recur locally and to remain in the pelvis; therefore, we may get a second chance at it. But distant metastasis occured in 341 of 2,220 patients treated at one hospital, according to CARLSON et al. (1967). They reported that single organs were involved in 110 instances and multiple sites in 231. Affected lymph nodes, if palpable, were generally inguinal or supraclavicular; and, although these were accessible for biopsy and excision, most often multiple sites were involved. The lungs were the second commonest distant site, and one third of the pulmonary metastases were solitary. Our feeling has been that if a chest film reveals a lung nodule, we first compare it with previous films. Then we try to exclude a primary bronchogenic lesion, and finally, before excising the nodule, we wait 2 to 3 months and recheck the patient. If no evidence of additional metastases has developed, the nodule is excised (DECKER et al., 1962).

Bony metastases pose a problem in that they may give severe symptoms without providing roentgenographic evidence of their location; therefore, no confirmatory biopsy is possible. When symptoms are severe, local radiation may be tried without a definitive diagnosis.

References

BREEN, J. L.: Personal communication to the author.
CARLSON, V., L. DELCLOS, and G. H. FLETCHER: Radiology **88**, 961—966 (1967).

Dalali, S. J., A. A. Plentl, and A. L. Bachman: Surg. Gynec. Obstet. **98**, 735—742 (1954).
Decker, D. G., J. W. Warren, O. T. Clagett, and D. C. Dahlin: Amer. J. Obstet. Gynec. **84**, 192—197 (1962).
Gary, R. K., J. M. Sala, and J. S. Spratt, Jr.: Radiology **83**, 208—218 (1964).
Howkins, J., and J. D. Andrews: J. Obstet. Gynaec. Brit. Emp. **62**, 870—871 (1955).
Kaplan, A. L., P. T. Hudgins, and J. A. Wall: Amer. J. Obstet. Gynec. **92**, 117—123 (1965).
Lipson, R. L., J. H. Pratt, E. J. Baldes, and M. B. Dockerty: Obstet. and Gynec. **24**, 78—84 (1964).
Paunier, J.-P., L. Delclos, and G. H. Fletcher: Radiology **88**, 555—562 (1967).
Suit, H., R. Wette, and R. Lindberg: Radiology **88**, 311—320 (1967).

Management of Recurrent Cervical Cancer

Eugene M. Bricker

In the United States in the past 20 years there has been an intensive study of the role of extended pelvic surgery in the treatment of advanced or recurrent carcinoma within the pelvis. The concept of ultraradical surgery sprang up simultaneously in several different clinics but was given impetus by the publications of Brunschwig and Appleby appearing in 1948 and 1950. Brunschwig reported his initial results of pelvic exenteration in the treatment of advanced carcinoma of the uterine cervix. Appleby reported on "proctocystectomy" in the treatment of advanced carcinoma of the rectum in males. One of Appleby's patients was a 7 year survivor of this operation, having been operated upon in 1943. My own initial excursion into this field of surgery occurred in 1940 and 1941 at the Ellis Fischel State Cancer Hospital in Columbia, Missouri, where a few patients were operated upon just before World War II. The results in these cases were not good because of poor selection of patients for the operation and because the problem of urinary diversion was not solved. These patients were never reported in the literature.

After World War II my interest in advanced pelvic cancer was resumed and a few male patients with advanced rectal cancer were operated upon successfully. It was not until after Brunschwig's report in 1948 that I became interested in advanced and recurrent cancer of the cervix and in doing pelvic exenteration on those patients who were referred to me by the gynecologists in our medical center. Since this time my colleagues and I have accumulated enough experience to enable us to crystalize our ideas regarding the indications for this type of ultraradical surgery and to allow us to give a fair estimate of the morbidity, mortality, and survival rates that may result. Our results are similar to those obtained in other medical centers, the differences in morbidity and mortality figures being chiefly an indication of the differing criteria used in the selection of patients for operation. The success of this type of surgery is dependent upon factors that pertain to both the patient's cancer and to the surgeon doing the operation. It is a biological characteristic of certain cancers of the cervix and of the rectum that they may remain localized to within the pelvis for a long period of time. Although quite large locally, with involvement of contiguous organs, there may be no regional lymphatic metastases. Such lesions theoretically are curable if operated upon radically enough. The surgeon must have judgment and skill. He must exercise judgment in the selection of patients for the ultraradical operation, in determining what is operable and what is inoperable, and he must have the necessary surgical skill to carry the rather complicated operation to a successful completion. This skill will be dependent upon adequate training and background in the various techniques of surgery involved.

An inseparable part of this clinical problem has been the development of a method of urinary diversion in the absence of a rectum. Various clinics approach this problem in different ways. The transplantation of both ureters to the remaining portion of the colon producing a so-called "wet colostomy" was the method used by BRUNSCHWIG and APPLEBY in their early cases. Bilateral skin ureterostomies were tresorted to in some patients. The use of the terminal ileum and cecum as a substitute for the urinary bladder was given a trial. During our own experience we tried several methods of substituting for the urinary bladder after pelvic exenteration but none were satisfactory until we developed the idea of transplanting the ureters to a segment of small intestine which acted merely as a conduit to convey the urine to the outside of the abdominal wall in a convenient location. We reported upon three cases of urinary diversion by this method in 1950, not realizing that essentially the same idea had been reported in the German literature by SEIFFERT in 1935, nor did we realize that MERSHEIMER and KOLARSICK were, at the time of our report, doing the same operation in laboratory dogs. The use of the ileal conduit for urinary diversion after pelvic exenteration has been so satisfactory that one of the chief objections to the operation has been removed. Indeed, the use of an ileal segment for this purpose has been widely accepted and has been used by many surgeons as the preferred method of substituting for bladder function in any age and for any reason. The acceptability of the ileal conduit is the result of the development of satisfactory external appliances that act as a receptacle for the urine when glued to the skin over the ileostomy stoma. The results of this operation have been published previously and show a most gratifying low instance of pyelonephritis (14%) and almost a complete absence of hyperchloremia and acidosis. These favorable results appear to be due to the separation of the segment from fecal contamination, the shortness of the segment which minimizes stagnation, back pressure, and ascending infection.

Selection of Patients for Operation

Since carcinoma of the cervix is the lesion most frequently requiring a decision regarding ultraradical surgery, the following comments will be limited to a consideration of this lesion. The suitability of carcinoma of the cervix for pelvic exenteration rests upon the fact that a rather high percentage of these lesions metastasize late and the patient may have advanced local carcinoma with no regional metastases. Various studies have shown that between one third and one half of the patients dying of cancer of the cervix do not have spread outside the pelvis, death having occurred from involvement of the lower urinary tract. Most of the patients that we have found to be operable have been those who have shown persistance or recurrence after irradiation therapy. Recurrence after Wertheim hysterectomy is very likely to be inoperable if the standard radical lamphadenectomy was done. The reason for inoperability in these cases is that it is impossible to get outside the previous plane of dissection and the recurrent cancer will usually be found to involve this plane. This does not mean that recurrence in the central pelvis involving the vaginal stump after hysterectomy may not be operable.

Although most of our patients have had irradiation, we feel that there is a place for ultraradical surgery as a primary method of treatment in selected patients with

Stage III and Stage IV carcinoma of the cervix. It is simply important to determine that less radical surgery will have no chance for cure and that there is indeed a chance for cure if ultraradical technique is used. We do not believe that the ultraradical technique should be used in any type of case unless the surgeon feels that there is a chance for cure by the extirpation of all tumor. In other words, we do not believe in this type of mutilating, ultraradical surgery for palliative reasons alone.

In view of the foregoing, it becomes apparent that the determination of inoperability (no chance for cure) becomes most important. All patients are very carefully searched for evidence of spread of tumor outside the pelvis. If none can be found, the patient is prepared for operation. It is most desirable that a positive histological diagnosis be made either before or at the time of operation. The adbomen and pelvis are carefully searched for evidence of metastases that would indicate no chance for cure. Special attention is paid to the paraaortic lymph nodes which are biopsied if metastatic involvement is suspected. If no spread outside the pelvis can be demonstrated, it becomes a matter of determining what is operable within the pelvis. This can be extremely difficult even for an experienced surgeon. Lateral fixation and induration can be due either to tumor or to inflammation and irradiation fibrosis. True tumor fixation to the lateral pelvis is probably incurable by any technique of removal. However, in our opinion true tumor fixation very rarely occurs, the fixation in most instances being due to irradiation fibrosis.

Determination of inoperability in the absence of remote metastases can sometimes be accomplished through a combination of subjective and physical findings. We have found most reliable to be the findings of 1. pain in the pelvis and leg on the same side showing evidence of advanced disease on physical examination; 2. edema of the leg on that side; and 3. obstruction of the corresponding ureter. These findings are so indicative of inoperability that we no longer explore patients presenting this picture.

Technique of Operation

The type of surgery being referred to here is an extended attempt at extirpation of advanced disease for which no other type of therapy can offer any hope of cure. The majority of our patients had what we refer to as a standard complete pelvic exenteration which involves the removal of all pelvic viscera and lymph nodes from the iliac blood vessels down, the levator muscles, and the perineum. This operation has been previously described and I will go into no further detail here. There are certain modifications of the operation which are done with some regularity. These modifications may be an extension of the operation by the inclusion of other abdominal viscera (cecum or small intestine) or by the inclusion of major vascular structures (iliac artery or vein). More frequently an alteration of the operation will be in the direction of preserving function. Occasionally it will be found that the entire rectum can be saved and the operation can be limited to resection of the pelvic viscera anterior to the rectum. Occasionally also, it may be found that the levator muscles and rectal stump may be saved and continuity of the intestinal tract established. In addition, in recent years, we find opportunities to preserve some degree of sexual function through vaginal reconstruction by the use of a colon segment in selected patients for whom this effort appears to be worthwhile.

The technical concept of pelvic exenteration is quite simple and is complicated by only two factors; 1. control of the lateral attachments and blood supply of the pelvic viscera during resection, and 2. the necessity for substituting for the urinary bladder.

Operative experience has greatly facilitated the control of lateral vascular attachments. The use of the ileal conduit has greatly simplified the matter of substituting for the urinary bladder.

Material and Results

Table 1 lists the lesions for which pelvic exenteration was done at our medical center in the 15 years between 1950 and 1965. Also listed are the operative mortality and the 5 year survival rates. Carcinoma of the cervix is by far the most frequent lesion for which this type of surgery is done.

Table 2 indicates the operative mortality broken down into 5 year time periods and demonstrating a progressive drop in mortality with improvement in the selection of patients and experience in performance of the operation.

Table 1[a]. *Exenteration of pelvic organs for advanced pelvic carcinoma, 1950 to 1965*

Indications	Number of patients	Operative mortality	5 year survival rate (based on those at risk 5 years)
A. Postirradiational carcinoma of cervix	207	16 (8%)	35%
B. Carcinoma of the:			
1) Rectum or sigmoid	43	7 (16%)	30%
2) Endometrium	12	2 (17%)	30%
3) Vagina	13	1 (8%)	
4) Bladder or urethra	6	0	
5) Ovary	8	1 (13%)	
6) Vulva or anus	5	0	
7) Small bowel	2	0	
C. Sarcoma prostate	1	1	
D. Palliative operation for cancer of cervix	2	1	
E. Irradiation necrosis	13	3 (23%)	
Total	312	32 (10%)	

[a] Tables 1—6 from Kiselow, M., H. R. Butcher and E. M. Bricker, Ann. Surg. **166**, 428 (1967).

Table 2. *Operative mortality rates following pelvic exenteration for carcinoma of the cervix by 5 year intervals*

Years operations performed	Number of patients	Number of operative deaths	Operative mortality rate
1950—1954	75	10	13.4%
1955—1959	78	5	6.4%
1960—1965	54	1	1.8%
Total	207	16	7.8%

Table 3. *Operative mortality rates following pelvic exenteration for all lesions*

Interval	Number of patients	Number of operative deaths	Operative mortality rate
1950 to 1960	222	26	12%
1960 to 1965	90	6	7%
Total	312	32	10%

Table 4. *Absolute survival rates of 153 patients following exenteration for carcinoma of the cervix 1950 to 1960*

Years after operation	Number of patients	Number dying	Lost to follow-up	Number alive	Absolute survival rate
2	153	66[a]	1[b]	86	56%
5	153	93[a]	7[b]	53	35%

[a] These figures include 15 operative deaths.
[b] Counted as dead.

Table 5. *Postoperative complications in 92 of 207 women after pelvic exenteration for persistent carcinoma of the cervix*[a]

Complication (postoperative)	Number of patients having each complication		Number of patients dying postoperatively	
1. Intestinal obstruction	24		6	
Treated by laparotomy		9		5
Treated without laparotomy		15		1
2. Hemorrhage	8		3	
3. Ileal stoma separation	4		1	
4. Colostomy stoma separation	2			
5. Ureteral obstruction or necrosis	3		1	
6. Fecal or urinary fistula	6			
7. Acute pyelonephritis	8		1	
8. Postoperative psychosis	4		1	
9. Wound infection, pelvic abscess, peritonitis	39			
10. Convulsions	5		1	
11. Thrombosis of iliac artery	1			
12. Thrombophlebitis	8			
13. Heart failure	2		1	
14. Cerebrovascular accident	1		1	
15. Acoustic nerve damage	2			
16. Miscellaneous (Tracheostomy, atelectasis, osteitis pubis, parotitis)	6			
Total complications	123		16	

[a] 115 patients had none, 67 had one, and 25 had more than one complication.

Table 3 presents the operative mortality when all lesions for which pelvic exenteration was done are included.

Table 4 presents the 2 and 5 year survival rates. Those patients surviving 2 years (56%) are considered to have had a good palliative result. Those patients not surviving 2 years include those dying of the operation and those whose lesion was probably unsuitable for the extended operation. It is this latter group that we try to minimize by the exercise of proper judgment in the selection of patients for operation. The 35% 5 year survival rate appears to more than justify the operation.

The early and late postoperative complications are included in Tables 5 and 6. The low incidence of pyelonephritis in the long term followup is particularly noteworthy.

Table 6. *Complications in 75 of 191 women who left the hospital after having had pelvic exenteration for carcinoma of the cervix*[a]

Complication (late)		Number of patients having each complication
1. Intestinal obstruction		12
Operation	10	
Tube only	2	
2. Progressive hydronephrosis requiring ileal bladder revision		3
3. Enteroperineal fistula		9
Due to recurrent carcinoma	2	
Without recurrent carcinoma	7	
4. Rectoperineal fistula		5[b]
Due to recurrent carcinoma	1	
Without recurrent carcinoma	4	
5. Pyelonephritis		12
6. Ileal stoma revision		14
7. Colostomy revision		16
8. Perineal sinus or abscess		7
9. Perineal hernia		4
10. Renal calculus		2
11. Serum hepatitis		1
12. Thrombophlebitis		1
13. Incisional hernia		1
14. Osteitis pubis		1
Total complications[c]		88

[a] 116 had no further complications referable to the operation.

[b] Rectoperineal fistulae occurred in 5 of 9 women having colo-anal anastomoses.

[c] Complications incident to recurrent cancer not included except as noted (3 and 4).

Conclusion

The treatment of advanced and recurrent carcinoma of certain pelvic viscera is now an established procedure and has been proved to provide a satisfactory 5 year salvage rate when done on properly selected patients. The lesions most suitable for this type of surgery include carcinoma of the uterus and cervix and carcinoma of the rectum. 207 patients with advanced or recurrent carcinoma of the cervix were operated upon by pelvic exenteration with an 8% mortality rate and a 35% 5 year survival rate. Satisfactory rehabilitation of these patients can be expected. The technique of the operation is varied to fit the individual case and it is possible in many instances to save rectal function, and at times, to provide a functional vaginal reconstruction.

Urinary diversion by the use of an ileal segment to act as a conduit for the urine to an external receptacle has proved to be a most advantageous method of substituting for the urinary bladder in those patients having exenteration of the pelvic organs. The low incidence of early and late complications that have followed this type of urinary diversion have given the surgeon more freedom to use ultraradical procedures when they seem indicated.

The magnitude, risk and other features of this type of surgery make it mandatory that it be done only in selected centers where there are facilities and personnel capable of developing the judgment and skill necessary to do it successfully. If this is not done, the complications, morbidity, and mortality will be prohibitive.

References

Appleby, L. H.: Amer. J. Surg. **79**, 57 (1950).

Bricker, E. M.: Total exenteration of the pelvic organs. In: J. V. Meigs, Surgical treatment of cancer of the cervix, pp. 349—374. New York: Grune & Stratton, Inc. 1954.

— The technique of ileal segment bladder substitution. In: J. V. Meigs, Progress in gynecology, Vol. III. New York: Grune & Stratton, Inc. 1957.

— Beckeneviszeration. In: Käser, O., u. F. A. Iklé, Atlas der gynäkologischen Operationen, S. 311. Stuttgart: Thieme 1965.

— Die radikale Evisceration des Beckens für fortgeschrittene und rezidivierende Carcinome. Arch. Gynäk. **204**, 1—19 (1967).

Brunschwig, A.: Cancer (Philad.) **1**, 177—183 (1948).

— J. Amer. med. Ass. **194**, 274 (1965).

Douglas, R. G., and W. J. Sweeney: Amer. J. Obstet. Gynec. **73**, 1169 (1957).

Jaffe, B. M., E. M. Bricker, and H. R. Butcher: Ann. Surg. **167**, 367 (1968).

Kiselow, M., H. R. Butcher, and E. M. Bricker: Ann. Surg. **166**, 428 (1967).

Mersheimer, W. L., A. J. Kolarskick, and M. Kammandel: Bull. N.Y. med. Coll. **13**, 71—77 (1950).

Parsons, L., and G. J. Friedell: Proc. nat. Cancer Conf. **5**, 241 (1964).

Ruttledge, F. N., and B. S. Burns: Amer. J. Obstet. Gynec. **91**, 692 (1965).

Seiffert, L.: Langenbecks Arch. klin. Chir. **183**, 569—574 (1935).

Smith, R. R., A. S. Ketcham, and L. B. Thomas: Cancer (Philad.) **16**, 1105 (1963).

The manufacturer's authorised representative in the EU is Springer Nature Customer Service Centre GmbH, Europaplatz 3, 69115 Heidelberg, Germany. If you have any concerns regarding our products, please contact ProductSafety@springernature.com

Printed and bound by CPI Group (UK) Ltd, Croydon, CR0 4YY

02/10/2026

02226631-0004